Modern Pharmaceutics

DRUGS AND THE PHARMACEUTICAL SCIENCES
A Series of Textbooks and Monographs

Executive Editor

James Swarbrick
PharmaceuTech, Inc.
Pinehurst, North Carolina

Advisory Board

Modern Pharmaceutics

Volume 2
Applications and Advances

edited by

Alexander T. Florence
The School of Pharmacy
University of London
London, UK

Juergen Siepmann
College of Pharmacy
Université Lille Nord de France
Lille, France

informa

healthcare

New York   London

Informa Healthcare USA, Inc.
52 Vanderbilt Avenue
New York, NY 10017

© 2009 by Informa Healthcare USA, Inc.
Informa Healthcare is an Informa business

No claim to original U.S. Government works
Printed in the United States of America on acid-free paper
10 9 8 7 6 5 4 3 2 1

International Standard Book Number-10: 1-4200-6566-1 (Hardcover)
International Standard Book Number-13: 978-1-4200-6566-4 (Hardcover)

Library of Congress Cataloging-in-Publication Data

Modern pharmaceutics / edited by Alexander T. Florence, Juergen Siepmann.—5th ed.
    p. ; cm.—(Drugs and the pharmaceutical sciences ; v. 188-)
  Includes bibliographical references and index.
  ISBN-13: 978-1-4200-6564-0 (hb : alk. paper)
  ISBN-10: 1-4200-6564-5 (hb : alk. paper) 1. Drugs—Dosage forms. 2. Pharmacy. 3. Biopharmaceutics. 4. Drugs–Administration. I. Florence, A. T. (Alexander Taylor) II. Siepmann, Juergen. III. Series: Drugs and the pharmaceutical sciences ; v. 188.
  [DNLM: 1. Dosage Forms. 2. Biopharmaceutics. 3. Drug Delivery Systems. 4. Pharmaceutical Preparations—administration & dosage. 5. Pharmacokinetics. W1 DR893B v.188 2009 / QV 785 M6895 2009]
  RS200.M63 2009
  615′.1—dc22

                2009002881

For Corporate Sales and Reprint Permissions call 212-520-2700 or write to: Sales Department, 52 Vanderbilt Avenue, 16th floor, New York, NY 10017.

Visit the Informa Web site at
www.informa.com

and the Informa Healthcare Web site at
www.informahealthcare.com

Preface

Modern Pharmaceutics edited by Gilbert Banker and Christopher Rhodes has become a classic in the field. It is well known and has been well received on an international basis, necessitating the publication of this fifth edition. The present editors took on the difficult task of following in the footsteps of the founding editors and their associates with some trepidation. It has been several years since the last edition, and on realizing that Dr. Banker and Dr. Rhodes wanted to pass on the editorship, we accepted the mantle.

Given the passage of time and the growth and change in the field, the book has been divided into two volumes: *Basic Principles and Systems* and *Applications and Advances*. There have been so many exciting developments which impinge on pharmaceutics that it was time to reconsider the content of the book.

Applications and Advances is principally a textbook and an advanced reference source of pharmaceutics, which focus on the core of the subject that is key to pharmacy. We define pharmaceutics as encompassing the design, formulation, manufacture, assessment and determination of the quality of pharmaceutical products, and also the quality of effect in patients as the guiding principles. We have therefore continued only with chapters that fall within these criteria.

It is of course difficult to separate an essentially applied subject into basic principles and applications, but we have chosen subjects that follow naturally from those in *Basic Principles and Systems*. In *Applications and Advances* we have added chapters on biotechnology-based pharmaceuticals, modern evaluation techniques for medicinal products, an overview chapter on pharmaceutical nanotechnology, as well as a chapter on aspects of pharmaceutical physics, a reflection of the still increasing molecular and quantitative basis of pharmaceutics. Expert chapters on bioequivalence, controlled release systems, transdermal delivery, delivery to the lung, and the design and evaluation of ophthalmic products cover most of the routes of administration. Pediatric and geriatric pharmaceutics are of increasing relevance not least due to its concurrence with the concept of personalized medicine. The chapter on veterinary pharmaceutical dosage forms discusses fascinating challenges and solutions that do not always exist in human medicine. Target-oriented drug delivery itself presents a whole gamut of challenges to the ingenuity of those that design both drugs and delivery systems. A chapter is devoted to this important aspect of pharmacy.

The editors have also speculated in the final chapter on dosage forms for specialized medicines. The human genome project should allow more precision in the medication of patient groups and, indeed, individuals in the coming era of personalized medicines. Personalized medicine is not only about the choice of an effective drug, but it is we argue about appropriate dosing and adapting systems for individuals. Pharmaceutics has clearly a part to play in devising systems with which to deliver more flexible doses in improved ways. We believe that this endeavor might engender new paradigms in pharmacy itself.

Many of these chapters are written by their original authors. We are grateful for their enterprise, enthusiasm, and time and also thank the authors who wished to stand down. They have allowed the new authors to draw heavily on their original material, which has eased the process and has allowed us to retain the essence of the earlier volumes.

We thank Sandra Beberman of Informa Healthcare USA for her patience with new editors and her encouragement, and all the staff at Informa Healthcare USA who have nursed these two volumes through to press. We also thank of course all who have devoted time in preparing material for this new edition of *Modern Pharmaceutics*.

We trust that *Applications and Advances* and its companion *Basic Principles and Systems* will satisfy a wide range of colleagues who have an interest or indeed passion for pharmaceutics, and encourage them in their studies and research and development.

Alexander T. Florence
Juergen Siepmann

Contents

Contributors

Göran Alderborn Department of Pharmacy, Uppsala University, Uppsala Biomedical Center, Uppsala, Sweden

Jörg Breitkreutz Institute of Pharmaceutics and Biopharmaceutics, Heinrich-Heine University, Düsseldorf, Germany

James Chastain Alcon Research, Ltd., Fort Worth, Texas, U.S.A.

Masood A. Chowhan Alcon Research, Ltd., Fort Worth, Texas, U.S.A.

Barry Crean L.B.S.A. and Formulation Insights Group in Drug Delivery, School of Pharmacy, The University of Nottingham, Nottingham, U.K.

Terry Dagnon Alcon Research, Ltd., Fort Worth, Texas, U.S.A.

Alexander T. Florence Centre for Drug Delivery Research, The School of Pharmacy, University of London, London, U.K.

Gordon L. Flynn College of Pharmacy, University of Michigan, Ann Arbor, Michigan, U.S.A.

Todd P. Foster Pfizer Animal Health, Kalamazoo, Michigan, U.S.A.

Göran Frenning Department of Pharmacy, Uppsala University, Uppsala Biomedical Center, Uppsala, Sweden

Sven Frokjaer Department of Pharmaceutics and Analytical Chemistry, Faculty of Pharmaceutical Sciences, University of Copenhagen, Copenhagen, Denmark

Anthony J. Hickey Dispersed Systems Laboratory, Division of Molecular Pharmaceutics, University of North Carolina at Chapel Hill, School of Pharmacy, Chapel Hill, North Carolina, U.S.A.

Rajni Jani Alcon Research, Ltd., Fort Worth, Texas, U.S.A.

Lene Jorgensen   Department of Pharmaceutics and Analytical Chemistry, Faculty of Pharmaceutical Sciences, University of Copenhagen, Copenhagen, Denmark

Vijay Kumar   Division of Pharmaceutics, College of Pharmacy, The University of Iowa, Iowa City, Iowa, U.S.A.

John C. Lang   Alcon Research, Ltd., Fort Worth, Texas, U.S.A.

Guang Wei Lu   Parenteral Center of Emphasis, Global Research & Development, Pfizer Inc., Groton, Connecticut, U.S.A.

Panos Macheras   Laboratory of Biopharmaceutics and Pharmacokinetics, Faculty of Pharmacy, National and Kapodistrian University of Athens, Athens, Greece

Heidi M. Mansour   Department of Pharmaceutical Sciences-Drug Development, College of Pharmacy, University of Kentucky, Lexington, Kentucky, U.S.A.

Colin D. Melia   Formulation Insights Group in Drug Delivery, School of Pharmacy, The University of Nottingham, Nottingham, U.K.

Paul J. Missel   Alcon Research, Ltd., Fort Worth, Texas, U.S.A.

Hanne Moerck Nielsen   Department of Pharmaceutics and Analytical Chemistry, Faculty of Pharmaceutical Sciences, University of Copenhagen, Copenhagen, Denmark

Samuel R. Pygall   Formulation Insights Group in Drug Delivery, School of Pharmacy, The University of Nottingham, Nottingham, U.K.

Michael J. Rathbone   Griffith University, Gold Coast Campus, Queensland, Australia

Christos Reppas   Laboratory of Biopharmaceutics and Pharmacokinetics, Faculty of Pharmacy, National and Kapodistrian University of Athens, Athens, Greece

Denise P. Rodeheaver   Alcon Research, Ltd., Fort Worth, Texas, U.S.A.

Florence Siepmann   Department of Pharmaceutical Technology, College of Pharmacy, Université Lille Nord de France, Lille, France

Juergen Siepmann   Department of Pharmaceutical Technology, College of Pharmacy, Université Lille Nord de France, Lille, France

Mira Symillides   Laboratory of Biopharmaceutics and Pharmacokinetics, Faculty of Pharmacy, National and Kapodistrian University of Athens, Athens, Greece

Catherine Tuleu   Department of Pharmaceutics and Centre for Paediatric Pharmacy Research, The School of Pharmacy, University of London, London, U.K.

Hywel D. Williams   Formulation Insights Group in Drug Delivery, School of Pharmacy, The University of Nottingham, Nottingham, U.K.

1

Time-Controlled Drug Delivery Systems

Juergen Siepmann and Florence Siepmann
Department of Pharmaceutical Technology, College of Pharmacy, Université Lille Nord de France, Lille, France

INTRODUCTION

The success of a pharmaco-treatment essentially depends on the availability of the drug at the site of action in the living body. It is mandatory that the *intact* drug reaches its target site (e.g., a specific receptor in the central nervous system) and to an extent that concentrations greater than the minimal effective concentration (MEC) are provided. If these two prerequisites are not fulfilled, the therapy fails in vivo, even if the drug has an ideal chemical structure to allow for optimal interactions with the target structure and pharmacodynamic effects. Some of the potential reasons for the inability of a drug to reach its site of action are (*i*) poor aqueous solubility, (*ii*) poor permeability across biological barriers, and (*iii*) rapid clearance out of the living body. In the first case, the drug remains at the site of administration or—in the case of oral administration—is not absorbed from the contents of the gastrointestinal tract (GIT). This is because only *dissolved* (individualized) drug molecules are able to diffuse and cross the major natural barriers in a living body (e.g., the GIT mucosa or blood-brain barrier). Poor *permeability* through biological barriers can, for example, be caused by a high molecular weight of the drug (hindering, for instance, diffusional mass transport), poor partitioning into the barrier (membrane), and/or effective efflux systems (e.g., *P*-glycoprotein pumps). Rapid *drug inactivation* can be due to fast drug metabolism and/or elimination and can also prevent many drugs from becoming active in vivo, despite of a great therapeutic potential. Furthermore, in various cases, the *undesired side effects* of a drug, caused in other parts of the living body, can be so severe that the administered dose must be limited, eventually to an extent that does not allow for therapeutic drug concentrations at the site of action. Also in these cases the therapy fails in vivo, since the drug is distributed throughout the living body, and not specifically delivered to the target site.

To overcome these restrictions, an *ideal drug delivery system* should be able (*i*) to release the drug at a *rate* that perfectly matches the real need in vivo for the duration of the therapy, and (*ii*) to deliver the drug exclusively to its target site. The term "controlled drug delivery" encompasses both aspects: time and spatial control of drug release. In this chapter, only time-controlled drug delivery systems are addressed; the reader is referred to chapter 9 of this volume ("Target-Oriented Drug Delivery Systems") for details on spatial-controlled drug delivery approaches.

The use of *time-controlled* drug delivery systems can provide tremendous advantages for a pharmaco-treatment including the following:

1. The *optimization of the resulting drug concentration–time profiles at the site of action* in the living body over prolonged periods of time (1–3). Each drug has a characteristic, so-called "minimal effective concentration" (MEC), below which no therapeutic effect occurs, even if the drug is present at the site of action. In addition, each drug has a so-called "minimal toxic concentration" (MTC), above which undesired side effects occur. The range in-between these two concentrations is called "therapeutic range," or "therapeutic window." Depending on the type of drug, this concentration range can be more or less narrow. Ideally, the drug concentration remains within the therapeutic window during the treatment period. However, if a conventional (immediate-release) dosage form is used to administer a highly potent drug exhibiting a narrow therapeutic range (e.g., an anticancer drug), the entire drug dose is generally rapidly released. In the case of oral administration, the drug is subsequently absorbed into the blood stream, distributed throughout the living body, and reaches its site of action. Depending on the administered dose and therapeutic range of the drug, the risk can be considerable to achieve toxic concentrations, which might necessitate the interruption/termination of the drug treatment (thin curve in Fig. 1). In addition, as the entire drug dose is rapidly released, there is no further drug supply. Thus, the elimination of the drug out of the living body leads to decreasing drug concentrations at the site of action. In many cases, therapeutic drug concentrations are achieved only during short periods of time (thin curve in Fig. 1). Importantly, time-controlled drug delivery systems can allow overcoming these restrictions: If the rate at which the drug enters the living body can be adjusted, the rate at which the drug appears at the site of action (and in the rest of the organism) can be controlled, avoiding both toxic as well as subtherapeutic drug concentrations. For instance, a constant drug supply might be provided, which compensates the drug elimination out of the body, resulting in about constant drug concentrations within the therapeutic range (thick curve in Fig. 1). However, it must be pointed out that constant drug levels

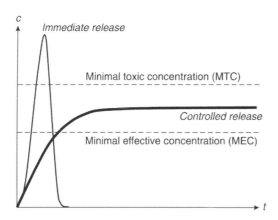

Figure 1 Schematic presentation of the "therapeutic window" of a drug and potential drug concentration–time profiles upon administration of oral *immediate-* and *controlled-release* dosage forms (*thin and bold curve*) (*c* denotes the drug concentration at the site of action in the living body, *t* the time after administration).

are not optimal for all types of pharmaco-treatments. For instance, due to circadian fluctuations in certain hormone concentrations, daytime-dependent drug concentrations might be needed (chrono-pharmacology).

2. The *reduction of the administration frequency* of the drugs. This is particularly important for drugs with short in vivo half-lives. In the case of oral administration, for instance, a three to four times daily administration might be replaced by a once-daily administration only. In the case of parenteral administration, the injection of a drug solution every day might be replaced by a once a month injection of a suspension only. These simplifications of the administration schedule do not only help save time and financial resources, but most importantly, *improve patient compliance*. The inappropriate/inaccurate administration of many drugs still limits the success of various pharmaco-therapies in practice. Many patients are elderly people with multiple, complicated drug treatments.

3. The *simulation of nighttime dosing*. Certain diseases require high drug concentrations at the site of action in the very early morning. For instance, the risk of asthma attacks is particularly elevated at this time of the day. Thus, the patient should wake up in the night and take a conventional dosage form to be protected in the very early morning. Alternatively, a controlled-release dosage form with a so-called "pulsatile" drug-release profile can be administered in the late evening, before going to bed. In the first part of the night, no drug is released, but after a predetermined lag time, the entire dose is rapidly released.

4. The *simulation of multiple dosing* of one or multiple drug(s). The combination of an immediate-release dosage form with a pulsatile drug delivery system, releasing the drug, for instance, six hours after swallowing, can provide two drug doses with only one administration. This again simplifies the administration schedule, which can significantly improve patient compliance. Furthermore, several different types of drugs might be combined and released at preprogrammed time points.

5. The *development of novel drug therapies*, which cannot be realized with immediate-release dosage forms. For instance, many drugs are not able to cross the blood-brain barrier due to limited passive diffusion and/or efficient efflux pumps (4,5). One possibility to overcome this restriction is to administer the drug dose directly into the brain tissue (intracranially). However, this type of administration includes a significant risk of serious infections, thus, frequent intracranial injections are not feasible. Using time-controlled drug delivery systems, a preprogrammed drug supply can be provided during several weeks or months, ideally reducing the number of administrations to only one. In the early drug discover phase, this type of advanced drug delivery systems can also be interesting to evaluate the potential of a novel drug candidate in animal models. If in vivo efficacy is shown, other strategies aiming at target-specific drug delivery across the blood-brain barrier might be envisaged. Thus, time-controlled drug delivery systems can provide fundamental advantages and significantly increase the therapeutic efficacy of a drug treatment.

Time-controlled drug delivery systems can be classified according to different principles, for example, with respect to the route of administration, field of application, and/or underlying drug-release mechanisms. In this chapter, the various types of devices that have been described so far in literature have been classified based on the major physical/chemical phenomenon, which controls the resulting drug-release rate: diffusion, swelling, osmosis, degradation/erosion, and "others." However, it should be kept in mind that, in practice, often several of these processes are simultaneously involved in the control of drug release. Thus, this classification system should not be seen as very rigid.

To be able to control the rate at which a drug leaves its dosage form, it is generally embedded within a polymeric (6–8) or lipidic material (9–11), which avoids immediate drug dissolution and release upon contact with aqueous body fluids. For parenteral administration, the matrix former is ideally biodegradable to avoid the necessity to remove empty remnants after drug exhaust. Upon administration of the device in vivo, the first step is often the wetting of the dosage form by water and subsequent water diffusion into the system. In the case of *polymeric* matrix formers, glassy-to-rubbery phase transitions with subsequent significant increases in the polymer chain and drug mobility might occur. Once the drug comes in contact with water, it dissolves (12), and the *dissolved* (individualized) drug molecules diffuse out of the dosage form. If the matrix former is a biodegradable polymer, the molecular weight of the macromolecules decreases with time, resulting in increased drug mobility. Also, the creation of water-filled pores (due to the dissolution of drug crystals and/or water-soluble excipients) can lead to time- and position-dependent drug diffusivities. In some systems, the involved mass-transport phenomena can be highly complex while others are relatively straightforward/mechanistically simple. If several physical/chemical phenomena are involved, their relative importance for the overall control of drug release might be very different. If, for instance, different processes occur in a sequence and one of them is much slower than all others, this process is dominant and the others can be neglected without introducing considerable errors.

It is always highly desirable to know at least which *major* physical-chemical processes are involved in the control of drug release (13–15). Otherwise, if the dosage form is treated like a "black box," device optimization is generally cumbersome, requiring time- and cost-intensive series of trial-and-error experiments. In addition, trouble shooting during production can be challenging and the safety of the drug treatment might be questionable. In an ideal case, the underlying mass transport mechanisms are known and mathematical models available, allowing for quantitative predictions of the device design parameters (e.g., shape and composition) and environmental conditions (e.g., diseased state) on the resulting drug-release kinetics (16–19). Yet, there is a significant lack of *mechanistic realistic* mathematical theories allowing for a quantitative description of drug release *within the dosage forms* as well as of the *subsequent drug transport within the living body* to the target site (20).

DIFFUSION-CONTROLLED DRUG DELIVERY SYSTEMS

Diffusion is one of the basic mass transport mechanisms, which is involved in the control of drug release from numerous drug delivery systems (14–16). Fick was the first to treat this phenomenon in a quantitative way (21), and the textbook of Crank (22) provides various solutions of Fick's second law for different device geometries and initial and boundary conditions. A very interesting introduction into this type of mass transport is given by Cussler (23).

Several types of species can diffuse in and out of controlled drug delivery systems, including water, drug, water-soluble excipients (e.g., polymers, plasticizers, and/or fillers), acids, and bases from the environmental bulk fluid as well as polymer degradation products. Often, the polymeric material is chosen in such a way that drug diffusion through the macromolecular network is the rate-limiting step. In these cases, the systems

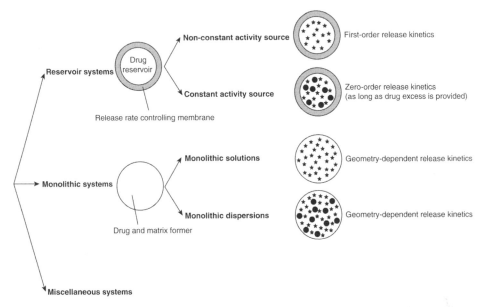

Figure 2 Classification scheme for predominantly diffusion-controlled drug delivery systems. Only spherical dosage forms are illustrated, but the scheme is applicable to any type of geometry. Stars represent dissolved (individual) drug molecules, whereas black circles represent undissolved drug excess (e.g., crystals and/or amorphous aggregates).

are called primarily "diffusion controlled." According to their inner structure, three types of diffusion-controlled drug delivery systems can be distinguished (Fig. 2): reservoir systems, monolithic systems, and miscellaneous systems.

Reservoir Systems

In these cases, the drug and the release rate–controlling material (generally a polymer or lipid) are physically separated: The drug is located at the center of the dosage form, constituting the "reservoir" or "drug depot," and the polymer or lipid surrounds this reservoir as a "release rate–controlling membrane." A clear "core-shell structure" is given. This can, for instance, be a coated pellet, capsule, or tablet. Please note that only spherical dosage forms are illustrated in Figure 2. However, this classification scheme is valid for any type of geometry. Depending on the ratio "initial drug concentration/drug solubility within the device," two types of systems can be distinguished (Fig. 2):

1. Reservoir devices with *non-constant activity source*: In this case, the initial drug loading is below drug solubility and drug molecules (or ions) that leave the dosage form are not replaced. Consequently, the resulting drug concentrations at the inner side of the release rate–controlling membrane decreases with time, resulting in decreasing drug-concentration gradients (which are the driving forces for diffusion). If the properties of the release rate–controlling membrane (in particular its thickness and permeability) do not change during drug release and if perfect sink conditions are provided throughout the experiment (negligible drug concentrations outside of the dosage form), first-order release kinetics result, irrespective of the geometry of the device.

2. Reservoir devices with *constant activity source*: In this case, the initial drug concentration is greater than drug solubility. Hence, *dissolved* and *undissolved*

drugs coexist within the reservoir. The drug excess can, for instance, be drug crystals and/or amorphous aggregates. Please note that in Figure 2, the dissolved drug molecules are represented by stars, whereas the drug excess by black circles. Importantly, only *dissolved* (individualized) drug molecules are able to diffuse, not large drug crystals and/or amorphous aggregates. If the diffusion of the drug through the surrounding polymeric or lipidic membrane is release-rate limiting (and drug dissolution is comparatively fast), released drug molecules (or ions) are rapidly replaced by the (partial) dissolution of drug excess. Hence, constant drug concentrations at the inner membrane's surface result (saturated drug solutions). If perfect sink conditions are provided outside the system, constant concentration differences result as long as the drug concentration in the reservoir exceeds drug solubility. If, in addition, the properties of the release rate–controlling membrane (in particular its thickness and permeability) do not change during drug release, the drug-concentration gradients remain constant, leading to constant drug-release rates (zero-order kinetics), irrespective of the geometry of the device.

Monolithic Systems

In these cases, the drug and matrix former are not clearly physically separated with a core-shell structure, but more or less homogeneously mixed (Fig. 2). Analogous to the reservoir systems, two types of devices can be distinguished according to the "initial drug concentration/drug solubility" ratio:

1. *Monolithic solutions*, in which the drug is molecularly dispersed within the matrix former. This type of controlled drug delivery system might, for instance, be highly suitable for poorly water-soluble drugs. Individualizing the drug molecules within a (often polymeric) matrix former avoids the dissolution step of the drug during drug release and might enhance the bioavailability. However, care must be taken that the systems are not metastable and poorly water-soluble drug crystals formed upon long-term storage.
2. *Monolithic dispersions*, which contain both dissolved and dispersed drug (stars and black circles in Fig. 2).

In contrast to the reservoir devices described above, the resulting drug-release kinetics depend on the device geometry in the case of monolithic systems. Under specific conditions (e.g., absence of polymer dissolution and polymer swelling, time- and position-independent diffusion coefficients), analytical solutions of Fick's second law can be derived, allowing for the calculation of the resulting drug-release kinetics as a function of the device geometry and dimensions (13,22). Also, easy-to-use (often short-time) approximations have been proposed (2). However, care must be taken not to violate any of the assumptions on which such simplified theories are based (14). One very interesting example for an easy-to-use approximation is the classical Higuchi equation (24,25). It has been derived for the geometry of thin ointment films with negligible edge effects and a significant initial excess of suspended drug particles (initial drug loading >> drug solubility in the ointment base). The equation states that the cumulative absolute amount of drug released at time t, M_t, is proportional to the square root of time:

$$\frac{M_t}{A} = \sqrt{D(2c_0 - c_s)c_s t} \qquad (1)$$

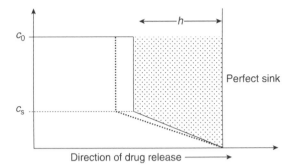

Figure 3 Scheme of the pseudo-steady-state approach, which is used for the derivation of the classical Higuchi equation. Assumed drug concentration–distance profiles in a thin ointment film initially containing a significant drug excess and in contact with a perfect sink.

where A is the surface area of the film exposed to the skin or release medium, D is the drug diffusivity in the ointment base, and c_0 and c_s represent the initial drug concentration and the solubility of the drug in the ointment base, respectively. A major advantage of this equation is its simplicity. Importantly, it can also be applied to other controlled drug delivery systems than thin ointment films (e.g., polymeric patches). However, great care must be taken that none of the assumptions on which the derivation of this equation is based is violated, including the following ones:

- The initial drug concentration in the system is significantly greater than drug solubility. This assumption is crucial, because it provides the basis for the justification of the applied *pseudo-steady-state approach* allowing for major simplifications. Figure 3 illustrates this concept. The concentration-distance profiles of a drug that is homogeneously suspended within an ointment are shown. The release medium (or skin) providing perfect sink is on the right-hand side. The solid line represents the concentration profile after exposure of the ointment to this sink for a certain time t. Importantly, a sharp discontinuity is observed at distance h from the release medium. For this distance h, the concentration gradient is essentially constant, provided the initial drug concentration within the system, c_0, is much greater than the solubility of the drug ($c_0 \gg c_s$) (pseudo steady state). The front, separating the ointment still containing both dissolved and dispersed drug from the ointment containing only dissolved drug, moves only very slowly inward (is virtually stationary), because it takes a long time for all the drug excess to be dissolved at a given position. After an additional time interval, Δt, the new concentration profile of the drug is indicated by the dashed line. Again, a sharp discontinuity and otherwise linear concentration profiles result.
- The device geometry is that of a thin film with negligible edge effects.
- The size of the drug particles is much smaller than the thickness of the film.
- The carrier material (e.g., ointment base) does not swell or dissolve.
- The diffusivity of the drug is constant (not dependent on time or position).
- Perfect sink conditions are maintained throughout the experiment.

Unfortunately, equation (1) is often misused and applied to controlled drug delivery systems, which do not fulfill all these assumptions. In these cases, any conclusion should be viewed with great caution. Even if the cumulative amount of drug that is released from a particular drug delivery system is proportional to the square root of time, this does not necessarily mean that the underlying drug-release mechanism is the same as in the ointment Higuchi studied. For example, the superposition of various other physicochemical phenomena (such as polymer swelling and dissolution, time- and position-dependent changes in the diffusion coefficients of water and/or drug) might result in an apparent square root of time kinetics. Later Higuchi also extended his classical equation to other geometries than thin films (26). However, these equations are *implicit* solutions and not as easy to apply as equation (1).

Miscellaneous Systems

This can, for instance, be a coated pellet, capsule, or tablet, containing the drug in the core as well as in the coating. Alternatively, the device might consist of a monolithic drug polymer/lipid core, which is surrounded by an additional polymer/lipid coating, with both the core as well as the coating being involved in the control of drug release.

SWELLING-CONTROLLED DRUG DELIVERY SYSTEMS

Various polymeric matrix formers show significant swelling once they come into contact with aqueous media. Hydroxypropyl methylcellulose (HPMC), which is often the first choice for oral controlled-release matrix tablets, is an example for a highly swellable polymer (14,27,28). The two most important consequences of polymer swelling for the resulting drug-release kinetics are:

1. The length of the diffusion pathways increases (increase in volume of the systems). This can lead to *de*creasing drug-concentration gradients and, thus, *de*creasing drug-release rates.
2. The polymer molecular mobility significantly *in*creases, resulting in *in*creasing drug diffusivities within the polymeric network (29,30). For example, in a dry HPMC tablet, the apparent drug-diffusion coefficient approaches zero, whereas in a fully swollen HPMC matrix, diffusivities can be achieved that are similar to those in aqueous solutions, in particular, in the case of small molecular weight drugs. This is due to the fact that the average mesh size of the fully swollen HPMC network is large in comparison to the drug molecule size. This increase in drug mobility can lead to *in*creasing drug-release rates.

Depending on the type of polymer and type of drug, one of these two effects (increase in diffusion pathway length and increase in drug mobility) might dominate, resulting in either *de*creasing or *in*creasing drug-release rates compared to a non-swellable drug delivery system.

Figure 4 schematically illustrates the phenomena that can be involved in the control of drug release from a highly swellable drug delivery system, for example, an HPMC matrix tablet. This can, for instance, be a schematic cross section through one-half of a cylindrical matrix tablet. On the left-hand side, the release medium (well-agitated bulk fluid) is shown, on the right-hand side, the still dry (non-swollen) tablet core. The curves represent the macromolecules, the stars *dissolved* (individualized) drug molecules, and the black circles drug excess (e.g., drug crystals and/or amorphous aggregates). Once the system comes into contact with aqueous body fluids, water diffuses into the device. With increasing water content, the mobility of the macromolecules increases (please note that the degree of polymer chain mobility is different in the dry tablet core compared to the

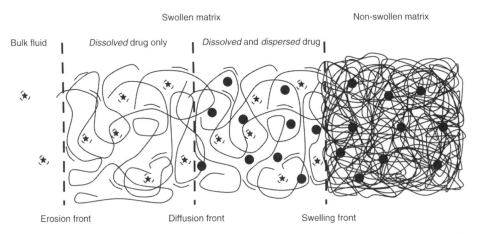

Figure 4 Schematic presentation of a swelling-controlled drug delivery system containing *dissolved* and *dispersed* drug (*illustrated by the stars and black circles, respectively*). Three moving boundaries can be distinguished: (*i*) an "erosion front," separating the bulk fluid from the delivery system; (*ii*) a "diffusion front," separating the swollen matrix containing *dissolved* drug only and the swollen matrix containing *dissolved* and *dispersed* drug; and (*iii*) a "swelling front," separating the swollen and non-swollen matrix.

rest of the tablet, Fig. 2). Certain polymers, including HPMC, show steep, sudden increases in their mobility as soon as a critical, polymer-specific water concentration is reached ("polymer chain relaxation"). The front at which this phenomenon occurs is called "swelling front" (Fig. 2). This front separates the region of the tablet in which the macromolecules (and, thus, also dissolved drug molecules) are highly mobile from the region in which the drug is efficiently trapped within a rigid polymeric system. In the non-swollen part of the tablet, the water concentration is generally very low and the amount of dissolved drug often negligible. In contrast, in the swollen part of the tablet, the macromolecules are much more mobile and often significant amounts of water available for drug dissolution. Due to concentration gradients, the individualized, *dissolved* drug molecules diffuse out of the system. If the initial drug concentration in the device is greater than the solubility of the drug in the swollen matrix, dissolved and undissolved drug coexist directly next to the swelling front. In case drug dissolution is rapid compared to drug diffusion, saturated drug solutions are maintained in these parts of the system (released drug molecules are replaced by the partial dissolution of undissolved drug). However, once all drug excess is dissolved, the concentration of dissolved drug, also in this part of polymeric network, decreases with time. The front separating the region containing both dissolved and dispersed drug from the region containing only dissolved drug, is called "diffusion front" (31,32) (Fig. 2). If the polymeric matrix former is water soluble, the third front is called "erosion" front, separating the bulk fluid from the swollen polymer network. Importantly, these three fronts are not stationary but moving, and the distances between them determine the length of the diffusion pathways for the drug and water. For a more detailed mechanistic analysis and quantitative mathematical treatment, the reader is referred to the literature (14,19,33,34).

OSMOTIC-CONTROLLED DRUG DELIVERY SYSTEMS

The release rate of a drug out of a pharmaceutical dosage form can also be controlled by the hydrostatic pressure, which is built up upon water influx into the system that is driven by osmosis (35–37). Figure 5 illustrates two types of systems: a one-chamber device and a

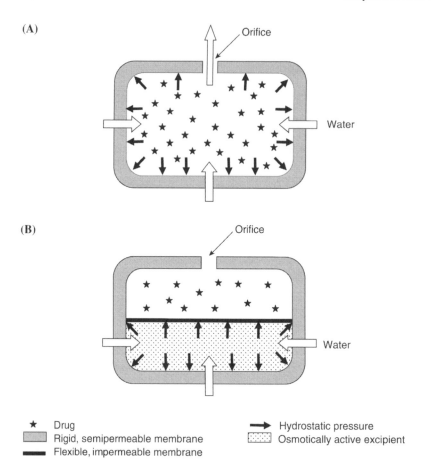

Figure 5 Schematic presentation of osmotic-controlled drug delivery systems: (**A**) one-chamber device; (**B**) two-chamber device. The osmotically driven influx of water creates considerable hydrostatic pressure within the system, which pushes the drug out into the bulk fluid.

two-chamber device. Both are surrounded by a rigid, semipermeable film coating, which is permeable for water, but not for the drug or excipients. Often, cellulose acetate is used for this purpose. Once the system comes into contact with aqueous body fluids, water penetrates into the device.

In the case of a *one-chamber device* (Fig. 5A), the water influx is driven by the difference in osmolarity of the surrounding bulk fluid and of the drug (and potentially excipient) solution inside the system. The generated hydrostatic pressure pushes the drug solution or suspension out of the dosage form, through one or more holes/orifices in the film coating. As the resulting drug-release rate strongly depends on the diameter of this/these hole(s), the latter(s) is/are often prepared with a laser. Importantly, the semipermeable membrane is rigid, so that the developed hydrostatic pressure fully serves to push out the drug and not to extend the systems' dimensions. If the aqueous solubility of the drug is insufficient to create the required osmotic pressure difference "inside-outside" to achieve the desired drug-release rate, freely water-soluble excipients might be added. The resulting drug-release from this type of dosage forms is constant (zero-order kinetics) as long as (*i*) the drug concentration inside the system is constant (e.g., saturated solution) and (*ii*) the osmotic pressure difference inside-outside is constant (e.g., saturated drug solution inside versus perfect sink outside).

In the case of a *two-chamber device* (Fig. 5B), the rigid semipermeable membrane surrounds two compartments: one filled with the drug (and eventually excipients) and the other filled with a freely water-soluble excipient, creating significant osmotic pressure upon contact with aqueous media. These two compartments are separated by an *impermeable, flexible* membrane. The water influx into this type of dosage forms is mainly driven by the osmotically active excipient located in the second chamber. The hydrostatic pressure that is created upon water penetration deforms the flexible, impermeable membrane and, thus, pushes the drug solution or suspension located in the other chamber out of device through the orifice(s) of this chamber. The resulting drug-release rate can be adjusted via the diameter of the hole(s) and the osmotic activity of the excipients (and drug). Again, zero-order release kinetics can be provided as long as the driving forces are constant.

DEGRADATION/EROSION-CONTROLLED DRUG DELIVERY SYSTEMS

Most degradable/erodible-controlled drug delivery systems are based on polymeric matrix formers. In the case of parenteral administration, they provide the major advantage to avoid the removal of empty remnants upon drug exhaust. Unfortunately, different definitions of the terms *erosion* and *degradation* are used in the literature (38). In this chapter, the term polymer *degradation* is understood as the chain scission process by which macromolecules are cleaved into shorter-chain molecules and finally oligomers and monomers. The term *erosion* is understood as the process of material loss from the polymer bulk. Such materials can include monomers, oligomers, parts of the polymer backbone, or even parts of the polymer bulk.

Depending on the relative velocities of water penetration into the drug delivery system and polymer chain cleavage, two erosion mechanisms can be distinguished: *surface* (heterogeneous) and *bulk* (homogeneous erosion) (39–41). The basic principles of these two mechanisms are illustrated in Figure 6. Exemplarily, schematic cross sections through erodible, cylindrical implants are shown. Before exposure to the release medium ($t = 0$) (schemes on the left-hand side), the drug is homogeneously distributed within the devices in the form of dissolved (individualized) molecules and undissolved drug excess (e.g., crystals and/or amorphous aggregates), represented by the stars and black circles, respectively. In the case of *surface*-eroding drug delivery systems (Fig. 6, top row), the rate at which the polymer chains are cleaved is much higher than the rate at which water penetrates into the device. Thus, polymer degradation is mainly restricted to the surface-near regions of the systems. Consequently, the device shrinks with time and the drug is released by the disappearance of the surrounding polymer matrix. The inner structure (e. g., porosity, relative drug content, and distribution) remains about unaltered. In contrast, the water-penetration rate is much greater than the polymer chain–cleavage rate in the case of *bulk*-eroding drug delivery systems (Fig. 6, bottom row). Thus, the entire device is rapidly wetted upon contact with aqueous media and polymer chain cleavage occurs throughout the system. Due to the presence of water, the drug becomes mobile and diffuses out of the device. In case of initial drug excess, released drug molecules are replaced by the (partial) dissolution of drug crystals/amorphous aggregates. Importantly, the device dimensions remain nearly constant, whereas the inner system structure significantly changes: the porosity increases and the drug concentration decreases. With decreasing average polymer molecular weight, the mobility of the macromolecules increases and, thus, also the drug mobility.

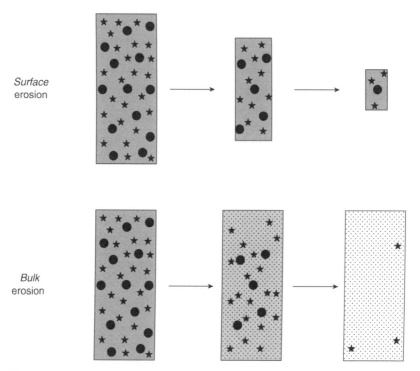

Figure 6 Schematic presentation of a *surface* and a *bulk*-eroding drug delivery system. Stars represent dissolved (individual) drug molecules, whereas black circles represent undissolved drug excess (e.g., crystals and/or amorphous aggregates).

Generally, polymers containing very reactive functional groups in their backbone degrade rapidly and show *surface* erosion, whereas polymers containing less reactive functional groups tend to be *bulk* eroding. Polyanhydrides are examples for predominantly surface-eroding polymers, while poly(lactic acid) (PLA) and poly(lacticco-glycolic acid) (PLGA) are examples for predominantly bulk-eroding materials. However, it has to be kept in mind that the absolute polymer degradation rate alone not only determines the type of erosion (surface or bulk), but also the ratio "rate of polymer chain cleavage:rate of water penetration." The rate at which water enters the system strongly depends on the device dimensions. Thus, in extreme cases, drug delivery systems based on polymers with very reactive functional groups might show *bulk* erosion, for example, nanoparticles consisting of polyanhydrides. In contrast, devices based on polymers, which generally show bulk erosion, can exhibit surface erosion if they are large enough. Von Burkersroda et al. (42) proposed a polymer-specific, critical device dimension ($L_{critical}$), above which the drug delivery system undergoes primarily surface erosion, and below which bulk erosion. For example, the $L_{critical}$ value is in the order of 100 µm for polyanhydrides, and in the order of 10 cm for PLGA. However, it has to be kept in mind that in the vicinity of the $L_{critical}$ values, *both* surface as well as bulk erosion are of importance and the overall erosion behavior of the system shows characteristics of both types of erosion.

Interesting mathematical theories have been proposed to quantify the involved physical and chemical phenomena in *surface*- (43) and *bulk*-eroding (38,40,44,45) drug delivery systems. As polymer chain cleavage is a random process, Monte Carlo simulations can effectively be used to simulate this phenomenon. The first to combine such Monte Carlo simulations with diffusional mass transport (based on Fick's second law) was A. Goepferich (46,47). This type of theories can, for instance, be applied to quantify drug release from PLGA-based microparticles (48,49). The basic idea is to divide a spherical microparticle into concentric rings of equal volume. One-quarter of a cross section of such a sphere is illustrated in Figure 7A. As it can be seen, a grid is used to divide this cross section into pixels. If this grid rotates around the z-axis, it describes half a sphere. If the drug and polymer are homogeneously distributed throughout the microparticles, there is a symmetry plane at $r = 0$, allowing for the calculation of the mass transport phenomena in the entire system. Each pixel shown in Figure 7A represents either drug or nondegraded polymer. This is the situation before exposure to the release medium ($t = 0$). Upon rotation around the z-axis, each pixel describes a ring. Importantly, the size of the two-dimensional pixels is not uniform and chosen in such as way that the volume of all three-dimensional rings is equal. This assures that the number of cleavable polymer backbone bonds in a ring representing nondegraded polymer is similar in all rings. Thus, the probability at which such a ring degrades upon first contact with water is similar. Since it is not possible to predict that at which time point which polymer backbone bond is cleaved, and as this process is random, Monte Carlo simulations can be used to describe this phenomenon. The idea is to randomly distribute "lifetime expectancies" to all pixels representing nondegraded polymer at $t = 0$. As soon as a particular pixel comes into contact with water, its "lifetime" starts to decrease. Once the latter expires, the pixel is assumed to be instantaneously transformed into a water-filled pore. Thus, the inner structure of the microparticles can be calculated at any time point (Fig. 7B). This information is crucial for the quantitative description of the resulting drug diffusion out of the system: The knowledge of the time- and position-dependent porosity of the device allows for the calculation of the time- and position-dependent drug-diffusion coefficients. Using Fick's second law of diffusion (22) and considering the given initial and boundary conditions, the resulting drug-release kinetics can be quantified and effects of processing and formulation parameters theoretically predicted (48,49).

As ester hydrolysis is catalyzed by protons, the underlying drug-release mechanisms from PLGA-based drug delivery systems can be even more complex (50,51). As described above, water penetration into these systems is much more rapid than the subsequent polymer chain cleavage. Thus, the entire device is rapidly wetted and ester hydrolysis occurs throughout the system. Figure 8 shows exemplarily a spherical microparticle, but these phenomena can also occur in other types of drug delivery systems, exhibiting different geometries. Due to concentration gradients, the generated shorter-chain acids diffuse out of the microparticles into the surrounding bulk fluid, where they are neutralized. In addition, bases from the environment diffuse into the system (again due to concentration gradients) and neutralize the generated acids. However, diffusional mass transport is generally slow and the rate at which the acids are generated via ester hydrolysis can be higher than the acid-neutralization rate, resulting in the local accumulation of acids and, thus, microenvironmental drops in the pH (52–54). This phenomenon is often most pronounced at the center of the device, because of the longer diffusion pathways. Importantly, ester hydrolysis is catalyzed by protons (55). Thus, polymer degradation is accelerated in the regions with low local pH. Consequently, drug release can be facilitated (50,51). In case of acid-labile drugs (e.g., proteins), care needs to be taken so that the biological activity is not lost. The importance of these phenomena essentially depends on the acid *generation* and *neutralization* rate. As the latter is a

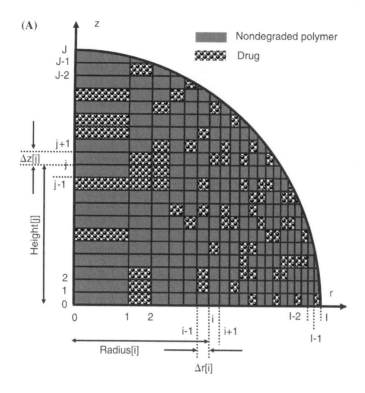

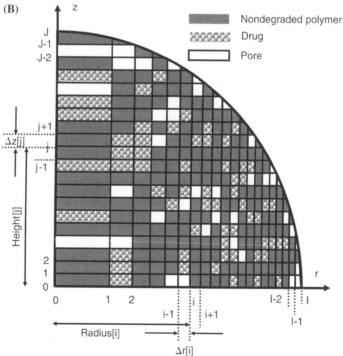

Figure 7 Principle of a Monte Carlo–based approach to mathematically model polymer degradation and drug diffusion in PLGA-based microparticles. Scheme of the inner structure of the system (one-quarter of a spherical cross section): (**A**) at time $t = 0$ (before exposure to the release medium); and (**B**) during drug release. Gray, dotted, and white pixels represent nondegraded polymer, drug and pores, respectively. *Source*: From Ref. 48.

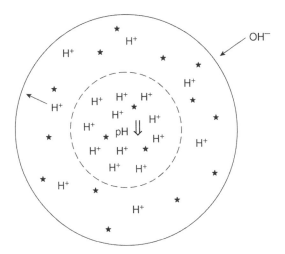

Figure 8 Scheme of a bulk-eroding PLGA-based microparticle exhibiting autocatalysis: Upon hydrolytic ester bond cleavage, generated shorter-chain acids diffuse out of the system, while bases from the surrounding bulk fluid diffuse in. As the relative acid-*neutralization* rate exceeds the acid-*generation* rate, the microenvironmental pH within the system drops (this is often most pronounced at the *center* of the microparticle because of the longer diffusion pathways). As hydrolytic ester bond cleavage is catalyzed by protons, this leads to accelerated polymer degradation (autocatalysis) and potentially to drug degradation. The stars represent drug molecules.

function of the device dimensions and mobility of the involved acids and bases, the system size and initial porosity strongly affect the extent in local acidification.

A practical example for a drug treatment with a biodegradable-controlled drug delivery system is illustrated in Figure 9. The delivery system is a disk-shaped wafer (flat cylinder, commercialized under the trade name "Gliadel") and contains 3.85% of the anticancer drug BCNU [1,3-bis(2-chloroethyl)-1-nitrosourea; carmustine] (56–60). Despite its lipophilicity and low molecular weight (and, thus, ability to cross the blood-brain barrier to a certain extent), a systemic treatment with BCNU is not feasible because of the severe, dose-limiting side effects (in particular bone marrow suppression and pulmonary fibrosis) combined with a relatively short half-life (<15 min) (61). The biodegradable matrix former in Gliadel is a polyanhydride: poly[bis(*p*-carboxyphenoxy) propane–sebacic acid] [p(CPP:SA)]. This advanced drug delivery system has been developed by Brem and coworkers and presented a major breakthrough in the field of controlled *local* brain delivery, which is highly challenging due to the blood-brain barrier. Gliadel got approved by the Food and Drug Administration (FDA) in 1996 for the treatment of recurrent glioblastoma multiforme. Figure 9A illustrates the basic principle of this treatment method: schematic cross sections of a human brain are shown. The black circle represents the tumor, the surrounding tissue being infiltrated by tumor cells. As the surgeon cannot remove large quantities of the surrounding tissue (due to the risk to affect vital brain functions), the probability that tumor cells remain within the brain is considerable. Consequently, many patients die due to local tumor recurrence in the direct vicinity of the primary tumor. To reduce this risk, up to eight BCNU-loaded wafers are placed into the resection cavity of the tumor, during the same operation, when the cranium is still open (Fig. 9A). The anticancer drug is then released in a time-controlled manner into the resection cavity and penetrates into the surrounding tissue. As the matrix-forming polymer is biodegradable, there is no need to remove empty remnants. In addition, the drug is released in the direct vicinity of the site of action, thus, systemic side effects are

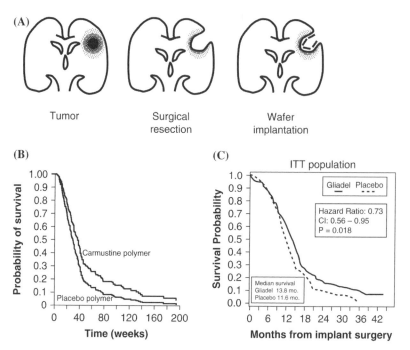

Figure 9 Treatment of operable brain tumors with BCNU-loaded, p(CPP:SA)-based wafers. (**A**) Schematic cross sections through a brain: The tumor is illustrated as a black circle; the surrounding tissue is infiltrated by cancer cells. Upon tumor resection, up to eight drug-loaded wafers (cylindrical disks) are placed into the resection cavity to minimize the risk of local tumor recurrence. (**B**) Overall survival of 222 patients with *recurrent* brain tumors (phase III clinical trial, after adjustment for prognostic factors). (**C**) Overall survival of 240 patients with *newly diagnosed* brain tumors (phase III clinical trial, including results from the long-term follow-up). *Abbreviation*: ITT, intent-to-treat. *Source*: From Refs. 58 and 63 (**B** and **C**).

reduced. In 1995, a multicentered, randomized, double-blinded, and placebo-controlled phase III clinical trial was conducted with 222 patients with recurrent malignant brain tumors (58). Importantly, the median survival time of the group of 110 patients who were treated with drug-loaded wafers was 31 weeks compared to only 23 weeks in the case of the 112 patients who received placebo disks. Figure 9B shows the overall survival of the patients (after adjustment for the examined prognostic factors). Furthermore, there were no clinically important side effects caused by the BCNU-loaded, p(CPP:SA)-based disks—neither locally within the brain, nor systemically. Later on, Gliadel was also used for the *initial* treatment of malignant gliomas (59,62). Upon surgical tumor resection, 240 patients received either BCNU-loaded or drug-free wafers. Both groups were postoperatively treated with external beam radiation. The median survival time in the intent-to-treat (ITT) group was 13.9 months for the Gliadel-treated patients and 11.6 months for the placebo group. The one-year survival rates were 59.2% and 49.6%, respectively. A long-term follow-up of this phase III clinical trial with 59 patients showed that 11 were alive at 56 months: 9 of them had been treated with Gliadel and only 2 with placebo wafers (63). The extended Kaplan–Meier curves for all 240 patients are shown in Figure 9C. Clearly, the survival advantage of the Gliadel-treated group was maintained even after one, two, and three years.

Another interesting example of the major benefits that a biodegradable, time-controlled drug delivery systems can offer is the delivery of growth factors and/or cytokines to proliferating/differentiating cells. This type of approach can be very useful for cell therapies: Up to now, the success of such advanced treatment methods, for instance, for neurodegenerative disease (e.g., Parkinson's disease) is limited because (*i*) the survival rate of transplanted cells within the brain tissue is low, and (*ii*) the integration of the cells in their new environment is poor. Generally, about 90% of the transplanted cells die within the first two weeks after administration. One strategy to overcome these restrictions is to combine controlled-release microparticles and cell transplantation (64). The microparticles can, for example, release specific growth factors and/or cytokines at a predetermined rate and, thus, help to reduce cell death and to improve cell integration into the brain tissue. An even more sophisticated strategy is the use of microparticles not only as time-controlled drug delivery systems, but at the same time as *microcarriers* for the transplanted cells (64–68). This type of devices are also called "pharmacologically active microcarriers (PAM)." Figure 10A illustrates the concept of this approach. The microparticles exhibit two characteristic features: (*i*) a coating with cell adhesion or extracellular matrix molecules, and (*ii*) time-controlled release of suitable biologically active agents at predetermined rates. Figure 10B, C show optical and scanning electron micrographs of such devices with PC12 cells adhering on their surfaces. Furthermore, the microparticles can additionally release drugs that are able to modify the microenvironment,

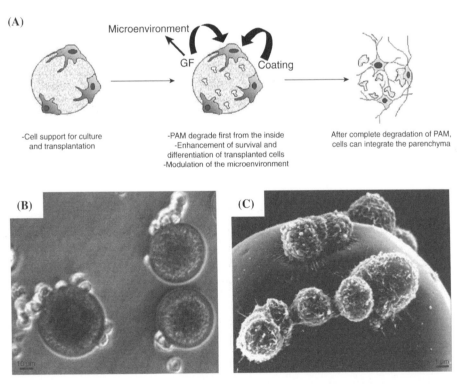

Figure 10 PAM used to improve the efficacy of cell therapies: (**A**) Schematic illustration of the principle of the approach. (**B** and **C**) Optical and scanning electron micrographs of cells adhering onto PAM. *Abbreviations*: GF, growth factor and/or cytokine; PAM, pharmacologically active microcarriers. *Source*: From Ref. 65.

for example, favor angiogenesis or local immunodepression. Upon complete microparticle degradation, the cells can integrate the parenchyma. Recently, nerve growth factor–releasing PAM conveying PC12 cells were transplanted into "Parkinsonian rats" (64). The idea is as follows: When PC12 cells expressing tyrosine hydroxylase (TH) are exposed to nerve growth factor, they stop cell division, extend long neuritis, become excitable, and after depolarization, can release significant amounts of dopamine (the neurotransmitter that is missing in Parkinson's Disease). Interestingly, first results showed that these nerve growth factor–releasing PAM can indeed reduce cell death and improve the amphetamine-induced rotational behavior of the rats.

OTHER TYPES OF CONTROLLED DRUG DELIVERY SYSTEMS

As mentioned above, the presented classification system for time-controlled drug delivery devices should not be viewed very strictly. There are various overlaps and other types of release rate–controlling mechanisms, including, for example, systems in which the drug is chemically bound to a matrix former (which is not necessarily biodegradable), coated solid dosage forms from which drug release occurs only upon crack formation within the surrounding membrane, and microchip-based drug delivery systems.

If the drug is covalently bound to an insoluble matrix former (e.g., polymer) via hydrolysable bondings, the latter are more or less rapidly cleaved upon water penetration into the device. The rate of this chemical reaction together with the rate of diffusion of water and drug through the polymeric network determine the overall drug-release rate (2).

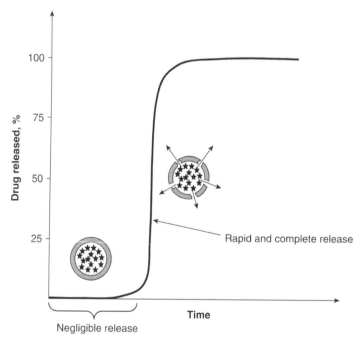

Figure 11 *Pulsatile* drug-release patterns: negligible release at early time points, followed by rapid and complete release after a predetermined lag phase. Exemplarily, a polymer-coated pellet is illustrated: The intact macromolecular membrane effectively hinders drug release until the steadily increasing hydrostatic pressure within the pellet core (caused by the influx of water) induces crack formation, resulting in rapid drug release through water-filled pores/channels.

Pulsatile drug-release patterns (negligible drug release at early time points combined with rapid and complete drug release after a predetermined lag phase) can, for instance, be provided with drug-loaded pellets, which are coated with a polymeric film that is impermeable for the drug as long as the film is intact. The principle of this type of approach is illustrated in Figure 11. Upon contact with aqueous media, water penetrates into the system, resulting in a steadily increasing hydrostatic pressure, which acts against the film coating. As soon as this pressure exceeds the mechanical stability of the polymeric membrane, crack formation is induced in the latter and drug release occurs through water-filled pores/channels.

Promising *microchip-based*, time-controlled drug delivery systems have been proposed by Langer and coworkers (69–71): Tiny reservoirs on a microchip are loaded with one or more drugs using, for example, inkjet printing techniques. The drug can be in the solid, liquid, or semisolid state. The reservoirs can, for instance, be sealed with thin gold layers (e.g., 50 μm × 50 μm and 0.3 μm in thickness), which serve as anodes. The microchip also contains a cathode. When applying a potential of +1.04 V, the gold membranes electrochemically dissolve and the drug is released. One of the fundamental advantages of this novel type of time-controlled drug delivery systems is the considerable number of drug reservoirs that can be located on one single microchip and the fact that each reservoir can be activated individually. Thus, virtually any type of drug-release patterns with one or multiple drugs can be provided. For more details, the reader is referred to chapter 12 of this volume ("Dosage Forms for Personalized Medicine: From the Simple to the Complex").

REFERENCES

1. Tanquary AC, Lacey RE, eds. Controlled Release of Biologically Active Agents. New York: Plenum Press, 1974.
2. Baker R., ed. Controlled Release of Biologically Active Agents. New York: John Wiley, 1987.
3. Langer RS, Wise DL, eds. Medical Applications of Controlled Release, Vol 1: Classes of Systems. Boca Raton: CRC Press, 1984.
4. Grieg NH. Optimizing drug delivery to brain tumors. Cancer Treat Rev 1987; 14:1–28.
5. Abott NJ, Romero IA. Transporting therapeutics across the blood-brain barrier. Mol Med Today 1996; 2:106–113.
6. Langer R. Polymeric delivery systems for controlled drug release. Chem Eng Commun 1980; 6: 1–48.
7. Langer R, Peppas NA. Chemical and physical structure of polymers as carriers for controlled release of bioactive agents: a review. Rev Macromol Chem Phys 1983; C23:61–126.
8. Rosen HB, Kohn J, Leong K, et al. Bioerodible polymers for controlled release systems. In: Hsieh D, ed. Controlled Release Systems: Fabrication Technology, Vol 2. Boca Raton: CRC Press, 1988:83–110.
9. Guse C, Koennings S, Kreye F, et al. Drug release from lipid-based implants: elucidation of the underlying mass transport mechanisms. Int J Pharm 2006; 314:137–144.
10. Kreye F, Siepmann F, Siepmann J. Lipid implants as drug delivery systems. Expert Opin Drug Deliv 2008; 5:291–307.
11. Herrmann S, Winter G, Mohl S, et al. Mechanisms controlling protein release from lipidic implants: effects of PEG addition. J Control Release 2007; 118:161–168.
12. Noyes AA, Whitney WR. Ueber die Aufloesungsgeschwindigkeit von festen Stoffen in ihren eigenen Loesungen. Z Physikal Chem 1897; 23:689–692.
13. Fan LT, Singh SK, eds. Controlled release. A Quantitative Treatment. Berlin: Springer-Verlag, 1989.

14. Siepmann J, Peppas NA. Modeling of drug release from delivery systems based on hydroxypropyl methylcellulose (HPMC). Adv Drug Deliv Rev 2001; 48:139–157.

15. Siepmann J, Goepferich A. Mathematical modeling of bioerodible, polymeric drug delivery systems. Adv Drug Deliv Rev 2001; 48:229–247.

16. Peppas NA. Mathematical modeling of diffusion processes in drug delivery polymeric systems. In: Smolen VF, Ball L, eds. Controlled Drug Bioavailability, Vol 1. New York: John Wiley, 1984:203–237.

17. Vergnaud JM, ed. Liquid Transport Processes in Polymeric Materials. Englewood Cliffs: Prentice-Hall, 1991:26–29.

18. Vergnaud JM, ed. Controlled Drug Release of Oral Dosage Forms. Chichester: Ellis Horwood, 1993.

19. Siepmann J, Siepmann F. Mathematical modeling of drug delivery. Int J Pharm 2008; 364:328–343.

20. Siepmann J, Siepmann F, Florence AT. Local controlled drug delivery to the brain: mathematical modeling of the underlying mass transport mechanisms. Int J Pharm 2006; 314:101–119.

21. Fick A. Ueber Diffusion. Ann Phys 1855; 94:59–86.

22. Crank J, ed. The Mathematics of Diffusion. Oxford: Clarendon Press, 1975.

23. Cussler EL, ed. Diffusion: Mass Transfer in Fluid Systems. New York: Cambridge University Press, 1984.

24. Higuchi T. Physical chemical analysis of percutaneous absorption process from creams and ointments. J Soc Cosmet Chem 1961; 11:85–97.

25. Higuchi T. Rate of release of medicaments from ointment bases containing drugs in suspensions. J Pharm Sci 1961; 50:874–875.

26. Higuchi T. Mechanisms of sustained action mediation. Theoretical analysis of rate of release of solid drugs dispersed in solid matrices. J Pharm Sci 1963; 52:1145–1149.

27. Colombo P. Swelling-controlled release in hydrogel matrices for oral route. Adv Drug Deliv Rev 1993; 11:37–57.

28. Doelker E. Water-swollen cellulose derivatives in pharmacy. In: Peppas NA, ed. Hydrogels in Medicine and Pharmacy, Vol 2. Boca Raton: CRC Press, 1986:115–160.

29. Siepmann J, Kranz H, Bodmeier R, et al. HPMC-matrices for controlled drug delivery: a new model combining diffusion, swelling and dissolution mechanisms and predicting the release kinetics. Pharm Res 1999; 16:1748–1756.

30. Siepmann J, Peppas NA. Hydrophilic matrices for controlled drug delivery: an improved mathematical model to predict the resulting drug release kinetics (the "sequential layer" model). Pharm Res 2000; 17:1290–1298.

31. Colombo P, Bettini R, Peppas NA. Observation of swelling process and diffusion front position during swelling in hydroxypropyl methyl cellulose (HPMC) matrices containing a soluble drug. J Control Release 1999; 61:83–91.

32. Colombo P, Bettini R, Santi P, et al. Swellable matrices for controlled drug delivery: gel-layer behaviour, mechanisms and optimal performance. Pharm Sci Technol Today 2000; 3:198–204.

33. Narasimhan B, Peppas NA. Disentanglement and reptation during dissolution of rubbery polymers. J Poly Sci Poly Phys 1996; 34:947–961.

34. Narasimhan B, Peppas NA. On the importance of chain reptation in models of dissolution of glassy polymers. Macromolecules 1996; 29:3283–3291.

35. Wright JC, Stevenson CL. Pumps/osmotic. In: Mathiowitz E, ed. Encyclopedia of Controlled Drug Delivery, Vol 2. New York: John Wiley, 1999.

36. Perkins L, Peer C, Fleming V. Pumps/osmotic—alzet system. In: Mathiowitz E, ed. Encyclopedia of Controlled Drug Delivery, Vol 2. New York: John Wiley, 1999.

37. Bittner B, Thelly T, Isel H, et al. The impact of co-solvents and the composition of experimental formulations on the pump rate of the ALZET osmotic pump. Int J Pharm 2000; 205:195–198.

38. Goepferich A. Polymer degradation and erosion: mechanisms and applications. Eur J Pharm Biopharm 1996; 42:1–11.

39. Goepferich A, Langer R. Modeling of polymer erosion. Macromolecules 1993; 26:4105–4112.

40. Goepferich A. Mechanisms of polymer degradation and erosion. Biomaterials 1996; 17:103–114.

41. Goepferich A. Polymer bulk erosion. Macromolecules 1997; 30:2598–2604.
42. von Burkersroda F, Schedl L, Goepferich A. Why degradable polymers undergo surface erosion or bulk erosion. Biomaterials 2002; 23:4221–4231.
43. Lee PI. Diffusional release of a solute from a polymeric matrix—approximate analytical solutions. J Membr Sci 1980; 7:255–275.
44. Goepferich A, Langer R. Modeling monomer release from bioerodible polymers. J Control Release 1995; 33:55–69.
45. Goepferich A, Langer R. Modeling of polymer erosion in three dimensions—rotationally symmetric devices. AIChE J 1995; 41:2292–2299.
46. Goepferich A. Bioerodible implants with programmable drug release. J Control Release 1997; 44:271–281.
47. Goepferich A. Erosion of composite polymer matrices. Biomaterials 1997; 18:397–403.
48. Siepmann J, Faisant N, Benoit JP. A new mathematical model quantifying drug release from bioerodible microparticles using Monte Carlo simulations. Pharm Res 2002; 19:1887–1895.
49. Faisant N, Siepmann J, Richard J, et al. Mathematical modeling of drug release from bioerodible microparticles: effect of gamma-irradiation. Eur J Pharm Biopharm 2003; 56:271–279.
50. Siepmann J, Elkharraz K, Siepmann F, et al. How autocatalysis accelerates drug release from PLGA-based microparticles: a quantitative treatment. Biomacromolecules 2005; 6:2312–2319.
51. Klose D, Siepmann F, Elkharraz K, et al. How porosity and size affect the drug release mechanisms from PLGA-based microparticles. Int J Pharm 2006; 314:198–206.
52. Shenderova A, Burke TG, Schwendeman SP. The acidic microclimate in poly(lactide-co-glycolide) microspheres stabilizes camptothecins. Pharm Res 1999; 16:241–248.
53. Brunner A, Maeder K, Goepferich A. pH and osmotic pressure inside biodegradable microspheres during erosion. Pharm Res 1999; 16:847–853.
54. Li L, Schwendeman SP. Mapping neutral microclimate pH in PLGA microspheres. J Control Release 2005; 101:163–173.
55. Lu L, Garcia CA, Mikos AG. In vitro degradation of thin poly(DL-lactic-co-glycolic acid) films. J Biomed Mater Res 1999; 46:236–244.
56. Brem H, Mahaley MS, Vick NA, et al. Interstitial chemotherapy with drug polymer implants for the treatment of recurrent gliomas. J Neurosurg 1991; 74:441–446.
57. Grossman SA, Reinhard C, Colvin OM, et al. The intracerebral distribution of BCNU delivered by surgically implanted biodegradable polymers. J Neurosurg 1992; 76:640–647.
58. Brem H, Piantadosi S, Burger PC, et al. Placebo-controlled trial of safety and efficacy of intraoperative controlled delivery by biodegradable polymers of chemotherapy for recurrent gliomas. The Polymer-brain Tumor Treatment Group. Lancet 1995; 345:1008–1012.
59. Brem H, Ewend MG, Piantadosi S, et al. The safety of interstitial chemotherapy with BCNU-loaded polymer followed by radiation therapy in the treatment of newly diagnosed malignant gliomas: phase I trial. J Neurooncol 1995; 26:111–123.
60. Moses MA, Brem H, Langer R. Advancing the field of drug delivery taking aim at cancer. Cancer Cell 2003; 4:337–341.
61. Green SB, Byar DP, Walker MD, et al. Comparisons of carmustine; procarbazine; and high-dose methylprednisolone as additions to surgery and radiotherapy for the treatment of malignant glioma. Cancer Treat Rep 1983; 67:121–132.
62. Westphal M, Hilt DC, Bortey E, et al. A phase 3 trial of local chemotherapy with biodegradable carmustine (BCNU) wafers (Glidel wafers) in patients with primary malignant glioma. Neuro-Oncology (serial online) 2003, 5, Doc. 02-023. Available at: http://neuro-oncology.mc.duke.edu.
63. Westphal M, Ram Z, Riddle V, et al. Gliadel wafer in initial surgery for malignant glioma: long-term follow-up of a multicenter controlled trial. Acta Neurochir (Wien) 2006; 148:269–275.
64. Menei P, Montero-Menei C, Venier MC, et al. Drug delivery into the brain using poly(lactide-co-glycolide) microspheres. Expert Opin Drug Deliv 2005; 2:363–376.
65. Tatard VM, Venier-Julienne MC, Benoit JP, et al. In vivo evaluation of pharmacologically active microcarriers releasing NGF and conveying PC12 cells. Cell Transplant 2004; 13:573–583.

66. Tatard VM, Venier-Julienne MC, Saulnier P, et al. Pharmacologically active microcarriers: a tool for cell therapy. Biomaterials 2005; 26:3727–3737.
67. Tatard VM, Menei P, Benoit JP, et al. Combining polymeric devices and stem cells for the treatment of neurological disorders: a promising therapeutic approach. Curr Drug Targets 2005; 6: 81–96.
68. Tatard VM, Sindji L, Branton JG, et al. Pharmacologically active microcarriers releasing glial cell line—derived neurotrophic factor: survival and differentiation of embryonic dopaminergic neurons after grafting in hemiparkinsonian rats. Biomaterials 2007; 28:1978–1988.
69. Santini JT, Cima MJ, Langer R. A controlled-release microchip. Nature 1999; 397:335–338.
70. Wang PP, Frazier J, Brem H. Local drug delivery to the brain. Adv Drug Deliv Rev 2002; 54: 987–1013.
71. Li Y, Shawgo RS, Tyler B, et al. In vivo release from a drug delivery MEMS device. J Control Release 2004; 100:211–219.

2

Bioequivalence

Panos Macheras, Christos Reppas, and Mira Symillides
Laboratory of Biopharmaceutics and Pharmacokinetics, Faculty of Pharmacy, National and Kapodistrian University of Athens, Athens, Greece

BACKGROUND

The realization of the importance of product formulation for the speed of onset, intensity, and duration of drug response occurred in the early 1960s. At that time, various scattered reports in the literature (1–5) indicated that formulation changes result in marked differences in maximum observed plasma concentration (C_{max}) and area under the concentration-time curve (AUC), and the term "bioavailability" was coined to describe the fraction of dose reaching the general circulation. A few years later, dramatic bioavailability problems were observed with formulations of phenytoin in Australia and New Zealand in 1968 (6,7) and digoxin in the United Kingdom and the United States in 1971 (8,9). Consequently, comparative bioavailability studies were introduced in the United States regulatory setting (10,11) and the term bioavailability was officially introduced by the Food and Drug Administration (FDA) (12) and defined as follows: "Bioavailability means the rate and extent to which an active drug ingredient or therapeutic moiety is absorbed from a drug product and becomes available at the site of drug action." Since the late 1970s, a test (T) formulation that meets statistical criteria for the measures of relative bioavailability is termed "bioequivalent" to, and therapeutically interchangeable with, the reference (R) formulation. For more details on the regulatory history of generic drug development the reader is referred to relevant publications (13–15).

According to the bioavailability definition given above and because of the (most frequently) linear relationship between AUC and the fraction, F, of dose reaching the systemic circulation, AUC is used as a measure of the amount of drug reaching the general circulation.

$$\text{AUC} = \frac{F \times \text{dose}}{\text{CL}} \qquad (1)$$

By expressing the parameters of equation (1) in terms of the T and R formulations, assuming that the drug clearance is the same after administration of the two products, i.e., $\text{CL}_T = \text{CL}_R$, and assuming that the two formulations contain the same dose, i.e., $(\text{dose})_T = (\text{dose})_R$, one can easily derive from equation (1) that the ratio of bioavailability coefficients F_T/F_R is equal to the ratio of AUCs.

$$\frac{F_T}{F_R} = \frac{(\text{AUC})_T}{(\text{AUC})_R} \qquad (2)$$

Equation (2) comprises the pharmacokinetic (PK) basis for the routine use of AUC in bioequivalence (BE) studies as a robust measure of the amount of drug reaching the general circulation.

The rate of appearance in the general circulation is the second component in the definition of bioavailability. Since most frequently the rate is a time-dependent parameter, comparisons of rates are based on C_{max} values, because they are supposed to reflect adequately the input rate constant of the drug. Simulations have shown that C_{max} is not only insensitive to changes in the rate of input, but it is also dependent on amount of drug reaching the general circulation, i.e., it is a hybrid parameter (16). Several other absorption rate metrics like C_{max}/AUC (17), partial area (18,19), and the intercept of ln (C/t) versus time curve (20) with more favorable kinetic sensitivity properties have been proposed in literature. However, C_{max} continues to be the unique measure for rate comparisons in the regulatory setting, since it is considered meaningful from a clinical point of view. Today, AUC and C_{max} are viewed as clinically relevant measures of total and peak exposure, respectively (21).

In the early stages of recognition of BE, physicians by general consensus recommended that a difference of 20% between the two formulations would have no clinical significance for many drugs. This recommendation was interpreted as an allowable difference of 20% in the means of PK variables, namely, AUC and C_{max}, measured after administration of the T and R formulations. However, this definition is a statement for the difference of relative bioavailability of the total production (or population) of the two formulations. Since the assessment of BE relies on a sample of the formulations administered to a limited number of human subjects, regulatory agencies developed methodologies for the assessment of BE based on statistical criteria.

AVERAGE BIOEQUIVALENCE: THE CLASSIC APPROACH

Classically, the assessment of BE relies on the concept of average bioequivalence (ABE) (22). Determination of the ABE of two drug products (T vs. R) is based on the comparison of the means of logarithmically transformed PK parameters, such as AUC and C_{max}. BE is accepted if the difference of the log means (μ_T and μ_R, for the T and the R formulations, respectively) falls between specific predefined values for the upper and lower BE limits (23). The current approach of ABE is based on constant BE limits (BEL_0) at a level set by the regulatory agencies (22,24), and usually $\text{BEL}_0 = \ln(1.25)$. Thus, the criterion applied for the determination of ABE is

$$-\text{BEL}_0 \leq \mu_T - \mu_R \leq \text{BEL}_0 \qquad (3)$$

In practice, the true population means (μ_T and μ_R) are estimated by the calculated sample averages of the logarithmic parameters of the two formulations (m_T and m_R). In this context, ABE is declared if the calculated 90% confidence interval (CI) for the difference of the log means lies within the preset BE limits (23). Assuming the classic two-treatment, two-period, crossover BE study design, with equal numbers of subjects in each sequence, the upper and lower limits of the 90% CI are calculated according to equation (4).

$$(\text{Upper, Lower limit of the 90\% CI}) = \exp\left(\text{Diff} \pm t_{0.05, N-2}\sqrt{\frac{s^2 2}{N}}\right) \quad (4)$$

where Diff is the difference of T and R means, i.e., $\text{Diff} = m_T - m_R$; t the student's statistic; s^2 the residual variance, calculated by the residual mean square error of ANOVA (reflecting within-subject variance); and N the number of subjects. The usual statistical approach for the evaluation of ABE consists of two one-sided t procedures (25) to determine if the PK measures of the T and R products are comparable. This definition of ABE ensures the consumer safety, since the probability of an erroneous acceptance of BE does not exceed the preset level of significance (22).

During the past three decades or so, significant contributions to the theoretical and practical aspects of BE have been made by professional associations such as the American Pharmaceutical Association, American Association of Pharmaceutical Scientists and regulatory bodies, e.g., FDA and European Medicines Evaluation Agency (EMEA). Also, international symposia (26–28) have contributed to the evolution of BE studies and methodology. During the last decade significant advances on scientific issues relating to BE assessment have been made in three areas: in the assessment of the BE of highly variable (HV) drugs and drug products (28), in identifying situations where BE could or should be based on the plasma levels of metabolites (28), and in identifying situations where an in vivo BE study could be waived (29).

HIGHLY VARIABLE DRUGS AND DRUG PRODUCTS

The Problem in Establishing Bioequivalence

A drug or drug product is usually characterized as HV if the within-subject coefficient of variation (CV) of its PK responses is $\geq$30% (30–35). It is worth mentioning that the CV is related to the residual variance s^2 in the log scale, calculated by ANOVA, with the formula: $s^2 = \ln(\text{CV}^2 + 1)$. For HV drugs, the 0.80 to 1.25 BE limits seem to be too restrictive, leading to high producer risks (30–32,36,37).

As can be seen from equation (4), the width of the 90% CI is proportional to the within-subject variability and inversely proportional to the number of subjects participating in the study. Consequently, as within-subject variability increases, a higher rejection rate of BE for truly equivalent drug products is observed. Therefore, for truly equivalent products, it becomes too difficult to establish BE unless a large number of subjects are recruited to achieve adequate statistical power.

The need for unusually large numbers of healthy volunteers for the assessment of BE of HV drugs can raise ethical and practical issues. The exposure of large numbers of healthy volunteers to a drug even if it is deemed to be "safe," to satisfy a traditional preset criterion, must be seriously considered (38). In addition, the increase in the cost of the investigations of HV drugs—with usually wide therapeutic indices (35,38)—may result in difficulties in the development of new or generic drug products.

In the case where the upper limit of the 90% CI (equation 4) falls exactly on the upper preset BE limit, Diff becomes equal to Diff_{max}, which is the maximum acceptable difference between means (25,39). Diff_{max}, and therefore the maximum acceptable geometric mean ratio (GMR_{max}) [$\text{GMR}_{\text{max}} = \exp(\text{Diff}_{\text{max}})$], for a given number of subjects, is related not only to the estimated intrasubject variance but also to the value of the preset upper BE limit.

The major feature of the definition of classic unscaled ABE relies on the fact that two constant "borderline" values (0.80 and 1.25) are assigned for BE limits. Under this condition, extreme geometric mean ratio (GMR) values, which ensure BE, converge at unity as intrasubject variability increases (25,40). In other words, when upper and lower BE limits are fixed, the demonstration of BE requires that the means of two products must be as close as possible as variability increases. Although setting constant the BE limits is conceptually fundamental, the 0.80 to 1.25 limits appear very "strict" in the case of HV drugs. To overcome the difficulties encountered in the assessment of the bioavailability of HV drugs with the currently used BE limits, several approaches have been proposed.

Approaches for the Evaluation of Bioequivalence

Multiple-Dose Studies

To reduce within-subject variability, multiple-dose steady-state studies have been considered (24,41). It has been shown that the observed variation of PK parameters is often lower at steady state than after single dosing (41–43). The reduced variation of C_{max} at steady state is probably due to its lower kinetic sensitivity in reflecting absorption rate (22,44). Nevertheless, under certain conditions, C_{max} was found to exhibit higher variation at steady state than after a single administration, and therefore multiple-dose designs were not considered to be the solution for the assessment of BE of HV drugs (43,45). Currently, the FDA approach recommends applicants to conduct single-dose studies rather than multiple-dose studies because "single-dose studies are generally more sensitive in assessing release of the drug substance from the drug product into the systemic circulation" (22).

Replicate Designs

For single-dose studies, replicate designs that reduce the total number of subjects required have been also proposed (22,24,32,41) for the assessment of BE for HV drugs. Roughly, about half as many volunteers are needed in a four-period study than in a two-period investigation to attain the same statistical power.

However, replicate designs (as multiple-dose studies) lead to increased duration of exposure to the drug and, moreover, potential practical problems may arise, e.g., increased incidence of subject withdrawals. In addition, in certain cases, e.g., for drugs with long half-lives, replicated designs are difficult to apply.

Consideration of Only the Point Estimate of the Mean Test/Reference Ratio

Another approach for the assessment of BE of HV products has been based on the point estimate of the mean T/R ratio. In this context, a relaxed requirement is adopted by the regulatory authority in Canada in the case of C_{max}. This PK parameter is a single-measure estimate and often shows higher variation than AUC. Therefore, Health Canada requires that only the point estimate of the GMR for C_{max}, and not its 90% CI, fall between the BE limits of 0.80 to 1.25 (46).

Individual Bioequivalence

Individual BE (23,47–52), a procedure relying on the concept of switchability between drug formulations, has been also proposed for the evaluation of HV drugs. According to this concept, the T-R difference is compared with the R-R difference within subjects using repeated measures. The individual BE criterion comprises the ratio of the sum of the contrast of the squared means of the two formulations, the contrast of their within-subject variances and the subject by formulation variance over the within-subject variance of the R formulation. While individual BE represents an attractive approach, several problems have limited its application in practice (38,51).

Widening of Acceptance Limits to Prefixed Constant Values

Widening the BE acceptance limits to prefixed constant values (0.70–1.43 or 0.75–1.33) (24,31,53) has been proposed, especially for PK parameters showing increased variation, e.g., C_{max}.

Expanded 0.75 to 1.33 or 0.70. to 1.43 BE limits for drugs meeting a "high variability criterion" Several questions may arise, indicative of the difficulties of the application of this approach: What is the high variability criterion? An intrasubject variability value, estimated from ANOVA? For example, when CV > 30% (33,34)? A problem may arise about the classification of drugs presenting borderline variability values (54). It was estimated that about 20% of the evaluated HV drugs constitute borderline cases (34). Nevertheless, the use of an extended region of acceptance reduces the producer risk at high CV values, but at the same time, large differences between the means are allowed (55) for drug products with moderate residual variability. This constitutes a potential problem of switchability for multisource formulations, each declared bioequivalent to the same R product (39,56). Consequently, an additional point estimate constraint criterion on GMR, e.g., $0.80 \leq GMR \leq 1.25$, may be needed.

Widening of BE limits only beyond a limiting, "switching" variability value (mixed model) It has been suggested to use either the classic 0.80 to 1.25, or the more "liberal" (e.g., 0.75–1.33 or 0.70–1.43) BE limits only beyond a switching variability value (24,53). However, apart from the fact that in this case two criteria are required, applying an arbitrarily chosen switching variability value can lead to unfair treatment of different formulations of the same drug evaluated in separate BE studies and presenting only minor differences in variability (57). For example, assuming a switching variability of CV = 30%, it seems rather unfair that a drug with broad therapeutic index and CV = 29.9% has to be evaluated using the classic 0.80 to 1.25 BE range, which allows a maximum accepted value of GMR, $GMR_{max} = 1.08$, while the same drug could be evaluated in a different BE study with CV = 30%, using the expanded 0.70 to 1.43 range, which allows a $GMR_{max} = 1.24$ (see Fig. 6B of Ref. 57). The major cause of this attribute is the inherent discontinuity when these two BE criteria are concomitantly applied (Fig. 1). Consequently, a question arises: How do we deal with BE studies with borderline variability values, i.e., BE trials presenting variability values very close to the switching variability?

Scaled Procedures

A method for expanding the limits for HV drugs, based on an estimate of intrasubject variation, was proposed: The BE limits are scaled according to a fixed multiple, of within-subject standard deviation, σ_W, on the log scale (58).

$$(\text{Upper, Lower BE limit}) = \exp(\pm k\sigma_W) \qquad (5)$$

where k is a multiplying factor.

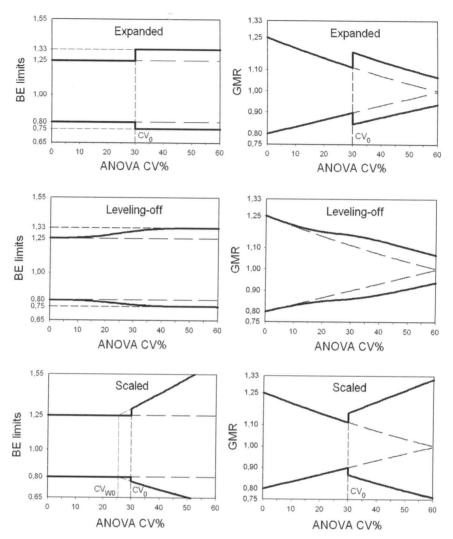

Figure 1 BE limits (*left side*) and extreme GMR values, which ensure BE (*right side*) as a function of within-subject variability (ANOVA CV), for the classic (0.80–1.25) limits (*dashed lines*) and three proposed procedures (*solid lines*): expanded BE limits beyond a switching variability $CV_0 = 30\%$ (24) (*top*); BE limits with levelling-off properties based on a sigmoid function (63) (*middle*); and scaled BE limits (equation 10) with a preset variability $CV_{W0} = 25.4\%$ and switching variability $CV_0 = 30\%$ (35,64) (*bottom*). A two-period crossover study with 36 subjects was assumed for the calculation of extreme GMR values. *Abbreviations*: BE, bioequivalence; GMR, geometric mean ratio; CV, coefficient of variation.

Thus, the acceptance criterion can be expressed as

$$-k\sigma_W \leq \mu_T - \mu_R \leq k\sigma_W \tag{6}$$

It has been also suggested that the regulatory criterion of ABE, in the case of HV drugs, could be scaled by a standard deviation, leading to an approach known as scaled average bioequivalence (ABEsc) (59,60). The acceptance criterion is then defined as

$$-k \leq \frac{\mu_T - \mu_R}{\sigma_W} \leq k \tag{7}$$

The scaling factor, σ_W, in the case of a two-period design is the residual standard deviation, σ_{Res}, estimated from ANOVA, while for a replicate design the within-subject standard deviation of the R formulation, σ_{WR}, is used.

An approach using the noncentral t distribution to calculate the confidence limits for ABEsc has been suggested (60). An alternative procedure consisting of a numerical approximation based on the method of Hyslop et al. (61) has been also proposed for the statistical evaluation of ABEsc.

It is worth mentioning that the model for ABEsc (equation 7) can be readily converted to that of the scaled BE limits (equation 6). Indeed, when investigated, the two approaches yielded very similar results (60).

Various suggestions have been made for the most appropriate proportionality factor, k, for scaled BE limits (39,58,62). The value of k affects the slope of the BE limits and therefore the degree of expansion.

Simple scaled BE limits When variability is low, very small deviations of GMR from unity are permitted to declare BE. Consequently, scaled BE limits appear to be very strict for drugs with low variability and probably inappropriate even for the evaluation of drugs with narrow therapeutic range. At a specific value of the variability ($\sigma_W = \sigma_0$), depending on the value of the proportionality factor k, scaled BE limits become equal to the classic BEL_0.

$$k\sigma_0 = BEL_0 = \ln(1.25) \tag{8}$$

As variability increases, scaled BE limits become very liberal, allowing GMR values higher than 1.25 (40). Therefore, a common drawback of the reported scaled BE limits (39,58,62) is their continuous increase with variability. This leads to very broad acceptance limits of BE. The GMR acceptance region has a nonconvex shape (40), similar to that for the Hauck and Anderson procedure as pointed out by Schuirmann (see Fig. 12 of Ref. 25), and gets wider and wider with increasing CV. Thus, BE studies with GMR deviating considerably from unity even at very high CVs could be accepted. Since large differences between the means can be accepted by scaled methods with substantial probabilities, an additional regulatory criterion was proposed to be imposed concomitantly with the CI test (53). This secondary criterion suggests that the estimated GMR should be constrained in the range 0.80 to 1.25. Nevertheless, even with the concomitant application of the above-mentioned additional criterion, the acceptance region still has a nonconvex shape, and BE studies with GMR values between 0.80 and 1.25 can be accepted, even at very high variability level.

Mixed model An interesting variant of the simple scaled procedure has been proposed (62). It involves the use of both the classic unscaled ABE (when drugs do not exhibit high variability) and the ABEsc for HV drugs (when a preset magnitude of the variability is exceeded) (62). The switching variability, σ_0, for the ABEsc was set to 0.20, and corresponds to a proportionality constant, $k = \ln(1.25)/\sigma_0 = 1.116$. This mixed model (62) for ABEsc can be converted to a mixed approach of scaled BE limits, using the classic unscaled criterion up to CV 20% and scaled BE limits with a proportionality factor of 1.116, for CV over 20%. When the mixed model is used, the boundaries of the GMR acceptance region converge to a minimum value as CV values increase up to 20%, and then start to spread apart, for values of CV higher than 20% (see Fig. 2 of Ref. 40). Consequently, this approach is less "permissive" for drugs with moderate variability (CV $\sim$ 20%) than for drugs with low or high variability. The nonmonotony of the extreme accepted GMR versus CV plots is an unfavorable property of the method, because it appears to "punish" drug products with moderate variability (40). Moreover, as the mixed model is a scaled procedure, it suffers also from the common drawback of the simple scaled BE limits mentioned previously, i.e., the continuous increase with variability leading to very broad acceptance BE limits. Again, the GMR acceptance region has a nonconvex shape and an additional (3rd) point estimate constraint criterion, e.g., $0.80 \leq GMR \leq 1.25$ may be needed. Nevertheless, BE studies with GMR deviating from unity can be accepted even at very high CVs.

Finally, if one uses a different value for k, e.g., $k = 0.760$ (39,62) for the mixed model, the switching variability, σ_0, is 0.294 (corresponding to a CV = 30%), and a stricter BE criterion is constructed.

Combined scaled criterion To improve the performance of the above-mentioned scaled procedures, a novel approach has been proposed, consisting of a combined criterion for evaluating BE (40). Scaled BE limits containing an effective constraint have been developed. The proposed BE limits scale with intrasubject variability but incorporate also a GMR-dependent criterion, which makes them less permissive as GMR values depart from unity (40,57).

Scaled BE Limits with Leveling-off Properties

A new rationale for the design of scaled BE limits has been developed (63) to improve the too restrictive behavior of the classic BE limits when truly bioequivalent HV drugs are compared, and concomitantly to avoid the drawbacks of the simple scaled or mixed methods, discussed previously. To this end, the BE limits developed scale with intrasubject variability but only until a "plateau" value and combine the classic (0.80–1.25) and expanded (0.75–1.33) BE limits into a single criterion (Fig. 1). To combine the above-mentioned desired properties into a single criterion, the upper BE limit is expressed as a function of intrasubject variability, which levels off at a predefined plateau value. Accordingly, this function has three controlling parameters, which are

1. the minimum (or starting) value of the upper BE limit,
2. the maximum (or plateau) value of the upper BE limit, and
3. the "rate" of the gradual change of the upper BE limit value as a function of variability.

The new scaled limits become more permissive than the classic unscaled BE limits as variability increases, and thus they require fewer subjects to prove BE. Nevertheless, the GMR acceptance region has a convex shape (Fig. 1), which is similar to that of the classic unscaled 0.80 to 1.25 limits (29,40). Undoubtedly, this is not only a desired property but also a unique characteristic for a scaled method. This finding is a consequence of the new structure of the BE limits with leveling-off properties.

One of the major advantages of the new scaled limits is their gradual expansion with variability until a plateau value. The gradual expansion of the BE limits is by far preferable than the use of expanded criteria only beyond an arbitrarily chosen, critical switching variability value (Fig. 1), as the discontinuity of the BE limits may lead to preferential treatment of drugs presenting only minor differences in variability. The gradual expansion from a strict to a permissive BE limit, apart from avoiding the discontinuity around a switching variability, makes the new BE limits also suitable for use at low CV levels. In fact, when variability is low, BE limits with leveling-off properties exhibit similar percentage of accepted BE studies as the classic BE limits (63). Therefore, these BE limits would be implemented in practice, e.g., in the case of C_{max} ratio, in lieu of a wider acceptance interval (23). It is also worthy to mention that leveling-off BE limits present a quite flexible structure, and therefore a variety of starting and plateau values for the upper BE limit can be considered. The flexibility, continuity, and leveling-off properties of these scaled BE limits in conjunction with their performance in simulation studies (63) make them suitable for the assessment of BE studies, without the need of a secondary criterion of constrained GMR value and irrespective of the level of variability encountered.

Current Thinking Within the FDA for the Evaluation of Highly Variable Drugs and Drug Products

For drugs with an expected within-subject variability of $\geq 30\%$, a BE study with three-period, R-replicated, crossover design has been proposed (34,35,64). The minimum number of subjects that would be acceptable is 24. The BE assessment comprises two parts: an ABEsc evaluation and a point estimate constraint. The BE criterion for both AUC and C_{max} is defined as

$$\frac{(\mu_T - \mu_R)^2}{\sigma_{WR}^2} \leq \theta \tag{9}$$

where $\theta = (\ln \Delta)^2/\sigma_{W0}^2$, with $\Delta = 1.25$ and $\sigma_{W0} = 0.25$ (the preset standard variability).

A 95% upper confidence bound for $(\mu_T - \mu_R)^2/\sigma_{WR}^2$ must be $\leq \theta$, or equivalently, a 95% upper confidence bound for $(\mu_T - \mu_R)^2 - \theta\sigma_{WR}^2$ must be ≤ 0. Additionally, the point estimate for GMR of T/R must fall within (0.80, 1.25).

In the original scale, the proposed BE limits are

$$(\text{Upper, Lower BE limit}) = \exp\left(\pm \frac{\ln(1.25)}{0.25}\sigma_{WR}\right) \tag{10}$$

According to this criterion, the value of the k factor chosen is $k = \ln(1.25)/0.25 = 0.892$, presenting an intermediate value between the too liberal approach of $k = 1.116$ (62) and the stricter one, $k = 0.760$ (39,62). However, the choice of this value (or equivalently the choice of $\sigma_{W0} = 0.25$) presents the demerit of an inherent discontinuity of the BE limits when applied for drugs with CV $\geq 30\%$ (i.e., with $\sigma_{WR} \geq 0.294$), (Fig. 1). The cause of this attribute is that the preset standard variability value ($\sigma_{W0} = 0.25$) is not the same as the switching variability value ($\sigma_0 = 0.294$). A relevant comment has been also made recently (65). Consequently, if the estimated within-subject CV of the R formulation is just above the changeover point of 30%, the BE limits will be much wider (i.e., > 1.30) than just below (i.e., 1.25).

Moreover, the proposed procedure suffers from the same drawbacks as all the mixed models of the scaled methods: The boundaries of the GMR acceptance region converge to a minimum at the switching variability value and then start to spread apart for higher values of CV, presenting a nonconvex shape (Fig. 1). Consequently, an *additional* point estimate constraint criterion on GMR is needed.

The EMEA Approach for the Evaluation of Highly Variable Drugs

EMEA in the Note for Guidance on the Investigation of Bioavailability and Bioequivalence (24) states that the 90% CI for AUC and C_{max} ratios should lie within an acceptance interval of 0.80 to 1.25. However, "in certain cases a wider interval may be acceptable" for C_{max} (Fig. 1), provided that there are no safety or efficacy concerns. Some points of this statement were furthermore clarified in a Questions & Answers document (33) as follows: The possibility offered by the guideline to widen the acceptance range "should be considered *exceptional* and *limited to a small widening* (0.75–1.33)." Furthermore, this possibility is restricted to those products for which at least one of the following applies: Safety and efficacy should be *clinically justified* [i.e., using adequate pharmacokinetic/pharmacodynamic (PK/PD) or clinical data], or should refer to a *defined HV drug* (i.e., an R product with intrasubject variability greater than 30%). Recently, EMEA has addressed more intensively the issue of HV drugs. In this context, the Committee for Medicinal Products for Human use (CHMP) has also released a concept paper for an addendum, focusing on scaled procedures for the evaluation of BE of HV drugs (66) and a recommendation document on the need for revision of the note for guidance (67).

METABOLITES IN BIOEQUIVALENCE ASSESSMENT

In the majority of cases assessment of BE relies on the plasma concentrations of the parent drug since this is either the only reported therapeutic moiety or it is not metabolized. Concern is raised, however, when the parent drug is metabolized and the metabolite(s) exhibit comparable therapeutic activity with the parent drug. On the other hand, obvious reasons for measuring the metabolite(s) are (*i*) whenever an inactive prodrug is metabolized to an active metabolite and (*ii*) the parent drug concentrations are too low, while metabolite(s) plasma levels are quantifiable. The reader can find several examples in the literature, whereas the target species for measurement is either the metabolite(s) or the parent drug and the metabolite(s) (68–76).

Computer-simulated BE studies are a powerful tool in this field of research since the modeling assumptions along with the values of the parameters are specified and the results can be contrasted with the assumptions used. The simulations are based on classical PK models with the formation of metabolite taking place during the presystemic absorption and/or during subsequent recirculation through the liver. The simulations try to explore which of the species is the most appropriate for BE decision making on the basis of statistical criteria such as the width of the relevant CIs. One should recall, however, that all these approaches are approximations of the reality because the complexity-variability in hepatic clearance can be also a function of the magnitude of alternative elimination processes for the drug and/or the metabolite. During the last 15 years or so, several simulation studies on the role of metabolites in BE have been published (77–82). Many of these studies have been reviewed by Midha and colleagues (83), and the use of metabolites in BE studies has been the subject of a recent Bio-International congress (28).

The first study (77) in this topic published in 1991 was based on a simple first-order one-compartment PK model, with exclusive formation of a metabolite during recirculation through the liver. The authors focused on the rate of metabolite elimination being either limited by its formation or its excretion. Simulated BE studies were carried out with random error added to the absorption rate constant values of the R and T formulation. The statistical analysis based on the comparison of variability (using 90% CIs) associated with the C_{max} values of parent drug and the metabolite revealed that the former was greater than the latter. Although their simulation results were contrasted with experimental BE studies of four drugs, caution should be exercised whether the drugs fulfill the modeling assumptions relevant to the metabolism of drug (83).

The second study by the same authors four years later (78) utilized a two-compartment model, with formation of the metabolite taking place either presystemically or during recirculation through the liver. Again, comparisons were based on the variability of C_{max} values for the parent drug and the metabolite as a function of the variabilities used for the absorption rate constant of the parent drug, k_a, as well as the first-pass formation of the metabolite, k_f. The variability of C_{max} values of the parent drug and the metabolite was found to follow the magnitude of variability associated with k_a and k_f, respectively.

The work of Tucker and colleagues (79) has been based on a model in which the formation of metabolite in the liver takes place both on first passage and on subsequent recirculation through the organ. The analysis was focused on AUC values derived from simulation studies of drug and metabolite kinetics. The PK parameters considered were intrinsic, CL_{int} and renal clearance, CL_r as well as the hepatic blood flow, Q_H. According to the authors, metabolite data have to be used for high extraction ratio drugs, namely, $CL_{int} \geq Q_H$. For low extraction ratio drugs ($CL_{int} < Q_H$), the parent drug data are preferred; however, when CL_r is low, one has to use metabolite data. The basic conclusion of the study is that the within-subject variabilities of metabolic and renal clearances are the basic determinants for the use of drug or metabolite data since they determine the sensitivity of AUC to the differences of fraction of dose reaching the general circulation.

In similar work, Rosenbaum and Lam (80) studied the sensitivities of the parameters AUC and C_{max} of the parent drug and the metabolite to variabilities associated with the intrinsic and hepatic clearance. A simple PK model was utilized with the formation of a single metabolite taking place during first passage. The statistical analysis of data revealed that the parent drug had wider 90% CIs around the point estimates for the ratio (T/R) of geometric means of AUC and C_{max} than the corresponding one for the single metabolite. In a similar vein, Rosenbaum (81) used a semiphysiological pharmacostatistical model to study the manner in which intraindividual variability in hepatic clearance is transferred to AUC of a drug and its metabolite. The model assumes the formation of metabolite in the liver both on first passage and on subsequent recirculation through the organ. The results indicated that as the drug's hepatic extraction ratio increased, the variability of the drug's AUC was increased, whereas that of the metabolite decreased.

Jackson (82) carried out simulations, focusing on the response of parent drug and metabolite 90% CIs for AUC and C_{max} to equivalent and inequivalent immediate release formulations. A linear first-pass model with random error added to the model parameters: renal clearance, hepatic clearance, systemic clearance, and liver blood flow. Specific values were assigned to the absorption rate constant and fraction absorbed to investigate problems associated with equivalent and nonequivalent immediate release formulations. According to Jackson (82), the C_{max} for the parent drug provided the most accurate assessment of BE. On the contrary, the metabolite C_{max} was found to be insensitive to changes related to rate of absorption. In addition, when the value of the intrinsic clearance is higher than the liver blood flow, the use of the metabolite C_{max} data can lead to a conclusion of BE for truly bioinequivalent products.

In parallel, the use of prodrugs in therapy is pertinent to the matter since most of them are rapidly absorbed from the gastrointestinal tract and rapidly biotransformed to the active metabolite. Prodrug blood levels tend to be very low and much more variable when compared with the active metabolite. It should be noted that many prodrugs (ACE inhibitors, some statins, valacyclovir, fenofibrate) were not quantified with analytical methods of high sensitivity in PK studies by the innovator because of their short residence time and low blood levels. However, the continuous evolution in mass spectrometry allows today for the reliable measurement of prodrugs for a reasonable period of time. Thus, the measurement of both the prodrug and the active metabolite for the assessment of BE remains to be further evaluated. To emphasize the contradictory approaches as well as the incoherence of the description of the current guidelines (22,24) for the role of metabolites in BE assessment, we quote below two characteristic extracts. The FDA guideline (22) states, "The moieties to be measured in biological fluids collected in bioavailability and bioequivalence studies are either the active dug ingredient or its active moiety in the administered dosage form (parent drug) and, when appropriate its active metabolite. . . . Measurement of a metabolite may be preferred when parent drug levels are too low to allow reliable analytical measurement in blood, plasma or serum for an adequate length of time. . . . If the metabolite contributes meaningfully to safety and/or efficacy, we also recommend that the metabolite and the parent drug be measured." The EMEA guideline (24) states, "In most cases evaluation of bioavailability and bioequivalence will be based upon the measured concentrations of the parent compound. In some situations, however, measurements of an active or inactive metabolite may be necessary instead of the parent compound. . . . Bioequivalence determinations based on metabolites should be justified in each case bearing in mind that the aim of a bioequivalence study is intended to compare the in vivo performance of T and R products. In particular if metabolites significantly contribute to the net activity of an active substance and the pharmacokinetic system is nonlinear, it is necessary to measure both parent drug and active metabolite plasma concentrations and evaluate them separately."

WAIVING AN IN VIVO BIOEQUIVALENCE STUDY

To date, comparison of the PKs of the drug in plasma to demonstrate BE is considered as the most commonly used and successful tool of similarity of two drug products in terms of safety and efficacy. However, since the initial proposal of the Biopharmaceutics Classification System (BCS) in 1995 (84), regulatory authorities worldwide may accept BE of two drug products based on in vitro data only (29,85) (Table 1), whereas there are ongoing discussions on defining additional situations where in vivo BE studies can be safely replaced with in vitro experiments. Compared with in vivo BE studies, in vitro studies are cheaper, faster, and not associated with ethical considerations. In addition, they provide a better opportunity for focusing at product performance, i.e., at the presentation of the drug to the intestinal epithelium.

Table 1 The Biopharmaceutics Classification System Arranges Drug Substances into Four Classes on the Basis of Their Biopharmaceutical Properties and Provides the Basis for Waving In Vivo BE Studies

	High solubility[a]	Low solubility
High permeability[a]	Class 1 High solubility[a] High permeability[b] Rapid dissolution and wide therapeutic index[c]	Class 2 Low solubility High permeability[b]
Low permeability	Class 3 High solubility[a] Low permeability	Class 4 Low solubility Low permeability

[a]Solubility is high when the highest dose strength is soluble in no more than 250 mL of aqueous media over the pH range 1 to 7.5.

[b]Permeability is considered high when total fraction absorbed is at least 90% or is measured in vitro to be higher than that of standard compounds.

[c]Class 1 drugs must have wide therapeutic index, and their dissolution must be rapid for an in vivo bioequivalence study to be waived. An immediate release product is considered rapidly dissolving when not less than 85% of the labeled amount of the drug substance is dissolved within 30 minutes of using USP Apparatus I at 100 rpm (or Apparatus II at 50 rpm) in a volume of 900 mL or less in each of the following media: 0.1N HCl or simulated gastric fluid USP without enzymes, in a pH 4.5 buffer, and in a pH 6.8 buffer or simulated intestinal fluid USP without enzymes (29).

Abbreviation: USP, U.S. Pharmacopeia.

Source: From Refs. 29 and 84.

The Biopharmaceutics Classification System

The concept of BCS is that immediate release drug products containing the same dose of the same drug substance, and having the same intralumenal dissolution and gut wall permeability profiles in vivo, will be bioequivalent. Although the concept has received wide acceptance worldwide, there are difficulties in measuring the parameters of interest, which most frequently refer to the small intestine, because drug absorption takes place primarily in this region.

Although both invasive (86) and noninvasive (87) methods have been proposed, measurement of dissolution intralumenally is not practical and, at best, existing methods require further validation. As a result, to date, intralumenal dissolution is mostly assessed with in vitro setups that simulate (to a certain degree) the intralumenal environment (29,88). Since direct correlation of in vitro dissolution data with intralumenal dissolution data is, to date, not practical to achieve, attempts are being made to estimate intralumenal dissolution from intralumenal solubility data that can be collected relatively easier (89–92). However, intralumenal solubility data may not be directly proportional to intralumenal dissolution data (89), because solubility is only one of the parameters affecting dissolution. For example, intralumenal hydrodynamics (that to date are only poorly simulated in vitro) play a significant role (93).

In regard to permeability of the epithelium of the small intestine, although it can be measured in humans (94), associated costs are extremely high. Thus, permeability estimations are typically based on in vitro data [most frequently collected by using cell monolayers developed from human colonic carcinoma epithelia (e.g., the Caco-2 cell lines)] or in situ animal data (most frequently collected by perfusing segments of rat small intestine). However, Caco-2 cell lines are associated with overexpression of certain transporters, and they do not allow for paracellular transport. In addition, correlations of either Caco-2 data with human data or rat perfusion data with human data are highly scattered. Alternative methodologies for assessing permeability are also not free of drawbacks. For example, decision on high or low permeability based on the total percentage of dose absorbed in humans (Table 1) has two weaknesses. First, the *extent* of absorption is used as surrogate of a *kinetic* parameter, permeability. Second is that if first pass metabolism is substantial, it would complicate the estimation of total percentage of dose absorbed. Recently, it has been suggested that drugs that are extensively metabolized are highly permeable drugs and regulatory agencies should add the extent of drug metabolism (i.e., >90% metabolized) as an alternate method for the extent of drug absorption (i.e., >90% absorbed) (95). Even this approach, however, has some drawbacks. For example, permeable drugs that are excreted unchanged into urine or bile may be incorrectly classified as lowly absorbed compounds, whereas drugs such as amoxicillin, chloroquine, lomefloxacin, trimethorpin, and zalcitabine that exhibit >90% oral bioavailability will also be listed as poorly absorbed drugs (96).

Biowaivers[a] Based on the Biopharmaceutics Classification System

Despite the problems associated with the correct classification of compounds according to the BCS, the current approach in deciding high solubility and high permeability compounds is considered a conservative and, therefore, safe approach (Table 1) (29,85). Using this approach, biowaivers could be granted for high solubility-high permeability

---

[a]Generic drug products approvals without in vivo bioequivalence studies.

drugs, whereas possible extensions of biowaivers in other classes are currently being considered.

According to the relevant guidance launched in 2000 by the FDA (29) and subsequently adapted by other regulatory bodies worldwide (85), biowaivers can be requested and granted for drug substances that do not have a narrow therapeutic index, belong to BCS class 1, and are housed in rapidly dissolving immediate release products (Table 1). If these criteria are met, the drug absorption process is controlled by gastric emptying and, therefore, formulation differences are not expected to play a role.

Class 1 drugs represent a subset of drugs that is decreasing with time: If the orally administered immediate release products in the List of Essential Medicines of the World Health Organization (WHO) are considered, approximately 30% can be considered as class 1 drugs (97,98). However, the proportion of class 1 compounds in the development phase for oral immediate-release formulations at AstraZeneca was less than 10% in 2001 (99), and is slightly less than 20% at GlaxoSmithKline (100).

The percentage of drugs belonging to class 2 is steadily increasing (96,100), and there is growing interest in identifying situations within this class that can be considered for waiving an in vivo BE study. It has been suggested that acidic drugs that belong to class 2 that show low solubility in the stomach and high solubility in the upper small intestine could be granted biowaivers (101,102). An approach for waiving an in vivo BE study of weakly acidic class 2 compounds has been recently proposed by the WHO on the basis of the rapid dissolution characteristics in slightly acidic pH values (simulating the pH conditions of the upper small intestine) (103). However, other studies suggest that, although in vitro testing of this type of drugs could predict differences between two products on the extent of absorption, differences on the maximum plasma concentration may not be predicted with in vitro testing as these may additionally be affected by intragastric solubility, gastric emptying, and type of formulation (104). Therefore, at present time, there are no widely accepted procedures for granting biowaivers to class 2 drugs.

Since permeability of a class 3 drug through the gut wall is the rate-determining step for the overall absorption process, formulation effects are expected to play a less important role in drug absorption, and, consequently, biowaivers have been suggested to be granted to compounds belonging to this class (105–107). For passively absorbed class 3 drugs, one issue is that permeability might be location dependent, i.e., it is likely that will fall to low values in the distal small intestine. This issue could be overcome with the development of rapidly dissolving formulations to obtain the best possible absorption (103). Another issue for passively absorbed drugs is the potential excipients' effects on permeability. Conventional excipients at commonly used amounts have been shown not to be critical with regard to the absorption of atenolol (108), cimetidine (109), and ranitidine (110) in humans. However, it should be underlined that other excipients can have pronounced effects on the absorption of these drugs (111,112). Finally, class 3 compounds for which their absorption in humans has been convincingly shown to involve the participation of certain carriers should be very cautiously considered for granting biowaivers, since excipients' effects on this type of transport may be even more difficult to predict (113).

REFERENCES

1. Morrison A, Chapman D, Campbell J. Further studies on the relation between in vitro disintegration time of tablets and the urinary excretion rates of riboflavin. J Am Pharm Assoc 1959; 48:634–637.
2. Morrison A, Campbell J. The relationship between physiological availability of salicylates and riboflavin and in vitro disintegration time of enteric coated tablets. J Am Pharm Assoc 1960; 49:473–478.

3. Levy G. Comparison of dissolution and absorption rates of different commercial aspirin tablets. J Pharm Sci 1961; 50:388–392.

4. Levy G. Effect of particle size on dissolution and gastrointestinal absorption rates of pharmaceuticals. Am J Pharm Sci Support Public Health 1963; 135:78–92.

5. Middleton E, Davies J, Morrison A. Relationship between rate of dissolution, disintegration time, and physiological availability of riboflavin in sugar-coated tablets. J Pharm Sci 1964; 53:1378–1380.

6. Tyrer JH, Eadie MJ, Sutherland JM, et al. Outbreak of anticonvulsant intoxication in an Australian city. Br Med J 1970; 4:271–273.

7. Bochner F, Hooper WD, Tyrer JH, et al. Factors involved in an outbreak of phenytoin intoxication. J Neurol Sci 1972; 16:481–487.

8. Lindenbaum J, Mellow MH, Blackstone MO, et al. Variation in biologic availability of digoxin from four preparations. N Engl J Med 1971; 285:1344–1347.

9. Fraser EJ, Leach RH, Poston JW. Bioavailability of digoxin. Lancet 1972; 2:541.

10. Federal Register 34: 2673 (1969).

11. Federal Register 35: 6574 (1970).

12. Federal Register 42: 1642 (1977).

13. Federal Register 54: 28873 (1989).

14. Strom BL. Generic drug substitution revisited. N Engl J Med 1987; 316:1456–1462.

15. Nightingale SL, Morisson JC. Generic drugs and the prescribing physician. JAMA 1987; 258:1200–1204.

16. Lacey LF, Keene ON, Duquesnoy C, et al. Evaluation of different indirect measures of rate of drug absorption in comparative pharmacokinetic studies. J Pharm Sci 1994; 83:212–215.

17. Endrenyi L, Fritsch S, Yan W. Cmax/AUC is a clearer measure than Cmax for absorption rates in investigations of bioequivalence. Int J Clin Pharmacol Ther Toxicol 1991; 29:394–399.

18. Chen ML. An alternative approach for assessment of rate of absorption in bioequivalence studies. Pharm Res 1992; 9:1380–1385.

19. Macheras P, Symillides M, Reppas C. The cut-off time point of the partial area method for assessment of rate of absorption in bioequivalence studies. Pharm Res 1994; 11:831–834.

20. Macheras P, Symillides M, Reppas C. An improved intercept method for the assessment of absorption rate in bioequivalence studies. Pharm Res 1996; 13:1753–1756.

21. Chen ML, Lesko L, Williams RL. Measures of exposure versus measures of rate and extent of absorption. Clin Pharmacokinet 2001; 40:565–572.

22. U.S. Department of Health and Human Services, Food and Drug Administration (FDA), Center for Drug Evaluation and Research (CDER). Guidance for Industry: Bioavailability and bioequivalence studies for orally administered drug products—General considerations, March 2003.

23. U.S. Department of Health and Human Services, Food and Drug Administration (FDA), Center for Drug Evaluation and Research (CDER). Guidance for Industry: Statistical Approaches to Establishing Bioequivalence, January 2001.

24. European Agency for the Evaluation of Medicinal Products (EMEA), Committee for Proprietary Medicinal Products (CPMP). Note for guidance on the investigation of bioavailability and bioequivalence. Doc. Ref. CPMP/EWR/QWP/1401/98, July 2001.

25. Schuirmann DJ. A comparison of the two one-sided tests procedure and the power approach for assessing the equivalence of average bioavailability. J Pharmacokinet Biopharm 1987; 15:657–680.

26. Blume HH, Midha KK. Bio-International 92, Conference on bioavailability, bioequivalence, and pharmacokinetic studies. J Pharm Sci 1993; 82:1186–1189.

27. Blume HH, McGilveray IJ, Midha KK. Bio-International '94 Conference on Bioavailability, Bioequivalence and Pharmacokinetic Studies and Pre-Conference Satellite on 'In Vivo/In Vitro Correlation.' Munich, Germany, June 14–17, 1994. Eur J Drug Metab Pharmacokinet 1995; 20:3–13.

28. Midha KK, Shah VP, Singh GJ, et al. Conference report: Bio-International 2005. J Pharm Sci 2007; 96:747–754.

29. US Department of Health and Human Services, Food and Drug Administration, Center for Drug Evaluation and Research (CDER). Guidance for Industry: waiver of in vivo bioavailability and bioequivalence studies for immediate-release solid oral dosage forms based on a biopharmaceutics classification system. Available at: http://www.fda.gov/cder/guidance/3618fnl.pdf. Accessed September 21, 2007.

30. Blume H, Midha K. Report of consensus meeting: Bio-International '92, Conference on Bioavailability, Bioequivalence and Pharmacokinetics studies, Bad Homburg, Germany, May 20–22, 1992. Eur J Pharm Sci 1993; 1:165–171.

31. Blume H, McGilveray I, Midha K. Report of consensus meeting: Bio-international '94, Conference on Bioavailability, Bioequivalence and Pharmacokinetics studies, Munich, Germany, June 14–17, 1994. Eur J Pharm Sci 1995; 3:113–124.

32. Shah V, Yacobi A, Barr W, et al. Evaluation of orally administered highly variable drugs and drug formulations. Pharm Res 1996; 13:1590–1594.

33. European Medicines Evaluation Agency, Committee for Medicinal Products for Human use (CHMP), Efficacy working party, therapeutic subgroup on pharmacokinetics (EWP-PK). Questions & Answers on the bioavailability and bioequivalence guideline. Doc. Ref. EMEA/CHMP/EWP/40326/2006, July 2006.

34. Davit B. Highly variable drugs – bioequivalence issues: FDA proposal under consideration. Meeting of FDA Committee for Pharmaceutical Science, October 6, 2006. Available at: http://www.fda.gov/ohrms/dockets/ac/06/slides/2006-4241s2_5_files/frame.htm. Accessed November 2007.

35. Haidar SH, Davit B, Chen ML, et al. Bioequivalence approaches for highly variable drugs and drug products. Pharm Res 2008; 25(1):237–241 [Epub September 22, 2007].

36. U.S. Food and Drug Administration (FDA), Advisory Committee for Pharmaceutical Science (ACPS), April 13–14, 2004. Available at: http://www.fda.gov/ohrms/dockets/ac/04/minutes/4034M1.htm. Accessed November 2007.

37. Midha K, Rawson M, Hubbard J. The bioequivalence of highly variable drugs and drug products. Int J Clin Pharmacol Ther 2005; 43:485–498.

38. Benet LZ. Why highly variable drugs are safer. Meeting of FDA Committee for Pharmaceutical Science, October 6, 2006. Available at: http://www.fda.gov/ohrms/dockets/ac/06/slides/2006-4241s2_2_files/frame.htm. Accessed November 2007.

39. Midha K, Rawson M, Hubbard J. Bioequivalence: switchability and scaling. Eur J Pharm Sci 1998; 6:87–91.

40. Karalis V, Symillides M, Macheras P. Novel scaled average bioequivalence limits based on GMR and variability considerations. Pharm Res 2004; 21:1933–1942.

41. Blume H, Elze M, Potthast H, et al. Practical strategies and design advantages in highly variable drug studies: multiple dose and replicate administration design. In: Blume H, Midha K, eds. Bio-international 2: Bioavailability, Bioequivalence and Pharmacokinetic studies. Stuttgart: Medpharm Scientific Publishers, 1995:117–122.

42. El-Tahtawy AA, Jackson AJ, Ludden TM. Comparison of single and multiple dose pharmacokinetics using clinical bioequivalence data and Monte Carlo simulations. Pharm Res 1994; 11:1330–1336.

43. El-Tahtawy AA, Jackson AJ, Ludden TM. Evaluation of bioequivalence of highly variable drugs using Monte Carlo simulations. Part I: Estimation of rate of absorption for single and multiple dose trials using C_{max}. Pharm Res 1995; 12:1634–1641.

44. Zha J, Tothfalusi L, Endrenyi L. Properties of metrics applied for the evaluation of bioequivalence. Drug Inf J 1995; 29:989–996.

45. El-Tahtawy AA, Tozer TN, Harrison F, et al. Evaluation of bioequivalence of highly variable drugs using clinical trial simulations. II: Comparison of single and multiple-dose trials using AUC and C_{max}. Pharm Res 1998; 15:98–104.

46. Health Canada, Ministry of Health. Guidance for Industry: Conduct and Analysis of bioavailability and bioequivalence studies. Part A: Oral Dosage Formulations Used for Systemic Effects, 1992.

47. Anderson S, Hauck WW. Consideration of individual bioequivalence. J Pharmacokinet Biopharm 1990; 18:259–273.
48. Schall R, Luus H. On population and individual bioequivalence. Stat Med 1993; 12:1109–1124.
49. Patnaik R, Lesko L, Chen ML, et al. Individual bioequivalence: new concepts in the statistical assessment of bioequivalence metrics. Clin Pharmacokinet 1997; 33:1–6.
50. Midha K, Rawson M, Hubbard J. Individual and average bioequivalence of highly variable drugs and drug products. J Pharm Sci 1997; 86:1193–1197.
51. Endrenyi L, Amidon G, Midha K, et al. Individual bioequivalence: attractive in principle, difficult in practice. Pharm Res 1998; 15:1321–1325.
52. Midha K, Rawson M, Hubbard J. Prescribability and switchability of highly variable drugs. J Control Release 1999; 62:33–40.
53. Tothfalusi L, Endrenyi L, Midha K. Scaling or wider bioequivalence limits for highly variable drugs and for the special case of C_{max}. Int J Clin Pharmacol Ther 2003; 41:217–225.
54. Haidar S. Bioequivalence of Highly Variable Drugs: Regulatory Perspectives. Meeting of FDA Committee for Pharmaceutical Science, April 13–14, 2004. Available at: http://www.fda.gov/ohrms/dockets/ac/04/slides/4034S2_07_Haidar.ppt. Accessed November 2007.
55. Hauck L, Parekh A, Lesko L, et al. Limits of 80%-125% for AUC and 70%-143% for C_{max}. What is the impact on the bioequivalence studies? Int J Clin Pharmacol Ther 2001; 39: 350–355.
56. Anderson S, Hauck W. The transitivity of bioequivalence testing. Potential for drift. Int J Clin Pharmacol Ther 1996; 34:369–374.
57. Karalis V, Macheras P, Symillides M. Geometric Mean Ratio–dependent scaled bioequivalence limits with leveling-off properties. Eur J Pharm Sci 2005; 26:54–61.
58. Boddy A, Snikeris F, Kringle R, et al. An approach for widening the bioequivalence acceptance limits in the case of highly variable drugs. Pharm Res 1995; 12:1865–1868.
59. Schall R. A unified view of individual, population, and average bioequivalence. In: Blume H, Midha K, eds. Bio-international 2: Bioavailability, Bioequivalence and Pharmacokinetic Studies. Stuttgart: Medpharm Scientific Publishers, 1995:91–106.
60. Tothfalusi L, Endrenyi L, Midha K, et al. Evaluation of the bioequivalence of highly-variable drugs and drug products. Pharm Res 2001; 18:728–733.
61. Hyslop T, Hsuan F, Holder DJ. A small sample confidence interval approach to assess individual bioequivalence. Stat Med 2000; 19:2885–2897.
62. Tothfalusi L, Endrenyi L. Limits for the scaled average bioequivalence of highly variable drugs and drug products. Pharm Res 2003; 20:382–389.
63. Kytariolos J, Karalis V, Macheras P, et al. Novel scaled bioequivalence limits with leveling-off properties based on variability considerations. Pharm Res 2006; 23:2657–2664.
64. Haidar SH. Evaluation of a scaling approach for highly variable drugs. Meeting of FDA Committee for Pharmaceutical Science, October 6, 2006. Available at: http://www.fda.gov/ohrms/dockets/ac/06/slides/2006-4241s2_4_files/frame.htm. Accessed November 2007.
65. Endrenyi L, Tothfalusi L. Determination of bioequivalence for highly-variable drugs. AAPS Annual Meeting, Current Issues and Advances in the Determination of Bioequivalence, San Diego, November 13, 2007.
66. European Medicines Evaluation Agency, Committee for Medicinal Products for Human Use (CHMP). Concept paper for an addendum to the note for guidance on the investigation of bioavailability and bioequivalence: Evaluation of bioequivalence of highly variable drugs and drug products. Doc. Ref. EMEA/CHMP/EWP/147231/2006, April 2006.
67. European Medicines Evaluation Agency, Committee for Medicinal Products for Human Use (CHMP). Recommendation on the need for revision of (CHMP) "Note for guidance on the investigation of bioavailability and bioequivalence". Doc. Ref. EMEA/CHMP/EWP/200943/2007, May 2007.
68. Eradiri O, Sista S, Lai JC, et al. Single- and multiple-dose bioequivalence of two once-daily tramadol formulations using stereospecific analysis of tramadol and its demethylated (M1 and M5) metabolites. Curr Med Res Opin 2007; 23:1593–1604.

69. Nirogi RV, Kandikere VN, Shukla M, et al. Simultaneous quantification of atorvastatin and active metabolites in human plasma by liquid chromatography-tandem mass spectrometry using rosuvastatin as internal standard. Biomed Chromatogr 2006; 20:924–936.

70. Timmer CJ, Verheul HA, Doorstam DP. Pharmacokinetics of tibolone in early and late postmenopausal women. Br J Clin Pharmacol 2002; 54:101–106.

71. Zimmermann T, Wehling M, Schulz HU. Evaluation of the relative bioavailability and the pharmacokinetics of chloral hydrate and its metabolites. Arzneimittel Forschung Drug Res 1998; 48:5–12.

72. Mascher HJ, Kikuta C, Millendorfer A, et al. Pharmacokinetics and bioequivalence of the main metabolites of selegiline: desmethylselegiline, methamphetamine and amphetamine after oral administration of selegiline. Int J Clin Pharmacol Ther 1997; 35:9–13.

73. Sun JX, Piraino AJ, Morgan JM, et al. Comparative pharmacokinetics and bioavailability of nitroglycerin and its metabolites from transdermnitro, nitrodisc, and nitro-dur II systems using a stable-isotope technique. J Clin Pharmacol 1995; 35:390–397.

74. Heinonen E, Anttila M, Lammintausta A. Pharmacokinetic aspects of l-deprenyl (selegiline) and its metabolites. Clin Pharmacol Ther 1994; 56:742–749.

75. Keller-Stanislawski B, Marschner JP, Rietbrock N. Pharmacokinetics of low-dose isosorbide dinitrate and metabolites after buccal or oral administration. Arzneimittelforschung 1992; 42:17–20.

76. Kwon HR, Green P, Curry SH. Pharmacokinetics of nitroglycerin and its metabolites after administration of sustained-release tablets. Biopharm Drug Dispos 1992; 13:141–152.

77. Chen ML, Jackson AJ. The role of metabolites in bioequivalency assessment. I. Linear pharmacokinetics without first-pass effect. Pharm Res 1991; 8:25–32.

78. Chen ML, Jackson AJ. The role of metabolites in bioequivalency assessment. II: Drugs with linear pharmacokinetics and first-pass effect. Pharm Res 1995; 12:700–708.

79. Tucker G, Rostami A, Jackson P. Metabolite measurement in bioequivalence studies: theoretical considerations. In: Midha KK, Blume HH, eds. Bio-International: Bioavailability, Bioequivalence and Pharmacokinetics. Stuttgart: Medpharm Scientific Publishers, 1993: 163–170.

80. Rosenbaum SE, Lam J. Bioequivalence parameters of parent drug and its first-pass metabolite: comparative sensitivity to sources of pharmacokinetic variability. Drug Dev Ind Pharm 1997; 23:337–344.

81. Rosenbaum SE. Effect of variability in hepatic clearance on the bioequivalence parameters of a drug and its metabolite: simulations using a pharmacostatistical model. Pharm Acta Helv 1998; 73:135–144.

82. Jackson AJ. The role of metabolites in bioequivalency assessment. III: Highly variable drugs with linear kinetics and first-pass effect. Pharm Res 2000; 17:1432–1436.

83. Midha KK, Rawson MJ, Hubbard JW. The role of metabolites in bioequivalence. Pharm Res 2004; 21:1331–1344.

84. Amidon GL, Lennernaes H, Shah VP, et al. A theoretical basis for a biopharmaceutic drug classification: the correlation of in vitro drug product dissolution and in vivo bioavailability. Pharm Res 1995; 12(3):413–420.

85. European Medicines Evaluation Agency, Committee for Medicinal Products for Human use (CHMP), Concept paper on BCS-based biowaiver. Doc. Ref. EMEA/CHMP/EWP/213035/2007, London May 24, 2007.

86. Bonlokke L, Hovgaard L, Kristensen HG, et al. Direct estimation of the in vivo dissolution of spironolactone, in two particle size ranges, using the single-pass perfusion technique (Loc-I-Gut) in humans. Eur J Pharm Sci 2001; 12(3):239–250.

87. Weitschies W, Wedemeyer RS, Kosch O, et al. Impact of the intragastric location of extended release tablets on food interactions. J Control Release 2005; 108(2–3):375–385.

88. Galia E, Nicolaides E, Hörter D, et al. Evaluation of various dissolution media for predicting in vivo performance of class I and II drugs. Pharm Res 1998; 15(5):698–705.

89. Persson EM, Gustafsson AS, Carlsson AS, et al. The effects of food on the dissolution of poorly soluble drugs in human and in model small intestinal fluids. Pharm Res 2005; 22(12): 2141–2151.

90. Kalantzi L, Persson E, Polentarutti B, et al. Canine intestinal contents vs. simulated media for the assessment of solubility of two weak bases in the human small intestinal contents. Pharm Res 2006; 23(6):1373–1381.

91. Clarysse S, Psachoulias D, Brouwers J, et al. Postprandial Changes in solubilizing capacity of human intestinal fluids for BCS Class II Drugs. Pharm Res 2009, in press.

92. Pedersen BL, Mullertz A, Brondsted H, et al. A comparison of the solubility of danazol in human and simulated gastrointestinal fluids. Pharm Res 2000; 17(7):891–894.

93. Dressman JB, Vertzoni M, Goumas K, et al. Estimating drug solubility in the gastrointestinal tract. Adv Drug Deliv Rev 2007; 59(7):591–602.

94. Winiwarter S, Bonham NM, Ax F, et al. Correlation of human jejunal permeability (in vivo) of drugs with experimentally and theoretically derived parameters. A multivariate data analysis approach. J Med Chem 1998; 41(25):4939–4949.

95. Benet L, Amidon GL, Barends D, et al. The use of BDDCS in classifying the permeability of marketed drugs. Pharm Res 2008; 25(3):483–488 [Epub January 31, 2008].

96. Takagi T, Ramachandran C, Bermejo M, et al. A provisional biopharmaceutical classification of the top 200 oral drug products in the United States, Great Britain, Spain, and Japan. Mol Pharm 2006; 3(6):631–643.

97. Kasim NA, Whitehouse M, Ramachandran C, et al. Molecular properties of WHO essential drugs and provisional biopharmaceutical classification. Mol Pharm 2004; 1(1):85–96.

98. Lindenberg M, Kopp S, Dressman JB. Classification of orally administered drugs on the World Health Organization model list of essential medicines according to the biopharmaceutics classification system. Eur J Pharm Biopharm 2004; 58:265–278.

99. Lennernas H, Abrahamsson B. The use of biopharmaceutic classification of drugs in drug discovery and development: current status and future extension. J Pharm Pharmacol 2005; 57(3):273–285 (review).

100. Baldoni J. Roles of BCS in Drug Development. AAPS Workshop on BE, BCS and Beyond, May 21–23, 2007, North Bethesda, MD, USA.

101. Yazdanian M, Briggs K, Jankovsky C, et al. The "high solubility" definition of the current FDA Guidance on Biopharmaceutical Classification System may be too strict for acidic drugs. Pharm Res 2004; 21(2):293–299.

102. Rinaki E, Dokoumetzidis A, Valsami G, et al. Identification of biowaivers among class II drugs: theoretical justification and practical examples. Pharm Res 2004; 21(9):1567–1572.

103. World Health Organization, Proposal to waive in vivo bioequivalence requirements for the WHO model list of essential medicines immediate release, solid oral dosage forms, Working document QAS/04.109/Rev.1. Available at: www.who.org. Accessed November 13, 2007.

104. Kortejarvi H, Urtti A, Yliperttula M. Pharmacokinetic simulation of biowaiver criteria: the effects of gastric emptying, dissolution, absorption and elimination rates. Eur J Pharm Sci 2007; 30(2):155–166.

105. Blume HH, Schug BS. The biopharmaceutics classification system (BCS): class III drugs–better candidates for BA/BE waiver? Eur J Pharm Sci 1999; 9(2):117–121 (review).

106. Yu LX, Amidon GL, Polli JE, et al. Biopharmaceutics classification system: the scientific basis for biowaiver extensions. Pharm Res 2002; 19(7):921–925.

107. Chen CL, Yu LX, Lee HL, et al. Biowaiver extension potential to BCS class III high solubility–low permeability drugs: bridging evidence for metformin immediate-release table. Eur J Pharm Sci 2004; 22(4):297–304.

108. Vogelpoel H, Welink J, Amidon GL, et al. Biowaiver monographs for immediate release solid oral dosage forms based on biopharmaceutics classification system (BCS) literature data: verapamil hydrochloride, propranolol hydrochloride, and atenolol. J Pharm Sci 2004; 93(8): 1945–1956.

109. Jantratid E, Prakongpan S, Dressman JB, et al. Biowaiver monographs for immediate release solid oral dosage forms: cimetidine. J Pharm Sci 2006; 95(5):974–984.

110. Kortejärvi H, Yliperttula M, Dressman JB, et al. Biowaiver monographs for immediate release solid oral dosage forms: ranitidine hydrochloride. J Pharm Sci 2005; 94(8):1617–1625.
111. Koch KM, Parr AF, Tomlinson JJ, et al. Effect of sodium acid pyrophosphate on ranitidine bioavailability and gastrointestinal transit time. Pharm Res 1993; 10(7):1027–1030.
112. Adkin DA, Davis SS, Sparrow RA, et al. The effect of mannitol on the oral bioavailability of cimetidine. J Pharm Sci 1995; 84(12):1405–1409.
113. Custodio JM, Wu C-Y, Benet LZ. Predicting drug disposition, absorption/elimination/ transporter interplay and the role of food on drug absorption. Adv Drug Del Reviews 2008; 60:717–733.

3

Cutaneous and Transdermal Delivery— Processes and Systems of Delivery

Guang Wei Lu
Parenteral Center of Emphasis, Global Research & Development, Pfizer Inc., Groton, Connecticut, U.S.A.

Gordon L. Flynn
College of Pharmacy, University of Michigan, Ann Arbor, Michigan, U.S.A.

INTRODUCTION

The skin forms the body's defensive perimeter against what is in reality the biologically hostile environment humans live in. As such, in the normal course of living, it suffers more physical and chemical insult than any other tissue of the body. It is inadvertently scraped, abraded, scratched, bruised, cut, nicked, and burned. Insects bite it, sting it, and occasionally furrow through it. It is exposed to detergents, solvents, and myriad other chemicals and residues. Bacteria, yeasts, molds, and fungi live on its surface and within its cracks and crevices. It is brushed, smeared, dusted, sprayed, and otherwise anointed with toiletries, cosmetics, and drugs. Any of these exposures can rile the skin and/or provoke allergy. In its intact state the skin is a formidable barrier, resistant to chemicals and tissue-harmful ultraviolet rays and virtually impenetrable to life-threatening microorganisms. To perform these necessary functions, the skin has to be tough and at the same time flexible, for it is stretched and flexed continually as we move around within it. In its healthy state it is thus a remarkable fabric, strong and far more complex than any artificial material (1).

Myriad medicated products are applied to the skin or readily accessible mucous membranes that in some way either augment or restore a fundamental function of the skin or pharmacologically modulate an action in the underlying tissues. Such products are referred to as *topicals* or *dermatologicals*. A topical delivery system is one that is applied directly to any external body surface by inuncting it (spreading and rubbing in a semisolid with the fingers), by spraying or dusting on it, or by instilling it (applying a liquid as drops). Thus, topical is frequently used in contexts where the application is to the surface of the eye (cornea and conjunctival membranes), the external ear, or the nasal mucosa or to the lining of the mouth (buccal mucosa) or even the rectum, the vagina, or the urethra. The term dermatological, on the other hand, describes products that are only to be applied to the skin or the scalp. An *external use only* label is used to denote such restricted use. The distinction between general topical use and external use is not trivial. Mucous membranes allow rapid absorption of many locally applied substances that do not pass at all readily through intact, normal skin. This raises the potential that both drugs and excipients have to be locally irritating and/or systemically toxic. Consequently, many drugs that can be applied to the external skin with impunity should not be placed in contact with moist mucosal surfaces. Upon applying an external use only label to a package, a pharmacist warns patients of such dangers. This chapter mainly deals with dermatological products, but general concepts and drug delivery rationale are applicable to other modes of topical therapy as well.

The distinctions pharmacists have to make concerning topical dosage forms and their suitability for use obviously go far deeper than merely appreciating the significance of external use only labels. Pharmacological, toxicological, and risk-benefit valuations must be made for every dispensed product. An attending physician usually has such issues in mind when prescribing. But even before the physician or pharmacist sees a product, the manufacturer has to establish its safety and effectiveness to FDA's satisfaction. As part of the process, the delivery system for the drug is subjected to intense FDA scrutiny. Despite this regulatory oversight, no system is fail-safe. Consequently, the lack of input into drug and drug delivery system development does not abrogate the dispensing pharmacist's responsibility for assuring that every dispensed pharmaceutical conforms to high standards. The consummate professional thus takes every opportunity to evaluate, by literature or by personal observation, how the various products dispensed measure up to established standards. A pharmacist should be continually asking the following questions. Is the drug bioavailable as administered? What safety concerns should patients be advised of? Are the drug and its dosage form stable? Is the formulation free of contamination? Is the product pharmaceutically elegant? Attribute particulars of course vary by dosage form type and the route of administration. Regardless, a *no* to any of the first four questions is reason to remove a product from distribution. Elegance is sometimes sacrificed relative to other function, but only in degree. A goal of this chapter is to elucidate the attributes of dermatological dosage forms that are helpful in evaluating and selecting products.

To answer questions regarding the therapeutic and cosmetic uses of the myriad dermatological concoctions that are available, a pharmacist must be knowledgeable about the anatomical structure and physiological functions of the skin and the chemical compositions and physicochemical properties of its constituent tissues. Some understanding of how its properties are affected by disease and damage is a must, as is knowledge of how the skin's physiology and function vary with age, race, environmental conditions, and other factors. Rational approaches to topical therapy rest on having such insights.

THE STRUCTURE OF SKIN

Let us consider how the skin is structured to better understand how this tissue performs some of its vital functions. Consider the cross-section of the skin sketched in Figure 1. This illustration shows the readily distinguishable layers of the skin, from the outside of the skin inward, are (*i*) the ≈ 10-μm-thin, fully differentiated, devitalized outer epidermal layer called the stratum corneum; (*ii*) the ≈ 100-μm-thin, live, cellular epidermis; and (*iii*) the ≈ 1000-μm-thin (1-mm-thin) dermis. Note that all the thicknesses specified here are representative only, for the actual thickness of each stratum varies severalfold from place to place on the body. Dispersed throughout the skin, varying in number and size

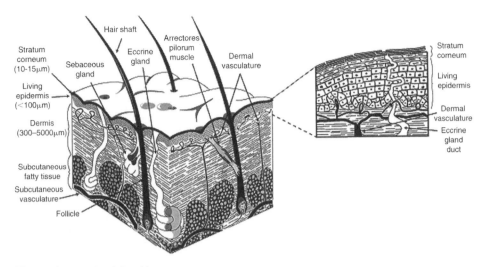

Figure 1 Sketch of the skin.

depending on body site, are several glands and appendages. These include (*i*) hair follicles and their associated sebaceous glands (pilosebaceous glands), (*ii*) eccrine sweat glands, (*iii*) apocrine sweat glands, and (*iv*) nails of the fingers and toes. Each appendage has its unique population densities and body distributions. The appendages also exhibit characteristic structural differences from one location to another on the body.

A highly complex network of arteries, arterioles, and capillaries penetrates the dermis from below and extends up to the surface of, but not actually into, the epidermis. A matching venous system siphons the blood and returns it to the central circulation. Blood flow through the vasculature is linked to the production and movement of lymph through a complementary dermal lymphatic system. The dermis is laced with tactile, thermal, and pain sensors.

Stratum Corneum

The outermost layer of the skin appearing in the exploded epidermal sketch of Figure 1 represents the stratum corneum (the *horny layer*). Stratum corneum, the principal barrier element of the skin, is an essentially metabolically inactive tissue that comprises acutely flattened, stacked, hexagonal cell-building blocks formed from once-living cells. These cellular building blocks are layered 15 to 25 cells deep over most of the body (2). At some sites, the cells appear to be stacked in neat columns. The stratum corneum exhibits regional differences in thickness, being as thick as several hundred micrometers on the friction surfaces of the body (palms and soles). However, over most of the body, the tissue measures only about 10 μm thick, dimensionally less than a fifth of the thickness of an ordinary piece of paper (2,3). It is a dense tissue, about 1.4 g/cm^3 in the dry state, a fact that has led it to also be referred to as the stratum compactum.

The stratum corneum is continuously under formation. Microscopic flakes (squama) dislodged from the surface through wear and tear are replaced with new cells from beneath, with complete turnover of the horny layer occurring roughly every two weeks in normal individuals (4). In humans the cells that give rise to the stratum corneum originate exclusively in the basal layer of the epidermis. Cell division in the basal layer begins an extraordinary process in which daughter cells are pushed outward, first to form a layer of so-called spinous or prickle cells and then, serially, the granular, lucid, and horny layers. As suggested in Figure 1, during their transit through the epidermal mass, the cells flatten acutely. The protein and lipid components that eventually characterize the fully differentiated horny layer are synthesized in transit, with the initial strands of the structural protein that will eventually fill the cell interior being formed in the basal layer. During their inexorable migration to the stratum corneum, the protein content of the cells expands to the point that massed proteins of several kinds are distinguishable as they merge into the granular layer. In culmination, the intracellular space of the fully differentiated horny cell is literally packed with structural protein, namely, semicrystalline α-keratin intermixed with more amorphous β-keratin. Nothing but keratin is visible inside the fully differentiated horny cell by electron microscope. The intracellular space is dense, offering little freedom of movement to organic molecules that may become dissolved within it. Moreover, because of its remarkable ionic character, the intracellular keratin mass borders on being thermodynamically impenetrable.

Lipid synthesized during a keratinocyte's epidermal transit is collected in small vesicles that become visible within the granular layer. These were designated membrane-coating granules long before their content and function were known. As granular cells undergo transformation, the "coating granules" gravitate to the outermost cell membrane and are passed exocytotically into the intercellular space. A lipid "mortar" is formed that seals the horny structure. Virtually all the lipid of the stratum corneum is in the interstitial space, much of it being present in liquid crystalline, bilayer assemblage (5). The densely packed keratin platelets caulked with intercellular lipid make the stratum corneum, pound for pound, an incredibly resistive moisture barrier. An exoskeleton (infrastructure) of residual cell membranes bound together by desmosomes and tonofibrils acts to separate the keratin and lipid domains. The lipid content of the horny layer represents about 20% of the stratum corneum's dry weight, while the endoskeleton contributes roughly 5% to the weight (Table 1) (2,4,6).

In its normal state at ordinary relative humidity, the stratum corneum takes up moisture to the extent of 15% to 20% of its dry weight (2). The ionic character of keratin is certainly a factor of consequence here. Should the skin become waterlogged, the water content of horny tissue covering the friction surfaces (callused surfaces) can rise to several multiples of the tissue's dry weight. The water content of stratum corneum appears to be less affected under the same circumstance. It appears that the stratum

Table 1 Composition of the Stratum Corneum

Tissue component	Gross composition	Percentage of dry weight
Cell membrane	Lipid, protein	≈5
Intercellular space	Mostly lipid, some protein, and polysaccharide	≈20
Intracellular space	Fibrous protein (≈65–70%), nonfibrous (soluble) protein (≈5–10%)	≈75
Overall protein	Water soluble (10%), keratin (≈65%), cell wall (≈5%)	70–80
Overall lipid	–	10–20
All other	–	Up to 10
Water (normal hydration)	–	15–20
Water (fully hydrated)	–	Upward of 300

Source: From Refs. 2 and 3.

corneum covering the greater part of the human body has less capacity to imbibe water. Nevertheless, all horny tissue becomes hydrated to some degree when the natural evaporation of water from the skin's surface, so-called insensible perspiration, is held in check upon applying an *occlusive dressing*. The horny tissue becomes more pliable. Consequently, molecules diffuse through it with greater facility. And it is likely that some substances may exhibit greater solubility within the hydrated horny mass, adding further to their ease of permeation. Conversely, the stratum corneum becomes brittle when it dries out. Ultradry, inelastic horny tissue splits and fissures when stretched, giving rise to the common conditions we know as chapped lips, windburn, and dishpan hands.

The stratum corneum is thus a dense, polyphasic epidermal sheathing made from dehydrated and internally filamented former cells held together by desmosomes, tonofibrils (intercellular anchors), and interstitial lipid. It has been estimated that it contains 10 times the fibrous material of the living epidermis in roughly one-tenth the space (7). The stratum corneum is in contact with the living epidermal mass at its undersurface. Its external surface interfaces the environment. Cells at the basement of the stratum corneum contain water at high thermodynamic activity of the physiological milieu, whereas air at the surface of the skin tends to have a far lower water activity. As a result, under ordinary circumstances, water diffuses out through the skin (*down* the implied activity gradient) and into the environment. This process is known as *insensible perspiration*. About 5 mL of water is lost this way per square meter of intact body surface per hour (or 0.5 mg/cm^2/hr) (8).

Viable Epidermis

The animate cells of the epidermis make a sharp, upper interface with the lifeless stratum corneum. They also have a well-demarcated, deep interface with the dermis (Figure 1). When physicochemically considered, the viable epidermis is nothing more than a wedge of tightly massed, live cells. Consequently, the whole of this live, cellular mass is regarded as a singular diffusional field (resistance) in percutaneous absorption models, although, when viewed under microscope, the tissue is clearly multilayered. The identifiable strata, bottom to top, are (*i*) the basal layer (stratum germinativum), a single layer of cubical or columnar cells that is unremarkable in appearance; (*ii*) the multicellular spinous or prickle layer (stratum spinosum) in which the cells exhibit sharp surface protuberances; and (*iii*) the granular layer (stratum granulosum), a thin layer that stains to yield a mottled appearance. In some histological displays, a fourth, upper transitional and translucent layer is also distinguishable (stratum lucidum). These layers reflect the progressive differentiation of the cells that eventuates in their death and placement as "bricks" within the horny structure. As elsewhere in the body, water found in the live epidermis has an activity equivalent to that of a highly dilute, isotonic NaCl solution (0.9% NaCl). The density and consistency of the live epidermal composite are only a little greater than those found for water.

The interface the viable epidermis makes with the stratum corneum is flat. However, the interface with the dermis is papillose (mounded). Myriad tiny bulges of the epidermis fit with exacting reciprocity over dermal depressions and ridges. It is these ridges that give the friction surfaces of the body their distinctive patterns (e.g., fingerprints). Importantly, since hair follicles and eccrine glands have epidermal origins, cells capable of regenerating the epidermis actually extend well into and through the dermis by way of these tiny glands (Figure 1). When the skin is superficially injured, surviving cells at the base of these glands regenerate a scar-free surface. Discounting these deep rootages, the epidermis is on the order of 100 to 250 μm thick (9).

Table 2 Cells of the Skin

Cell type	Principal function
Cells of the epidermis	
Keratinocytes	Formation of keratinized structures
Langerhans cells	Antigen presentation
Melanocytes	Pigment synthesis
Macrophages, lymphocytes	Migrant cells, immune responses
Cells of the dermis	
Fibroblasts	Fiber synthesis
Mast cells	Making of ground substance, histamine
Blood cells	
Endothelial cells	Formation of blood vessels
Nerve cells and endings	Sensors

Source: From Refs. 2 and 11.

Keratinocytes account for most of the cells of the epidermis. One also finds Langerhans cells of white blood cell progeny here. The latter well-dispersed cells function as antigen-presenting cells (APCs) in the skin's immunological responses. Yet another group of cells, melanocytes, are strategically placed in the epidermis just above the epidermal-dermal junction (Table 2). Acting under the influence of melanocyte-stimulating hormone (MSH), they synthesize and deposit the pigment granules into skin, which give the races of human beings their unique skin coloration. Melanocytes are also set into action by ultraviolet radiation. Their activities in this circumstance lead to sun tanning. Migrant macrophages and lymphocytes are occasionally found in skin sections. Such cells can be numerous in traumatized skin.

Dermis

The dermis appears in Figure 1 as a nondescript region lying between the epidermis and a region of subcutaneous fat. In reality it is a complex structure held together by a meshwork of structural fibers, for example, collagen, reticulum, and elastin. Most of the space between fibers is filled with a mucopolysaccharidic gel called the ground substance (2). Approximate proportions of these phases are indicated in Table 3. The dermis ranges from about 0.3 mm (300 μm) on the eyelids to about 3 mm in thickness on the back (10). The upper one-fifth or so of the wedge of tissue, the papillary layer by name, is finely structured and provides the support for the delicate capillary plexus that nurtures the epidermis. The papillary dermis merges into a far coarser fibrous matrix, the reticular dermis. This deepest layer of the true skin is the main structural element of the skin. Of considerable importance, the microcirculation that subserves the skin is entirely located in

Table 3 Composition of the Dermis

Component	Approximate % composition
Collagen	75.0
Elastin	4.0
Reticulin	0.4
Ground substance	20.0

Source: From Refs. 2 and 10.

the dermis. The dermis is also penetrated by sensory nerve endings (pressure, temperature, and pain) and houses an extensive lymphatic network. Fibroblasts, cells that synthesize the structural fibers, are found here (2), and one also finds mast cells scattered about (Table 2). The latter are thought to synthesize the ground substance. They are known to be a source of histamine that is released when the skin is immunologically provoked.

Skin's Circulatory System

Arteries entering the skin arise from more substantial vessels located in the subcutaneous connective tissue. These offshoots form a plexus just beneath the dermis (10). Branches from this subcutaneous network directly supply blood to the hair follicles, the glandular appendages, and the subcutaneous fat. Branches to the upper skin from this deep plexus divide again within the lower dermis, forming a deep subpapillary network. Arterioles reaching the upper dermis out of this plexus are on the order of 50 μm in diameter. They exhibit arteriovenous anastomoses, shunt-like connections that link the arterioles directly to corresponding venules. The dermal arterioles then further branch to form the shallower subpapillary plexus of capillary loops that bring a blood supply up into the papillae at the dermal-epidermal interface. The epidermis itself is avascular.

The veins of skin are organized along the same lines as the arteries in that there are both subpapillary and subdermal plexuses (10). The main arteriole communication to these is the capillary bed. Copious blood is passed through capillaries when the core body is either feverish or overheated, far more than needed to sustain the life force of the epidermis, and this rich perfusion lends a red coloration to fair skin. The vascular surface available for exchange of substances between the blood and the local tissue has been estimated to be of the same magnitude as that of the skin, that is, 1 to 2 cm^2 per square centimeter of skin. At room temperature, about 0.05 mL of blood flows through the skin per minute per gram of tissue. This perfusion increases considerably when the skin is warmed (3,11). Sufficient blood courses to within 150 μm of the skin's surface to efficiently draw chemicals into the body that have percutaneously gained access to this depth (6). Blood circulation at this level is turned off by vasoconstrictors (e.g., glucocorticoids) and turned up by vasodilators (e.g., nicotine). These vasoactivities are so reliable that vasoconstriction (blanching) has become an FDA-sanctioned measure of the penetration of corticosteroids through the skin (12,13). The relationships between capillary blood flow and local clearances of percutaneously absorbed drugs, including the influences of vasoconstriction and vasodilation, are not well drawn.

The lymphatic system of the skin extends up and into the papillary layers of the dermis. A dense, flat meshwork of lymphatic capillaries is found here (10). Lymph passes into a deeper network at the lower boundary of the dermis. Serum, macrophages, and lymphocytes readily negotiate through the skin's lymphatic and vascular networks.

Skin Appendages

Hair follicles and their associated sebaceous glands (pilosebaceous glands), eccrine glands, apocrine glands, and finger and toenails are all considered skin appendages. Hair follicles are found everywhere within the skin except for the soles of the feet, the palms of the hand, the red portion (vermilion border) of the lips, and the external genitalia. All are formed from fetal epidermal cells. Hair differs markedly in its prominence from place to place over the body. Delicate primary hair is found on the fetus; secondary hair or *down* covers the adult forehead; terminal hair ordinarily blankets the scalp and is found as pubic and axillary (underarm) hair (2). A hair (hair shaft) emerges from a *follicle*, as shown in Figure 1. Each follicle is set within the skin at a slight angle. Each consists of concentric layers of cellular and noncellular components, and each is anchored to the surrounding connective tissue by an individual strand of smooth muscle, the arrector pilorum. Contraction of this muscle causes the hair to stand upright, merely raising *goose pimples* on human skin. The hair shaft is formed continuously by cell division, differentiation, and compaction within the bulb (base) of each active hair follicle, a process that is completed deep in the follicle. Hair, like stratum corneum, is thus a compact of fused, keratinized cells. Collectively, hair follicles occupy about one-thousandth of the skin's surface with about 100 follicles per square centimeter of skin (9,14), a factor that sets a limit on the role that follicular orifices can play as a route of penetration. Each hair follicle possesses one or more flask-like sebaceous glands (Figure 1). These have ducts that vent into the open space surrounding the hair shaft just below the skin's surface. The cells of sebaceous glands, *sebocytes* by name, are programmed to divide, differentiate, and die. Before they die and disintegrate, they pack themselves full of lipid-containing vesicles. The residue left behind at their death is mixed with other follicular debris below the follicular orifice to form an oily substance called sebum. Sebum is then forced upward around the hair shaft and onto the skin surface. The follicular outlets for sebum exhibit diameters ranging from 200 to 2000 μm (2 mm) depending on body location (10). Glands with the largest openings are found on the forehead, face, nose, and upper back. These large follicles contain an almost microscopic hair, if they contain one at all, and are therefore referred to as sebaceous follicles.

Eccrine glands (salty sweat glands) are found over the entire body except the genitalia and lips. They appear as tubes extending from the skin surface all the way to the footings of the dermis. Here the tube coils into a ball roughly 100 μm in diameter (Figure 1) (10). By anatomical count, there are between 150 and 600 glands per square centimeter of body surface depending on body site (15). They are particularly concentrated in the palms and soles, attaining densities in these locations well in excess of 400 glands/cm^2. However, since many of these glands remain dormant, estimates of their numbers are appreciably lower if based on actual sweating units. Each gland has an approximately 20 μm diameter orifice at surface of the skin from which its secretions are spilled. In total, these glandular openings represent approximately one-ten-thousandth of the skin's surface (9). Eccrine sweat is a dilute (hypotonic), slightly acidic (pH ≈ 5.0 due to traces of lactic acid) aqueous solution of salt. Its secretion is stimulated when the body becomes overheated through warm temperatures or exercise. Evaporation of the water of the sweat cools the body's surface and thus the body. Since the gland is innervated by the autonomic nervous system, eccrine sweating is also stimulated emotionally (the *clammy* handshake).

Apocrine glands are found only in the axillae (armpits), in the anogenital region, and around the nipples. Along with other secondary sexual characteristics, these glands develop at puberty. We know that they are innervated emotionally and through concupiscence. In the mature female, they exhibit cyclical activities in harmony with the menstrual cycle. Like eccrine glands, they are coiled tubular structures, but the coils are roughly 10 times larger. They extend well into the subcutaneous layer beneath the skin (2,10). Each gland is paired with a hair follicle; its secretion is vented into the sebaceous duct of the follicle beneath the surface of the skin. Because this secretion is minor in amount and combines with sebum before reaching the skin's surface, its exact chemical makeup remains an enigma. What is not a mystery is that bacterial decomposition of the secretion is responsible for human body odor.

SKIN FUNCTIONS

Among the skin's main physiological roles the chemical barrier function is central to the use of topical drugs because deposition of a topical drug into the deeper, living strata of skin is a prerequisite for achieving its pharmacological effect. An outline of the functions follows. Degeneration in some of the functions can be pathognomonic of disease. Even where specific functions do not relate materially to the skin's state of health, they are tied in with cosmetic practices and thereby are of interest to pharmacists.

Containment

The containment function relates specifically to the ability of the skin to confine underlying tissues and restrain their movements. The skin draws the strength it needs to perform this mechanical role from its tough, fibrous dermis (2). Ordinarily, the skin is taut even when under resting tension, yet it stretches easily and elastically when the body is in motion, quickly returning to normal contours when the stretching ceases. This extensibility of the skin is attributable to an alignment of collagen fibers under tension and in the direction of a load, which are otherwise nonaligned in the ground tension state. If the skin becomes stretched beyond its ability to elastically restore its initial condition, it folds over itself or *wrinkles*. Lost elasticity is advanced through extended exposure to ultraviolet radiation (sunlight) and thus wrinkling is often pronounced on dedicated sunbathers.

   The behavior of the epidermis when distended is also of importance. It is the stratum corneum's role to fend against tearing (2). This tissue is actually stronger per unit mass than the dermal fabric and, as a rule, is sufficiently elastic to adjust to stretching. Its pliability, however, is conditional, and it fissures and cracks if stretched when excessively dry. Arid atmospheres alone can produce this condition (windburn). Detergents and solvents, which extract essential, water-sequestering lipids from the stratum corneum, and diseases such as psoriasis associated with a malformed horny structure render the stratum corneum brittle and prone to fissuring.

   Although much is still to be learned about the factors that contribute to the pliability of the stratum corneum, it is generally accepted that its elasticity is dependent on a proper balance of lipids, hygroscopic, water-soluble substances, and water, all in conjunction with its keratin proteins. Water is its principal plasticizer, or softening agent, and it takes roughly 15% moisture to maintain adequate pliability. The capacity of the stratum corneum to bind and hold onto water is greatly reduced by extracting it with lipid solvents such as ether and chloroform. Amino acids, hydroxy acids, urea, and inorganic ions, cosmetically referred to as the skin's *natural moistening factor*, and the stratum corneum's lipids assist the stratum corneum in retaining moisture necessary to plasticize its mosaic, filamented matrix. In effect, the water makes the tissue less *crystalline* through its interposition between polymer strands.

Microbial Barrier

Normal stratum corneum, taken in its entirety, is a dense molecular continuum penetrable only by molecular diffusion. It is virtually an absolute barrier to microbes, preventing them from reaching the viable tissues and an environment suitable for their growth. The outermost stratum corneum is continuously being shed in the form of microscopic scales (natural desquamation) and, to a limited depth, is laced with tiny crevices. Many microorganisms, pathogens and harmless forms alike, are found in these rifts. The microorganisms residing on and in the skin can and do initiate infections if seeded into living tissues as a result of abrasive or disease-induced stratum corneum damage. Consequently, antiseptics and antibiotics are widely used to chemically sanitize wounds.

Beyond physical barrier protection, several natural processes lead to skin surface conditions unfavorable to microbial growth. Both sebaceous and eccrine secretions are acidic, lowering the surface pH of the skin below that welcomed by most pathogens. This *acid mantle* (pH $\approx$ 5) (15) is moderately bacteriostatic. Sebum also contains a number of short-chain fungistatic and bacteriostatic fatty acids, including propanoic, butanoic, hexanoic, and heptanoic acids (16). That the skin's surface is dry also offers a level of protection. Glandular orifices provide possible entry points for microbes. The duct of the eccrine sweat gland is tiny and generally evacuated. Experience tells us that this is not an easy portal of entry, although localized infection is seen occasionally in infants suffering prickly heat. Pilosebaceous glands seem more susceptible to infection, particularly those on the forehead, face, and upper back referred to as sebaceous follicles. Sebaceous gland infections are usually localized. However, if the infected gland ruptures and spews it contents internally, deep infection is possible. For example, the destruction of cystic acne is deep, so much so that facial scarring is associated with it.

Chemical Barrier

The intact stratum corneum also acts as a barrier to chemicals brought into contact with it. Its diffusional resistance is orders of magnitude greater than that found in other barrier membranes of the body. Externally contacted chemicals can, in principle, bypass the stratum corneum by diffusing through the ducts of the appendages. The ability of each chemical to breach the skin and the diffusional route or routes it takes are dependent on its own physicochemical properties and the interactions it has within the skin's various conduit regimes. Being central to the effectiveness of dermatological products, exposition of the skin's barrier properties is made in the following sections.

Radiation Barrier

Exposure to ultraviolet light, UVA or UVB, from sunlight has substantial effect on the skin, causing premature skin aging, skin cancer, and other skin changes. Ultraviolet wavelengths of 290 to 310 nm from the UVB band of radiation and of 320 to 400 nm from the UVA constitute the principal tissue-damaging rays of the sun that are not fully atmospherically *filtered.* An hour's exposure to the summer sun and its damaging rays can produce a painful burn with a characteristic erythema. The skin has natural mechanisms to prevent or minimize such sun-induced trauma, but it takes time to set these into place. Upon stimulation by ultraviolet rays, particularly longer, lower-energy rays above 320 nm, melanocytes at the epidermal-dermal junction produce the pigment melanin. Melanin's synthesis begins in the corpus of the melanocyte, with forming pigment granules migrating outward to the tips of the long protrusions of these *starlike* cells. Adjacent epidermal cells endocytotically engulf these projections. Through this cellular cooperation melanin, which absorbs and diffracts harmful ultraviolet rays, becomes dispersed throughout the epidermis and a person *tans,* with the person's capacity to sunburn declining accordingly. It should be realized that tanning takes time, several days in fact, and is incapable of protecting a person on first exposure. Damaging ultraviolet exposure also stimulates epidermal cell division and thickening of the epidermis (acanthosis). Such thickening, too, takes several days. When affected, it also lends protection to the underlying tissues.

Pharmacists should tell their sun-deprived, fair-skinned patrons not to spend more than 15 to 20 minutes in the midday sun (10:00 a.m. to 3:00 p.m.) on first exposure when traveling to vacation spots such as Florida (17). This is ample, safe exposure to initiate the tanning response in those who are able to tan. Exposures can be increased incrementally by 15 minutes a day until a 45-minute tolerance is developed, which is generally an adequate level of sun protection in conjunction with the use of sunscreens. It should be obvious that dark-skinned people are already heavily pigmented and thus far less susceptible to burning. Other individuals do not tan at all and must apply sunscreens with high protection factors before sun bathing.

Electrical Barrier

Dry skin offers high impedance to the flow of an electrical current (18). Stripping the skin by successively removing layers of the stratum corneum with an adhesive tape reduces the electrical resistance about sixfold, which tells us that the horny layer is the skin's prime electrical insulator. Its high impedance complicates the measurement of body potentials, as is done in electroencephalograms and electrocardiograms. Consequently, electrodes having large contact areas are used to monitor the brain's and the heart's electrical rhythms. Granular salt suspensions or creams and pastes containing high percentages of electrolytes are placed between the electrode surface and the skin to assure that the electrical conductance is adequate to make the measurements.

Thermal Barrier and Body Temperature Regulation

The body is basically an isothermal system fine-tuned to 37°C (98.6°F). The skin has major responsibility in temperature maintenance. When the body is exposed to chilling temperatures that remove heat faster than what the body's metabolic output can replace, changes take place in the skin to conserve heat. Conversely, when the body becomes overheated, physiological processes come into play that lead to cooling.

The skin's mechanism of heat conservation involves its very complex circulatory system (2,18). To conserve heat, blood is diverted away from the skin's periphery by way of the arteriovenous anastomoses. Blood's external-most circulation is effectively shut down, leading to a characteristic blanching of the skin in fair-skinned individuals. When the body is faced with the need to cast out thermal energy, the circulatory processes are reversed and blood is sent coursing through the skin's periphery, maximizing radiative and convective heat losses. This process produces a reddening in light skin, a phenomenon that is particularly noticeable following strenuous exercise. Exercise also leads to profuse eccrine sweating, a process which is even more efficient in heat removal. Watery sweat evaporates, with the heat attending this process (heat of vaporization) cooling the skin's surface. Pharmacists should be aware that eccrine sweating is a vital process not to be tampered with. Coverage of the body with a water-impermeable wrapping, as has occasionally been done in faddish weight control programs, may result in hyperthermia, particularly if there is concurrent exercise. In its extreme, hyperthermia can be fatal.

RATIONALE FOR TOPICALS

One's grasp of topical dosage forms and their functioning can be nicely organized into several broad usage categories. For instance, many products exist to augment the skin barrier. Sunscreens and anti-infective drugs obviously do this. The barrier is made pliable and restored in function by emollients. Pastes are sometimes used to directly block out sunlight and at other times to sequester irritating chemicals that would otherwise penetrate into the skin. Even insect repellants add function to the barrier. A second general purpose of topical application involves the selective access drugs have to epidermal and dermal tissues when administered this way. Penetration of the skin can drench the local tissues with the drug prior to its systemic dissemination and dilution. As a result, the drug's systemic levels are kept low and pharmacologically inconsequential. In contrast, systemic treatment of local conditions bathes highly blood-perfused tissues with the drug first, with the drug's systemic effects or its side effects sometimes overpowering the actions sought for it in the skin.

In a few instances, drugs are applied to the skin to actually elicit their systemic effects. This is called transdermal therapy. Transdermal therapy is set apart from local treatment on several counts. It is only possible with potent drugs that are also highly skin permeable. To be used transdermally, compounds must be free of untoward cutaneous actions as well. When these demanding conditions are met, transdermal therapy offers an excellent means of sustaining the action of a drug. Transdermal delivery also skirts frequently encountered oral delivery problems such as first-pass metabolic inactivation and gastrointestinal upset. Transdermal therapy is actually an old medical strategy, as compresses and poultices have been used for centuries, although never with certainty of effect. The current, effective use of small adhesive patches to treat systemic disease or its symptoms has revolutionized the practice.

Therapeutic Stratification of the Skin

How does a person best organize his or her thinking relative to these different rationales? One can start by asking what the topical drug is supposed to do: Is it to be applied to suppress inflammation; eradicate infectious microorganisms; provide protection from the sun; stop glandular secretions; or provide extended relief from visceral pain? Regardless of which feat the drug is to perform, the answer to the question directs us to where and sometimes how the drug must act to be effective or to a *target* for the drug. Once knowing the locus of action, one can then consider its accessibility. Clearly, if the drug cannot adequately access its target, little or no therapeutic benefit will be realized.

Sundry drug targets exist on, within, or beneath the skin. These include (*i*) the skin surface itself (external target); (*ii*) the stratum corneum; (*iii*) any one of several levels of the live epidermis; (*iv*) the avascular, upper dermis; (*v*) any one of several deeper regions of the dermis; (*vi*) one or another of the anatomically distinct domains of the pilosebaceous glands; (*vii*) eccrine glands; (*viii*) apocrine glands; (*ix*) the local vasculature; and, following systemic absorption, (*x*) any of numerous internal tissues. As these targets become increasingly remote, delivery to them becomes sparser, and as a result dilution via tissue distribution and, consequently, adequacy of delivery become less certain. Moreover, the specific properties of these targets and their negotiability are very much determined by the state of health of the skin. Disease and damage alter the barrier characteristics of the skin and therefore target accessibility itself.

Causes of skin damage and/or eruptions are diverse and may alternatively be traced to damage, irritant or allergic reactions, an underlying pathophysiological condition, or an infection. Depending on the problem, the entire skin or only a small part of it may be involved. Moreover, disease may be manifest in one part of a tissue as a consequence of a biochemical abnormality in another. For instance, the cardinal expression of psoriasis is its thickened, silvery, malformed stratum corneum (psoriatic scale), but the disease actually results from maverick proliferation of keratinocytes in the germinal layer of the epidermis. Humankind suffers many skin problems like this, each unique in expression to the well-trained eye. The pharmacist will, from time to time, be called upon to examine an eruption or condition and make recommendation for treatment. If and only if the condition is unmistakable in origin, delimited in area, and of modest intensity, should the pharmacist recommend an over-the-counter (OTC) remedy for its symptomatic relief. Physicians neither need nor want to see inconsequential cuts, abrasions, or mosquito bites, or unremarkable cases of chapped skin, sunburn, or poison ivy eruption, and so on. However, if infection is present and is at all deep seated or if expansive areas of the body are involved, otherwise minor problems can pose a serious threat and physician referral is mandatory. Patients should also be directed to counsel with a physician whenever the origins of a skin problem are in question.

Surface Effects

Of the many possible dermatological targets mentioned above, the skin surface is clearly the easiest to access. Surface treatment begins at the fringe of cosmetic practice. Special cosmetics are available to hide unsightly blemishes and birthmarks. These lessen self-consciousness and are psychologically uplifting. Applying a protective layer over the skin is sometimes desirable. For example, zinc oxide pastes are used to create a barrier between an infant and its diaper that adsorbs irritants found in urine, ameliorating diaper rash. These same pastes literally block out the sun and at the same time hold in moisture, protecting the ski enthusiast from facial sun and windburns on the high slopes. Transparent films containing ultraviolet light–absorbing chemicals are also used as sunscreens. Lip balms and like products lay down occlusive (water-impermeable) films over the skin, preventing dehydration of the underlying stratum corneum and thereby allaying dry skin and chapping. The actions of calamine lotion and other products of the kind are limited to the skin's surface. The suspended matter in these purportedly binds urushiol, the hapten (allergen) found in poison ivy and oak. However, these may best benefit the patient by drying up secretions, relieving itchiness. In all these instances where the film itself is therapeutic, bioavailability has little meaning.

Bioavailability does matter with topical antiseptics and antibiotics, even though these also act mainly at the skin's surface. These anti-infectives are meant to stifle the growth of surface microflora, and thus formulations that penetrate into the cracks and fissures of the skin where the microorganisms reside are desirable. The extent to which the surface is sanitized then depends on uptake of the anti-infective by the microbes themselves. Slipshod formulation can result in a drug being entrapped in its film and inactivated. For instance, little to no activity is to be expected when a drug is placed in a vehicle in which it is highly insoluble. Ointment bases that contain salts of neomycin, polymyxin, and bacitracin are suspect in this regard in that hydrocarbon vehicles are extremely poor solvents for such drugs. A pharmacist should seek evidence that such formulations are effective before recommending them. Inunction (rubbing in) may release such drugs, the sebum on skin surface may dissolve a fraction of lipophilic drugs, and sweating may make the water-soluble drug available for absorption. Particularly, application of cosmetic products, insect repellents, sunscreens on the sites where topical drug applied, either before or after, may have profound effect on percutaneous absorption of drugs from dermatological products.

Deodorants are also targeted to the skin surface to keep microbial growth in check. Here, they slow or prevent rancidification of the secretions of apocrine glands found in and around the axillae (armpits) and the anogenital regions. Medicated soaps also belong to this family.

Stratum Corneum Effects

The stratum corneum is the most easily accessed part of the skin itself, and there are two actions targeted to this tissue, namely, emolliency, the *softening of the horny tissue*, which comes about through remoisturizing it, and keratolysis, the chemical digestion and removal of thickened or scaly horny tissue. Tissue needing such removal is found in calluses, corns, and psoriasis and as dandruff. Common agents as salicylic acid and, to a lesser extent, sulfur, cause lysis of the sulfhydral linkages holding the keratin of the horny structure together, leading to its disintegration and sloughing.

It has been mentioned that elasticity of the stratum corneum depends on its formation and on the presence of adequate natural lipids, hygroscopic substances, and moisture (19,20). Simply occluding the surface and blocking insensible perspiration can induce remoisturization (emolliency). However, it is best accomplished by lotions, creams, and/or waxy formulations (e.g., lip balms), which replenish lost lipid constituents of the stratum corneum. The fatty acids and fatty acid esters these contain in part fill the microscopic cracks and crevices in the horny layer, sealing it off, stabilizing its bilayer structures, allowing it to retain moisture. Many emollient products also contain hygroscopic glycols and polyols to replenish and augment natural moisturizing factors of this kind, also assisting the stratum corneum in retaining moisture.

The introduction of moisturizing substances into the stratum corneum is ordinarily a straightforward process. Deposition of keratolytics, on the other hand, is not as easily achieved, as these agents must penetrate into the horny mass itself. Some salicylic acid–containing corn removers are therefore made up as concentrated nonaqueous solutions in volatile solvents. As these volatile solvents evaporate, drug is concentrated in the remaining vehicle and thereby thermodynamically driven into the tissue. These many examples illustrate the fact that when the therapeutic target is at the skin's surface or is the stratum corneum, the therapeutic rationale behind the treatment usually involves enhancing or repairing or otherwise modulating barrier functions.

Drug Actions on the Skin's Glands

A few products modulate operation of the skin's appendages. These include antiperspirants (as opposed to deodorants), which use the astringency of chemicals such as aluminum chloride so as to reversibly irritate and close the orifices of eccrine glands (21) to impede the flow of sweat. Astringents also decimate the population of surface microbes, explaining their presence in deodorants. The distinction between antiperspirants and deodorants is legally significant, as antiperspirants alter a body function and are regulated as drugs, while deodorants are classified as cosmetics. Thus, the antiperspirant action has to be scientifically proven to before it can be claimed for a product. Nevertheless, given the similarities in the compositions of deodorants and antiperspirants, they are likely functionally equivalent. Since eccrine glands are mediated by cholinergic nerves, sweating also can be shut off by anticholinergic drugs administered systematically (22) or topically. However, such drugs are too toxic for routine use as antiperspirants even when administered topically.

Acne is a common glandular problem arising from hyperproliferative closure of individual glands in the unique set of pilosebaceous glands located in and around the face and across the upper back. Both local and systemic antibiotics and antiseptics suppress the formation of lesions. It is believed these attenuate the population of anaerobic microorganisms that are deep seated in the gland, the metabolic byproducts of which irritate the lining of the gland, setting off lesion formation. Mild cases of acne improve and clear under the influence of astringents, possibly for the same reason. Retinoids, oral and topical, reset the processes of epidermal proliferation and differentiation. Through such dramatic influences on cell growth patterns, they actually prevent the formation of lesions. However, because of concerns over toxicity, they tend to be used only in the most severe cases of acne and thus are prescribed for those patients whose acne lesions progress to cysts.

Hair is a product of the pilosebaceous apparatus and in this sense is glandular. It often grows out visibly in places where such display is unwanted. It may be shaved but chemical hair removers (depilatories) along with other products are also used to remove it. In the main, the use of depilatories is cosmetic rather than therapeutic. Thioglycolate-containing, highly alkaline creams generally dissolve hair in short order without doing great harm to surrounding tissues. Facial skin is delicate, however, and depilatories must be used carefully here.

Effects in Deep Tissues

Local, Regional, and Systemic Delivery
When the target of therapy lies beneath the stratum corneum, topical drug delivery is more difficult and becomes more uncertain. Therefore, many potentially useful drugs find no place in topical therapy because of their inability to adequately penetrate the skin. Nevertheless, a number of pathophysiological states can be controlled through local administration and subsequent percutaneous absorption. For example, most skin conditions are accompanied by inflammation of the skin; topical corticosteroids and nonsteroidal anti-inflammatory drugs alike are used to provide symptomatic relief in such instances. Corticosteroids are also used in psoriasis where, in addition to suppressing inflammation, they somehow act on the basal epidermal layer to slow proliferation and restore the skin's normal turnover rhythm (23). Pain originating in the skin can be arrested with locally applied anesthetics. OTC benzocaine and related prescription drugs are used for this purpose. Hydroquinone is applied to the skin to lighten excessively pigmented skin by oxidizing melanin deep within the surface. Another treatment that involves percutaneous absorption is the application of 5-fluorouracil (5-FU) for the selective eradication of premalignant and basal cell carcinomas of the skin (22). In all these examples, the key to success is the ability that we have to get therapeutic amounts of the drugs through the stratum corneum and into the viable tissues.

Systemic actions of some drugs can also be achieved via local application, in which case their delivery is known as transdermal delivery. Just past the middle of the 20th century, improvements in analytical instrumentation made it possible to measure the exceedingly low circulating levels of drugs that build up in the body during the course of therapy. Novel delivery systems involving nontraditional routes of administration were subsequently conceived, constructed, and put to test. The possibilities for transdermal delivery might have been seen long ago in the systemic toxicities of certain topically contacted chemicals. As long as a century ago, it was known that munitions workers who handle nitroglycerine suffer severe headaches and ringing in the ears (tinnitus). These same effects are experienced to a degree by those taking nitroglycerine to alleviate angina. The association between therapy and the inadvertent percutaneous absorption of nitroglycerine was finally made in the 1970s and a nitroglycerine ointment was introduced, producing peak blood levels comparable to those attained upon sublingual administration of traditional tablet triturates, but levels that were also sustained. Consequently, a nitroglycerine ointment became the first commercially successful, therapeutically proven transdermal delivery system. But ointments are *greasy* and suffer variability in their dosing, even with dose titration, as a result of the fact that different patients apply semisolids more or less thinly and therefore over lesser or greater areas.

As shown in Table 4, sophisticated adhesive patches for transdermal delivery of scopolamine (motion sickness), nitroglycerine (anginal symptoms), clonidine (regulation

Table 4 Adhesive Drug Delivery Systems

Drug molecular weight; melting point	Product name(s)	Main use(s)	Available strengths[a] (dosing rates)	Customary duration of wear	Available sizes (cm²)[b]
Transdermal					
Clonidine 230.1; 130°C	Catapres-TTS[®]	Lower blood pressure	0.1, 0.2, 0.3 mg/day	7 days	3.5, 7, 10.5
17-β-Estradiol 272.4; 176°C	Alora[®]	Treat menopausal symptoms, prevent osteoporosis	0.05, 0.075, 0.1		18, 27, 36
	Climara[®]		0.05, 0.075, 0.1	34 days	12.5, 18.75, 25
	Estraderm[®]		0.05, 0.1		10, 20
	Fempatch[®]		0.025		30
	Vivelle[®]		0.0375, 0.050, and 0.075, 0.1	7 days	11, 14.5, 22, 29
	Menostar[®]		0.014 mg/day[c]	3–4 days	3.25
				7 days	
Ethinyl estradiol 296.4; 183°C	Ortho Evra[®]	Prevent pregnancy	0.75 mg/7 day[d]	7 days	20
Norelgestromin 327.5			6.00 mg/7 day[d]		
Estradiol, levonorgestrel 312.4; 240°C	Climara Pro[®]	Treat vasomotor symptoms and prevent postmenopausal osteoporosis	0.045 mg/day 0.015 mg/day	7 days	22
Fentanyl 336.5; 84°C	Duragesic[®] Ionsys[TM]	Block visceral pain	0.6, 1.2, 1.8, 2.4 mg/day[e] 40 µg/10 min/dose[f]	Up to 3 days Up to 80 doses	10, 20, 30, 40
Methylphenidate 233.3; 224–226°C	Daytrana[TM]	Treat attention deficit hyperactivity disorder	1.1, 1.6, 2.2, 3.3 mg/hr	9 hr	12.5, 18.75, 25, 37.5
Nicotine 162.2; liquid	Habitrol[®] Nicoderm[®] Nicotrol[®] ProStep[®] *generic* (Par)	Assist in smoking cessation	7, 14, 21 7, 14, 21 15 11, 22 mg/day[g]	16–24 hr	10, 20, 30 Unspecified Unspecified 3.5, 7
Nicotine polacrilex					
Nitroglycerine 227.1; liquid	Deponit[®]	Obviate and/or relieve anginal pain	4.8, 9.6	12–14 hr "on", 10–12 hr "off"	16, 32

	Brand name (manufacturer)	Use	Delivery rate	Wear time	Strengths
	Minitran®		2.4, 4.8, 9.6, 14.4		3.3, 6.7, 13.3, 20
	Nitro-Dur®		2.4, 4.6, 7.2, 9.6, 14.4, 19.6		5, 10, 15, 20, 30, and 40
	Transderm-Nitro® generics (Mylan, Warner Chilcott)		2.4, 4.8, 9.6, 14.4 mg/day[h]		5, 10, 20, 30
Oxybutynin 357.5; 129–130°C	Oxytrol®	Treat overactive bladder	3.9 mg/day	3–4 days	39
Rotigotine 315.5	Neupro®	Treat Parkinson's	2, 4, 6 mg/day	24 hr	10, 20, 30
Scopolamine 303.4; 59°C	Transderm-Scop®	Prevent motion sickness	0.33 mg/day	3 days	2.5
Selegiline 187.3; 141–142°C	Emsam®	Treat depressive disorder	6, 9, 12 mg/day	24 hr	20, 30, 40
Testosterone 288.4; 155°C	Androderm®	Supplement androgen (general), treat hypogonadism	2.5, 5	1 day	7.5, 15
	Testoderm TTS®		5		60
	Testoderm®[i]		4, 6 mg/day		40, 60[j]
Topical					
Lidocaine–prilocaine	EMLA Anesthetic Disk®	Local anesthetic prior to office surgery	Lidocaine and prilocaine each at 2.5% in cream	≈3 hr to deaden tissue	10 (contains 1 g EMLA cream)

a"Strengths" are based on delivery rates which are, in turn, proportional to the area of the patch. This can be seen upon comparing the information in column 3 with that in column 5.

bIf no size is given in the current package insert, the size is "unspecified." Areas relate to the brand name products listed in column 2. In some cases, the areas given are "active areas" and do not include the additional area of a ring of peripheral adhesive.

cThe strengths here may be expressed in µg/day and, in this unit, are 25, 37.5, 50, and 75 µg/day.

dThe number is the drug loading in patches.

eDose rates for fentanyl are usually expressed in units of g/hr and range from 25 to 100 µg/hr (0.6–2.4 mg/day).

fThis is a patient-controlled iontophoretic transdermal system.

gThe products in this category vary widely in dosing rate. Habitrol, Nicoderm, and generic offer patches that deliver 7, 14, and 21 mg/day; Nicotrol is a one-strength patch at 15 mg in 16 hours. ProStep provides patches that deliver 11 and 22 mg/day. In many cases, patches may not be worn at night (while in bed).

hThese strengths amount to delivery rates of 0.1, 0.2, 0.3, 0.4, 0.6 mg/hr, respectively. Nitroglycerine patches are put on in the morning and taken off in the evening and therefore worn for 12 to 14 hours. The 10- to 12-hour hiatus in dosing, the so-called washout period, is necessary to reactivate enzymes that convert nitroglycerine to its active nitrous oxide (NO) metabolite.

iTestoderm TTS is applied to body skin, while Testoderm forms are applied to scrotal skin only.

jOne Testoderm scrotal form comes with an adhering surface (adhesive).

of blood pressure), β-estradiol (menopausal symptoms), fentanyl (cancer pain), nicotine (smoking cessation), testosterone (hypogonadism), and others have been introduced into medicine since about 1980 (24–26). These patches, affixed to an appropriate body location, deliver drug continuously for periods ranging from about half a day (nitroglycerine) to a week (clonidine, β-estradiol). It is obvious from the above that the skin is a formidable barrier irrespective of whether therapy is to be local, regional, or systemic, and the first concern in topical delivery is sufficiency of delivery. With local therapy, the aim is to get enough drug into the living epidermis or its surroundings to effect a pharmacological action there without producing a systemically significant load of the drug. The latter is actually a rare occurrence except when massive areas of application are involved (overdose of methyl salicylate). Regional therapy involves effects in musculature and joints deep beneath the site of application. To be successful, this requires a greater delivery rate because an enormous fraction of the drug that passes through the epidermis is routed systemically via the local vasculature. Indeed, the levels of drug reached in deep local tissues have proven to be only a few multiples higher than those obtained upon systemic administration of the drug (27). Even more drug has to be delivered per unit area to transdermally effectuate a systemic action.

Factors Affecting Functioning of the Skin Barrier

A matter of considerable consequence in topical delivery is the variability in skin permeability between patients, which may be as much as 10-fold. This, however, has more to do with some patients having unusually impermeable skin rather than the reverse. Literature data suggest that the most permeable human skins are only twice the average in comparative studies, while the least permeable skins are fivefold below the average. The underlying sources of this high degree of variability are thought to be many and diverse. Humans differ in age, gender, race, and health, all of which are alleged to influence barrier function. Yet, insofar as can be told, a full-term baby is born with a barrier-competent skin and, barring damage or disease, the skin remains so through life. There is little convincing evidence that senile skin, which tends to be dry, irritable, and poorly vascularized, is actually barrier compromised (28). However, premature neonates have inordinately permeable skins. The incubators used to sustain such infants provide a humidified environment, which abates insensible perspiration, and a warm one, conditions that not only make the baby comfortable but also forestall potentially lethal dehydration and hypothermia (29).

Gender too affects the appearance of human skin. Nevertheless, there is little evidence that the skins of male and female differ greatly in permeability. However, there are established differences in the barrier properties of skin across the races of humans. While the horny layers of Caucasians and Blacks are of equal thickness, the latter population has more cell layers and is measurably denser (30). As a consequence, black skin tends to be severalfold less permeable (30,31).

Humidity and temperature also affect permeability. It has long been known that skin hydration, however brought about, increases skin permeability. Occlusive wrappings are therefore placed over applications on occasion to seal off water loss, hydrate the horny layer, and increase drug penetration. Temperature influences skin permeability in both physical and physiological ways. For instance, activation energies for diffusion of small nonelectrolytes across the stratum corneum have been shown to lie between 8 and 15 kcal/mole (3,32). Thus, thermal activation alone can double the rate of skin permeability when there is a 10°C change in the surface temperature of the skin (33). Additionally, blood perfusion through the skin in terms of amount and closeness of approach to the skin's surface is regulated by its temperature and also by an individual's need to maintain the body's 37°C isothermal state. Since clearance of percutaneously absorbed drug to the systemic circulation is sensitive to blood flow, a fluctuation in blood flow might be expected to alter the uptake of chemicals. Above all else, the health of the skin establishes its physical and physiological condition and thus its permeability. Consequences attributable to an unhealthy condition of skin can be subtle or exaggerated. *Broken skin* represents a high permeability state, and polar solutes are several log orders more permeable when administered over abrasions and cuts. Irritation and mild trauma tend to increase the skin's permeability even when the skin is not broken, but such augmentation is far less substantial. Sunburn can be used to illustrate many of the barrier-altering events that occur in traumatized skin. Vasodilation of the papillary vasculature with marked reddening of the skin is among the first signs that a solar exposure has been overdone. In its inflamed state, the skin becomes warm to the touch. After a day or two, epidermal repair begins in earnest and the tissue is hyperproliferatively rebuilt in its entirety. It doubles in thickness, and a new stratum corneum is quickly laid down (34). Because the newly formed stratum corneum's anchorage to existing tissues is faulty, the preexisting horny layer often eventually peels. Of more importance, hyperplastic repair leads to a poorly formed horny structure of increased permeability to water (as measured by transepidermal water loss) and presumably other substances. Given these events surrounding irritation, since many chemicals found in the workplace and home are mildly irritating, including the soaps we use to bathe and the detergents we use to clean house and clothes, is it really a wonder that the permeability of human skin is so demonstrably variable?

Some chemicals have prompt, destructive effects on the skin barrier. Saturated aqueous phenol, corrosive acids, and strong alkali instantly denature the stratum corneum and destroy its functionality even as their corrosive actions stifle the living cells beneath. Though the stratum corneum may appear normal following such damage, the skin may be only marginally less permeable than denuded tissue (35). Other chemicals are deliberately added to formulations to raise the permeability of skin and improve drug delivery. For obvious reasons, these are referred to as skin penetration enhancers. More will be said of these later.

Thermal burning produces comparably high states of permeability immediately following burning, providing that the surface temperature of the skin is raised above 80°C, a temperature on the lower side of temperatures able to denature keratin (36). However, burning temperatures below 75°C, though fully capable of deep tissue destruction in seconds, leave the structure of the stratum corneum itself relatively unscathed. Burn wounds of this kind remain impermeable until tissue repair and restructuring processes get under way and the necrotic tissue with its horny capping is sloughed. In the later stage, all such wounds remain highly permeable until covered over again with a healthy, fully differentiated epidermis.

As with burns, physical disruption of the stratum corneum opens the skin in proportion to the extent of damage. Cuts and abrasions are associated with high permeability at and around such injuries. Eruption of the skin in disease has a similar effect to the extent that the stratum corneum's integrity is lost. The skin over eczematous lesions should be regarded as highly permeable. Not all skin diseases raise permeability, however. The states of permeability of ichthyosiform, psoriatic, and lichenified skin have not been well characterized, but in all likelihood are low for most drugs. It has been proven difficult to get potent corticosteroids through psoriatic plaque, for instance, and occlusive wrapping is often called for.

Percutaneous Absorption—The Process

The process of percutaneous absorption can be described as follows. When a drug system is applied topically, the drug diffuses passively out of its carrier or vehicle and, depending on where the molecules are placed down, partitions into either the stratum corneum or the sebum-filled ducts of the pilosebaceous glands. Inward diffusive movement continues from these locations to the viable epidermal and dermal points of entry. In this way, a concentration gradient is established across the skin up to the outer reaches of the skin's microcirculation where the drug is swept away by the capillary flow and rapidly distributed throughout the body. The volume of the epidermis and dermis beneath a 100-cm^2 area of application, roughly the size of the back of the hand, is approximately 2 cm^3. The total aqueous volume of a 75 kg ($\approx$ 165 lb) person is about 50,000 cm^3, yielding a systemic-to-local dilution factor well in excess of 10,000. Consequently, systemic drug levels are usually low and inconsequential. Thus, selectively high epidermal concentrations of some drugs can be obtained. However, if massive areas of the body ($\geqq$ 20% of the body surface) are covered with a topical therapeutic, systemic accumulation can be appreciable. For instance, corticosteroids have produced serious systemic toxicities on occasion when they have been applied over large areas of the body (37). Moreover, as has already been pointed out, if the stratum corneum is not intact, many chemicals can gain systemic entrance at alarming rates. Together these factors may place a patient at grave risk and should always be taken into account when topical drugs are put in use. The pharmacist should therefore carefully measure how topical systems are to be applied and be on alert for untoward systemic responses when body coverages are unavoidably extensive.

The events governing percutaneous absorption following application of a drug in a thin vehicle film are illustrated in Figure 2. The important processes of dissolution and

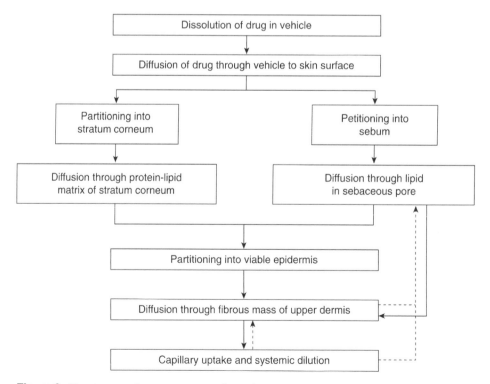

Figure 2 Events governing percutaneous absorption.

diffusion within the vehicle are cataloged. These will be discussed later. Two principal absorption routes are indicated in the sketch: (*i*) the transepidermal route, which involves diffusion directly across the stratum corneum, and (*ii*) the transfollicular route, where diffusion is through the follicular pore. Much has been written concerning the relative importance of these two pathways. Claims that one or the other of the routes is the sole absorption pathway are groundless, since percutaneous absorption is a spontaneous, passive diffusional process that takes the path of least resistance. Therefore, depending on the drug in question and the condition of the skin, either or both routes can be important. There are temporal dependencies to the relative importance of the routes too. Corticosteroids breach the stratum corneum so slowly that clinical responses to them, which are prompt, are reasoned to be due to follicular diffusion (3).

Sight should not be lost of the fact that the chemical barrier of the skin actually consists of all skin tissues between the surface and the systemic entry point. While it is true that the stratum corneum is a source of high diffusional resistance to most compounds and thus the skin's foremost barrier layer, exceptional situations exist where it is not the only or even the major resistance to be encountered. For example, extremely hydrophobic chemicals have as much or more trouble passing across the viable tissues lying immediately beneath the stratum corneum and above the circulatory bed, because such drugs have little capacity to partition into these tissues. Backing for the latter assertion comes from extensive clinical experience as well as from physical modeling of percutaneous absorption. Consider that ointments can be used safely over open wounds for their hydrocarbon constituents are not transported significantly across even denuded skin. Similarly, the whole skin is considerably more impermeable to octanol and higher alkanols than is the stratum corneum alone because of the presence of the viable tissue layer beneath.

Model of the Skin Barrier

The percutaneous absorption picture can be qualitatively clarified by considering Figure 3, where the schematic skin cross-section is placed side by side with a simple model for

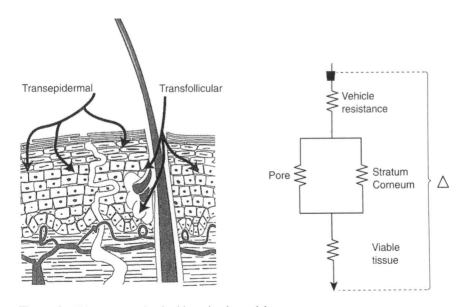

Figure 3 Skin cross-section beside a simple model.

percutaneous absorption patterned after an electrical circuit. In the case of absorption across a membrane, the current or flux is in terms of matter or molecules rather than electrons, and the driving force is a concentration gradient (technically, a chemical potential gradient) rather than a voltage drop (38). Each layer of a membrane acts as a *diffusional resistor*. The resistance of a layer is proportional to its thickness (symbol $= h$), inversely proportional to the diffusive mobility of a substance within it as reflected in a diffusion coefficient (D), inversely proportional to the capacity of the layer to solubilize the substance relative to all other layers as expressed in a partition coefficient (K), and inversely proportional to the fractional area of the membrane occupied by the diffusion route (f) if there is more than one route in operation (39). In general, an individual resistance in a set may be represented by

$$R_i = \frac{h_i}{f_i D_i K_i} = \frac{(\text{thickness})}{(\text{fractional area})(\text{diffusion coefficient})(\text{partition coefficient})} \qquad (1)$$

The overall phenomenon of percutaneous absorption is describable upon recognizing that the resistances of phases in series (phases encountered serially) are additive and that diffusional currents (fluxes) through routes in parallel (differing routes through a given phase) are additive. Such considerations applied to skin allow one to explain, in semiquantitative terms, why percutaneous absorption through intact skin is slow for most chemicals and drugs and why disruption of the horny covering of the skin profoundly increases permeability of the ordinary run of solutes.

At the steady state and under sink conditions, the following equation describes that drug transport through the skin is primarily by parallel transepidermal (stratum corneum is the primary barrier) and follicular pathways:

$$J_{\text{total}} = J_{\text{sebum}} + J_{\text{sc}} = \text{APC}_{\text{sebum}} + \text{APC}_{\text{sc}} \qquad (2)$$

where J_{total} is the total flux and J_{sebum} and J_{sc} are fluxes through independent pathways (sebum/hair follicles and stratum corneum). A is the total area of application, P is the permeability coefficient, and C is the concentration of drug in the application. It follows that

$$J_{\text{total}} = \left(A_{\text{sebum}} \frac{D_{\text{sebum}} K_{\text{sebum}} C}{h_{\text{sebum}}} \right) + \left(A_{\text{sc}} \frac{D_{\text{sc}} K_{\text{sc}} C}{h_{\text{sc}}} \right) \qquad (3)$$

In these equations, A_{sebum} and A_{sc} are the actual areas of the sebum and stratum corneum routes. D_{sebum} and D_{sc} are the effective diffusion coefficients (composite diffusion coefficients for heterogeneous phases) for the drug in question through sebum and the stratum corneum, while K_{sebum} and K_{sc} are the drug's partition coefficients in sebum/water and stratum corneum/water, respectively. The terms, h_{sebum} and h_{sc}, refer to the functional thicknesses of the sebum and stratum corneum, respectively.

First, consider the transepidermal route. The fractional area of this route is virtually 1.0, meaning the route constitutes the bulk of the area available for transport. Molecules passing through this route encounter the stratum corneum and then the viable tissues located above the capillary bed. As a practical matter, the total stratum corneum is considered a singular diffusional resistance. Because the histologically definable layers of the viable tissues are also physicochemically indistinct, the set of strata represented by viable epidermis and dermis is handled comparably and treated as a second diffusional resistance in series.

Estimated diffusion coefficients in the stratum corneum are up to 10,000 times smaller than that found anywhere else in the skin, reflecting in part the considerable density of this tissue. If diffusion is almost exclusively through the intercellular lipid regime within the horny tissue, as most experts believe, then the estimates, which range between 1×10^{-13} cm^2/sec and a low of 1×10^{-9} cm^2/sec, have to be tempered with the knowledge that path tortuosity (nonlinearity) and excluded volume were not taken into account in calculating these values. Regardless, such low values still speak to the high resistance of the horny tissue (3), particularly given that the thickness of the stratum corneum is only about 1×10^{-3} cm (10 μm). The parameter exhibiting the most variability relative to the stratum corneum's diffusion resistance is the partition coefficient, K_{sc}, where the subscript sc denotes this specific tissue. The partition coefficient can take values several log orders less than 1 with highly polar molecules, for example, glucose, or values several log orders greater than 1 for hydrophobic molecules, for example, β-estradiol. The wedge of living tissue lying between the stratum corneum and the capillaries is on the order of 100 μm thick (1×10^{-2} cm). Permeation of this element of the barrier is facile and without great molecular selectivity. Where measured, diffusion coefficients through this cellular mass have proven to be no less than one-tenth of the magnitude of those found for the same compounds passing through water (40).

The follicular route can be analyzed similarly. The fractional area available for penetration by this route is on the order of one-one-thousandth (3), clearly a restricting factor. Here, partitioning is into sebum, and the distance that has to be traveled through sebaceous medium filling the follicular duct can be estimated as 200 to 500 μm, which is much greater than the thickness of the stratum corneum (41). Diffusion coefficients in the quasi-liquid sebum can be reasoned to be more than thousand times greater than found for the stratum corneum, however (3,9,42).

Net chemical penetration of the skin is simply the sum of the accumulations by each of the mentioned routes and by other routes, for instance, eccrine glands, where these contribute. The latter tiny glands are ubiquitously distributed over the body but are generally discounted in importance because of the limited fractional area they occupy and their unfavorable physiological states, either empty or profusely sweating.

For reasons that need not be elaborated here, water is invariably the solvent medium used to experimentally access permeability coefficients. Accordingly, water is assumed to be the vehicle used to apply a drug to the skin. This choice of vehicle effectively sets the partition coefficients between the aqueous tissues and the vehicle roughly to unity. Choosing water as the vehicle of consideration does not in any way invalidate insights that can be drawn from the model as long as saturated solutions, which operate at the thermodynamic activity of the solid drug, are brought into the analysis. Barring specific solvent-induced changes in the physical chemistry of the tissue, from the thermodynamic perspective, all saturated solutions should deliver drug at the maximal rate. Some parameter estimates are given in Table 5. The listed fractional areas, diffusion coefficients, and strata thicknesses reported in the table are based on the best information that is available.

Some scientists, including the authors, believe that the stratum corneum harbors a minor polar (aqueous pore) pathway,[a] mostly because of evidence that suggests that the stratum corneum offers higher fluxes to polar solutes the likes of methanol, ethanol, propylene glycol, glycerol, and glucose than one would otherwise expect. In this regard, it is also relevant that ions diffuse through the stratum corneum with deceptive ease considering their solution attributes. Sebum is generally taken to be an oily composite, which consists of wax esters, triglycerides, squalene, cholesterol/cholesteryl esters, and fatty acids. If the latter portrayal were apt, then sebum would have a thermodynamically limited ability to dissolve polar compounds. On these admittedly flimsy grounds, an argument can be mounted that the transepidermal route dominates the transfollicular route with respect to the permeation of small, polar nonelectrolytes and ions (3,7,9,42,43).

---

[a]This supposition is hotly debated in scientific circles.

Table 5 Representative Parameters to Probe Model

	Diffusion coefficient, D (cm^2/sec)[a] (4,8)
Stratum corneum	10^{-9}–10^{-13}
Water	$\approx 10^{-9}$
n-Alkanols (hydrated tissue)	$\approx 10^{-9}$
n-Alkanols (dry tissue)	$\approx 10^{-10}$
Small nonelectrolytes	10^{-9}–10^{-10}
Progesterone	$\approx 10^{-11}$
Cortisone	$\approx 10^{-12}$
Hydrocortisone	$\approx 10^{-13}$
Follicular pore (sebum)	10^{-7}–10^{-9}
Viable tissue	$\approx 10^{-6}$

	Tissue thickness, h (μm) (2,7,10)
Stratum corneum	
Dry (normal state)	~10
Hydrated (as by occlusion) state	20–30
Pore diffusional length	Approximately 2 to 5 times greater than the stratum corneum thickness
Viable tissue stratum	150–2000[b] (200)

	Fractional area of the routes, F (3,7)
Transepidermal	~1
Transfollicular	~10^{-3}
Transeccrine	<10^{-4c}

	Tissue/vehicle partition coefficient, K
Stratum corneum	From <1 to ≫1[d]
4-Hydroxybenzoate esters and topicals	10^1–10^4 (43)
Sebum	From ≪1 to ≫1[d]
4-Hydroxybenzoate esters and topicals	10^1–10^3 (43)
Viable tissue	
Aqueous vehicle	~1
Nonaqueous vehicle	From ≪1 to ≫1[d]

[a]These diffusivities are estimates obtained by in vitro experiment (stratum corneum) or by comparison with small tissues in which diffusivities have been measured (all others). They do not account for regional variations across the body surface, so on both counts must be considered highly approximate.
[b]Highly approximate and variable, depending on blood flow patterns.
[c]This is sufficiently small to discount transeccrine diffusion contributions in the general treatment.
[d]All depend on the physicochemical nature of the drug and vehicle as well as the physicochemical mature of respective tissues.

It is thought that both the stratum corneum and the sebum are, to first good approximations, lipoidal routes. Consequently, drug substances of diminishing polarity should partition out of water into the key transport regimes within these routes to increasing extents. Homologues formed by extending the length of an alkyl chain provide a means for testing this hypothesis because of the fact that oil/water (o/w) partition coefficients of alkyl homologues grow exponentially. One can therefore probe the fundamental physical behaviors of lipid membranes as long as (in the permeability domain where) permeability coefficients are directly related to o/w partitioning. The slope of log (partition coefficient) against alkyl chain length plot indicates the sensitivity of partitioning between the phases in question to the addition of a methylene group (a $-CH_2-$ group). The value of $d[\log (K_{o/w})]/dn$, the slope, is referred to as the π-value for the partitioning system in question. The π-value for the partitioning of homologues between octanol and water is very close to 0.5. Thus, regardless of the homologous series in question, octanol/water partition coefficient increases by a factor of about 10 for every two methylene units added to an alkyl chain. With a π-value of greater than 0.6, hexane/water partitioning evidences an even greater lipoidal sensitivity. On the basis of permeation of n-alkanols through human skin (and the permeability partitioning relationship), human stratum corneum appears have a π-value slightly less than 0.3 (3). The low partitioning sensitivity to the addition of a methylene group suggests that the stratum corneum's lipoidal phase is considerably more polar than the reference organic solvents. This still means that, all else equal, partition coefficients increase rapidly by this route. The follicular route in seemingly more nonpolar than the route through the stratum corneum. This suggests that the region of direct partitioning dependency of permeability by this route would be narrower than found for the transdermal pathway (44,45). Recent studies have demonstrated that the correlation between partition coefficients of octanol/water, artificial sebum/water, and stratum corneum/water is somewhat complicated (41,42). A good linear relationship exists between the partition coefficient of sebum/water and the carbon chain length in the 4-hydroxybenzoate series compounds, but not for compounds with more diverse structures. The partition coefficient between stratum corneum/water is relatively higher for methyl-4-hydroxybenzoate, lower for ethyl-4-hydroxybenzoate, and then exponentially increases with the increase in alkyl chain length, reflecting the polar and nonpolar matrix property of stratum corneum. The permeability of the lipophilic compounds is much higher across sebum than across the stratum corneum, indicating that the transfollicular permeation could play a measurable role in the initial phase of percutaneous absorption, even though the relative permeation area is much smaller than for transepidermal permeation. However, the water-rich dermis functions as a primary barrier for lipophilic permeates. Excellent linear relationships between sebum permeability and log P for the 4-hydroxybenzoates homologues and hydrocortisone esters were observed, though the slopes were different (41,42). Within the tested compounds, the sebum permeability of an ionizable compound, lidocaine HCl, is six orders of magnitude lower than that of hydrocortisone 21-caprylate, demonstrating an extremely wide range of permeability of molecules across sebum plugs. Clearly, sebum serves an almost impermeable barrier to highly polar compounds but a friendly pathway to lipophilic compounds. This mechanism is critical when sebaceous glands and follicles are targeting sites and the lipophilic therapeutic agents are applied on sebaceous follicle-rich area, such as facial and scalp skin. It is well documented that molecules at log P of 2 to 3 are desirable for transdermal delivery because skin flux decreases at higher log Ps. However, the decrease in sebum flux with increased lipophilicity occurred in a more lipophilic range compared to that of skin flux. In case of the 4-hydroxybenzoic acid ester compounds, the decline in sebum flux was shown at clog $P > 4$ or the alkyl side chain $> C_6$. Figure 4 demonstrates a window between hexyl 4-hydroxybenzoate and nonyl 4-hydroxybenzoate (C_6-C_9) in which the skin flux of these compounds is extremely low but the sebum flux and sebum partition remain high. Molecules falling into this window would be ideal candidates for sebum or follicular-targeted delivery because of lower systemic exposure and higher localization in the pilosebaceous unit.

So far only steady-state conditions for permeation have been considered. But in all phenomena involving the mass transport of substances across membranes, one also has to consider the time it takes for gradients to be set up across the membranes by molecules moving randomly within the substance of the membranes. This early period of permeation

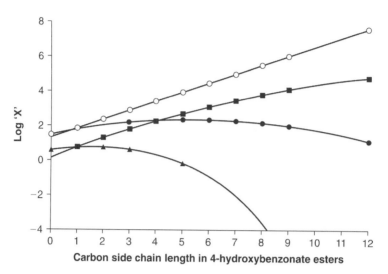

Figure 4 Relationship of carbon side chain length of 4-hydroxbenzoic acid esters with log J_s (sebum flux), log K_{sebum} (sebum partition coefficient), clog P (calculated octanol/water partition coefficient), and log J_{hs} [human skin flux from the literature by Pozzo and Pastori (46)]. ○, clog P; ■, log K_{sebum}; ◆, log (sebum flux); ▲, log (skin flux).

is referred to as the non-stationary-state period. The duration of this period is characterized by a lag time, as illustrated in Figure 5.[b] The non-stationary-state period may be of some importance in the instance of skin permeation (47). Where independent parallel pathways exist, as they seem to do through the skin, compounds may gain access to underlying tissues far more readily by one pathway than by the other. We can consider this point in terms of the lag time, t_L, that one expects to obtain for a compound diffusing through a simple isotropic field of a membrane:

$$t_L = \frac{h^2}{6 \times D} \qquad (4)$$

Here, h identifies the membrane's thickness and D is the compound's diffusion coefficient. The equation teaches us that the lag times for parallel routes should differ to the extents that h and D are different for the routes. We can crudely estimate the respective lag times for the transepidermal and transfollicular routes from the diffusion coefficient and thickness estimates tabulated in Table 5. Taking this approach, lag times for the transepidermal route are projected to range from minutes for small nonelectrolytes to multiple days for molecules of the size and properties of the corticosteroids. On the other hand, the lag times for breaching the transfollicular route should range from seconds to minutes. Though relatively few molecules reach the living tissues via the transfollicular route because of the limited fractional area of this pathway, it appears that the first lipophilic molecules to reach the viable epidermis actually get there via this path. This comparison has led scientists to suggest that the early clinical responses seen with drugs as large as steroids are the result of follicularly transported molecules. However, if the lag time for passage directly through the stratum corneum is also very brief, the follicular shunt diffusion is far less likely to be clinically meaningful. These non-stationary-state considerations do not apply at all when the horny barrier is impaired. Under this circumstance, transepidermal lag times can be so brief that they cannot be easily measured.

---

[b]The lag time is the intercept that results by extrapolating the steady-state line of a plot of cumulative amount of drug penetrated versus time to the time axis.

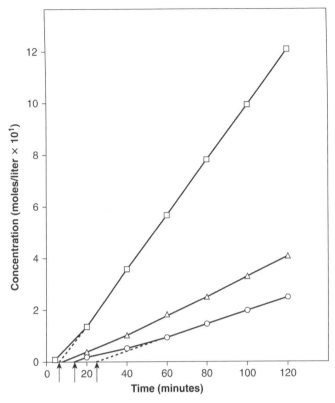

Figure 5 Generalized permeation profile. From left to right the data are for *n*-butanol permeating hairless mouse skin at 20°C, 25°C, and 30°C, respectively. Increasing temperature raises the flux (*slope*) and shortens the lag time.

Equations (1) and (2) point to the fact that the amount of drug delivered through the skin is proportional to the area of application of a topical dosage form or a transdermal patch. Nitroglycerine and other patches are available in different sizes (areas) to take advantage of this proportionality in dosing. Pharmacists have to be cognizant of this area dependency for another important reason, this being that the systemic accumulations, and thus systemic toxicities, of topically applied drugs are proportional to application area. Indeed, excessive areas of application are the most frequent cause of the untoward systemic actions seen with topically applied drugs. Tiny infants have been fatally poisoned following all too liberal applications of borate-containing talcum powders. As a result, borates are no longer used as lubricants in powder formulations. Babies have also been poisoned upon bathing them with a hexachlorophene-containing soap. Bathing, of course, is virtually synonymous with whole body coverage. Hexachlorophene is no longer used as an antiseptic soap. Diaper dermatitis tends to be expressed over large areas. Anti-inflammatory corticosteroids have occasionally been used too liberally to remedy this condition, again eventuating in serious toxicity. And systemic toxicities have at times accompanied the application of salicylic acid, a keratolytic agent or substance that breaks down keratin, to large psoriatic lesions. There are documented cases of abuse of transdermal patches, including a case in which a patient, confused about the manner of usage, succumbed to fentanyl by wearing four patches simultaneously. A pharmacist must realize that, in the instance of topical therapy, area is dose!

Phenomenological Considerations in Percutaneous Delivery

While the model helps us understand the chemical structure dependencies of skin permeability, it is not all that useful for calculating permeability coefficients because of the many iffy assumptions it contains. A different tack has to be taken to gain a sense of the limits, especially the upper limit, of cutaneous drug delivery. There is no lower limit. Even proteins penetrate intact skin to some extent. Some idea of the upper limit can be gained upon examining the rates of delivery of nitroglycerine and like facile penetrants of the skin. Nitroglycerine, a liquid at room temperature, is a lipophilic nonelectrolyte of 227 Da molecular weight. These physical properties make this drug about as good a skin penetrant as can be found. It is formulated in transdermal systems virtually as a neat liquid and thus near its upper attainable thermodynamic activity. It diffuses through the skin at between 0.02 and 0.04 mg/cm^2/hr from the transdermal reservoirs it is placed in. These rates equate with a delivery of 0.5 to 1.0 mg/cm^2/day (24). Consequently, 20 cm^2 patches provide a daily delivery of between 10 and 20 mg of the drug (24). Nicotine, another low molecular weight, substantially hydrophobic, liquid compound at 25°C, permeates human skin from its transdermal delivery systems with comparable ease. Selegiline is yet another drug with properties as these that is a facile skin penetrator. Putting all of this together, it appears that a percutaneous delivery rate of about 1 mg/cm^2/day is near the upper achievable limit for "skin delivery." Now it is true that water diffuses out through the skin far faster than any of these compounds diffuse in the reverse direction. To be specific, we typically loose about 0.5 mg/cm^2/hr of water through the skin into a dry external atmosphere, a flux that exceeds that of the referenced compounds by more than an order of magnitude. However, water is a very unique molecule both with respect to its size and its interactions within the horny layer. It appears that its diffusion is not constrained to the intercellular domain of the stratum corneum but, rather, some water almost certainly works its way into and up through keratin amassed in the intracellular space. A major fraction of insensible perspiration exits the skin this way. By way of contrast, permeation of nitroglycerine and the other drugs mentioned is thought to mainly take place through the intercellular domain of the stratum corneum.

If all nonpolar drugs were as skin permeable as nitroglycerine, many more transdermal delivery systems might exist. Why are there so few transdermally delivered drugs? The crystallinity of compounds is one important answer for, in a general way, the level of crystallinity sets a limit on solubility and thus the activity gradient that can be expressed across the skin.

Since most drugs are quite crystalline, the delivery of 1 mg of drug per day through a 20-cm^2 area (roughly the area of a Ritz cracker) can be feat. This is one of the main reasons why only exceptionally potent drugs are taken seriously for transdermal delivery. The dose limit results from the fact that, irrespective of the solvent, drug solubilities are lowered over what they would otherwise be by crystallinity. In other words, a drug's solubility ordinarily sets the upper limit on a drug's driving force and therefore on its achievable dosing rate. It is particularly important to give serious weighing to the crystallinity factor when selecting compounds for topical or transdermal purposes from the many that may be available. Everything else equal, low-melting compounds are far easier to deliver in therapeutically adequate amounts.

Crystallinity aside, the two physical attributes of a drug that most control its skin permeability are its physical size and its lipophilicity (48,49). All extant human permeability coefficients (at the time over 90 compounds) were subjected to multiple linear regressions by Potts and Guy using the following semiempirical equation (49):

$$\log_{10}(P) = \log_{10}\left(\frac{D^\circ}{h}\right) + \alpha \log_{10}(K_{\text{oct/w}}) - \beta^{(\text{MW})} \qquad (5)$$

They found that almost 70% of the variation exhibited by human skin permeability coefficients is explained by differences in their molecular sizes and partitioning coefficients. $D°$ in equation (14) is the hypothetical diffusivity of a molecule having zero molecular volume (the molecular size influence appears in the molecular weight term). As before, h is meant to represent the length of the diffusion pathway. $K_{oct/w}$ is the octanol/water partition coefficient of each compound. $K_{oct/w}$ is a general measure of the relative lipophilicity of each compound and also something of a surrogate for a compound's stratum corneum/water partition coefficient, $K_{sc/w}$. α is a proportionality factor relating $K_{sc/w}$ to $K_{oct/w}$, while β is a constant arising from the dependency of diffusion coefficients on molecular size. The computer-determined expression that best fit all the permeability coefficient data is (48)

$$\log_{10}(P) = -6.3 + 0.71(K_{oct/w}) - 0.0061^{(MW)} \tag{6}$$

Equation (6) ostensibly allows one to estimate permeability coefficients in units of cm/ sec. However, as with any parameter calculated from statistically drawn relationships, such estimates have to be "taken with a grain of salt" for the absolute error of estimation for a single compound can be large.

UNIQUE PHYSICOCHEMICAL SYSTEMS USED TOPICALLY

As one scans the products at the drug counter, one finds an enormous variety of formulation types available for topical therapy or for cosmetic purposes. Solutions are commonly found. They come in packages that allow them to be rubbed on, sprayed on by aerosol and atomizers, painted on, rolled on, swabbed on by premoistened pledgets, and dabbed on from applicators. Assorted medicated soaps are available for a range of purposes. Emulsions for the skin are found in the form of shampoos and as medicated lotions. Powders to soothe and lubricate are placed in sprinkling cans, while others containing drugs are formulated into aerosols to be sprayed on the skin. There are numerous fluid suspensions to be used as makeup or for therapeutic purposes. Clear and opaque gels are also to be found in both cosmetic and therapeutic spheres as are assorted semisolid creams, ointments, and pastes. The physical natures of these latter systems range from soft semisolids that are squeezed out of tubes to hardened systems suitable for application in stick form. There are therapeutic and cosmetic oils for the bath. The list of products and formulation types is nearly endless.

Of all these formulations, it is the diverse semisolids that stand out as being uniquely topical. Semisolid systems fulfill a special topical need as they cling to the surface of the skin to which they are applied, generally until being washed off or worn off. In contrast, fluid systems have poor substantivity and readily streak and run off the desired area. Similarly, powders have poor staying properties. Importantly, the fundamental physicochemical characteristics of solutions, liquid emulsions and suspensions, and powders are independent of their route of application, which are discussed adequately elsewhere in this text and need not be reconsidered. This is not to say the compositions of such systems cannot be uniquely topical, for there are chemicals that can be safely applied to the skin but are unsafe to use systemically]. There is need to elaborate the properties of semisolids.

General Behavior of Semisolids

The term semisolid infers a unique rheological character. Like solids, such systems retain their shape until acted upon by an outside force, whereupon, unlike solids, they are easily deformed. Thus, a finger drawn through a semisolid mass leaves a track that does not fill up when the action is complete. Rather, the deformation made is for all practical purposes permanent, an outcome physically characterized by saying semisolids deform plastically. Their overall rheological properties allow them to be spread over the skin to form films that cling tenaciously.

To be semisolid, a system must have a three-dimensional structure that is sufficient to impart solid-like character to the undistributed system that is easily broken down and realigned under an applied force. The semisolid systems used pharmaceutically include ointments and solidified water-in-oil (w/o) emulsion variants thereof, pastes, o/w creams with solidified internal phases, o/w creams with fluid internal phases, gels, and rigid foams. The natures of the underlying structures differ remarkably across all these systems, but all share the property that their structures are easily broken down, rearranged, and reformed. Only to the extent that one understands the structural sources of these systems does one understand them at all.

Ointments

Unless expressly stated otherwise, ointments are hydrocarbon-based semisolids containing dissolved or suspended drugs. They comprise fluid hydrocarbons, C_{16} to perhaps C_{30} straight chain and branched, entrapped in a fine crystalline matrix of yet higher molecular weight hydrocarbons. Upon cooling, the high molecular weight fraction precipitates out substantially above at room temperature, forming interlocking crystallites (50). The extent and specific nature of this structure at room temperature determine the stiffness of the ointment. It follows directly from this that hydrocarbon-based ointments liquefy upon heating for the crystallites melt. Moreover, when cooled very slowly, they assume fluidity much greater than when rapidly cooled because slow cooling leads to fewer and larger crystallites and therefore less total structure. Ordinary white and yellow petrolatums are examples of such systems.

Several alternative means of forming hydrocarbon ointments illustrate their structural properties. Ointments can be made by incorporating high-melting waxes into mineral oil (liquid petrolatum) at high temperature. Upon cooling, interlocking wax crystallites form and the system sets up. Polyethylene too can gel mineral oil if dissolved into this vehicle at high temperature and then the solution force cooled (51). A network of polyethylene crystallites provides the requisite solidifying matrix. This polyethylene-gelled system is more fluid on the molecular level than are the semisolid petroleum distillates while at the same time macroscopically behaving as an ointment. Consequently, diffusion of drugs through this vehicle is more facile and drug release is somewhat greater than are found with petrolatum-based systems (52). Plastibase (Squibb, New Brunswick, NJ) is the commercially available base of polyethylene-gelled mineral oil. It is useful for the extemporaneous preparation of ointments by cold incorporation of drugs. Pharmacists should not melt down this base to incorporate drugs for its gelled state cannot be restored without special processing equipment.

If a material other than a hydrocarbon is used as the base material of an ointment-like system, the *ointment* bears the name of its principal ingredient. There are silicone ointments that contain polydimethylsiloxane oil in large proportion. These reportedly act as excellent water barriers and superior emollients. Some are actually used to protect skin from undesirable influences of long immersion in water.

Ointments of the specific kinds mentioned above are taken to be good vehicles to apply to dry lesions but not to moist ones. All above are also greasy and stain clothes. The principal ingredients forming the systems, hydrocarbons and silicone oils, are generally poor solvents for most drugs, seemingly setting a low limit on the drug delivery capabilities of the systems. This solubility disadvantage can be offset somewhat if hydrocarbon-miscible solvents are blended into the systems to raise solvency. Alternatively, they can be made over into emulsions to raise their abilities to dissolve drugs. Along these lines, absorption bases are conventional ointments that contain w/o emulsifiers in appreciable quantity. A w/o emulsion is formed when an aqueous medium, perhaps containing the drug in solution, is worked into the base. Such emulsions are still ointments, as structurally defined, for it is the external phase of the formed emulsion that imparts the structure. It is important to note that the term absorption base refers to a water incorporation capacity and infers nothing about bioavailability. This is not to say that it is not better to have water-soluble drugs emulsified than as suspended solids in such systems from a bioavailability standpoint. In this regard, for optimum results, the internal, presumably aqueous phase should be close to saturated. Diverse additives are used to emulsify water into these systems, including cholesterol, lanolin (which contains cholesterol and cholesterol esters and other emulsifiers), semisynthetic lanolin derivatives, and assorted ionic and nonionic surfactants, singularly or in combination.

Polyethylene glycol *ointment* is a water-soluble system that contains fluid, short-chain polyoxyethylene polymers (polyethylene glycols) in a crystalline network of high-melting, long-chain polyoxyethylene polymers (Carbowaxes, Union Carbide Corp., Danbury, Connecticut, U.S.). The structure formed is totally analogous to that of the standard ointment. In one variation, this system functions well as a suppository base. Liquid polyethylene glycols are fully miscible with water, and many drugs that are insoluble in petroleum vehicles readily dissolve in the polar matrix of this base. In fact, with some drugs, delivery (bioavailability) can be compromised by an excessive capacity of the base to dissolve substances, resulting in poor vehicle-into-skin partitioning. Since polyethylene glycols are highly water soluble, bases formed from them literally dissolve off the skin when placed under a stream of running water.

Pastes

Pastes are basically ointments into which a high percentage of insoluble particulate solids have been added—as much or more than 50% by weight in some instances. This extraordinary amount of particulate matter stiffens the systems through direct interactions of the dispersed particulates and by adsorbing the liquid hydrocarbon fraction within the vehicle onto the particle surfaces. Insoluble ingredients such as starch, zinc oxide, calcium carbonate, and talc are used as the dispersed phase. Pastes make particularly good protective barriers when placed on the skin for, in addition to forming an unbroken film, the solids they contain can adsorb and thereby neutralize certain noxious chemicals before they ever reach the skin. This explains why they are used to ameliorate diaper rash, for when spread over the baby's *bottom*, they adsorb irritants formed by bacterial action on urine. Like ointments, pastes form an unbroken, relatively water-impermeable film on the skin surface and thus are emollients; unlike ointments, the film is opaque and therefore an effective sun block. Thus, skiers apply pastes around the nose and lips to gain a dual protection. Pastes are actually less greasy than ointments because of the adsorption of the fluid hydrocarbon fraction to the particulates.

Creams

Creams are semisolid emulsion systems having a *creamy* appearance as the result of reflection of light from their emulsified phases. This contrasts them with simple ointments, which are translucent. Little agreement exists among professionals concerning what constitutes a "cream," and thus the term has been applied both to absorption bases containing emulsified water (w/o emulsions) and to semisolid o/w systems, which are physicochemically totally different, strictly because of their similar creamy appearances. Logically, classification of these systems should be based on their physical natures, in which case absorption bases would be ointments and the term cream could be reserved exclusively for semisolid o/w systems, which in all instances derive their structures from their emulsifiers and internal phases.

The classical o/w cream is a vanishing cream that contains only 15% stearic acid or its equivalent as the internal phase. Vanishing cream and its variants are first prepared as ordinary liquid emulsions at high temperature; the structure that gives them their semisolid character forms as the emulsions cool. Both the aqueous and stearic acid phases are heated above the point where the waxy components liquefy and then are emulsified. Sufficient emulsifier is either formed in situ or added in to create a substantial micellar phase to exist in equilibrium with the liquefied internal phase of the hot emulsion. In the instance of the classical vanishing cream, about 20% of the stearic acid it contains is neutralized with strong alkali to form the surfactant. Portions of the waxy alcohols and/or undissociated waxy acids are solubilized within such micelles. As these systems are then cooled, their emulsion droplets solidify and the micellar structures linking all together take on a liquid crystalline character (53). The latter three-dimensional matrix has been referred to as *frozen micelles* and is what actually solidifies such creams. The compositions and amounts of both the internal phase and emulsifiers determine the extent and qualities of the structure. Creams like this are more or less stiff, depending on the level of micellar solubilization and the melting properties of the internal waxy component (53). Within the family of such creams, the internal phase ranges in composition from about 12% to 40% by weight.

Stiff o/w emulsions can also result from droplet interactions of the internal phase, but this requires emulsifying such a huge amount of internal phase that the droplets exceed close spherical packing. In this state the emulsified particles are squashed together, losing their sphericities, producing large interfacial areas of contact at the sites where the droplets come into contact. A fragile structure is obtained somewhere between that of a highly viscid liquid and a true semisolid. This cream type is far less common than systems built around frozen micellar structures.

A semisolid cream of the o/w type containing a solidified, liquid crystalline internal phase is an elegant topical system preferred by many for general purposes. Such o/w systems are readily diluted with water and thus easily rinsed off the skin and are generally nonstaining. Upon application, volatile components of the cream, which may comprise as much as 80% of the total system, evaporate, and the thin application shrinks down into an even thinner layer. Stearic acid creams are particularly interesting in this regard. The small amount of internal phase they contain causes them to evaporate down to near nothingness. The dry, nontacky, translucent nature of the stearic acid crystals left on the skin contributes to the sense of their lack of discernibleness. Most hand lotions and creams and foundation creams used to make face powders adherent to the face are variants of the vanishing cream formula.

Through evaporation, the drug in a cream is concentrated in its forming film, a process that can be orchestrated to program drug delivery. If no thought is given to the consequences attending drying out of the formulation, however, the drug is just as likely to precipitate out, in which instance drug delivery comes to an abrupt stop. One must therefore ensure that the formed film has some capacity to dissolve its drug. To this end, low-volatility, water-miscible solvents such as propylene glycol are added to many cream formulations. When ingredients like water and alcohol evaporate, the film left upon applying such creams becomes a rich concentrate of the drug, the internal phase, and its less volatile external phase components. One strives to add just enough cosolvent to keep the drug solubilized in the equilibrium film but also near saturation. It should be kept in mind that, unless the internal phase liquefies at body temperature, the waxy constituents cannot act as a solvent for the drug and thus do not lend the film much capacity for delivery.

The typical cream, a soft, emulsified mass of solidified particles in an aqueous, micelle-rich medium, does not form a water-impermeable (occlusive) film on the skin. Nevertheless, creams contain lipids and other moisturizers that replace substances lost from the skin in the course of everyday living. Creams thus make good emollients because, by replenishing lipids and in some instances also polar, hygroscopic substances, they restore the skin's ability to hold onto its own moisture.

The oleaginous phases of creams differ compositionally from hydrocarbon ointments. Many creams are patterned after vanishing cream and contain considerable stearic acid, but not all. In lieu of some or all of the stearic acid, creams sometime contain long-chain waxy alcohols (cetyl, C_{16}; stearyl, C_{18}), long-chain esters (myristates, C_{14}; palmitates, C_{16}; stearates, C_{18}), other long-chain acids (palmatic acid), vegetable and animal oils, and assorted other waxes of both animal and mineral origin.

Properly designed o/w creams are elegant drug delivery systems, pleasing in both appearance and feel post application. They are nongreasy and are easily rinsed off the skin. They are good for most topical purposes and are considered particularly suited for application to oozing wounds.

Gels (Jellies)

Gels are semisolid systems in which a liquid phase is trapped within an interlocking, three-dimensional polymeric matrix of a natural or synthetic gum. A high degree of physical or chemical cross-linking of the polymer is involved. It only takes from 0.5% to 2.0% of the most commonly used gelants to set up the systems. Some of these systems are as transparent as water, an aesthetically pleasing state. Others are turbid, as the polymer is present in colloidal aggregates that disperse light. Clarity of the latter ranges from slightly hazy to a whitish translucence not unlike that observed with petrolatum.

Agarose gels admirably illustrate the properties and to an extent the structural characteristics of most gels. Agarose solutions are water-thin when warm but solidify near room temperature to form systems that are soft to rubbery depending on the source and concentration of the agarose. A three-dimensional structure arises from the entwining of the ends of polymer strands into double helices. Kinks in the polymer mark the terminal points of these windings. Because individual polymer strands branch to form multiple endings, a three-dimensional array of physically cross-linked polymer strands is formed. The process of physical cross-linking is actually a crystallization phenomenon tying polymeric endings together, fixing the strands in place, yielding a stable, yet pliant structure (54). Less extensive structure than that found in agar growth media results in a spreadable semisolid suitable for medical application. The structure should persist to temperatures exceeding body temperature for the gelled systems to be the most useful. It is important to note that gelation is never a result of mere physical entanglement of polymer strands or otherwise the systems would only be highly viscid. The polymers used to prepare pharmaceutical gels include natural gums such as tragacanth, pectin, carrageen, agar, and alginic acid and synthetic and semisynthetic materials such as methylcellulose, hydroxyethylcellulose, carboxymethylcellulose, and carboxypolymethylene (carboxy vinyl polymers sold under the name Carbopol, B. F. Goodrich, Co., Cleveland, Ohio, U.S.).

Gels or jellies are used pharmaceutically as lubricants and also as carriers for spermicidal agents to be used intravaginally with diaphragms as an adjunctive means of contraception. Since the fluid phase of a gel does not have to be strictly water, gels offer a wide range of uses for, by blending solvents, it is possible to form films that exhibit a range of evaporation rates, solvency, and other release-determining attributes (55). Gel products containing anti-inflammatory steroids are used to treat inflammations of the scalp because this is an area of the body where creams and ointments are too greasy for patient acceptance.

Rigid Foams

Foams are systems in which air or some other gas is emulsified in a liquid phase to the point of stiffening. As spreadable topical systems go, medicated foams tend toward the fluid side, but, like some shaving creams, they can be stiffer and approximate to a true semisolid. Like the second type of o/w emulsion that only borders on semisolidity, these derive structure from an internal phase, bubbles of an entrapped gas, so voluminous that it exceeds close spherical packing. Consequently, the bubbles interact with their neighbors over areas rather than points of contact. The interactions are sufficient in many cases to provide a resistance to deformation and something approaching semisolid character. Whipped cream is a common example of this type of system. Here, air is literally beaten into the fluid cream until it becomes stiff. Aerosol shaving creams and certain medicated quick-breaking antiseptic foams are examples of the foams currently found in cosmetic and therapeutic practice. These are supplied in pressurized cans that have special valves capable of emulsifying a gas into the extruded preparations.

Common Constituents of Dermatological Preparations

So many materials are used as pharmaceutical necessities and as vehicles in topical systems that they defy thorough analysis. The pharmacist should nevertheless make some effort to learn of the more common constituents and their principal functions. The compositions of formulations as presented on product labels are the main source of such information. The compositions presented in Table 6 offer a glimpse into the compositional natures of semisolids.

Because of the large number of materials that are used in topical preparations and the diverseness of their physical properties, the formulation of topical dosage forms tends to be something of an art perfected through experience. Only by making myriad recipes does one eventually gain insight about the materials and their use in the design of new formulations. Such insight allows the experienced formulator to manipulate the properties of existing formulations to gain a desired characteristic. Often one finds good recipes to use as starting points for formulations in the trade literature. Two factors have to be kept in mind when *borrowing* the compositions of such trade formulations. First, the trade recipes (recipes supplied with advertising material touting specific components) are often inadequately tested in terms of their long-term stability. Second, the dominant features used in judging the merits of trade-promoted formulas tend to be their initial appearances and overall elegance. Little to no attention can be paid to the drug delivery attributes of the prototypical systems when they are first prepared in the suppliers laboratories because the drug delivery attributes are so compound specific. Thus, it is left up to the pharmacist (industrial research pharmacist) to make adjustments in the formulas, which are consistent

Table 6 Prototype Formulations

I. Ointment (white ointment, USP)

White petrolatum	95% (w/v)
White wax	5%

Melt the white wax and add the petrolatum; continue heating until a liquid melt is formed. Congeal with stirring. Heating should be gentle to avoid charring (steam is preferred), and *air incorporation* by too vigorous stirring is to be avoided.

II. Absorption ointment (hydrophilic petrolatum, USP)

White petrolatum	86% (w/w)
Stearyl alcohol	3%
White wax	8%
Cholesterol	3%

Melt the stearyl alcohol, white wax, and cholesterol (steam bath). Add the petrolatum and continue heating until a liquid melt is formed. Cool with stirring until congealed.

III. Water-washable ointment (hydrophilic ointment, USP)

White petrolatum	25% (w/w)
Stearyl alcohol	25%
Propylene glycol	12%
Sodium lauryl sulfate	1%
Methylparaben	0.025%
Propylparaben	0.015%
Purified water	37%

Melt the stearyl alcohol and white petrolatum (steam bath) and warm to about 75°C. Heat the water to 75°C and add the sodium lauryl sulfate, propylene glycol, methylparaben, and propylparaben. Add the aqueous phase and stir until congealed.

IV. Water-soluble ointment (polyethylene glycol ointment, USP 14)

Polyethylene glycol 4000 (Carbowax 4000)	50%
Polyethylene glycol 400	50%

Melt the PG 4000 and add the liquid PG 400. Cool with stirring until congealed.

V. Cream base, w/o (rose water ointment, NF 14)

Oleaginous phase	
Spermaceti	12.5%
White wax	12.0%
Almond oil	55.58%
Aqueous phase	
Sodium borate	0.5%
Stronger rose water, NF	2.5%
Purified water, USP	16.5%
Aromatic	
Rose oil, NF	0.02%

Melt the spermaceti and white wax on a steam bath. Add the almond oil and continue heating to 70°C. Dissolve the sodium borate in the purified water and stronger rose water, warmed to 75°C. Gradually add the aqueous phase to the oil phase with stirring. Cool to 45°C with stirring and incorporate the aromatic (rose oil).

Note: This is a typical cold cream formulation. The cooling effect comes from the slow evaporation of water from the applied films. The aromatic is added at as low a temperature as possible to prevent its loss by volatilization during manufacture.

Continued

Table 6 Prototype Formulations (*Continued*)

VI. Cream base, o/w (general prototype)

Oleagenous phase	
Stearyl alcohol	15%
Beeswax	8%
Sorbitan monooleate	1.25%
Aqueous phase	
Sorbitol solution, 70% USP	7.5%
Polysorbate 80	3.75%
Methylparaben	0.025%
Propylparaben	0.015%
Purified water, q.s. ad	100%

Heat the oil phase and water phase to 70°C. Add the oil phase slowly to the aqueous phase with stirring to form a crude emulsion. Cool to about 55°C and homogenize. Cool with agitation until congealed.

VII. Cream base, o/w (vanishing cream)

Oleagenous phase	
Stearic acid	13%
Stearyl alcohol	1%
Cetyl alcohol	1%
Aqueous phase	
Glycerin	10%
Methylparaben	0.1%
Propylparaben	0.05%
Potassium hydroxide	0.9%
Purified water, q.s. ad	100%

Heat the oil phase and water phase to about 65°C. Add the oil phase slowly to the aqueous phase with stirring to form a crude emulsion. Cool to about 50°C and homogenize. Cool with agitation until congealed.

Note: In this classic preparation, the stearic acid reacts with the alkaline borate to form the emulsifying stearate soap.

VIII. Paste (zinc oxide paste, USP)

Zinc oxide	25%
Starch	25%
Calamine	5%
White petrolatum, q.s. ad	100%

Titrate the calamine with the zinc oxide and starch and incorporate uniformly in the petrolatum by levigation in a mortar or on a glass slab with a spatula. Mineral oil should *not* be used as a levigating agent, since it would soften the product. A portion of the petrolatum can be melted and used as a levigating agent if so desired.

IX. Gel (lubricating jelly)

Methocel 90 H.C. 4000	0.8%
Carbopol 934	0.24%
Propylene glycol	16.7%
Methylparaben	10.015%
Sodium hydroxide, q.s. ad	pH 7
Purified water, q.s. ad	100%

Disperse the Methocel in 40 mL of hot (80–90°C), water. Chill overnight in a refrigerator to effect solution. Disperse the Carbopol 934 in 20 mL of water. Adjust the pH of the dispersion to 7.0 by adding sufficient 1% sodium hydroxide solution (about 12 mL is required per 100 mL) and bring the volume to 40 mL with purified water. Dissolve the methylparaben in the propylene glycol. Mix the Methocel, Carbopol 934, and propylene glycol fractions using caution to avoid the incorporation of air.

with good delivery of specific drugs. Each drug requires unique adjustments in accord with its singular physicochemical properties.

General Methods of Preparation of Topical Systems

Irrespective of whether the scale of preparation is large or small, ointments, pastes, and creams tend to be produced by one or the other of two general methods. Some are made at high temperature by blending liquid and melted-solid components together and then dispersing all other ingredients within the hot, oily melt. Alternatively, drug and/or adjuvants can be dispersed or dissolved within one of the phases or a fraction of one of the phases of an emulsion prior to forming the emulsion. The drug can be mixed into a freshly formed, still molten emulsion while it is still warm. Finally, a drug can be incorporated into an already solidified base via cold incorporation. As earlier pointed out, the first of these methods is commonly used to make o/w creams of the vanishing cream type. The fusion method is used to prepare many ointments as well. Cold incorporation comes into play in large-scale manufacture when the systems in preparation contain heat-labile drugs. In this instance, the drug is first crudely worked into an ointment or cream base by serial dilution and then distributed uniformly with the aid of a roller mill. Cold incorporation is also necessary when a base is destroyed by heat, as happens with Plastibase (Squibb).

In the fusion method for ointments, mineral oil, petrolatum, waxes, and other ingredients as belong in the formulation are heated together to somewhere between 60°C and 80°C, depending on the components, and mixed to a uniform composition while in the fluidized state. Cooling is then effected using some sort of a heat exchanger. To prevent decomposition, drugs and certain delicate adjuvants are added sometime during the cooling process. If insoluble solids need to be dispersed, the system is put through a milling process (colloid mill, homogenizer, ultrasonic mixer, etc.) to disperse them fully. A hand homogenizer works well at the prescription counter for small volume, extemporaneously prepared systems. Systems in preparation are always cooled with mild stirring until they are close to solidification. The rate of cooling is important, for rapid cooling, as mentioned, imparts a finer, more rigid structure. Stirring should be set to minimize vortexing and thereby prevent air incorporation into the solidifying system. Representative formulations with more system-specific, detailed directions are given in Table 6 for ointments and the other semisolid systems of note.

The fusion method for preparing creams is a bit more complex. In this instance, the aqueous and oil phases are heated separately to somewhere between 60°C and 80°C. As a general rule, the oil phase is heated to 5°C above the melting point of the highest-melting waxy ingredient and the water phase is heated to 5°C above the temperature of the oil phase, the latter to prevent premature solidification during the emulsification process. Water-soluble ingredients are dissolved in the heated aqueous phase and oil-soluble ingredients are dissolved in the oily melt, but only as long as they are heat stable and not too volatile. If an o/w system is to be made, the emulsifiers are added to the aqueous phase, and the emulsion is formed by slow addition of the oil phase. In the industry, the crude emulsion is then passed through a high-shear mixer to form a finely divided emulsion state. Following this, the emulsion is cooled with gentle stirring until congealed, again taking care not to whip air into the formulation. Typically, the emulsions solidify between 40°C and 50°C. If a w/o emulsion is to be made, the addition steps are usually reversed. Therefore, and generally, the discontinuous phase is added to the continuous, external phase containing the emulsifier. However, methods vary here, and for a particular formula the reverse order of addition may work best. Any means that reliably leads to a good emulsion is obviously acceptable.

As outlined when discussing absorption bases, the drug may also be dissolved in water to form a solution to be levigated into an ointment base or cream. Such addition softens creams even to the point of converting them to thick lotions. The chosen vehicle, of course, must have an inherent capacity to emulsify or otherwise take up the solution. Aromatic materials such as essential oils, perfume oils, camphor, and menthol, which volatilize if added when the base is hot, are incorporated into these semisolids while they are still being mixed but near the temperature where a particular system starts to congeal. Volatile materials are often introduced into the formulation as hydroalcoholic solutions.

The preparation of gels can involve high-temperature processing too. It is easier to disperse methylcellulose in hot than in cold water, for instance. The polymer then goes into solution and thickens or sets up as the temperature is lowered. Adding the hot methylcellulose dispersion to ice water gets one quickly to the final equilibrium state. Tragacanth gels, on the other hand, must be prepared at room temperature because of the extreme heat lability of this natural gum. A little alcohol or propylene glycol can be mixed into this gum before adding water to it to facilitate wetting of the gum prior to its dispersion. By way of contrast, Carbopol-containing systems are gelled by neutralizing the medium they have been dispersed in with alkali. Neutralization induces carboxyl groups found on the polymer backbone to ionize, instantaneously drawing these polymers into solution. Organic solvents can be gelled with Carbopol polymers as well, in such instances using soluble amines for the neutralization step.

Several prototype gel formulations are given in Table 6 to illustrate general compositional requirements and manufacturing methods. The design of specific systems tailored to meet predetermined, demanding performance criteria, particularly with respect to bioavailability, generally requires modification of published formulations or a totally original approach.

PERFORMANCE OF TOPICAL THERAPEUTIC SYSTEMS

Topical preparations, like all other dosage forms, must be formulated, manufactured, and packaged in a manner that assures that they meet general standards of bioavailability, physical (physical system) stability, chemical (ingredient) stability, freedom from contamination, and elegance. Like all other pharmaceuticals, these factors must remain essentially invariant over the stated shelf life of the product, and they must be reproducible from batch to batch.

Bioavailability

Chemical Structure, Delivery, Clinical Response
Much has already been said concerning the chemical structural dependencies of skin permeation. However, the goal of all treatment is successful therapy, not delivery per se, and consequently the intrinsic activities of the drugs must also be taken into account when selecting compounds for dermatological and transdermal development. The pharmacological response depends on delivering sufficient drug of a given activity to the target zone. Clearly, the more potent a compound is, the less of it needs to be delivered. Since topical delivery is difficult at best, potency often dictates which of the compounds found within a family of drugs should be developed, for the highly potent analog, reasonably formulated, offers the best chance of obtaining clinically sufficient delivery. Conversely, marginally potent analogs, even when expertly formulated, often fail because of inadequate delivery. An excellent example of this principle is found with the narcotic

analgesics. Because of its extraordinary potency, fentanyl, with a daily palliative requirement of 1 mg, and not morphine, which requires between 60 and 120 mg to alleviate pain over the course of a day, is what has made its way into transdermal use. The fact that fentanyl is also physicochemically more suited to transdermal delivery than morphine does not controvert this axiom.

Unlike mass transport across membranes, which relates to chemical structure in predictable ways, the potencies of drugs as seen in pharmacological, pharmacodynamic, or other tests are highly structurally specific within a class of drugs and are without commonality across classes. A drug's activity involves a complex merging of these separate structural influences, with bioavailability always one of the concerns. Such concern is minimal when a truly superficial effect is involved, however. For example, the most potent antiseptic as measured in the test tube is likely to have near the highest topical potency as well. The intrinsic activities of compounds may be poor indicators of relative topical potentials when deep skin penetration is required, however, because the structural features benefiting the biological response are often distinct from those that favor permeation. Thus, tissue permeability can be an important and sometimes a dominant factor in the clinical structure-activity profile.

We have seen that the determinants of skin permeation are the activity (concentration) of a drug in its vehicle, the drug's distribution coefficients between the vehicle and the skin and across all phases of the skin, and the drug's diffusion coefficients within the skin strata. Congeners, if comparably sized, exhibit little variance in their diffusion coefficients. However, the structural differences seen within congeneric families profoundly affect the solubility, partitioning, and in transit binding tendencies of the family members in addition to determining their binding with receptors. Drug delivery and resulting clinical effectiveness are captive of the former phenomena (56). For example, the 21-ester of hydrocortisone is more hydrophobic than its parent, its ether/water partition coefficient being about 18 times hydrocortisone's (57). Given the strong parallels in partitioning behaviors that exist across partitioning systems, it stands to reason that similar order-of-magnitude increases exist with respect to the acetate's stratum corneum/water and sebum/water partition coefficients. At the same time, acetylating hydrocortisone at the 21-position increases the melting point by 12°C. Consequently, not only does derivatization drop the aqueous solubility precipitously but it depresses solubility in all other solvents as well (58). While the increase in partition coefficient raises the permeability coefficient relative to hydrocortisone, this impact is more than offset by reduced solubility and far less of the acetate derivative can be delivered through the skin from respective saturated solutions (59). However, as the alkyl chain length of the ester is methodically extended (C3, C4, ..., C7), the growing bulkiness of alkyl group increasingly interferes with crystalline packing. Consequently, melting points fall incrementally from the 224°C peak of the acetate ester to 111°C when a chain length of seven, the heptanoate ester, is reached (58). An especially sharp drop of 69°C is experienced between chain lengths five and six. Because of declining crystallinity beyond the chain length of two, solubilities of the esters in organic solvents rise markedly. Moreover, aqueous solubilities, though methodically depressed by increasing hydrophobicity, remain many times higher than they otherwise would be. The net effect of these concerted forces is that the hexanoate and heptanoate esters of hydrocortisone are well over an order of magnitude more skin permeable than hydrocortisone when they are administered as saturated solutions (58,59).

Armed with the above insight, we can examine the pharmacological ramifications of esterifying hydrocortisone. In Figure 6, the ability of hydrocortisone esters to suppress inflammation induced by tetrahydrofurfural alcohol, which acts simultaneously as an

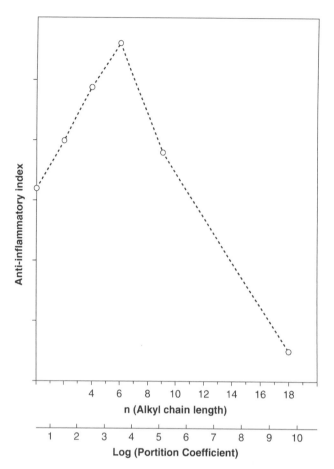

Figure 6 Ability of hydrocortisone esters to suppress inflammation.

irritant and a vehicle, is shown as a function of the alkyl chain length of the esters (60). An optimum chain in effect is seen at an alkyl chain length of six (hexanoate), with substantially longer and shorter esters being measurably less effective. The behavior is exactly what would be predicted from partitioning and solubility considerations. That this is not an isolated behavioral pattern with corticosteroids can be seen in Figure 7 where vasoconstriction data of McKenzie and Atkinson for three betamethasone ester families, 21-esters, 17,21-ortho-esters, and 17-esters, are shown as functions of the ether/water partition coefficients of the compounds (61). Vasoconstriction, blanching of the skin under the site of steroid application, is a proven index of a steroid's combined potency and ability to permeate through skin. Maxima are apparent in the data for the first two of these series, and the indications are that the 17-ester series is also peaking. Both maxima lie between ether/water partition coefficients of 1000 and 10,000 (57) as, interestingly and probably significantly, does the optimum ether/water partition coefficient of the hydrocortisone esters. The differing shapes and heights of the curves are not readily quantitatively explained but reflect differences in intrinsic vasomotor activities of each ester type. The coincidence of the maxima on the partitioning scale, on the other hand, seemingly relates to an optimum lipophilicity for delivery.

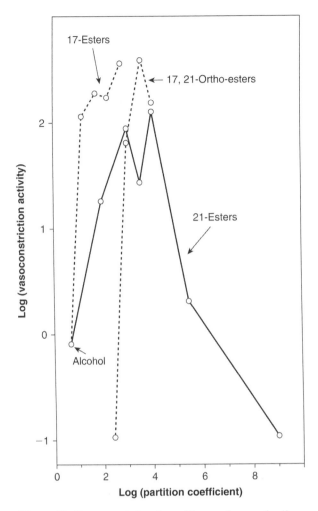

Figure 7 Vasoconstriction data of betamethasone family.

The decline in activity at the longer chain lengths (Figure 7) also has a plausible explanation. Two factors are reasoned to be operative here, declining solubilities coupled with changes in the absorption mechanism associated with stratification of the barrier. Aqueous solubilities of homologues decline exponentially as alkyl chain length is extended (62,63). While melting points are negatively impacted and depressed early in the series, the crystalline structure eventually accommodates the alkyl chain, whereupon further increases in chain length reverse the trend, reducing all solubilities (63). Through all of this, o/w partition coefficients, which are unaffected by crystallinity, increase exponentially, which has the effect of exponentially increasing the ability of the stratum corneum and sebum phases to transport of steroids relative to that of the viable tissue layer. In other words, the resistance of the stratum corneum drops precipitously without a commensurate drop in the resistance of the viable tissue layer. As a result, the latter takes control of the permeation process (9,37,64). Once this change in mechanism is manifest, the permeation of homologues from their saturated solutions mirrors the downward trend in aqueous solubilities, with further increases in chain length (hydrophobicity) marked with exponential declines in steady-state fluxes. The homologues quickly become inactive

(64). In effect, the homologues become so insoluble in water that they are thermodynamically restrained from partitioning into the viable tissues upon breaching the stratum corneum (or pore lipids). These features are in total agreement with expectations drawn from the earlier presented skin permeability model.

Clearly, the physicochemical properties of a drug are a decisive factor in its overall activity. Where possible, molecular structures should be optimized to obtain best clinical performance. Rarely does an oral drug have physicochemical features suitable for topical or transdermal therapy, and it can take a great deal of systematic research to identify where the best balance of activity and permeability lies. Experience with the corticosteroids suggests that as much as a 100-fold improvement in clinical activity may be attainable through molecular design, for today's most potent topical corticosteroids are more active than hydrocortisone by a factor at least this large.

Vehicle Properties and Percutaneous Absorption

The role solubility plays relative to maximal flux across membranes is clear from the preceding paragraphs. To kinetically reach the skin's surface, an appreciable fraction of a drug must also be in solution in the vehicle designed around it. Otherwise, diffusion of the drug through the vehicle to its interface with the skin may not completely compensate for the drug lost through partitioning into the skin, kinetically dropping the drug's activity within this critical juncture of formulation and skin below saturation, lowering the drug's release into the surface tissues. Taken to an extreme, low vehicle solubility sets up a situation in which drug dissolution within and diffusion through the vehicle becomes delivery rate controlling (65,66). In instances where a drug's pharmacological activity depends on getting as much drug as possible into the tissues, this is a problem. The outcome is similar when the drug is formulated in a highly unsaturated state in the first place. Again, it will not partition into the skin to the fullest possible extent, resulting in less than maximal bioavailability. Assuming maximal delivery is the goal, the optimum between these extremes is achieved by adjusting the solvency of the vehicle so that all or most all the drug is in solution but at the same time the vehicle is saturated or close thereto. This has the effect of balancing the kinetic and thermodynamic factors. It is for this reason that solvents like propylene glycol are added to topical formulations. Slowly evaporating propylene glycol provides a chemical environment in which drugs dissolve or remain dissolved, facilitating delivery. Therefore, one frequently finds propylene glycol (5–15%) in topical corticosteroid creams and other formulations.

These principles, which have been clinically validated, establish the critical role the vehicle plays in a drug's activity. While pharmacists do not have the wherewithal to actually test products at the dispensing counter, they nevertheless should be aware of these principles to select and dispense products from manufacturers who can demonstrate that such formulation factors have been given due consideration. These delivery dependencies also stand to caution the pharmacist. Extemporaneous mixing of commercial products, for example, one containing a steroid and another an antibiotic, and the diluting of products with homemade vehicle are suspect practices because the compositional changes associated with such blending are likely to adversely affect the delivery attributes of otherwise carefully designed systems (67,68).

There is another way vehicles can influence percutaneous absorption, which is by altering the physicochemical properties of the stratum corneum. In the main, modification of the barrier results in increased skin permeability, but a buttressing effect is also achievable with substances having the capacity to solidify the horny structure. To repeat a point, simply hydrating the stratum corneum promotes absorption. This may be accomplished by covering the skin with a water-impermeable bandage or other wrapping (an occlusive dressing). The blockage of evaporative water loss leads to hydration of the stratum corneum, softening it and increasing the diffusive mobility of chemicals through it. The occlusive covering also prevents evaporation of volatile vehicle components, compositionally stabilizing a spread film, maintaining its solvency for the drug. It is estimated that occlusive hydration increases percutaneous absorption about fivefold, an enlargement that is often clinically significant (69). The technique has been used with corticosteroids in refractory dermatoses such as psoriasis.

The following interesting phenomena associated with the occlusion of corticosteroids are enlightening. When applied under an occlusive dressing, corticosteroids induce vasoconstriction at lower concentrations than when applied in the open. When the dressing is removed, vasoconstriction subsides in a few hours. However, as many as several days later, blanching can sometimes be restored simply by rewrapping the area of application (70). This suggests that steroid molecules somehow bottled up in the stratum corneum are released when occlusion is reestablished. It appears that, as the stratum corneum dehydrates and returns to its normal state, substances as the corticosteroids that may be present are entrapped within one of its physical domains, freezing them in place until either the stratum corneum is sloughed or until occlusive hydration is reinstated. The phenomenon is referred to as the skin's *reservoir effect*. The application of drugs dissolved in volatile solvents such as acetone and ethanol also creates reservoirs in the stratum corneum for, as the solvents evaporate, the concentrating drug is driven into the skin's surface. Certain solvents also momentarily increase the solvency of the stratum corneum (71).

A few water-miscible organic solvents are taken up by the stratum corneum in amounts that soften its liquid crystalline, lipoidal domain (71), particularly when applied in concentrated form. If used very liberally (under laboratory conditions), these so-called skin penetration enhancers even elute interstitial lipids and denature keratin (72,73). Under admittedly artificial research conditions, the increases in percutaneous absorption resulting from their actions can be dramatic. Dimethyl sulfoxide (DMSO), dimethylacetamide (DMA), diethyltoluamide (DEET), oleic acid, and oleic alcohol are key examples. It has long been known that certain surfactants (e.g., sodium lauryl sulfate) are skin irritants even when in relatively diluted states, in part because they impair the barrier function of the stratum corneum, facilitating their own absorption. Concern over irritation precludes serious consideration of agents as this as enhancers. However, certain weaker amphiphilic substances (e.g., methyl oleate, glyceryl monolaurate, propylene glycol monolaurate), some of which have long been used as ingredients in cosmetics if not therapeutic systems, are showing that they have an unrealized potential as enhancers. Amphiphilic molecules penetrate into and blend with the stratum corneum's own lipids, which themselves are polar, amphiphilic substances. Thermoanalytical and spectroscopic evidence indicates that, in doing so, they relax the ordered structure of the stratum corneum's natural lipids, facilitating diffusion through existing channels and perhaps freeing up new channels (74–76). These emerging structural requirements of enhancement have launched a quest for new, even more powerful enhancers. Several potent amphiphilic compounds have surfaced from this pursuit that, at their worst, are only mildly tissue provocative, key examples being N-dodecylazacycloheptan-2-one (Azone[®]) and decyl methyl sulfoxide. Each of these example compounds contains a short alkyl chain (Azone = C_{12}; decyl methyl sulfoxide = C_{10}) attached to a highly water-interactive but nonionic head group. Neither compound is at all water soluble by itself, indicating that neither has the amphiphilic balance to form its own micelles. Of the two compounds, Azone has been the most scrutinized. It promotes the absorption of polar solutes at surprisingly low percentage concentrations. Its effects on animal skins have been especially profound; up to several hundred fold improvements in the in vitro permeation rates of highly polar cyclic nucleosides through hairless mouse skin have been reported (77), for example. Azone does not appear to be comparably effective on human skin, however, but those actions it has are effected at low concentration (78). As with any agent of the kind, its actions are dependent on the formulation and how this affects the thermodynamic activity of the enhancer in the delivery system. Concern over toxicity and the availability of alternative substances with established safety pedigrees have become impediments to the introduction enhancers having new, totally unfamiliar chemical structures.

The effects of skin penetration enhancers on the stratum corneum may or may not be lasting, depending on the degree of chemical alteration of the stratum corneum, which is experienced. Irreversibility is a perceived problem to the extent that the skin is left vulnerable to the absorption of other chemicals that come in contact with the conditioned area for as long at the area remains highly permeable. The fear is that such vulnerability will stay high until the greater part of the stratum corneum is renewed through mitosis, which minimally takes several whole days. Moreover, the enhancing solvents are themselves absorbed to some degree, another source toxicological concern. DMSO, for instance, is known to increase intraocular pressure. DMA has been associated with liver damage. Azone may irritate, but its real liability is that its chemical structure is totally novel and without toxicological precedent. While worry over toxicity may be out of proportion with actual degrees of exposure attending the ordinary circumstances of clinical use of dermatological products, concern is nevertheless warranted, given the occasional use of products over expansive areas. Consequently, compounds of proven safety, and their structural kind, have factored out as the enhancers of today's use.

Transdermal Delivery—Attributes of Transdermal delivery Systems

We are learning more and more that the conditions of use of topical delivery systems have profound influence on their performance. In this regard, transdermal systems, specifically the adhesive patches that are used to treat systemic disease and dermatological products are subject to very different operating environments and conditions (79). Transdermal delivery is aimed at achieving systemically active levels of a drug. A level of percutaneous absorption that leads to appreciable systemic drug accumulation is absolutely essential. Ideally one would like to avoid any buildup of a drug within the local tissues, but buildup is nevertheless unavoidable for the drug is driven through a relatively small diffusional area of the skin defined by the contact area (absorption *window*) of the application. Consequently, high accumulations of drug in the viable tissues underlying the patch are preordained by the nature of the delivery process. Irritation and sensitization can be associated with such high levels, and therefore careful testing is done to rule out these complications before a transdermal delivery system gets far along in development.

Table 7 outlines general expectations associated with transdermal delivery and compares with those associated with topical delivery. The water-impermeable backing materials of present and presumably most future transdermal systems make them occlusive. Impermeable polymer or foil backings also block the diffusive transport of body water to the atmosphere by way of the patch. Insensible perspiration at the site of the patch is thus held in check, but not without creating a substantially moist environment at the interface the patch has with the skin. Consequently, if given enough time, organisms already in the skin can colonize within this interface.

Table 7 General Norms of Operation of Transdermal Patches and Dermatological Formulations

Norms	Transdermal patches	Dermatological formulations
Occlusive application	Occluded	Open
Composition and phase changes in use	Relatively invariant	Experience profound composition shift and maybe phase changes
Application area	Predetermined	Variable
Application site	Specific site prescribed, healthy skin	In the disease's location, maybe damaged skin
Application technique	Highly reproducible	Highly individualized
Amount applied	Reproducible	Individualized
Delivery	Zero order, steady state, sustained	Nonstationary state kinetics, relative short action
Efficacy	Relevant to serum levels	Relevant to local tissue levels
Bioavailability and bioequivalent	Blood level as endpoint, based on pharmacokinetics	No easy endpoint
Safety	System toxicity based on blood levels, local irritation undesirable	Systemic exposure undesirable
Dose interruption	Removing patches	Washing residuals
Delivery efficiency	Relatively low, <60%	Low, <20%

Other than possibly for the insensible perspiration they absorb, transdermal patches tend to operate as thermodynamically static systems, meaning as compositionally fixed systems, from the moment they are applied until their removal. Compositional steadfastness is still the rule, however, and it is this feature that bestows the zero-order delivery attribute on the ordinary transdermal patch. Drug is present within the patches in reservoir amounts irrespective of whether or not the reservoir compartment is easily distinguished for there must be enough drug to sustain delivery over the full course of patch wear.

In some prototypes, for example, the nitroglycerine transdermal systems, huge excesses of drug are placed in the patch to assure that the drug's activity remains essentially level during the patch's wear. Only a small fraction of the drug, well under 50% of the patch's total content, is actually delivered during the prescribed time the patch is to be worn. Part of the inherent stability of the delivery environment of patches results because their main materials of construction are polymers, fabricating laminates and adhesives, all of which tend to be chemically robust. Solubilizing solvents (e.g., ethanol) and skin penetration enhancers (e.g., propylene glycol monolaurate) may also be present and their absorption into the skin may change compositions, but even here the processes are carefully orchestrated to gain a stable delivery environment over the long term.

A transdermal patch is a self-contained system that is applied as it is packaged, with its only manipulation being removal of the release liner to expose and ready its adhesive surface. The size of a patch, meaning its area of contact with the skin, is determined even before it is made. All of this area or only an inner portion of it may actually be involved in drug delivery, but, either way, the area is fixed. Since absorption is proportional to the area, to meet the differing drug requirements of individual patients, patches of different sizes are generally made available. The application site is also a constant of therapy in that a specific site or sites are recommended for use (not always for scientifically supportable reasons, e.g., nitroglycerine patches are worn over the heart!). Users tend to follow such dictates. Beyond this, the manner of application is also highly reproducible. Thus, there is as tight a control over absorption area and application site variables here as can be found in all of therapy. The only variability not customarily controlled for is that associated with the skin's permeability itself, but even here attempts have been made to make the systems operate with high delivery precision by incorporating rate-controlling membranes into them. However, with the possible exception of the antinauseant patch containing scopolamine, the rate-controlling membranes do not actually control the rate of delivery, the stratum corneum does. Regardless, the manner of function of the systems is highly reproduced from one application to the next.

Measures of function of transdermal systems distinguish them among the systems we use topically. Since systemic actions are sought, blood levels of the drug in question must reach and remain within therapeutic bounds. More often than not the requisite blood level is known from a drug's use by other routes of administration. Thus, a clear systemic target level usually exists, and an absolute rate of delivery commensurate with reaching this is a built-in feature of the patch. Bioequivalency of different systems built around a specific drug is easily measured in terms of the blood levels they produce. And if therapy is not going well, one can bring delivery to a reasonably abrupt halt by simply removing a patch.

Topical Delivery—Attributes of Topical Delivery Systems

Despite the fact that often less than 1% and almost never more than 15% of the drug in a dermatological application is systemically absorbed (systemically recoverable), topical delivery nevertheless allows one to achieve drug levels in local tissues far in excess of those that can be achieved by other means of administration. At the same time, systemic toxicities of the drug are rarely encountered with topical administration, with the exceptions occurring when dermatological formulations are used liberally over extensive areas. Because of only small amounts of a drug being ordinarily applied topically, in most instances the amounts absorbed are so limited that one has trouble even measuring them.

As shown in Table 7, we tend to think of topical dosage forms being much the same as transdermal delivery systems, but the functioning of semisolid dermatological products stands in stark contrast with that of transdermal delivery systems. To begin with, most topical applications are left open to the atmosphere. Amounts applied per unit area depend on the individual making the application. Of singular importance with respect to system function, extraordinary physicochemical changes accompany the evaporative concentration of these formulations, possibly including the precipitation of the drug or other substances that were comfortably in solution at the moment of their application. Evaporative concentration can also upset the oil-to-water balance of emulsions, destabilizing them, at times causing them to break or invert. In a matter of hours, if not just minutes, a surface film or dry residue having a totally different delivery faculty than the bulk formulation may be all that is left of the application. Such precipitous changes, if out of control, can bring drug delivery to an abrupt halt.

The amounts of semisolids people apply are highly individualized, and so are the techniques of application. Some patients vigorously rub semisolid formulations into the skin, while others just spread films until they are more or less uniform over the desired area. For many diseases, disease manifestation can be anywhere on the body. Moreover, from individual to individual, it varies in intensity and vastness. Thus, more area may be involved in one case than in another, and the barrier function of the skin may be more or less intact in any instance. The net of this creates a set of imponderables with respect to delivery, efficacy, and safety.

The removal of the dermatological applications is rarely deliberate. Rather, some substance is usually transferred to clothing, etc., some is absorbed, some is evaporated, and some is inadvertently removed by activities such as bathing. Of course, applications can be deliberately washed from the skin if one wishes to terminate the therapy. Partly because of their temporal inhabitancy, local applications tend to be short acting relative to transdermal delivery systems. Other factors here are the finite doses that are actually administered and the oftentimes rapid evaporative concentration of such films to compositions that cease supporting dissolution of the drug and its diffusion to the skin's surface. Such finite doses do not sustain delivery, and thus delivery wanes after several hours irrespective of the wearability of the application and of processes attending its evaporative shrinkage. Since all these attending processes defy quantification, there is precious little existing information to guide one concerning a fitting regimen of application for most topical dosage forms. Rather, dosing regimens evolve historically from collective clinical experience. All in all, topical therapy is an extraordinarily complex operation.

Compositional changes following the application of certain topical systems are unavoidable. Many o/w creams contain as much as 80% to 85% external phase, usually primarily water. Lotions and gels also contain volatile constituents in large proportion. All rapidly evaporate down after their application and, consequently, the drug delivery system is the formed, concentrated film that develops on the skin and not the medium as packaged in the tube, jar, or bottle. Ingredients should be chosen to assure that compositional changes as invariably occur interfere as little as possible with delivery and therapy. In this regard, the rate at which the volatile components evaporate to form the equilibrium film can itself be a factor in bioavailability (80). It has been reported, for instance, that a thinly applied corticosteroid preparation produced greater vasoconstriction than did thicker applications of the same material (81). Though the total amount of drug per unit area was greater with the thick films, responses were less in their case because evaporative concentration of the steroid in the applied medium proceeded more slowly. Even without knowing the mechanistic details, we can conclude from this that less steroid was driven into the skin from the thick applications in the course of the test. It has also been demonstrated that vasoconstriction is more pronounced at low concentrations when steroid is applied in volatile ethanol than when applied in propylene glycol (60). While differences in solvency play their role here, it is also clear that the rapid evaporation of solvents as ethanol drives drug into the skin. Such observations emphasize the importance of distinguishing between the system as packaged and the transitional system following application. Unfortunately, this distinction is not always made, and much topical delivery research aimed at assessing the relative abilities formulations have to deliver drug has been performed by placing extraordinarily thick layers of formulation over the skin. Such thick applications do not even remotely simulate the clinical release situation, especially when it comes to creams and gels. This area of drug delivery is in need of much research.

In summary, the way a topical drug is formulated has a great deal to do with its clinical effectiveness, a nonsurprising conclusion, given what is known about the relationships between bioavailability and formulation for other modes of administration. Yet in the area of topical drug performance, antiquated concepts and approaches to system design linger on. In days when topical bioavailability was little understood and therefore ignored, formulators concentrated on vehicle elegance and stability. Attempts were made to design vehicles compatible with all types of drugs, so-called universal vehicles. Universal vehicles are still discussed in many standard texts. Today's technology and science clearly indicate that the universal vehicle is akin to a unicorn, beautiful but totally mythical. In the real world, each system must be designed around the drug it contains to optimize the clinical potential of the active ingredient. The duration of action will depend on how long the drug remains appreciably in solution within its spread film. These matters

Table 8 Factors for Evaluation of Semisolids

Stability of the active ingredient(s)
Stability of the adjuvants
Visual appearance
Color
Odor (development of pungent odor or loss of fragrance)
Viscosity, extrudability
Loss of water and other volatile vehicle components
Phase distribution (homogeneity or phase separation, bleeding)
Particle size distribution of dispersed phases
pH
Texture, feel upon application (stiffness, grittiness, greasiness, tackiness)
Particulate contamination
Microbial contamination and sterility (in the unopened container and under conditions of use)
Release and bioavailability

are carefully examined when a drug delivery system, topical or otherwise, reaches the FDA as an Investigational New Drug Application (IND), New Drug Application (NDA), or Abbreviated New Drug Application (ANDA) (82).

Aspects of Physical and Chemical Stability

Concern for the physical and chemical integrity of topical systems is no different from that for other dosage forms. However, there are some unique and germane dimensions to stability associated with semisolid systems. A short list of some of the factors to be evaluated for semisolids is given in Table 8. All factors must be acceptable initially (within prescribed specifications) and all must remain so over the stated lifetime for the product (the product's *shelf life*).

The chemical integrities of drug, preservatives, and other key adjuvants must be assessed as a function of time to establish a product's useful shelf life from the chemical standpoint. Semisolid systems provide us two special problems in this regard. First, semisolids are chemically complex to the point that just separating drug and adjuvants from all other components is an analyst's nightmare. Many components interfere with standard assays, and therefore difficult separations are the rule before anything can be analyzed. Also, since semisolids undergo phase changes upon heating, one cannot use high-temperature kinetics for stability prediction. Thus, first estimates of stability have to be evaluated at the storage temperature of the formulation, and this of course takes a long time. Under these circumstances, problematic stability may not be evident until studies have been in progress for a year or more. Be this as it may, stability details are worked out in the laboratories of industry, the pharmacist ordinarily accepting projected shelf lives as fact. Some qualitative indicators of chemical instability that the pharmacist might look for are the development of color (or a change in color and/or its intensity) and the development of an off odor. Often products yellow or brown with age as a result of the oxidative reactions occurring in the base. Discolorations of the kind are commonly seen when natural fats and oils, for example, lanolins, are used to build the vehicle. Extensive oxidation of natural fatty materials (rancidification) is accompanied by development of a disagreeable odor. One may also notice phase and texture changes in a suspect product. Pharmacists should take note of the appearances of the topical products they dispense, removing all those from circulation that exhibit color changes or become fetid. Changes in product pH also indicate chemical decompositions, most probably of a hydrolytic nature, and if somehow detected are reason to return a product.

Time-variable rheological behavior of a semisolid may also signal physical and/or chemical change. However, measures such as spreadability and feel upon application are probably unreliable indicators of a changing rheology, and more exacting measurements are necessary. A pharmacist does not ordinarily have the tools at hand to make accurate rheological assessments, but the equipment to do so is generally available and used within the development laboratories of the industry. Here, one may find exquisitely sensitive plate and cone research viscometers that in principle precisely quantify viscosity and also utilitarian rheometers that put viscosities on a relative scale. The latter include extrusion rheometers, which measure the force it takes to extrude a semisolid through a narrow orifice; penetrometers, which characterize viscosity in terms of the penetration of a weighted cone into a semisolid; and Brookfield viscometers with spindle and helipath attachments. The latter measure the force it takes to drive a spindle helically through a semisolid. As used with semisolids, the utilitarian rheometers only provide relative, although quite useful, measures of viscosity. Increases (or decreases) in viscosity by any of these measuring tools indicate changes in the structural elements of the formulation. The gradual transformations that take place in semisolid structure are more often than not impermanent, in which case the systems are restored to their initial condition simply by mixing them. Substantial irreversible rheological changes are a sign of poor physical stability.

Changes in the natures of individual phases of or phase separation within a formulation are reasons to discontinue use of a product. Phase separation may result from emulsion breakage, clearly an acute instability. More often it appears more subtly as *bleeding*, the formation of visible droplets of an emulsion's internal phase in the continuum of the semisolid. This problem is the result of slow rearrangement and contraction of internal structure. Eventually, here and there, globules of what is often clear liquid internal phase are squeezed out of the matrix. Warm storage temperatures can induce or accelerate structural crenulation as this; thus, storage of dermatological products in a cool place is prudent. The main concern with a system that has undergone such separation is that a patient will not be applying a medium of uniform composition application after application. Because of unequal distribution between phases (internal partitioning), one phase will invariably have a higher concentration of the drug than the other. Therefore, since semisolid emulsions, unlike liquid emulsions, cannot be returned to an even distribution by shaking, formulations exhibiting separation are functionally suspect and should be removed from circulation.

Pharmacists should also take a dim view of changes in the particle size, size distribution, or particulate nature of semisolid suspensions. They are the consequence of crystal growth, changes in crystalline habit, or the reversion of the crystalline materials to a more stable polymorphic form. Any crystalline alteration can lead to a pronounced reduction in the drug delivery capabilities and therapeutic utility of a formulation. Thus, products exhibiting such changes are seriously physically unstable and unusable.

A more commonly encountered change in formulations is the evaporative loss of water or other volatile phases from a preparation while it is in storage. This can occur as a result of inappropriate packaging or a flaw made in packaging. Some plastic collapsible tubes allow diffusive loss of volatile substances through the container walls. One will find this phenomenon occasionally in cosmetics, which are hurried to the marketplace without adequate stability assessment, but rarely in ethical pharmaceuticals, which are time tested. However, a bad seal may occur in any tube or jar irrespective of its contents, with eventual loss of volatile ingredients around the cap or through the crimp. Such evaporative losses cause a formulation to stiffen and become puffy and its application characteristics change noticeably. There is corresponding weight loss. Under this influence, the contents of a formulation may shrink and pull away from the container wall. These phenomena are most likely to be seen in creams and gels because of the high fractions of volatile components that characterize them. Problems here are exacerbated when products are stored in warm locations.

Gross phase changes are detectable by eye upon close inspection of products. The package of course gets in the way of such analysis, but if a product is truly suspect, it should be closely examined by opening and inspecting the full contents of the container. A jar can be opened and its contents probed with a spatula without wrecking the container. Close inspection of the contents of a tube requires destruction of the package, however. The easy way to do this is to cut off the seal along the bottom of the tube with scissors and then make a perpendicular cut up the length of the tube to the edge of the platform to which the cap is anchored. Careful further trimming a quarter of the way around the platform in each direction creates left and right panels that can be pealed back with tweezers to expose the tube's contents. Textural changes such as graininess, bleeding, and other phase irregularities are easily seen on the unfolded, flat surface. Normally it takes a microscope to reveal changes in crystalline size, shape, and/or distribution, but palpable grit is a sure sign a problem of the kind exists. Weight loss of a product, which is easily checked at the prescription counter, clearly indicates the loss of volatile ingredients (the weight of a suspect tube can be directly compared to the weight of a fresh tube, etc.). On the rare occasions when a deterioration as this is noted by a pharmacist in the course of handling products or is reported to the pharmacist by a knowledgeable patient, the suspect package should be removed from circulation and the manufacturer informed of the action. If a problem seems general rather than isolated, that is, to a single bad package, FDA should be notified as well to best safeguard the public. This agency will determine if a product has gone bad and general recall is warranted.

Freedom from Contamination

Particulates

Numerous topical preparations contain finely dispersed solids. Pastes, for example, contain as much or more than 50% solids dispersed in an ointment medium. Powders themselves are used topically. Many dermatological liquids and semisolids contain suspended matter. However present, the particles should be impalpable, that is, incapable of being individually perceived by touch, so that the formulations do not feel gritty. The palpability of a particle is a function of its hardness, shape, and size. The pharmacist can only manipulate the latter, and thus it is important to prepare or use finely subdivided solids when making topical dosage forms. Individual particles greater than 50 μm in their longest dimension can be individually perceived by touch. The surface of the eye is substantially more sensitive and a 10 μm particle can be distinguished here. Clearly, the presence of hard, palpable particulates in semisolids makes them abrasive, particularly when applied to disease or damage-sensitized skin. Severe eye irritation is possible if ophthalmic ointments contain them. One particularly troublesome source of particulate contamination is flashings (tiny metal slivers and shavings) left over from the production of tin and aluminum-collapsible tubes. These often adhere electrostatically and tenaciously to tubing walls following cutting of the containers down to a particular size. Some escape removal in washing and rinsing done to cleanse the empty containers. Consequently, a jet of exceedingly high velocity air is blown into the open end of tubes just prior to their filling to remove all particulates. If this precaution is not taken, tiny metal slivers may be packaged with the product, posing the threat that they will become dislodged and instilled into the eye while the product is in use. For reasons as this, the

United States Pharmacopoeia/National Formulary (USP/NF) has a particulate test for ophthalmic ointments. In this test, the ointments are liquefied in a petri dish at high temperature, 85°C, for two hours, and then solidified by cooling. Particles that have settled to the bottom of the shallow glass container are counted by microscopic scanning at 30 times magnification. The requirements are met if the total number of particles 50 μm or larger in any dimension does not exceed 50 in the 10 tubes tested and if not more than eight particles are found in a single tube. Products that are put into the distribution channels have to meet this test. Nevertheless, the pharmacist should be on the lookout for particulate problems associated with commercial products. The pharmacist must also take measures to ensure that extemporaneously compounded formulations are free of particulates. Particular attention must be paid to the cleaning of collapsible tubes and other package parts prior to their use.

Microbial Specifications and Sterility

As of the USP XIX, ophthalmic ointments have to be prepared and dispensed as sterile products (until opened for use). Presently in the United States, nonophthalmic topical preparations do not need to be sterile, although they cannot contain pathogens and must have low microbe counts. The reasons ophthalmic sterility requirements were broadened to cover ointments are enlightening. In the mid-1960s, there was an outbreak of extremely serious *Pseudomonas* eye infections in the Scandinavian block of countries, in some instances with loss of sight. The source of the contamination was traced to antibiotic-containing ophthalmic ointments made by a regional manufacturer known for its high standards of manufacturing and quality control (83). Pathogenic *Pseudomonas* organisms were found in both the products and in the manufacturing facilities where the ointments were prepared. It was widely believed up until this time that pathogens could not and would not survive and grow in ointments and similar media. The presence of antibiotics in the preparations could only have added to the false sense of security this company had. This incident sent shock waves throughout the pharmaceutical world and spawned revisions in all world compendia. In the United States, ophthalmic ointments have to be sterile when dispensed. In Europe, dermatological products that are to be used over broken skin also have to be sterile.

The foregoing incident has special meaning to the dispensing pharmacist. Unopened ophthalmic ointments should be dispensed for each condition and should be given very short shelf life datings. Patients should be advised to discard unused quantities of old preparations and to return for fresh supplies if and when chronic symptoms reappear. Similar advice and precautions are good practice with dermatological products like ointments that do not ordinarily contain microbial preservatives. Lotions, creams, and topical solutions that contain preservatives tend to remain pathogen free after their packages have been opened, providing an extra measure of safety.

Preservatives have an important purpose in topical medications. Systems containing them tend to remain aseptic. Even if a few organisms subsist in the presence of the preservatives, these tend to be nonvegetative. Importantly, no pathogenic forms survive to cause problems. Preservatives are necessary for systems that have an aqueous phase, for water offers an environment that is particularly conducive for microbial growth. Therefore, all emulsions and aqueous solutions and suspensions should be preserved. However, choosing a preservative is no easy task, for the physical systems tend to be compositionally complex and polyphasic, affording many possible means for specific preservatives to be inactivated. In mass-produced products, the effectiveness of the preservation system of formulations is checked by the USP preservative challenge tests.

Pharmaceutical Elegance

There are a number of attributes of topical drug systems that may be classified as cosmetic that make patients more or less willing to use their medications (compliant). These include the ease of application, the feel of the preparation once it is on the skin, and the appearance of the applied film. Ideally, the application should be undetectable to the eye and neither tacky nor greasy. Certain items, such as ointments and pastes, are of course intrinsically greasy, and suspensions of all types tend to leave an opaque, easily detectable film. Thus, the extent to which the cosmetic features can be idealized is dependent on the nature and purpose of the dosage form.

The ease of application and method of application of a formulation depend on the physicochemical attributes of the system involved. Solutions and other highly fluid systems may be swabbed on, sprayed on, or rolled on. A cotton pledget or other applicator is often necessary to obtain an even application. Soft semisolid systems, on the other hand, may be spread evenly and massaged into the skin with the fingers, a procedure technically referred to as inunction. The spreadability is a rheological quality related to the nature and degree of internal structure of the formulation. Formulations such as pastes that are very stiff tend to be hard to apply; their application over broken or irritated skin can be disagreeable. The stiffness of a preparation can be upregulated or downregulated by manipulating the amounts of structure-building components of a vehicle and in some instances by adjusting the phase/volume ratio of semisolid emulsions. Thus, for ointments, increased spreadability can be obtained by decreasing the ratio of the waxy components (waxes and petrolatum) to fluid vehicle components (mineral oil, fixed oils). Greasiness of such preparations goes in the opposite direction. For o/w creams, decreasing the ratio of the internal phase to the external phase tends to make the systems more fluid. Substitution of more liquid oils for some of the high-melting waxy components of creams achieves the same end.

Tackiness and greasiness are determined by physicochemical properties of the vehicle constituents that comprise the formed film on the skin. A sticky film is extremely uncomfortable and, generally, considerable effort is directed to minimizing this inelegant feature. Where creams are concerned, waxy ingredients such as stearic acid and cetyl alcohol produce noticeably nontacky films. Stearic acid is the principal internal phase component of vanishing creams, systems that are virtually undetectable visually or by touch after inunction. On the other hand, propylene glycol, which may be added to creams and gels to solubilize a drug, tends to make systems as these tacky. The synthetic and natural gums used as thickening and suspending agents in gels and lotions tend to increase their tackiness and, therefore, these materials are used as sparingly as function allows.

Creams tend to be invisible on the skin. The same is true for ointments, although the oiliness of ointments causes them to glisten to an extent. Whatever opacity creams and ointments have is due primarily to the presence of insoluble solids. These often imbue applications with a powdery or even crusty appearance. Dispersed solids are usually functional, as in calamine lotion, zinc sulfide lotion, zinc oxide paste, and so on, and are an implacable feature of these preparations. However, at times insoluble solids are added as tints to match the color of the skin and to impart opacity. Since individual skins vary widely in hue (pigmentation) and texture, tinting to a single color and texture is generally unsuccessful.

Evaluation of the cosmetic elegance of topical preparations can be accomplished scientifically, but it is questionable whether physical experiments on system rheology and the like offer appreciable advantage over the subjective evaluations of the pharmacist, the formulator, or other experienced people. Persons who use cosmetics are particularly adept and helpful as evaluators.

Skin Sensitivity—A Specific Toxicological Concern

One further problem of topical formulations associated with many ingredients and of special concern with preservatives is the development of skin sensitivity (84). The skins of some individuals are particularly susceptible to an allergic conditioning to chemicals known as type IV contact hypersensitivity. Haptens (chemicals like urushiol found in poison ivy) are absorbed through the skin and, while in the local tissues, chemically react with local proteins. Langerhans cells, the local cells involved in immunological surveillance, identify these now denatured proteins as foreign (nonhost). The Langerhans cells then leave the dermis by way of the lymphatics and enter the draining lymph node, where they complete the sensitization process by passing the allergen message on to resident lymphocytes (antigen presentation). Once sensitized, subsequent contact with the offending chemical (hapten) leads to inflammation and skin eruption. Many of the preservatives used in pharmacy are phenols and comparably reactive substances, compounds that have a high propensity to sensitize susceptible individuals. The pharmacist should be alert to this possibility and prepared to recommend discontinuance of therapy and physician referral when allergic outbreak is evident or suspected. Moreover, the pharmacist should be ready to recommend alternative products that do not contain an allergically offending substance once it has been identified, assuming of course that therapeutically suitable alternatives exist.

Allergic incidents are widespread and, from an allergy standpoint, it is useful that the ingredients of dermatological medications are listed on the package or in the package insert. This allows the pharmacist to screen products for their suitability for individuals with known sensitivities. OTC medications and cosmetics also contain a qualitative listing of their ingredients. The pharmacist thus has access to critical information he or she needs to safeguard patients relative to their known hypersensitivity.

Interpersonal Transfer of Topical-Applied Medicines

The number of topically applied therapeutic agents, either for local treatment or systemic delivery, has substantially increased over last decades. Millions of baby boomers use transdermal estradiol or testosterone for hormone replacement. However, the safety of these therapies over full lifetimes needs to be evaluated and addressed from a public health perspective. In general, only 1% to 20% of medicines topically applied to the skin surface are absorbed into living cutaneous tissue or the systemic circulation during a 24-hour period. The efficiency of transdermal delivery on balance is better, but still more drug is usually left in patches than is actually therapeutically used. The rest of the medicine stays on the skin surface, within the superficial layers of skin, in the applied patches, or is transferred to clothing, etc., when semisolids and patches are applied. Therefore, the fate and safety of nonabsorbed medicine on the skin surface has to be evaluated not only for patients but also for the others who might have close or direct skin contact with them. Several studies have showed the measurable transfer of topically applied testosterone and estradiol gels (85,86). As a consequence of the public safety concern, the potential for testosterone transfer has been included in the new labeling of products that contain this ingredient. It is important for physicians, nurses, pharmacists, and patients to understand that pharmacological significant or clinically undesirable transfer of topically applied therapeutic agents can occur and should be avoided. The same is true for patches as these have been transferred from patient to a loved one following intimate contact, with very serious ill effects. The used patches should be collected and kept away from children. The application sites of patches, gels, creams, or ointments should be thoroughly washed before having contact with partners, children, and others. Furthermore, the environmental impact of nonabsorptable medicines and hormones following the massive and long-term use of topical products has not been fully investigated and understood.

ACKNOWLEDGMENT

We acknowledge the assistance provided by K. Carlson and B. Selvamani for figures.

REFERENCES

1. Lemberger AP. Eczema and psoriasis remedies. In: Griffernhagen GB, Hawking LL, eds. Handbook of Non-Prescription Drugs. Washington, DC: American Pharmaceutical Association, 1973:161–166.
2. Wilkes GL, Brown IA, Wildnauer RH. The biomechanical properties of skin. CRC Crit Rev Bioeng 1973; 1(4):453–495.
3. Scheuplein RJ, Blank IH. Permeability of the skin. Physiol Rev 1971; 51(4):702–747.
4. Montagna W. Parakkal PF. The Structure and Function of Skin. 3rd ed. New York: Academic Press, 1974.
5. Elias PM, Grayson S, Lampe MA, et al. The intercorneocyte space. In: Marks R, Plewig G, eds. Stratum Corneum. New York: Springer-Verlag, 1983:53–67.
6. Tingstad JE, Wurster DE, Higuchi T. Investigation of human skin lipids II. J Am Pharm Assoc 1958; 47(3 pt 1):192–193.
7. Scheuplein RJ. Mechanism of percutaneous adsorption. I. Routes of penetration and the influence of solubility. J Invest Dermatol 1965; 45(5):334–346.
8. Baker H, Kligman AM. Measurement of transepidermal water loss by electrical hygrometry. Instrumentation and responses to physical and chemical insults. Arch Dermatol 1967; 96(4): 441–452.
9. Scheuplein RJ. Mechanism of percutaneous absorption. II. Transient diffusion and the relative importance of various routes of skin penetration. J Invest Dermatol 1967; 48(1):79–88.
10. Woodburne RT. Essentials of Human Anatomy. New York: Oxford University Press, 1967:6.
11. Rothman S. Percutaneous absorption. In: Rothman S, ed. Physiology and Biochemistry of the Skin. Chicago: University of Chicago Press, 1954:26–59.
12. McKenzie AW. Percutaneous absorption of steroids. Arch Dermatol 1963; 86:611–614.
13. Stoughton RB. Percutaneous absorption. South Med J 1962; 55:1134–1138.
14. Szabo G. The number of eccrine sweat glands in human skin. Adv Biol Skin 1962; 3:1–5.
15. Katz M, Poulsen BJ. Absorption of drugs through the skin. In: Brodie BB, Gillette J, eds. Handbook of Experimental Pharmacology, New Series. Vol 28. New York: Springer-Verlag, 1972:103.
16. Peck SM, Russ WR. Propionate-caprylate mixtures in the treatment of dermatomycoses. Arch Dermatol Syph 1947; 56:601–608.
17. Liggins MR. Help for your sunburn prone patientsPatient Care 1974:56.
18. Rushmer RF, Buettner KJ, Short JM, et al. The skin. Science 1966; 154(747):343–348.
19. Idson B. Water and the skin. J Soc Cosmet Chem 1973; 24(3):197–212.
20. Laden K. Natural moisturizing factors in skin. Am Perfum Cosmet 1967; 82(10):77–79.
21. Robinson JR. O-T-C deodorants and antiperspirants. J Am Pharm Assoc 1967; 7(2):75–77, 93.
22. Stoughton RB. Status of topical therapy. Clin Pharmacol Ther 1974; 16(5 pt 2):869–872.
23. Voorhees JJ, Duell EA, Stawiski M, et al. Molecular and clinical pharmacology of psoriasis. Clin Pharmacol Ther 1974; 16(5 pt 2):919–921.
24. Good WR. Transdermal drug-delivery systems. Med Device Diagn Ind 1986:34–42.
25. Cleary GW. Transdermal controlled release systems. In: Langer RS, Wise DL, eds. Medical Applications of Controlled Release. Vol 1. Boca Raton, FL: CRC Press, 1983:203–251.
26. Chien YW. Transdermal drug delivery and delivery systems. In: Chien YW, ed. Novel Drug Delivery Systems. New York: Marcel Dekker, 1982:149–217.

27. Marty JP, Guy RH, Maibach HI. Percutaneous penetration as a method of delivery to muscle and other tissues. In: Bronaugh RL, Maibach HI, eds. Percutaneous Absorption. 2nd ed. New York: Marcel Dekker, 1989:511–529.

28. Behl CR, Bellantone NH, Flynn GL. Influence of age on percutaneous absorption of drug substances. In: Bronaugh RL, Maibach HI, eds. Percutaneous Absorption. New York: Marcel Dekker, 1985:183–212.

29. Fisher LB. In vitro studies on the permeability of human skin. In: Bronaugh RL, Maibach HI, eds. Percutaneous Absorption. New York: Marcel Dekker, 1985:213–222.

30. Weingand DA, Haygood C, Gaylor JR, et al. Racial variations in the cutaneous barrier. In: Drill VA, Lazar P, eds. Current Concepts in Cutaneous Toxicity. New York: Academic Press, 1980:221–235.

31. Weigand DA, Haygood C, Gaylor JR. Cell layers and density of Negro and Caucasian stratum corneum. J Invest Dermatol 1974; 62(6):563–568.

32. Durrheim H, Flynn GL, Higuchi WI, et al. Permeation of hairless mouse skin I: experimental methods and comparison with human epidermal permeation by alkanols. J Pharm Sci 1980; 69:781–786.

33. Flynn GL, Linn EE, Kurihara-Bergstrom T, et al. Parameters of skin condition and function. In: Kydonieus AF, Berner B, eds. Transdermal Delivery of Drugs. Vol 2. Boca Raton, FL: CRC Press, 1987:3–17.

34. Mathias CGT. Clinical and experimental aspects of cutaneous irritation. In: Marzulli FN, Maibach HI, eds. Dermatotoxicology. 3rd ed. New York: Hemisphere Publishing, 1987:173–189.

35. Roberts MS, Anderson RA, Swarbrick J, et al. The percutaneous absorption of phenolic compounds: the mechanism of diffusion across the stratum corneum. J Pharm Pharmacol 1978; 30(8):486–490.

36. Baden HP, Goldsmith LA, Bonar L. Conformational changes in the fibrous protein of epidermis. J Invest Dermatol 1973; 60(4):215–218.

37. Keipert JA. The absorption of topical corticosteroids, with particular reference to percutaneous absorption in infancy and childhood. Med J Aust 1971; 1(19):1021–1025.

38. Flynn GL. Mechanisms of percutaneous absorption from physicochemical evidence. In: Bronaugh RL, Maibach HI, eds. Percutaneous Absorption: Mechanisms–Methodology–Drug Delivery. 2nd ed. New York: Marcel Dekker, 1989:27–51.

39. Flynn GL, Yalkowsky SH, Roseman TJ. Mass transport phenomena and models: theoretical concepts. J Pharm Sci 1974; 63(4):479–510.

40. Scheuplein RJ, Bronaugh RL. Percutaneous absorption. In: Goldsmilh LA, ed. Biochemistry and Physiology of the Skin. Vol 2. New York: Oxford University Press, 1983:1255–1295.

41. Toll R, Jacobi U, Richter H, et al. Penetration profile of microspheres in follicular targeting of terminal follicles. J Invest Dermatol 2004; 123(1):168–176.

42. Valiveti S, Lu GW. Diffusion properties of model compounds in artificial sebum. Int J Pharm 2007; 345(1/2):88–94.

43. Valiveti S, Wesley J, Lu GW. Investigation of drug partition property in artificial sebum. Int J Pharm 2008; 346(1/2):10–16.

44. Higuchi T, Davis SS. Thermodynamic analysis of structure–activity relationships of drugs. Prediction of optimal structure. J Pharm Sci 1970; 59(10):1376–1383.

45. Davis SS, Higuchi T, Rytting JH. Determination of thermodynamics of functional groups in solutions of drug molecules. Adv Pharm Sci 1974; 4:73–261.

46. Pozzo DA, Pastori N. Percutaneous absorption of parabens from cosmetic formulations. Int J Cosmet Sci 1996; 18:57–66.

47. Scheuplein RJ, Blank IH, Brauner GJ, et al. Percutaneous absorption of steroids. J Invest Dermatol 1969; 52(1):63–70.

48. Flynn GL. Physicochemical determinants of skin absorption. In: Gerrity TR, Henry CJ, eds. Principles of Route-to-Route Extrapolation for Risk Assessment. New York: Elsevier, 1990:93–128.

49. Potts RO, Guy RH. Predicting skin permeability. Pharm Res 1992; 9(5):663–669.

50. Erdi NZ, Cruz MM, Battista OA. Rheological characteristics of polymeric microcrystal-gels. J Colloid Interface Sci 1968; 28(1):36–47.

51. Thau P, Fox C. A new procedure for the preparation of polyethylene–mineral oil gels. J Soc Cosmet Chem 1965; 16(6):359–363.

52. Foster S, Wurster DE, Higuchi T, et al. A pharmaceutical study of Jelene ointment base. J Am Pharm Assoc 1951; 40(3):123–125.

53. Barry BW. Control of oil-in-water emulsion consistency using mixed emulsifiers. J Pharm Pharmacol 1969; 21(8):533–540.

54. Arnott S, Fulmer A, Scott WE, et al. Agarose double helix and its function in agarose gel structure. J Mol Biol 1974; 90(2):269–284.

55. Physician's Desk Reference. 28th ed. Oradell, NJ: Medical Economics, 1974:1460.

56. Flynn GL, Roseman TJ. Membrane diffusion. II. Influence of physical adsorption on molecular flux through heterogeneous dimethylpolysiloxane barriers. J Pharm Sci 1971; 60(12):1788–1796.

57. Flynn GL. Structural approach to partitioning: estimation of steroid partition coefficients based upon molecular constitution. J Pharm Sci 1971; 60(3):345–353.

58. Hagen TA. Physicochemical Study of Hydrocortisone and Hydrocortisone n-Alkyl-21 Esters (thesis). University of Michigan, 1979.

59. Smith WM. An Inquiry into the Mechanism of Percutaneous Absorption of Hydrocortisone and Its n-Alkyl Esters (thesis). University of Michigan, 1982.

60. Schlagel CA. Penetration and action of glucocorticoids. Adv Biol Skin 1972; 12:339–356.

61. Mckenzie AW, Atkinson RM. Topical activities of betamethasone esters in man. Arch Dermatol 1964; 89:741–746.

62. Saracen G, Elena Spaccamela M. Influence of the C-atom chain on the solubility of a homologous series in water. Ann Chim (Rome, Italy) 1958; 48:1357–1370.

63. Yalkowsky SH, Flynn GL, Slunick TG. Importance of chain length on physicochemical and crystalline properties of organic homologs. J Pharm Sci 1972; 61(6):852–857.

64. Flynn GL, Yalkowsky SH. Correlation and prediction of mass transport across membranes. I. Influence of alkyl chain length on flux-determining properties of barrier and diffusant. J Pharm Sci 1972; 61(6):838–852.

65. Wurster DE. Some factors related to the formulation of preparations for percutaneous absorption. Am Perfum Cosmet 1965; 80(1):21–29.

66. Higuchi T. Physical chemical analysis of percutaneous absorption process from creams and ointments. J Soc Cosmet Chem 1960; 11:85–97.

67. Burdick KH, Poulsen B, Place VA. Extemporaneous formulation of corticosteroids for topical usage. JAMA 1970; 211(3):462–466.

68. Schaefer H, Redelmeier TE. Skin Barrier—Principles of Percutaneous Absorption. Basel, Switzerland: Karger, 1996:213–223.

69. McKenzie AW, Stoughton RB. Method for comparing percutaneous absorption of steroids. Arch Dermatol 1962; 86:608–610.

70. Vickers CFH. Stratum corneum reservoir for drugs. Adv Biol Skin 1972; 12:177–189.

71. Stoughton RB. Dimethylsulfoxide (DMSO) induction of a steroid reservoir in human skin. Arch Dermatol 1965; 91(6):657–660.

72. Scheuplein RJ, Ross L. Effects of surfactants and solvents on the permeability of epidermis. J Soc Cosmet Chem 1970; 21(13):853–873.

73. Elfbaum SG, Laden K. Effect of dimethyl sulfoxide on percutaneous absorption. Mechanistic study. II. J Soc Cosmet Chem 1968; 9(3):163–172.

74. Goodman M, Barry BW. Action of penetration enhancers as assessed by differential scanning calorimetry. In: Bronaugh RL, Maibach HI, eds. Percutaneous Absorption. 2nd ed. New York: Marcel Dekker, 1989:567–593.

75. Abraham W, Downing DT. Factors affecting the formation, morphology and permeability of stratum corneum lipid bilayers in vitro. In: Scott RC, Guy RH, Hadgraft J, eds. Prediction of Percutaneous Penetration. London: IBC Technical Services, 1990:110–122.

76. Anderson BD, Higuchi WI, Raykar PV. Heterogeneity effects on permeability–partition coefficient relationships in human stratum corneum. Pharm Res 1988; 5(9):566–573.

77. Higuchi WI, Shannon WM, Fox JL, et al. Topical delivery of antiviral agents: in vivo/in vitro correlations. In: Anderson JM, Kim SW, eds. Recent Advances in Drug Delivery Systems. New York: Plenum Press, 1984:1–7.
78. Hou SYE, Flynn GL. Azone enhanced permeation of skin. Mediation of penetration of benzoic acid as a function of pH. Pharm Res 1986; 3(suppl):52S.
79. Flynn GL, Weiner ND. Topical and transdermal delivery—provinces of realism. In: Gurny R, ed. Dermal and Transdermal Drug Delivery. Stuttgart: APV, 1993:33–65.
80. Coldman MF, Poulsen BJ, Higuchi T. Enhancement of precutaneous absorption by the use of volatile–nonvolatile systems as vehicles. J Pharm Sci 1969; 58(9):1098–1102.
81. Poulsen BJ, Young E, Coquilla V, et al. Effect of topical vehicle composition on the in vitro release of fluocinolone acetonide and its acetate ester. J Pharm Sci 1968; 57(6):928–933.
82. Shah VP, Ludden TM, Dighe SV, et al. Bioavailability and bioequivalence of transdermal drug delivery systems. Regulatory considerations. In: Shah VP, Maibach HI, eds. Topical Drug Bioavailability, Bioequivalence, and Penetration. New York: Plenum Press, 1993:415–424.
83. Kallings LO, Ringertz O, Silverstolpe L. Microbiological contamination of medical preparations. Acta Pharm Suec 1966; 3(3):219–228.
84. Fisher AA, Pascher F, Kanof NB. Allergic contact dermatitis due to ingredients of vehicles. A "vehicle tray" for patch testing. Arch Dermatol 1971; 104(3):286–290.
85. Mazer N, Fisher D, Fischer J, et al. Transfer of transdermal applied testosterone to clothing: a comparison of a testosterone patch versus a testosterone gel. J Sex Med 2005; 2(2):227–234.
86. Wester RC, Hui X, Maibach HI. In vivo human transfer of topical bioactive drug between individuals: estradiol. J Invest Dermatol 2006; 126(10):2190–2193.

4

Design and Evaluation of Ophthalmic Pharmaceutical Products

Paul J. Missel, John C. Lang, Denise P. Rodeheaver, Rajni Jani,
Masood A. Chowhan, James Chastain, and Terry Dagnon
Alcon Research, Ltd., Fort Worth, Texas, U.S.A.

INTRODUCTION

Any modern text on the design and evaluation of therapeutic products must place into unique perspective the nature of the eye and requirements of ophthalmic dosage forms. The eye, perhaps better than any other bodily organ, serves as a model structure for the evaluation of drug activity. In no other organ can a practitioner, without surgical or mechanical intervention, so well observe the activity of an administered drug. With such modern instrumentation as the biomicroscope, optical coherence tomography (OCT) instrument (Fig. 1), confocal microscope capable of viewing the single-layered corneal endothelium, and various devices for measuring intraocular pressure (IOP), blood flow, and electroretinal response, the ophthalmologist can readily track changes in ocular structures from the cornea to the retina and monitor their function and physiology (1) (Fig. 2). In so doing, the ophthalmologist and diagnostic scientist often detect signs of ocular or systemic disease long before sight-threatening or certain general health-threatening disease states become intractable. With such specialized instrumentation, the practitioner can view the activity of the drug product on the entire eye or the activity or effect on a cell, a group of cells, or entire tissues for products administered to the internal structure of the eye.

Ophthalmic pharmaceutical dosage forms serve as delivery vehicles for a wide range of drugs with pharmacological activity in the eye. The most commonly employed ophthalmic dosage forms are solutions, suspensions, and ointments. The essential characteristics for each of these dosage forms have been generally defined in the United States Pharmacopeia (USP) and will be expanded on in this chapter. Also included are the newest dosage forms for ophthalmic drug delivery—gels, gel-forming solutions, ocular inserts or systems, and intravitreal injections and implants. Common to all ophthalmic dosage forms is the critical requirement for sterility of the finished product as well as appreciation for the sensitivity of ocular tissue to irritation and toxicity and the inherent

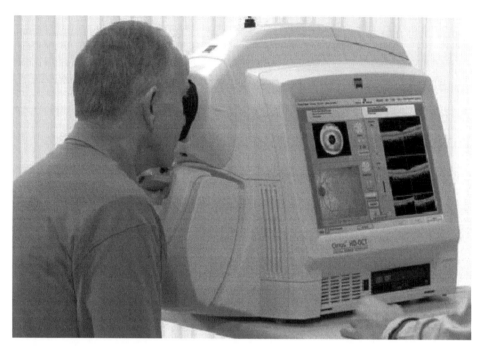

Figure 1 The Cirrus HD-OCT high-definition optical coherence tomography instrument, Carl Zeiss Meditec AG, is capable of feature resolutions in ocular tissue on the order of 5 to 25 μm.

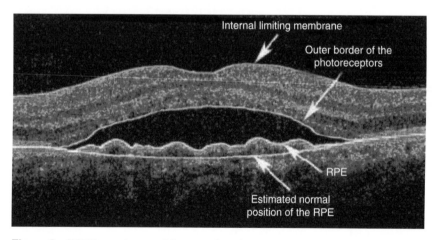

Figure 2 OCT B-scan image of the central portion of the retina. The large central dark region of subretinal fluid is an unnatural feature resulting from AMD. *Abbreviation*: AMD, age-related macular degeneration. *Source*: From Ref. 1. Courtesy of Association for Research in Vision and Ophthalmology.

limitations in topical ocular absorption of most drugs. As will be seen, these are primary factors in the design and evaluation of all ophthalmic pharmaceutical products.

The USP has numerous requirements. For example, "Ophthalmic solutions . . . [need be] . . . essentially free from foreign particles, suitably compounded and packaged for instillation into the eye," or "Ophthalmic suspensions . . . [need contain] . . . solid particles dispersed in liquid vehicle intended for application to the eye" (2). Ophthalmic suspensions are required to be made with the insoluble drug in a micronized form to prevent irritation or scratching of the cornea. A finished ophthalmic ointment must be free from large particles and must meet the requirements for Leakage and for Metal Particles under Ophthalmic Ointments ⟨771⟩. These and other requirements will be discussed further in the subsequent sections.

Behind the relatively straightforward compositional nature of ophthalmic solutions, suspensions, and ointments, however, lie many of the same physicochemical parameters that affect drug stability, safety, and efficacy, as they do for most other drug products. But additionally, specialized dosage forms present the ophthalmic product designer with some extraordinary compositional and manufacturing challenges. These range from concerns for sterility and consistency of parenteral-type ophthalmic solutions for intraocular, subtenon, and retrobulbar use, to resuspendability of such insoluble substances as dexamethasone or fluorometholone, to reconstitution, creating for the patient an apparently conventional solution for compounds such as acetylcholine chloride and epinephrine bitartrate, whose shelf life depends on storage conditions. More recently, the challenge to formulate with consistency highly potent actives present in diminishingly low concentrations raised the bar for formulations another significant notch. Procedures and devices for safe intravitreal implantation of sustained antiviral medication have grown from the advent of new therapies for a life- and eye-threatening new disease, HIV-AIDS.

Like most other products in the medical armamentarium, ophthalmic products are currently undergoing optimization. New modes of delivering a drug to the eye are being actively explored, ranging from solid, hydrophobic, or hydrophilic devices that are inserted into the ophthalmic cul-de-sac to conventionally applied dosage forms that, owing to their formulation characteristics, markedly increase the drug residence time in the fornix of the eye, thereby providing drug for absorption for prolonged periods and reducing the frequency that a given drug product must be administered. Intermediate between these alternatives, in both their physical state and effect on duration, are responsive polymeric systems that undergo transitions from liquid to gel or semisolid (3–7).

Inasmuch as products for the diagnosis and treatment of ocular disease the spectrum of practically all dosage forms are covered and, thus, the same pharmaceutical sciences are required for their development. In this chapter, we discuss the entire scope of considerations involved in the development of ophthalmic products, ranging from regulatory and compendial requirements, through physicochemical, safety, and efficacy considerations, to a discussion of types of dosage forms currently used by the medical practitioner. Because ocular health is not dependent only on treating disease, a section is provided that describes nutritional approaches to supporting ocular health or retarding progression of disease.

The final consideration, but by no means a minor one, is the design and evaluation of contact lens care products, which are regulated by the Food and Drug Administration (FDA) as medical devices, since they are accessory products necessary for the safe and effective use of contact lenses to correct visual acuity. These products include formulations for rinsing, storing, cleaning, and disinfecting contact lenses with specialized compositions for each major type of lens material, that is, hard, soft hydrophilic, and rigid gas-permeable (RGP) lenses. Also, lens care products for use in the eye as comfort drops while wearing contact lenses have been developed from similar products using lubricating polymers for treatment of minor eye irritation and tear deficiency (dry eye). The pharmaceutical scientist designing lens care products and improved ophthalmic drug dosage forms have taken advantage of advances in polymer and biomaterial sciences evident in the following sections.

HISTORICAL BACKGROUND

"If a physician performed a major operation on a seignior [a nobleman] with a bronze lancet and has saved the seignior's life, or he opened the eye socket of seignior with a bronze lancet and has saved the seignior's eye, he shall receive ten shekels of silver." But if the physician in so doing "has caused the seignior's death, or has destroyed the seignior's eye, they shall cut off his hand." The foregoing excerpts are from 2 of 282 laws of King Hammurabi's Code, engraved about 100 BC in a block of polished black igneous stone about 2.7 m high, now permanently preserved at the Louvre (8).

The code of Hammurabi is mentioned only to place that period in history when reference to eye medicines or poultices was beginning to appear. The Sumerians, in southern Mesopotamia, are considered to be the first to record their history, beginning about 3100 BC The Egyptians used copper compounds, such as malachite and chrysocalla, as green eye makeup with, no doubt, some beneficial effect against infection, owing to the antibacterial properties of copper (8, pp. 112–114). The standard wound salve of the Smith Papyrus (approximately 1700 BC)—grease, honey, and lint—probably served as one of the earliest ointments or ointment bases for the treatment of eye disease or wounds. The Greeks expanded on this basic salve to arrive at a typical enaimon (enheme), a drug for fresh wounds, which might have contained copper, lead, or alum, in addition to myrrh and frankincense (8, p. 154). The use of the aromatic substance myrrh in the form of sticks, blocks, or probes has been documented and attributed to the Romans and Greeks. Such sticks were called collyria and were dissolved in water, milk, or egg white for use as eyedrops. The Latin word collyrium is a derivative of the Greek word, kollyrien (in turn derived from kollyra, a roll of coarse bread), meaning a glutinous paste made from wheat and water that was rolled into thin cones, rods, or blocks. Often the physician's name was inscribed on these bodies (8, p. 216, 359). Pliney the Elder (ca. AD 23–79) advocated the use of egg whites to "cool" inflamed eyes, and lycium, one of the most popular of the plant extracts of India, was recommended especially for "eye troubles" (8, p. 348, 377).

After having placed the origin of at least two dosage forms (solution and ointment) for treating disorders or wounds of the eye between approximately the first and second millennium BC, we can readily reflect on the progress that the designers of dosage forms for eye products have made down through the ages—until relatively recently, little or none. Over the past two decades, however, we have begun to see new concepts emerging, some receiving the enthusiastic support of the ophthalmologist and optometrist, whereas others, not so fortunate, have been relegated to the status of little-used novelties.

ANATOMY OF THE EYE AND ADNEXA

In-depth discussions of the anatomy of the eye and adnexa have been adequately covered elsewhere in the pharmaceutical literature (9–13) and in recent texts on ocular anatomy. Here a brief overview is presented of the critical anatomical features that influence the nature and administration of ophthalmic preparations. In this discussion, consideration will be given primarily to drugs applied topically; that is, onto the cornea or conjunctiva or into the palpebral fornices. Increasingly, drugs are being developed for administration by parenteral-type dosage forms subconjunctivally into the anterior and posterior chambers, vitreous chamber, Tenon's capsule, or by retrobulbar injection. Because some of the dosage forms described may be considered as adjunctive to ophthalmic surgical procedures, those procedures and the concomitant use of the drug are described in section

Table 1   Anatomical Structures of the Eye

Conjunctiva	Posterior chamber
Inferior conjunctival sac	Lens
Superior conjunctival sac	Zonules of Zinn
	Vitreous humor
Cornea	Retina
Epithelium	
Bowman's membrane	Uvea
Stroma (substantia propria)	Ciliary body
Descemet's membrane	Iris
Endothelium	Choroid
Anterior chamber	Sclera
Schlemm's canal	Tenon's Capsule
Spaces of Fontana	Meibomian glands

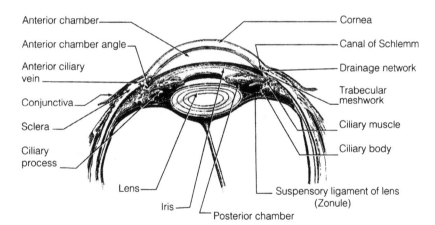

Figure 3   Anatomical cross-section of the human eye.

"Intraocular Dosage Forms." For orientation, readers are encouraged to familiarize themselves with the anatomical structures of the eye (Table 1), some of which are shown in Figure 3.

The eye is essentially a globe suspended in the ocular orbit, specialized for sight through an arrangement of multiple tissues that function to focus, transmit, and detect incoming light. There is a central path that light travels to the retina with all intervening tissues (cornea, aqueous humor, pupil, lens, and vitreous humor) being transparent. All surrounding tissues serve to nourish, support, and protect these essential structures.

The cornea composes only one-sixth of the outer surface of the eye, yet is the first and one of the most important barriers to external materials. The cornea is composed of three layers of tissue of varying structural and chemical properties. The presence and type of intercellular junctions regulate molecular diffusion around the cells, while the hydrophilic or lipophilic characteristic of each layer controls diffusion across and along the cell membrane. The cornea itself has no blood vessels, so it relies on passive diffusion of nutrients from surrounding tissues and aqueous humor.

The outermost layer, the epithelium, is composed of five to seven layers of stratified epithelial cells that make up only 10% (50 μm) of the total corneal thickness. Basal cells of the epithelium are mitotically active to replace the outer cells lost through normal sloughing or injury. The tight junctions and lipophilic composition of the epithelium combine to form an effective barrier to molecules and foreign substances that are hydrophilic or of high molecular weight. The tears, composed of mucin, aqueous and lipid phases, serve to hydrate the epithelium, prevent adhesion of bacteria and other foreign materials, and influence the distribution and toxicity of foreign materials (14). Finally, the epithelium is metabolically highly active, which is protective against toxic substances but may also significantly affect drug bioavailability and therapeutic index. Bowman's membrane separates the epithelium from the stroma, the layer that comprises 90% of the cornea.

In contrast to the epithelium, the stroma is 76% to 80% water and composed mostly of collagen fibrils in a highly organized array with interstices filled with glucosamino-glycan ground substance and a scattering of keratocytes. No junctions are present, yet the hydrophilic composition presents a significant barrier to lipophilic molecules. The stroma is susceptible to swelling, and water content must be actively controlled to prevent opacification. This is a primary function of the endothelium, a single layer of hexagonally arranged cells separated from the stroma by Decemet's membrane. Endothelial cells have discontinuous tight junctions to permit diffusion of essential nutrients into the cornea from the adjacent aqueous humor. Cellular ion pumps maintain proper hydration by active transport of ions back into the aqueous humor, drawing excess water out through passive diffusion along the ionic gradient. These "leaky" junctions present little or no barrier to drug penetration, but the overall lipophilic nature of the endothelium limits diffusion of hydrophilic molecules. The human endothelium has a fixed number of cells that are not mitotically active and compensates for cell loss only through migration and hypertrophy of remaining cells. Inability to compensate for cell loss will result in loss of function and corneal opacification; any ophthalmic preparation that could contact these cells must be carefully evaluated for biocompatibility.

The cornea is connected at the limbus to the opaque sclera, the tough fibroelastic capsule that encloses the eye and provides support and protection to the interior structures. The visible area of the sclera is generally referred to as the conjunctiva. The stroma has loosely packed collagen fibrils with scattered fibrocytes and few blood vessels, except in the limbal area. No junctional complexes are present, so the sclera presents only a lipophilic barrier to foreign materials. The limbus is rich in blood vessels, and systemic absorption of topically applied drugs occurs here primarily.

The interior of the eye is divided into three chambers by the iris and the lens. The iris, a ring of muscular tissue that regulates light entry into the back of the eye through the pupil, is located in front of the lens and physically forms the division between the anterior chamber and the posterior chamber. The lens is essentially a flattened sphere that is held in place and connected by fiber-like strands, the zonules of Zinn, to the ciliary body, a tissue that controls lens accommodation. Behind the lens is the vitreous chamber that contains vitreous humor, a transparent gelatinous material that has no turnover and is in direct contact with the retina. The iris, lens, and adjoining tissues serve to regulate light entry, focus light on the retina, regulate the turnover of aqueous humor within the eye, and provide structural support. At the junction of the iris and sclera, the trabecular meshwork and canal of Schlemm drain aqueous humor from the anterior chamber to prevent fluid accumulation, increased IOP, and glaucoma. The aqueous humor itself is produced by the anterior portion of the ciliary body and circulates through the posterior chamber through the pupil to the anterior chamber for a continual turnover of fluid. The iris itself can be affected by mydriatic or miotic agents that control the pupillary opening. The avascular lens has a single layer of epithelial cells on the anterior surface and is surrounded by a thin but tough capsule that conveniently provides the support for an intraocular lens (IOL) once a cataractous lens has been removed. The lens epithelial cells have some mitotic activity, and older cells progressively lose their cellular contents and migrate to form concentric layers of crystalline fibers that comprise the bulk of the lens. The lens is flexible and changes shape to adjust focal length for near objects (accommodation), an ability that is lost with age. Since there is little exchange of materials in the lens and no loss of cells, drug accumulation should be investigated for ophthalmic preparations that are absorbed into the eye.

Lining the back of the eye is the retina, a bilayered highly metabolically active tissue that transforms light to an electrical signal that is processed and transmitted as electronic images to the brain. The retina is isolated from the systemic circulation by the blood-retinal barrier, a combination of endothelial cell tight junctions lining the retinal blood vessels and tight junctions between the retinal pigmented epithelium (RPE) cells that restricts diffusion. A complex arrangement of photoreceptor cells (rods and cones) overlies the RPE. The retina connects to the optic nerve at the optic disk, a highly vascularized area that is susceptible to ocular hypertension and drug effects. The choroid is a highly vascularized collagenous tissue lying between the retina and the sclera from the ciliary body to the optic nerve. Finally, several accessory tissues (adnexa) are essential to proper functioning of the eye. Tenon's capsule, a thin membrane surrounding the sclera, separates the eye from the surrounding socket for freedom of movement. The lacrimal and meibomian glands provide essential tear and lipid components while the eyelids assist in tear distribution and protect against mechanical injury.

From this discussion, the reader can appreciate the intricacy of the eye and the care required in devising ophthalmic preparations to provide safe and effective therapy.

OCULAR PHARMACOKINETICS AND PHARMACOLOGY

Pharmacokinetics generally encompasses the process of absorption, distribution, metabolism, and excretion (ADME) of drugs. For the most part, ADME deals with systemically administered drugs that reach their pharmacological target by way of the systemic circulation, that is, blood, following oral or parenteral administration. Ocular pharmacokinetics embraces many features of ADME, but on a smaller scale and specifically applied to the eye. However, owing to the previously discussed unique anatomic, physiological, and barrier properties of the eye and surrounding tissue, ocular pharmacokinetics often can be as difficult to describe and predict as its systemic counterparts. The task is further confounded by the myriad of formulations, routes, and dosing regimens typically encountered in ophthalmology. For a more comprehensive discussion of ocular pharmacokinetics the reader is referred to various review articles (11,15–23). An overview of the principles regulating drug distribution is provided in section "Ocular Drug Transport and Delivery," but first we summarize the phenomenology.

While pharmacokinetics or ADME is often described as the action of the body on a drug, pharmacodynamics is the action of the drug on the body. More specifically, pharmacodynamics is the measurement of pharmacological response relative to dose or concentration. The pharmacological response induced by a drug in the eye can vary greatly from individual to individual because of differences in factors such as eye pigmentation, pathological state of the eye, tearing, and blink rate. The application of pharmacological endpoints is particularly useful in the study of drugs in the human eye, where, for obvious reasons, the ability to determine the ocular pharmacokinetics based on ocular tissue concentrations is severely limited.

Ocular Pharmacokinetics

Topical Ocular Instillation

The general process of ocular absorption from an eyedrop is surprisingly complex considering the simplicity of the administration method. Transcorneal absorption involves a series of events, including drug instillation, dilution in tear fluid, diffusion through the tear mucin layer, corneal penetration (epithelium, stroma, and endothelium), and transfer from cornea to aqueous humor. Parallel absorption via the conjunctiva/sclera also occurs; however, for the majority of drugs, this pathway is minor compared with the transcorneal route. In addition, nonproductive, competing pathways (e.g., nasolacrimal drainage or systemic absorption via the conjunctiva) operate to clear drug from the eye, thereby narrowing the time window during which absorption occurs (normally around 5–10 minutes).

Corneal Penetration

Transcorneal drug absorption is highly dependent on a drug's physicochemical properties, including its partition coefficient, molecular weight, solubility, and state of ionization. For most ophthalmic drugs, which are water soluble, the layers of stratified epithelial cells present the greatest barrier to penetration. The influence of the corneal epithelium on ocular absorption is clearly demonstrated by studying corneal penetration following removal of the epithelium. For rabbits administered topical ocular ^{14}C-dexamethasone, radioactivity is detected in the cornea and aqueous humor only after removal of the corneal epithelium (24,25). Stroma and endothelium offer resistance only to highly lipophilic drugs. Penetration through the lipophilic epithelium and hydrophilic stroma exhibits a parabolic relationship between log corneal permeability coefficients and log octanol-water coefficients (26,27), with an optimal log octanol-water coefficient of 2.9. Huang et al. refined the parabolic model by demonstrating in vitro a sigmoidal relationship between permeability coefficient and partition coefficient (25, p. 308).

A drug's transport and distribution can be influenced by the dosage form, such as solution versus suspension, and by its pH, buffering capacity, viscosity, or presence of a penetration enhancer. Burstein and Anderson evaluated the effects of preservatives, vehicles, adjunct agents, and anatomy, and developed model systems for selecting the best formulations for preclinical evaluation and clinical use (15). For example, by adjusting pH so that the drug is mostly unionized, corneal penetration was greatly enhanced. Conversely, buffering that increases the portion of drug ionized can be expected to reduce the portion absorbed.

Some excipients, such as the preservative benzalkonium chloride (BAC), can also act as penetration enhancers. Madhu et al. studied the influence of BAC/EDTA (disodium edetate) on ocular bioavailability of ketorolac tromethamine following topical ocular instillation onto normal and de-epithelialized rabbit corneas in vitro and in vivo (28), demonstrating its ability to disrupt epithelial cell tight junctions, and so enhance penetration.

Noncorneal, "Productive" Ocular Absorption

Ahmed and Patton investigated corneal versus noncorneal penetration of topically applied drugs in the eye (29,30), and identified a "productive" noncorneal route with penetration through the conjunctiva and underlying sclera. This pathway, previously thought only to eliminate drug from the eye ("nonproductive" absorption), parallels the corneal route and may be particularly important for drugs with low corneal permeability, such as inulin. Moreover, this pathway, which bypasses the anterior chamber, can distribute drug to the uveal tract and vitreous humor.

Evaluating drug diffusion employing in vitro barrier models of the conjunctiva, sclera, and cornea, Ahmed et al. demonstrated higher permeability in sclera and conjunctiva than cornea (31). Permeability coefficients of evaluated β-blockers ranked as follows: propranolol > penbutolol > timolol > nadolol for cornea, and penbutolol > propranolol > timolol > nadolol for the sclera. Permeability was higher in cornea versus conjunctiva for inulin, but similar in the case of timolol. Similarly, Chien et al. studied the ocular penetration pathways of three α2-adrenergic agents in rabbits both in vitro and in vivo (32). The predominant pathway for absorption was the corneal route, with the exception of *p*-aminoclonidine, the least lipophilic, which followed the conjunctival/scleral route. The results suggest that the absorption pathway may be determined in part by lipophilicity and that hydrophilic compounds may prefer the conjunctival/scleral route.

In a study by Schoenwald et al., the conjunctival/scleral pathway yielded higher iris-ciliary body concentrations for all compounds evaluated with the exception of lipophilic rhodamine B (33). Romanelli et al. demonstrated the absorption of topical ocular bendazac into the retina-choroid via the conjunctival-scleral pathway (34). Noncorneal absorption was influenced more by physicochemical properties of the drug than characteristics of the formulation, whereas conversely transcorneal absorption could be influenced more by characteristics of the formulation.

Noncorneal, Nonproductive Absorption and Precorneal Drainage

Routes of absorption that lead to the removal of drug from the precorneal area, and do not result in direct ocular uptake, are referred to as nonproductive. These noncorneal pathways, which are in parallel with corneal absorption and include conjunctival uptake and drainage via the nasolacrimal duct, lead to systemic absorption by way of conjunctival blood vessels in the former case and removal through the nasal mucosa and gastrointestinal tract in the latter. As discussed, drug can penetrate the conjunctiva, and, via the sclera, enter the eye; however, blood vessels within the conjunctiva can also lead to systemic absorption.

Nonproductive, noncorneal absorption and drainage greatly impact precorneal residence time, and thereby ocular absorption. Drainage, in particular, is generally rapid and limits ocular contact at the site of absorption to 3 to 10 minutes (21). For most drugs, however, the lag time for drug to traverse the cornea and appear in the aqueous humor extends exposure to maximal concentration in the aqueous to between 20 and 60 minutes. Interestingly, rapid loss of drug from the precorneal region results in ocular absorption of less than 10%, and more typically, less than 1% to 2% of a topical dose. Therefore, conventionally most of the topical dose is unavailable for local efficacy, with greater than 90% absorbed into the systemic circulation. As an example, Ling et al. demonstrated ocular bioavailability of topical ocular ketorolac in anesthetized rabbits to be 4% and systemic absorption to be nearly complete (35). Tang-Liu et al., for topical ocular administration of levobunolol in rabbits, found that ocular bioavailability was only 2.5% while systemic bioavailability reached 46% (36).

A number of factors can influence drainage and noncorneal absorption, and include, for example, anesthesia, instillation volume, formulation viscosity, and the status of the nasolacrimal duct. Using a radioisotopic method, Chrai et al. evaluated the effect of instilled volume on drainage loss using miosis data in albino rabbits (37) and showed that unanesthetized rabbits had lacrimal volume of 7.5 μL, whereas anesthetized rabbits had a slightly larger volume of 12.0 μL. Moreover, lacrimal turnover was slower in anesthetized rabbits. In a separate study, using 99mTc (technetium), Chrai et al. demonstrated that drug loss through drainage increased with drop volume (38), and five-minute spacing between drops was optimal for minimizing loss attributable to drainage. A volume of no more than 5 to 10 μL, containing a larger concentration of drug, was recommended, with at least a five-minute time gap between drops. By contrast, most commercial ophthalmic droppers deliver 30 to 70 μL. Also, for two drugs given as two separate drops, the second drop will negatively influence the first, arguing for combination therapy. Significantly, Keister et al. showed that for drugs with high corneal permeability, ocular bioavailability is relatively unaffected by drug volume (39).

Viscosity is another factor that can regulate nonproductive absorption, as well as ocular absorption. Increasing vehicle viscosity may decrease drainage rate, prolong precorneal residence time, and increase ocular absorption. However, there appears to be a finite limit to the extent of the influence of viscosity. Zaki et al. using γ-scintigraphy studied precorneal drainage with formulations containing radiolabeled polymers, either polyvinyl alcohol or hydroxymethylcellulose, in both rabbit and human (40). Significant retardation of drainage in humans was observed at higher polymer concentrations. Patton and Robinson also used polyvinyl alcohol, along with methylcellulose, to evaluate the relationship between viscosity and contact time or loss attributable to drainage (41). The optimum viscosity for rabbits ranged from 12 to 15 cP (centipoise). The relationship, however, was not proportional, and this was presumed to be related to increased shear forces from solutions of higher viscoelasticity. Chrai and Robinson also demonstrated, using methylcellulose vehicle, that increasing viscosity of an ophthalmic solution results in decreased drainage, and over the range of 1 to 15 cP, there was a threefold change in drainage rate constant and another threefold change over the range of 15 to 100 cP (42).

Occlusion of the nasolacrimal duct also is a means of controlling tear drainage and prolonging residence time. This highly effective means of increasing ocular bioavailability and concurrently decreasing systemic exposure, however, is not commonly employed as a clinical modality for increasing bioavailability. A few examples illustrate its efficacy. Kaila et al. studied the absorption kinetics of timolol following topical ocular administration to healthy volunteer subjects with eyelid closure, nasolacrimal occlusion (NLO), or normal blinking (43). NLO reduced total timolol systemic absorption, although, in some subjects, the initial absorption was enhanced. In another example, Zimmerman et al. showed that there were lower fluorescein anterior chamber levels and a shorter duration of fluorescein in the absence of NLO or eyelid closure (44). Systemic drug absorption in normal subjects was reduced more than 60% with these techniques. Linden and Alm studied the effect of tear drainage on intraocular penetration of topically applied fluorescein in healthy human eyes using fluorophotometry (45). Upper and lower punctal plugs in one eye caused a significant ($p < 0.025$) increase in aqueous humor fluorescein concentrations one to eight hours postdose of 20 μL of 2% solution of sodium fluorescein in the lower conjunctival sac. Compressing the tear sac and/or closing the eyelids for one minute after application had no effect on corneal or aqueous levels of fluorescein. Lee et al. evaluated the effect of NLO on the extent of systemic absorption following topical ocular administration of various adrenergic drugs (46). Table 2 summarizes the results of this study (see page 135). Hydrophilic atenolol and lipophilic betaxolol, which were not absorbed into the circulation as well as timolol and levobunolol, were not affected in their systemic absorption by five minutes of NLO. However, systemic bioavailability decreased 80% by prolonging precorneal retention of the dose to 480 minutes. It was concluded that modest formulation changes will have little effect on systemic absorption for extremely hydrophilic drugs. Drugs similar in lipophilicity to timolol will be well absorbed systemically, while extremely hydrophilic drugs or extremely lipophilic drugs will be absorbed to a lesser extent. The most likely explanation that NLO is not used more widely as a clinical strategy is the uncertainty of patient compliance, and hence the additional variability in efficacy.

As alluded to earlier in this chapter, the rate and extent of systemic absorption via the conjunctiva relative to corneal absorption is dependent on the physicochemical properties of a drug or its formulation. Ahmed and Patton showed that the conjunctival pathway is particularly important for drugs with low corneal permeability and that noncorneal permeation is limited by nonproductive loss to the systemic circulation (30). Hitoshe et al. demonstrated that drugs and prodrugs could be designed to reduce conjunctival absorption selectively and thus suppress systemic exposure (47). This can be accomplished by taking advantage of the effectively lower lipophilicity of the conjunctiva versus that of the cornea. Ashton et al. studied the influence of pH, tonicity, BAC, and EDTA on conjunctival and cornea penetration of four β-blockers: atenolol, timolol, levobunolol, and betaxolol (48). Isolated pigmented rabbit conjunctiva and cornea were used. The conjunctiva was more permeable than cornea, and formulation changes had greater influence on corneal versus conjunctival penetration. This was particularly true for the hydrophilic compounds; therefore, changes in formulation can affect both ocular and systemic absorption.

Ocular Pharmacodynamics

It is not the purpose of this text to present an in-depth review of the pharmacodynamics of ophthalmic drugs. For this purpose the reader is referred to one of the authoritative treatments of this subject (49–51). However, since this topic is not commonly covered in pharmacy school curricula, a brief treatment is presented here. For the most part, drugs used in the eye fall into one of several categories, including miotics, mydriatics (with or without cycloplegic activity), cycloplegics, anti-inflammatories, anti-infectives (including antibiotics, antivirals, and antibacterials), antiglaucoma drugs, surgical adjuncts, diagnostics, and a category of drugs for miscellaneous uses. The intended ophthalmic use will define more precisely what drug or combination of drugs are to be used, the appropriate dosage form, and route of administration. For example, the practitioner will, with knowledge of certain contraindications, use mydriatic drugs specifically for their pupillary and accommodative effects, both in the process of refraction and in the management of iridocyclitis, iritis, accommodative exotropia, and so on. Atropine, homatropine, scopolamine, tropicamide, and cyclopentolate are examples of para-sympathomimetic drugs possessing mydriatic and cycloplegic activity, whereas phenyl-ephrine and epinephrine are examples of sympathomimetic drugs possessing only mydriatic activity.

Drugs that may be chosen for use in the management of glaucoma may be topically applied miotics, such as pilocarpine hydrochloride or nitrate, carbachol, echothiophate iodide, or demecarium bromide; epinephrine prodrugs like dipivefrin hydrochloride, nonselective β-adrenergic blocking agents such as timolol maleate and bunolol hydrochloride, and selective β-adrenergic blocking agents such as racemic- or the more potent L-betaxolol hydrochloride, compounds devoid of pupillary effect; topically administered carbonic anhydrase inhibitors, such as dorzolamide and brinzolamide; prostaglandin analogs of the class $PGF_{2\alpha}$, such as latanoprost and travoprost, capable of lowering IOP significantly with little or no inflammatory or vasodilatory response; or, they may be orally administered drugs to present an osmotic effect that will lower IOP, such as 50% glycerin or 45% isosorbide. Other drugs administered orally to lower IOP are the carbonic anhydrous inhibitors acetazolamide and methazolamide. Furthermore, the miotic drugs may be chosen to reverse the effect of mydriatics after refraction or during surgical procedures such as cataract removal. There is now available an antimydriatic drug devoid of pupillary activity, dapiprazole hydrochloride, which is gaining importance in the reversal of the effect of mydriatics.

Depending on the location of ocular inflammation, a specific corticosteroid in a specific dosage form may be chosen. For instance, a corticosteroid of high potency, such as prednisolone acetate, fluorometholone, or dexamethasone, may be chosen for deep-seated inflammation of the uveal tract. Further treatment of such inflammation may take the form of subtenon injections or oral (systemic) administration of selected corticosteroids, depending on the indication and the dosage forms available. For inflammation of a more superficial nature, the lower strengths of prednisolone acetate or the lower-potency corticosterioids, such as hydrocortisone or medrysone, will usually be chosen.

Drugs used for the treatment of ocular infection will generally be chosen on the basis of the presumptive diagnosis of the causative agent by the ophthalmologist. Laboratory confirmation by microbial culture and identification is routinely conducted concurrently with the initiation of therapy. This is generally necessary because of the severity and sight-threatening nature of some type of infections. For example, if a patient has a foreign body lodged in the cornea originating from a potentially contaminated environment, the physician may choose to begin treatment of the eye, after foreign body removal, with a single or combination antibiotic, such as gentamicin, tobramycin, chloramphenicol, and a neomycin-polymyxin combination. This is considered appropriate, since an infection with *Pseudomonas aeruginosa* can destroy a cornea in 24 to 48 hours, generally the time it takes to identify an infectious agent. Less fulminating, but no less dangerous, are infections caused by various staphylococcal and streptococcal organisms. For superficial bacterial infections of the conjunctiva and eyelids, sulfonamides, such as sodium sulfacetamide, are usually prescribed, as are yellow mercuric oxide and mild silver protein. Prophylactic therapy for ophthalmia neonatorum is nearly universally required in the United States, with silver nitrate, penicillin G, or erythromycin as the primary anti-infectives used. Pre- and postsurgical prophylaxis is becoming more commonplace with the popularity of surgically corrected vision, and combinations of anti-infectives with anti-inflammatory agents are frequently used to reduce surgical trauma to the eye.

For fungal and viral infections, there are a very few agents that the ophthalmologist can prescribe. These organisms' resistance and similarity to mammalian tissue make it difficult to find effective and safe therapies. For instance, idoxuridine, a selective metabolic inhibitor, has been shown to be useful against herpes simplex virus infection of the cornea. For the trachoma virus and viruses that cause inclusion conjunctivitis [i.e., TRIC (the single largest cause of blindness worldwide)], no specific antiviral agent has demonstrated satisfactory activity, and the secondary bacterial ramifications of this disease are managed by conventional antibiotics, such as tetracycline, chloramphenicol, and erythromycin. The trachoma virus itself seems to be somewhat susceptible to these antibiotics; however, up to six weeks of treatment, antibiotics are required three times per day to achieve an 80% cure rate (52,53).

A similar situation exists for the treatment of fungal keratitis. The antifungal antibiotic drugs nystatin and natamycin have been effective to varying degrees in superficial fungal infection, as have copper sulfate and sodium sulfacetamide (54,55). For both of these drugs iontophoresis of the topically administered drug produces enhanced activities.

Drugs used as surgical adjuncts are primarily irrigating solutions, solutions of proteolytic enzymes, viscoelastics and miotics employed in cataract removal, intraocular lens placement, vitrectomy, and procedures to preserve retinal integrity. These drugs are considered true parenteral dosage forms, the design and evaluation of which are discussed in greater detail elsewhere in this chapter.

Diagnostic drugs, such as sodium fluorescein, are administered topically or intravenously to aid in the diagnosis of such conditions as corneal abrasions or ulceration and various retinopathies. This agent has become the most widely used diagnostic agent in the practice of ophthalmology and optometry. Rose bengal has also been used topically, although to a far lesser degree than sodium fluorescein, which is available as well-preserved alkaline solutions in concentrations ranging from 0.5% to 2.0% (56,57), as fluorescein-impregnated absorbent sterile paper strips (58), or as unpreserved, terminally sterilized intravenous injections in concentrations ranging from 5% to 25% (59).

Several topically applied local anesthetics are routinely used by the eye care specialist in certain routine diagnostic procedures and for various relatively simple surgical procedures such as insertion of punctal plugs and surgical vision correction. The first of these to be used was cocaine, in concentrations ranging from 1% to 4% (60). However, more modern local anesthetics, such as tetracaine hydrochloride and proparacaine hydrochloride, have replaced cocaine as drugs of choice in these procedures. For surgical procedures of a more complex nature, lidocaine hydrochloride and similar local anesthetics as retrobulbar injections have been used (61).

The foregoing overview has presented the major classes of ophthalmic drugs. One additional class of drugs that merits brief discussion includes drugs used for the treatment of various dry eye syndromes. The most severe of these, keratoconjunctivitis sicca, involves diminished secretion of mucins, consisting of glycoproteins and glycosaminoglycans and their complexes. These materials serve to coat the corneal epithelium with a hydrophilic layer that uniformly attracts water molecules, resulting in even hydration of the corneal surface. Diminished secretion of these substances causes dry spots to develop on the cornea, resulting in corneal dehydration, which can lead to ulceration, scarring, or corneal opacities (62). Modern pharmaceutical products are available (Hypotears, Tears Naturale Forte) that contain mucomimetic high molecular weight polymers that serve to resurface the cornea temporarily, thereby preventing the aforementioned dehydration and affording the dry eye sufferer with a degree of relief previously unavailable (63,64). These agents are not pharmacologically active although recent research leads to the promise of drugs that will stimulate tear production for longer-term relief.

GENERAL SAFETY CONSIDERATIONS

Sterility

Every ophthalmic product must be manufactured under conditions validated to render it sterile in its final container for the shelf life of the product (65,66). Sterility testing is conducted on each lot of ophthalmic product by suitable procedures, as set forth in the appropriate pharmacopoeia and validated in each manufacturer's laboratory. While the majority of topical ophthalmic preparations contain preservatives for multiple-dose use, sterile preparations in special containers for individual use on a single patient must also be made available and are more common in the European Union. This availability is especially critical for every hospital, office, or other installation where accidentally or surgically traumatized eyes are treated, as well as for patients intolerant to preservatives.

The USP recognizes six methods of achieving a sterile product: (*i*) steam sterilization, (*ii*) dry-heat sterilization, (*iii*) gas sterilization, (*iv*) sterilization by ionizing radiation, (*v*) sterilization by filtration, and (*vi*) aseptic processing (67). For ophthalmic products packaged in plastic containers, typical for ophthalmic products, a combination of two or more of these six methods is routinely used. For example, for a sterile ophthalmic suspension, bottles, dropper tips, and caps may be sterilized by ethylene oxide or γ-radiation; the suspended solid may be sterilized by dry heat, γ-radiation, or ethylene oxide; and the aqueous portion of the composition may be sterilized by filtration. The compounding is completed under aseptic conditions.

One can see by the complexity of these types of manufacturing procedures that much care and attention to detail must be maintained by the manufacturer. This sterile manufacturing procedure must then be validated to prove that no more than three containers in a lot of 3000 containers (0.1%) are nonsterile. Ultimately, it is the manufacturer's responsibility to ensure the safety and efficacy of the manufacturing process and the absence of any adverse effect on the product, such as the possible formation of substances toxic to the eye, an ever-present possibility with gas sterilization or when using ionizing radiation. For ophthalmic products sterilized by terminal sterilization (sterilization in the final sealed container, e.g., steam under pressure), the sterilization cycle must be validated to ensure sterility at a probability of 10^6 or greater.

In addition to process controls the USP has specific product sterility testing criteria for solutions, suspensions, ointments, and parenteral products. The two other major global compendia the Japanese Pharmacopoeia and the European Pharmacopoeia have similar testing criteria to assure the sterility of ophthalmic products. Unfortunately, the three major global compendia are not harmonized (68,69).

Ocular Toxicity and Irritation

Assessment of the potential for ocular irritation and toxicity of ophthalmic solutions represents an extremely important step in the development of both over-the-counter (OTC) and prescriptive pharmaceuticals. Excellent reviews of procedures describing these evaluations have been published (70–73). Refinements in procedures, study design, use of objective measures, and standardization of noninvasive methods such as specular microscopy have resulted in greater reliability, detection, and predictability. In addition, the incorporation of structure-activity relationship (SAR) evaluations provides an early assessment of probable toxic effects of the chemical moieties under consideration. The historical evaluation of these procedures can be traced through the literature (74–83), as can an understanding of the mechanisms of ocular response to external materials based on examination of the conjunctiva (84–87), the cornea (75,88–90), or the iris (49,75,91). Advances in design and use of ophthalmic drugs and devices have brought ocular toxicity into sharper focus. Many interior structures of the eye adjacent to target tissues, or which are targets of newer therapies themselves, can suffer irreversible damage, so safety evaluations must be comprehensive. In general, also, consideration must be given to the use of various ophthalmic preparations with other drugs and devices. Testing, therefore, must be based on risk analysis to include both the intended uses of the product as well as reasonably foreseeable misuse.

Albino rabbits have been the primary species used to test ocular toxicity and irritation of ophthalmic formulations. While recent debate has centered on the use of rabbits or other species as predictors for human responses, there is consensus that there is no more reliable model that captures the full complexity of the eye and the ocular response of its intricate biochemical and physiological processes. In addition, the rabbit has obvious advantages due to its availability, ease of handling and maintenance, and large prominent unpigmented eye that facilitates observation of ocular structures (71). Compared with the human eye, rabbits exhibit differences in the tear layer (decreased tearing and blinking rate, presence of lipid from the species-specific Harderian gland), adnexa (loosely attached eyelids and presence of a nictitating membrane (86,92–94), cornea (i.e., structure of Bowman's membrane, slower corneal re-epithelialization (75), and endothelium (regenerative). The corneal differences result in increased ocular response to irritants in the rabbit. The primate has gained in popularity as an ocular model for the evaluation of drugs and chemicals because it is more similar to human eye (92,93). However, due to the difficulty and risk inherent in their care and handling, primates are used secondarily and in cases where other species may not provide an accurate assessment. This is especially true for drugs with melanin-binding characteristics that may accumulate in a pigmented iris, although species such as pigmented rabbits and minipigs provide some alternatives.

Various governmental agencies have published guidelines for ocular irritancy studies (93–95). These guidelines are directed toward ophthalmic formulations, chemicals, cosmetics, extractables from ophthalmic containers, and other materials that may intentionally or accidentally contact the eye during use. It is the manufacturer's responsibility to determine those studies specifically appropriate for testing the safety of the ophthalmic formulation, yet abiding by governmental requirements and guidelines regarding ophthalmic preparations and excipients as well as biocompatibility of the packaging.

As a part of the Federal Hazardous Substances Act (FHSA), a modified Draize test was adopted (96–98) as the official method for evaluation of acute ocular irritancy (99). It is a pass/fail determination that remains in effect today. The test may use a small volume more consistent with the capacity of the inferior conjunctival sac (100), and incorporate biomicroscopic slit-lamp examination and/or fluorescein staining to assess ocular changes (71,97,98). While various in vitro tests have been proposed to replace this in vivo evaluation and a U.S. interagency committee has recommended certain in vitro tests to detect severe irritants and corrosives, none has yet been officially accepted or validated (101–104).

Current U.S. and international guidelines for toxicity evaluation of ophthalmic formulations involve both single and multiple applications to the eye, dependent on the proposed clinical use (71). The multiple applications may extend up to a 12-month period and incorporate evaluations of ocular irritation and toxicity, systemic toxicity, and determination of systemic exposure (toxicokinetics). In many cases, systemic exposure from the ocular route is less than by parenteral administration, information that will assist in determining the studies needed to establish safety of the ophthalmic preparation. Evaluations must assess the drug substance itself as well as the drug product, since excipients and preservatives may significantly influence the length of exposure and tissue absorption and directly affect toxicity. U.S. and international guidance documents are available (105,106), and regulations and tests have been summarized for ophthalmic preparations (71,107,108).

As mentioned previously (and discussed in detail in section "Contact Lens Care Products"), contact lens products have specific guidelines that focus on compatibility with the contact lens and biocompatibility with the cornea and conjunctiva (109). These solutions are viewed as new medical devices and require testing with the contact lenses with which they are to be used. Tests include a 21-day ocular study in rabbits, and may include other solutions that might be used with the lens. Additional tests to evaluate cytotoxicity, acute toxicity, sensitization potential (allergenicity), and risks specific to the preparation are also required (99,109,110). These tests are sufficient to meet requirements in the majority of countries, though testing requirements for Japan are currently much more extensive.

While systemic exposure is rarely encountered in intraocularly administered drug products, there are safety concerns related to the biocompatibility of these products with ocular tissues. These products have special design and evaluation concerns, since they may have prolonged contact with essential and delicate tissues, such as the endothelium and trabecular meshwork (111). For such drug products, it is mandatory to design specific testing that mimics the proposed clinical exposure. Methods may include ex vivo models that perfuse the anterior chamber of excised rabbit eyes with the product and assess compatibility with the corneal endothelium using specular microscopy (112) and histopathology. These materials can also be evaluated against specific cell lines in tissue culture, particularly corneal endothelial tissue. As tissue culture technology progresses, cell lines for the other ocular tissues are being established and will become useful in compatibility testing as well.

The sensitivity of the intraocular tissues places certain restrictions on intraocular dosage forms. In general, preparations that incorporate fewer ingredients in a properly balanced solution will have less likelihood of tissue incompatibility. This is not to say that a simple solution of drug in water is optimal, as even a simple isotonic solution of sodium chloride may be toxic to human corneal epithelial, endothelial, iris, and conjunctival cells. In the electron photomicrographs of human corneal endothelium presented in Figures 4 to 6, the effect of solution composition on tissue integrity is illustrated. Human corneal endothelial tissue perfused for three hours with lactated Ringer's solution shows cell darkening and swelling (Fig. 4), while normal cell confluence is retained in the same tissue perfused for three hours with Ringer's solution containing glutathione, adenosine, and bicarbonate (Fig. 5). A three-hour perfusion with a solution devoid of ingredients essential for normal cell confluence results in marked discontinuity of cell structure (Fig. 6).

Some agents commonly used in topical ocular drugs can be used only sparingly or not at all for intraocular use, and pH and buffering capacity must be taken into account. Most preservative agents commonly used in topical ophthalmic preparations are not compatible with the tissues of the anterior segments of the eye (113). The USP recognizes this problem and specifically warns against their use in intraocular solutions (2,114). Drug stabilizers, such as antioxidants and chelating agents, must be used with care and should be used in absolutely minimal quantities only when necessary. Occasionally, it may seem desirable to solubilize an otherwise sparingly soluble ingredient. Only fairly low concentrations of typical cosolvents such as glycerin and propylene glycol can be employed because of their osmotic effect on the surrounding tissues. Hyperosmotic solutions may elicit some transient desiccation of the anterior chamber tissues whereas hypotonic solutions may cause edema that could lead to corneal clouding. There appears to be little or no experience with these or other common cosolvents in products of this type, and their use in solubilizing solution ingredients should be avoided.

Additionally, since the anterior chamber fluid (aqueous humor) contains essentially the same buffering systems as the blood, products with a pH outside the physiological range of 7.0 to 7.4 are converted to this range by the buffering capacity of the aqueous

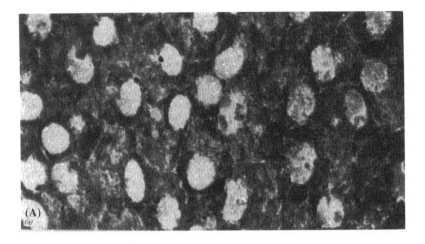

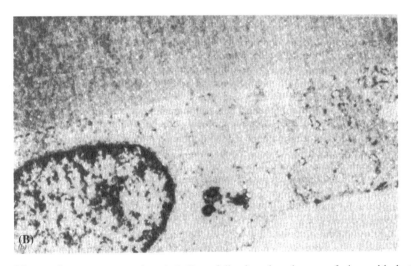

Figure 4 Human corneal endothelium following three-hour perfusion with lactated Ringer's solution: (**A**) scanning electron micrograph (2100×), (**B**) transmission electron micrograph (9100×). *Source*: Courtesy of H. Edelhauser.

humor if a relatively small volume of the solution is introduced. Often, however, aqueous humor is lost in the procedure or the volume of solution is relatively large; therefore, drug products should be formulated as closely as possible to this physiological pH range, although the use of buffering agents should be avoided if possible.

The question of particulate matter is also of great importance, and the European Pharmacopoeia includes specific guidance on the size and number of particles allowable in ophthalmic formulations. Particles administered topically have the potential to damage the epithelial layer, which may lead to infection and scarring. Although the total effect of particulates on intraocular tissue is not completely known, some possible results in the anterior chamber have been postulated (2). Certain amounts of iritis and uveitis might be expected, as well as the production of granulomas similar to the type reported for pulmonary tissue that results from particulates in large-volume parenterals. The possibility is equally important that particulate matter can block the canals of Schlemm, disrupting the outflow mechanism for the aqueous humor and leading to a rapid increase

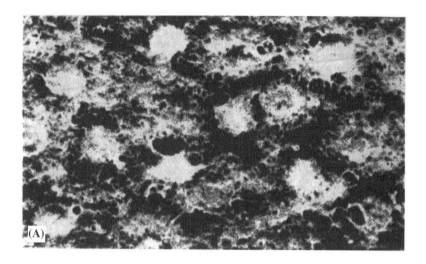

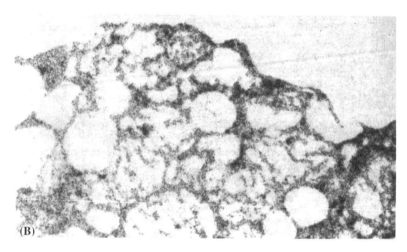

Figure 5 Human corneal endothelium following three-hour perfusion with glutathione bicarbonated Ringer's solution: (**A**) scanning electron micrograph (1950×), (**B**) transmission electron micrograph (8450×). *Source*: Courtesy of H. Edelhauser.

in IOP and the onset of an acute attack of glaucoma. The formulator should be aware that particulates may originate from raw materials as well as glass fragments produced in glass ampoule fracture or elastomeric particles generated during stopper penetration. Very specialized stopper design, cleaning procedures, and lubrication should be considered when the latter type of packaging is used.

To provide a complete assessment of all these variables, the final evaluation of the safety of ophthalmic products must be made in the in vivo model using the preparation under the proposed conditions for use, following tissue compatibility with many of the techniques already discussed. Irrigating solutions of low viscosity may have limited contact, while the gel-like viscoelastic materials, which maintain the corneal dome, or the solutions and gases used as vitreous replacements to prevent retinal detachment, may have prolonged contact with delicate ocular tissues or the retina. A recent therapy involves treatment for neovascularization of the retina, a disease in which proliferation of blood vessels can lead to blindness. The treatment combines a systemic chemical that localizes

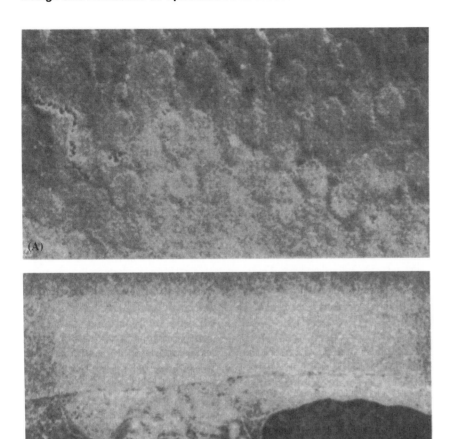

Figure 6 Human corneal endothelium following three-hour perfusion with solution devoid of essential nutrients: (**A**) scanning electron micrograph (2100×), (**B**) transmission electron micrograph (9100×). *Source*: Courtesy of H. Edelhauser.

in the new blood vessels followed by laser treatment to destroy the vessels. Such new therapies and new routes of administration require special care in their design and evaluation.

During the application of the various guidelines for ophthalmic, contact lens and intraocular products, ocular examination and biomicroscopic examination of rabbit eyes are completed with objective reproducible grading for conjunctival congestion, conjunctival swelling, conjunctival discharge, aqueous (humor) flare, iris involvement, corneal cloudiness, pannus, and fluorescein staining (71,115). Other available methods measure IOP, corneal thickness, endothelial cell changes, cells in the aqueous humor, and posterior segment changes. As part of improved design and responsible uses of animal models, in vivo methods that incorporate new noninvasive technology, such as confocal microscopy, and reduced numbers of animals have also been developed. Since international regulations specify the minimum number of animals that must be used, the latter are most useful in early development of these products.

As alternatives to in vivo testing of ophthalmic preparations, numerous in vitro methods have been developed over the past few years as alternatives to in vivo ocular testing (73,116–124). Particular attention has been given recently to evaluation of preservative effects on corneal penetration (125,126), cytotoxicity (127–131), and effects on wound healing (132–134). These methods have been able so far to mimic only acute ocular dosing regimens, and validation efforts have not substantiated the correlation of any in vitro method with rabbit or human responses. However, these methods are useful for comparing relative toxicity under controlled conditions or preliminary evaluations prior to lengthy in vivo testing, and several manufacturers currently are using in vitro toxicity tests at early stages in the development of ophthalmic solutions.

Preservation and Preservatives

In 1953, the FDA required that all ophthalmic solutions be sterile (135). Preservatives are included as a major component of all multiple-dose eye solutions for the primary purpose of maintaining sterility in the opened product through its shelf life. Packaging ophthalmic solutions in the popular plastic eyedrop container has reduced, but not completely eliminated, the chances of inadvertent contamination. There can be a "suckback" of an unreleased drop when pressure on the bottle is released. If the tip is allowed to touch a nonsterile surface, contamination may be introduced. Therefore, it is important that the pharmacist instruct the patient on the proper method of dispensing from a plastic eyedrop container to minimize the hazards of contamination. The hazard is magnified in the busy clinical practice of the eye care professional where a diagnostic solution—there are many, including cycloplegics, mydriatics, and dyes—may be used for many patients from the same container. The cross-contamination hazard can be eliminated by the use of packages containing small volumes designed for single application only (i.e., unit dose). Since preservatives are not included in solutions packaged in unit-dose containers, and because these single-use packages still contain (as a large-scale manufacturing necessity) an amount in excess of the several drops (0.05–0.20 mL) required, patient and physician alike should be cautioned to avoid exhausting their entire contents in a multiuse application that will increase the hazard of contamination and defeat the purpose of this special packaging.

Preservative effectiveness testing is defined in both United States and European Pharmacopoeias, and global regulatory agencies require an evaluation and control of the effectiveness of the preservative against various microbial strains from the four major classes of eye pathogens, namely gram-positive cocci (*Staphylococcus aureus*), gram-negative rods (*P. aeruginosa*), yeasts (*Candida albicans*), and fungi (*Aspergillus niger*) (136).

In the ophthalmic literature, because of reports of loss of eyes from corneal ulcerations caused by eye solutions contaminated with *P. aeruginosa*, considerable emphasis is placed on the effectiveness of preservatives against *Pseudomonas* species. This organism is not the most prevalent cause of bacterial eye infections, even though it is a common inhabitant of human skin, but it is the most opportunistic and virulent. *S. aureus* is responsible for most bacterial infections of the eye. The eye seems to be remarkably resistant to infection when the corneal epithelium is intact due to the barrier properties discussed previously as well as the antimicrobial activity of lysozyme and other enzymes present in tears. When there is a corneal epithelial abrasion, organisms can enter freely and *P. aeruginosa* can grow readily in the cornea, rapidly producing an ulceration and loss of vision. This microorganism has been found as a contaminant in a number of studies on sterility of ophthalmic solutions, particularly in sodium fluorescein solutions used to detect corneal epithelial damage. The chances for serious infections and cross-contamination are greatly enhanced by multiple use of this dye solution—a danger that has led to the practice by the ophthalmologist of using sterile disposable applicator strips of fluorescein.

Recently, preclinical and clinical studies have reported that the long-term use of preserved topical medications in chronic ophthalmic conditions, such as glaucoma, may adversely affect the ocular surface at the expense of corneal health (137). Consequently, preservatives are thought to be partially responsible for ocular side effects, for chronic ophthalmic diseases manufacturers are developing products with either reduced preservatives or preservative-free formulations (138). Alternative packaging for multidose nonpreserved preparations and drugs administered in dry form (139) may offer nonpreserved choices for the formulator, but efficacy and compatibility of each drug with these systems must be investigated. Because experimental results reported in the literature have shown a somewhat higher incidence of adverse effects with preserved solutions compared with unpreserved, there is some question of the necessity for preservatives in some applications (140,141). However, preservatives can enhance drug efficacy, chemically balance a preparation, and enable a dosing form that promotes patient compliance. While some ophthalmic drugs may be formulated in an unpreserved form, many drugs cannot, and it is the challenge of the formulator to provide an acceptable balance of safety and effectiveness.

Choice of Preservative

Although this chapter is directed toward ophthalmic products, it is largely applicable to parenteral and even nonsterile products (solutions, emulsions, and suspensions). The choice of preservative is limited to only a few chemicals that have been found, over the years, to be safe and effective for this purpose. These are benzalkonium chloride, thimerosal, methyl- and propylparaben, phenylethanol, chlorhexidine, polyquaternium-1, and polyaminopropyl biguanide. The chelating agent, EDTA, is sometimes used to increase activity against certain *Pseudomonas* strains, particularly solutions preserved with BAC. Chlorhexidine—as the hydrochloride, acetate, or gluconate salts—is used widely in the United Kingdom and Australia, but was not introduced into the United States until 1976, and only then for solutions intended for disinfection of soft contact lenses. This limited choice of preservative agents is further narrowed by the requirements of chemical and physical stability and compatibility with drugs, packaging, and contact lens materials. Many times it is necessary to design the formula to fit the requirements of the chosen preservative system since the buffer system and excipients can alter preservative action significantly. While it is recognized that excipients themselves may produce toxicity, and their use need be controlled, the large variety and number of available excipients prohibits discussion here, and the reader is referred to a pharmaceutical text that provides an excellent review (142).

Several guidelines are available in the literature for the pharmacist who must extemporaneously prepare an ophthalmic solution. The USP contains a section on ophthalmic solutions, as do other compendia and several standard textbooks. Since the pharmacist does not have the facilities to test the product, he or she should dispense only small quantities, with an expiration date of no more than 30 days. Refrigeration of the product should also be required as a precautionary measure. To reduce the largest potential source of microbial contamination, only sterile purified water should be used in compounding ophthalmic solutions. Sterile water for injection (WFI), USP, from unopened IV bottles or vials is the highest-quality water available to the pharmacist. Prepackaged sterile water with bacteriostatic agents should not be used.

Benzalkonium chloride The most widely used preservative remains BAC, which often is supplemented with disodium edetate. The BAC defined in the USP monograph is the quaternary ammonium compound alkylbenzyldimethylammonium chloride in which the alkyl portion is composed of a mixture of chain lengths ranging from C_8 to C_{16}. This compound's popularity is based, despite its compatibility limitations, on its being the most effective and rapid-acting preservative with excellent chemical stability. It is stable over a wide pH range and does not degrade even under excessively hot storage conditions. It has pronounced surface-active properties, and its activity can be reduced by adsorption. It is cationic, which unfortunately can lead to a number of incompatibilities with large negatively charged molecules with the potential for producing salts of lower solubility and possibly precipitation. For example, it cannot be used with nitrates, salicylate, anionic soaps, and large anionic drugs, such as sodium sulfacetamide and sodium fluorescein. When feasible, it is usually advisable to design the formula to avoid these incompatible anions, rather than to substitute a less effective preservative. There are a number of helpful lists of incompatibilities of BAC in the literature, but they should not be relied upon entirely. Compatibility is determined by the total environment in which the drug molecules exist (i.e., the total product formula). The pharmaceutical manufacturer can sometimes design around what appears to be an incompatibility, whereas the extemporaneous compounder may not have this option, or more importantly, the ability to test the final product for its stability, safety, and efficacy.

The conventional concentration of BAC in eyedrops is 0.01%, with a range of 0.004% to 0.02% (143). While uptake of BAC itself into ocular tissues is limited (144), even lower concentrations of BAC have been reported to enhance corneal penetration of other compounds, including therapeutic agents (125,145,146). The differential effect of this preservative on the cornea compared with the conjunctiva can be exploited to target a drug for corneal absorption and delivery to the posterior segment of the eye (147). Its use has been proposed as a means of delivering systemic doses by an ocular route of administration (148).

Richards (149), Mullen et al. (150), and the American College of Toxicology (151) have summarized the literature of BAC. The conclusion drawn was that BAC, up to 0.02%, has been well substantiated as being suitable for use in topical ophthalmic solutions when the conditions of its use are properly controlled.

Numerous studies comparing BAC with other preservatives have been described in the literature. Many of the articles give conflicting results, not surprising considering the many different test methods, formulas, and criteria used to arrive at these diverse conclusions. However, adequate information is available in the literature to permit the manufacturer to select appropriate tests for nearly any product. Generally, the USP (or similarly validated) test can be employed to decide which preservative system is most compatible with a specific composition. While multiple reports show BAC to have a somewhat higher incidence of ocular effects (152–154), this preservative remains one of the most effective available and generally assures an adequate level of preservative efficacy.

Some strains of *P. aeruginosa* are resistant to BAC and, in fact, can be grown in solutions concentrated in this agent. This has caused great concern because of the virulent nature of this organism in ocular infections, as discussed previously. Thus, it was an important finding in 1958 that the acquired resistance could be eliminated by the presence of ethylenediaminetetraacetic acid (sodium edetate; EDTA) in the formulation. This action of EDTA has been correlated with its ability to chelate divalent cations and is commonly used as a preservative aid (155). The use of EDTA, where it is compatible, is recommended in concentrations up to 0.1%.

Other quaternary ammonium germicides, benzethonium chloride and benzalkonium bromide, have been used in several ophthalmic solutions. While these have the advantage of not being a chemical mixture, they do not possess the bactericidal effectiveness of BAC and are subject to the same incompatibility limitations. In addition, the maximum concentration for benzethonium chloride is 0.01%.

Organic mercurials When BAC cannot be used in a particular formulation of a therapeutic agent—for example, pilocarpine nitrate, serine salicylate, or fluorescein sodium (because of potential anion-cation association)—one of three organic mercurials, phenylmercuric nitrate, phenylmercuric acetate, and thimerosal, had, until recent years, been used. Because of environmental concerns, however, the use of organic mercurials has fallen into disfavor. Although organic mercurials have not been implicated in classical mercurial toxicity, several countries have banned their use entirely, and other countries require its rigorous defense based on the absence of any suitable alternative. In those situations for which the use of an organic mercurial is the only avenue available, the usual range in concentration for the phenylmercuric compounds is 0.002% to 0.004% and for thimerosal 0.02% to 0.1%. Although they can be used effectively in some products, the mercurials are relatively weak and slow in their antimicrobial activity. The organic mercurials are generally restricted to use in neutral to alkaline solutions; however, they have been used successfully in slightly acid formulations. The phenyl mercuric ion can react with halide ions to form salts of lower solubility, reducing their effectiveness. Thimerosal has a greater solubility and is relatively more stable than the phenylmercuric compounds and has not been shown to deposit in the lens of the eye. The latter phenomenon has been observed with phenylmercuric compounds.

Ocular sensitization to thimerosal has been well documented over the years (156–162). Although thimerosal had at one time been referred to as the preservative of choice for soft contact lens care products (163–165), its use has been supplanted almost completely by the polyquaternium-1 and polybiguanide preservatives.

Since the organic mercurials offer an alternative to quaternary ammonium preservatives and since preservative efficacy of ophthalmic solutions is essential, the choice among these alternatives should be based on a benefit-to-risk analysis so long as a ban is not imposed on the use of these organometallic preservatives.

Chlorobutanol This aromatic alcohol has been an effective preservative and is still used in several ophthalmic products. Over the years, it has proved to be a relatively safe preservative for ophthalmic products (166) and has produced minimal effects in various tests (131,167,168). In addition to its relatively slower rate of activity, it imposes a number of limitations on the formulation and packaging. It possesses adequate stability when stored at room temperature in an acidic solution, usually about pH 5 or below. If autoclaved for 20 to 30 minutes at a pH of 5, it will decompose to about 30%. The hydrolytic decomposition of chlorobutanol produces hydrochloric acid (HCl), resulting in a decreasing pH as a function of time. As a result, the hydrolysis rate also decreases. Chlorobutanol is generally used at a concentration of 0.5%. Its maximum water solubility is only about 0.7% at room temperature, which may be lowered by active or excipients, and is slow to dissolve. Heat can be used to increase dissolution rate, but will also cause some decomposition and loss from sublimation. Concentrations as low as 0.125% have shown antimicrobial activity under the proper conditions.

Methyl- and propylparaben These esters of *p*-hydroxybenzoic acid have been used primarily to prevent growth of molds, but in higher concentrations possess some weak antibacterial activity. Their effective use is limited by low aqueous solubility and by reports of stinging and burning sensations related to their use in the eye. They bind to a number of nonionic surfactants and polymers, thereby reducing their bioactivity. They are used in combination with the methyl ester at 0.03% to 0.1% and the propyl ester at 0.01% to 0.02%. Parabens have also been shown to promote corneal absorption (133).

Phenylethyl alcohol This substituted alcohol has been used at 0.5% concentration, but in addition to its weak activity, it has several limitations. It is volatile and will lose activity by permeation through a plastic package. It has limited water solubility, can be "salted out" of solution, and can produce burning and stinging sensations in the eye. It has been recommended primarily for use in combination preservative systems.

Polyquaternium-1 (POLYQUAD®) This preservative is still comparatively new to ophthalmic preparations and is a polymeric quaternary ammonium germicide. Its advantage over other quaternary ammonium seems to be in its inability to penetrate ocular tissues, especially the cornea. It has been used at concentrations of 0.001% to 0.01% in contact lens solutions as well as dry eye products. At clinically effective levels of preservative, POLYQUAD is approximately 10 times less toxic than BAC (120,169). Various in vitro tests and in vivo evaluations substantiate the safety of this compound (169,170,171). This preservative has been extremely useful for soft contact lens solutions because it has the least propensity to adsorb onto or absorb into these lenses, and it has practically a nonexistent potential for sensitization. Its adsorption/absorption with high water and high ionic lenses can be resolved by carefully balancing formulation components (172).

Chlorhexidine Chlorhexidine, a bisbiguanide, has been demonstrated to be somewhat less toxic than BAC and thimerosal at clinically relevant concentrations (120,122,127, 173,174). This work was confirmed in a series of in vitro and in vivo experiments (169,175–177).

Polyaminopropyl biguanide This preservative is also comparatively new to ophthalmic formulations and has been used as a disinfectant in contact lens solutions. Polyaminopropyl biguanide (polyhexamethyl biguanide) also is a polymeric compound that has a low toxicity potential at the concentrations generally used in these solutions (170,178,179).

Cetrimonium chloride This preservative has been used in a dry eye treatment and was shown in a clinical study to have the same biocompatibility as another marketed preparation (180). Cetrimonium chloride (0.01%) produced the same corneal and conjunctival changes after one-month ocular administration in rats as the effective levels of other major preservatives (141).

Purite This preservative is a stabilized oxychloro complex and is used in brimonidine purite 0.1% and 0.15% and purite-preserved artificial tears. Purite has demonstrated antimicrobial efficacy and is reported to induce less corneal epithelial damage than BAC in a rabbit model (181,182). Clinical trials have also reported purite-containing formulations to be well tolerated (183,184).

SofZia This preservative system has been formulated in both OTC pharmaceuticals and in TRAVATAN Z® solution, an IOP-lowering medication. SofZia contains boric acid, propylene glycol, sorbitol, and zinc chloride. It has been reported that SofZia is less irritating than BAC (185–187).

OCULAR DRUG TRANSPORT AND DELIVERY

Modes of Transport

Passive transport or simple diffusion of molecules is a transport process dependent on water and lipid solubility, size of the molecule, and concentration gradient across the cellular membrane. No energy is expended in the process, and transport will cease when the concentrations of the molecules on both sides of the membrane are equal. Passive transport is not inhibited by metabolic inhibitors (inhibiting ATP production or utilization) or by competitive substrates. In general, hydrophilic molecules pass through proteinaceous pores in the cellular membrane, and lipophilic molecules diffuse through the lipid portion of the membrane. Transport through the pores is limited by the pore size that is specific to each tissue. The low lipid solubility of ionized molecules may be increased by altering the degree of ionization with changes in solution pH. Passive transport is important in diffusion of drugs across the cornea and in nutrient uptake across the corneal endothelium.

Active transport is an energy-dependent process requiring ATP, is carrier mediated, and is capable of transporting substrates against a concentration gradient. Macromolecular carriers are membrane bound and have varying degrees of substrate specificity. The carrier reversibly binds to the substrate, transports and releases the molecule on the other side of the membrane and returns to the original state. These characteristics also make active transport subject to metabolic inhibitors, competitive inhibition from other similar substrates, and saturation at high substrate concentrations. Active transport in the corneal endothelium is essential to maintain proper stromal hydration.

Facilitated transport combines some properties of both mechanisms discussed above. This type of transport is carrier mediated so that there is substrate specificity, a transport maximum, and competitive inhibition. However, facilitated transport is not energy dependent and is unable to transport a substrate against a concentration gradient.

Biological Barriers and Fundamentals of Passive Transport

Membranes as Barriers

In a very general sense, biological membranes serve an extremely useful function, effectively walling off the body from invasive and destructive pathological microorganisms as well as noxious influences of the environment. They allow tissues to customize their environments. Dosage forms are therefore devised so that either the therapeutic agent is introduced by a physical or chemical means that penetrates the barrier and introduces the drug behind the impediment or the drug design or dosage form itself enables the therapeutic agent to penetrate the barrier. If the latter is the preferred means, both the drug and the vehicle need to avoid producing a significant toxic insult to the barrier, lest that barrier be compromised in its ability to prevent intrusion of foreign chemical or biological agents or be rendered sufficiently uncomfortable that neither the delivery is effective nor the patient compliant.

The significance of the barrier function of membranes has been the topic of considerable research. The blood-brain barrier and the blood-retinal barrier are well understood, and the microscopic structures imparting and controlling barrier properties have been quite thoroughly investigated and the science reviewed (11,188,189). The structures and functions of ocular membranes specific to transport associated with ophthalmic drug administration also have been topics of extensive research (11,190,191).

The most common means of administering drugs to the eye is by topical administration of agents capable of penetrating the cornea and targeting the appropriate tissue for either physiological or medicinal effect (192,193). The trilaminar structure of the transparent avascular cornea has been described previously. The corneal epithelium exposes a hydrophobic barrier to hydrophilic therapeutic agents and a hydrophilic corneal stromal barrier to hydrophobic agents. Nonetheless, as the models considered below rationalize, low-molecular-weight therapeutic agents of modest hydrophobicity and high water solubility are often capable of penetrating the eye and may be effective ocular therapeutic agents if their potency, or receptor affinity if that is appropriate, can be maintained in the accommodation to these requirements.

More recently alternative routes of drug administration have been sought and utilized. Scientists are developing technologies to circumvent the constraints imposed on molecular weight, water solubility, and modest hydrophobicity by the conventional transcorneal route. Patents exist for ophthalmically acceptable penetration enhancers. More water-soluble therapeutic agents now in use for glaucoma appear to achieve approximately equal access by both scleral-limbal and transcorneal routes of administration (194,195). Research is ongoing to understand and utilize scleral administration of therapeutic agents; the role of hydrostatic pressure on the transport of both water and drug has been investigated to determine the classes of therapeutic agent for which this mode of delivery may be utilized (196–199). One consequence will be the determination of the diminished transport constraints imposed by a barrier from which the hydrophobic layer is absent. Both academic and industrial investigations have led to technologies for scleral implants and sustained release.

Role of Hydrodynamics

Basic hydrodynamic phenomena govern the duration of exposure of corneal and conjunctival membranes to the therapeutic agents. Rapid clearance provides a temporal barrier to drug delivery.

Drainage of the drop through the nasolacrimal system into the gastrointestinal tract begins immediately on instillation. This takes place when either reflex tearing or the dosage form causes the volume of fluid in the cul-de-sac and precorneal tears to exceed the normal lacrimal volume of 7 to 10 μL. Reference to Figure 7 indicates the pathway for this drainage. The excess fluid volume enters the superior and inferior lacrimal puncta, moves

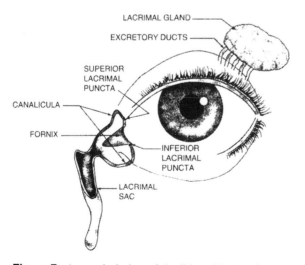

Figure 7 Anatomical view of the lids and lacrimal systems.

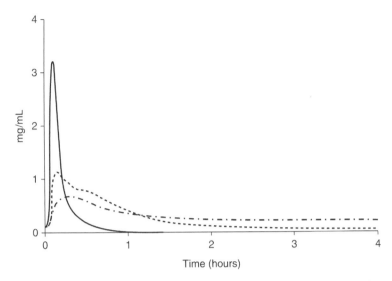

Figure 8 Comparison of time-release profiles from three different preparations of betaxolol: (- - - -) drug solution representing marketed product, (- - - -) suspension formulation, (- - - -) gel formulation.

down the canaliculi into the lacrimal sac, and continues into the gastrointestinal tract. It is due to this mechanism that significant systemic effects for certain potent ophthalmic medications have been reported (200–202). This also is the mechanism by which a patient may occasionally sense a bitter or salty taste, typical of therapeutic ammonium salts, following the use of eyedrops. The influence of drop size on bioavailability has been investigated thoroughly for conventional formulations and is significant (203). Even for nonconventional viscoelastic formulations, drop volume can be expected to influence efficacy and needs to be optimized (204). The clinical significance of drainage is so well recognized that manual NLO has been recommended as a means of improving the therapeutic index of antiglaucoma medications (205). Once the dynamics of tear-flow excess have taken their course, steady-state hydrodynamics can be expected.

Loss of drug from a precorneal volume has been investigated both in vivo and in vitro. These studies relate to both design of dosage forms as well as investigations of transport, bioavailability, and pharmacokinetics. Simultaneous release profiles of drugs and adjuvant from an artificial in vitro reservoir, designed with its volume to be characteristic of the eye, can be correlated simply with exposure for transmembrane transport (206). An example of release profiles and the influence of dosage form from one of these models, the Controlled Release Analytical System (CRAS) model, is shown in Figure 8.

Simple hydrodynamic analysis of the in vitro mechanism indicates that the elution concentration, in the absence of absorption, is a linear kinetic process, with a release profile that scales as the ratio of the tear production to the volume of the tear reservoir, $\dot{V}_T/V_T$. Specifically

$$N_E(t) = N_I \left[1 - \exp\left(\frac{-\dot{V}_T \cdot t}{V_T} \right) \right] \tag{1}$$

where $N_E(t)$ is the time-dependent total amount eluted from volume in time t, V_T the volume of the reservoir, $\dot{V}_T$ the flow rate through reservoir (alternatively Q_T), and N_I the

Design and evaluation of ophthalmic products

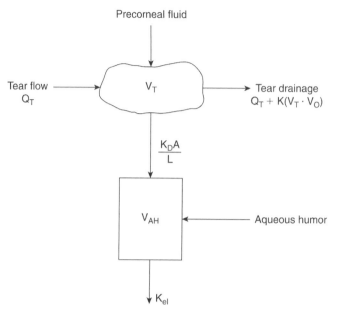

Figure 9 Pharmacokinetic scheme for ocular absorption, distribution, and elimination.

amount of drug in reservoir at time zero, and where the complementary amount, the amount of drug in the reservoir, is defined as

$$N_T(t) \equiv N_I - N_E(t) \text{ is the amount contained in reservoir at time } t \qquad (2)$$

which is characteristic of the stirred-tank chemical reactor models (207–209). Combining these containment profiles, $N_T(t)$, with diffusional transmembrane transport, yields expected tissue profiles. The time-dependent concentrations are dictated by both containment profile and tissue affinities, and the magnitude is often dominated by transmembrane flux (see "Mechanisms and Models of Transmembrane Transport"). A pictorial representation of the processes is shown in Figure 9. Pharmacokinetic modeling with this scheme has been successful in fitting the aqueous humor levels of pilocarpine following topical administration (Fig. 10) (203). Although this type of data fitting has been quite successful, there have not been a sufficient number of systematic studies to determine the role of every molecular and physiological property influencing each of the various pharmacokinetic parameters. The pharmacokinetic consequences of these competing transport processes have been reviewed recently (210). Elaborate analyses of such data using Green's function solutions, for responses to unit impulse, can be integrated as a means of generating responses to more complicated dosage regimens (211,212). Alternatively, and more simply, the differential equations representing the coupled effects of instillation, hydrodynamics and drainage, and membrane transport can be readily integrated numerically to provide predictions of the impact of drug and dosage form on bioavailability (11).

Mechanisms and Models of Transmembrane Transport

At a physical level, the description of the cornea is as a transparent, avascular tissue that, with the adherent precorneal tear film, is the first refracting surface operant in the process of sight. At a morphological and chemical level, the description is of a three-layered

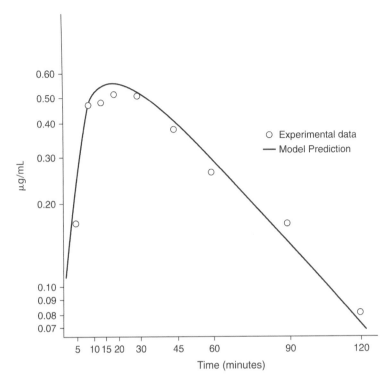

Figure 10 Comparison of predicted and experimental aqueous humor concentrations following topical administration of pilocarpine.

structure: a multilayered, lipid-rich epithelium, a well-hydrated and lipid-poor stroma, and a lipid-rich endothelium of one-cell-layer thickness. Differential studies of the relative lipid densities for these three corneal layers have shown that the densities of lipid in epithelium and endothelium are approximately 40 times as large as that in the stroma (213), although more recent studies suggest that the disparity may be less (214). This can be a primary physiological factor influencing drug penetration through the cornea and into the aqueous humor. For a topically administered drug to traverse an intact cornea and to appear in the aqueous humor, it must possess dual or differential solubility. But as evermore explicit descriptions have been developed by histologists, microscopic anatomists, and electron microscopists, increasingly detailed mechanisms of transport through these tissues have been envisioned and tested.

The multilayered corneal epithelium consists of cells attached by microstructural junctions of well-established morphology and function and separated by water-filled intercellular spaces. Drug transport through such an environment can be imagined to consist of two competing pathways. Predominantly water-soluble compounds presumably pass through the tortuously connected aqueous channels, establishing a path through the maze from epithelial surface to stroma, a paracellular pathway. Predominantly lipid-soluble compounds presumably pass by surface diffusion along the lipid surfaces, passing in a tortuous path from adjacent cell to cell, the transcellular pathway. In either case boundaries of lipid junctions for water-soluble compounds or aqueous channels for lipid-soluble compounds would be more readily surmounted by compounds with shared functionality. The characteristics of diffusion through and along such well-defined structures are well known, and the statistical mechanics of percolation phenomena governing such random paths has been well investigated.

For example, several recent studies have attempted to provide a molecular basis for the earlier largely empirical observations and essentially macroscopic continuum analyses (215,216). For the stroma and sclera, much is known about their structure and composition. These tissues consist primarily of water, collagen, and glycosaminoglycans wherein the lamellar order is derived primarily from collagen, which has a fivefold organizational hierarchy. The collagen molecule consists of three α-chains of peptides. These α-chains are organized into ordered, relatively stiff collagen fibrils, typically 50 nm in diameter. Many fibrils, along with proteoglycan-rich ground substance, compose collagen fibers, which are about a half-micron in diameter and in stroma and sclera are organized into nearly lamellar sheets (217–219). These membranes, over which there will be hydrodynamic pressure gradients, will be barriers to fluid flow. With the administration of drugs, these membranes, over which there will be concentration gradients, will be barriers to molecular diffusional flow. The effects of fibrous obstructions on both fluid flow and solute diffusion have been the topic of intense research in chemical engineering and physics. The flow and diffusional characteristics have been related to the relative dimensions and volume fractions of the fibers and the permeabilities (which is influenced by the state of hydration) of the different materials to the solvent and solutes, respectively. The diffusional characteristics of solute molecules will be influenced by the relative solubilities of these molecules in the different environments; more water-soluble solutes will diffuse more rapidly through the highly hydrated stroma.

These effects, specialized for the geometries and materials properties of the collagen-rich stroma and sclera, have been calculated in a recent paper by Edwards and Prausnitz (215). They also modeled diffusion across the corneal endothelium assuming that the major path was between cells and that this was governed by the most restrictive portion, the diffusion through the tight junctions. The diffusional flow was predicted based on the density and width of these parallel channels. These authors generalized this description for both corneal endothelium and epithelium by allowing a balance between the paracellular and transcellular pathways. The only difference between the epithelial and endothelial paracellular pathways was the geometry of the junctions and their number, larger for the multilayered epithelium. The transcellular pathway was modeled from the known geometry of the cells, which determined the length of the diffusional pathway and the partitioning characteristics of the molecules.

The cumulative effects of these barriers, and the resistance to flow they produce, were computed, and it was demonstrated that these macroscopically derived laws applied at molecular dimensions were able to provide semiquantitative agreement with the available data. While further tests of these models will undoubtedly provide refinements to our understanding, the agreement supports our understanding of the basic phenomena regulating transport of therapeutically active substances through these barriers, and the role of disease states that impact hydrodynamic pressure on the efficacy of drug delivery.

Passive Absorption and Intraocular Delivery

Considerations Influencing Drug Design for Topical Administration
From the perspective of drug design for conventional topical delivery, several requirements need to be satisfied by ophthalmic therapeutic agents. The drug must be (*i*) both biochemically and pharmacologically potent, (*ii*) nontoxic to both ocular and systemic tissues, (*iii*) sufficiently stable, so that neither significant loss in potency from diminished availability nor increase in toxicity from by-products of degradation arises, (*iv*) targetable either to tissues and location of primary disease-state etiology or to sites responsible for

symptomatic response, and (v) sufficiently compatible with the dosage form, and with the tissues exposed to it, to achieve an effective pharmacokinetic tissue profile.

Often the demand for such a complement of properties requires a hierarchical strategy in which only the broadest possible limits are satisfied by the less demanding design requirements. For example, topical administration assists in limiting toxicity while improving targeting and pharmacokinetic response. On the other hand, the requirements for effective absorption of such topical ophthalmic medications often place significant demands on the physical, chemical, and transport characteristics of the drug, which in most cases was designed primarily to satisfy more stringent biological, physiological, and pharmacological criteria. Simple guidelines can be appreciated readily by examining the factors influencing absorption of an antiglaucoma agent administered in the conventional manner as drops into the cul-de-sac, discussed in the next section (220).

Efficacy is also influenced by minimizing factors that diminish availability. The first factor reducing drug availability is loss of drug from the palpebral fissure. This takes place by spillage of drug from the eye and its removal by the nasolacrimal drainage. The normal volume of tears in the human eye is estimated to be approximately 7 μL, and if blinking occurs, the human eye can accommodate a volume of up to 30 μL, without spillage from the palpebral fissure. With an estimated drop volume of 50 μL, 70% of the administered volume of two drops can be seen to be expelled from the eye by overflow. If blinking occurs, the residual volume of 10 μL indicates that 90% of the administered volume of two drops will be expelled within the first several minutes (38,221).

Many technologies have been devised, some discussed below, for modifying the dosage form as a means of slowing the escape of drug from the precorneal location from which it can be transported to tissues influencing ocular physiology. In addition, other approaches have also been recommended. For example, temporary manual punctal occlusion immediately after instillation of drug transiently prevents drainage of the enriched tears from the puncta. For patients with dry eye, often permanent occlusion, which is implemented either by cautery or one of several designs of punctal plug, results in a diminished rate of tear clearance. Transient occlusion can be expected to influence drug delivery only modestly and be effective only in rather specific circumstances, when either the molecular weight or the aqueous solubility of the therapeutic agent is high. For circumstances in which the therapeutic agent is reasonably lipophilic, the kinetics of absorption by transepithelial transport can be quite rapid (see "A Generalized Phenomenological Transport Model and Simple Consequences").

A second factor reducing drug availability is the drainage associated with hydrodynamic flow of tears through the precorneal space and cul-de-sac, discussed earlier. A third and more difficult problem for delivery by nondirectional technologies and devices is the undesirable adsorption and absorption by nearby noncorneal tissues competing for therapeutic agents. These include absorption by adjacent palpebral and bulbar conjunctiva, with concomitant rapid removal from ocular tissues by peripheral blood flow. For example, the extensive vascularity of the uvea underlies the bulbar conjunctiva, a mucous membrane, and the sclera, a white tissue providing a tough outer covering (222). Binding of drug to either external sites, like the tear polymers such as mucins or lysozyme, or internal tissues, like the sclera, can be detrimental to efficacy.

To the extent that these competing and detrimental effects can be controlled, delivery can be enhanced. But their control is inconsequential if the molecular properties regulating transmembrane transport are not selected in a manner to facilitate corneal permeation, the topic of the next section. Finally, in competition with the three foregoing forms of therapeutically ineffective drug removal from the palpebral fissure is the transcorneal absorption of drug, often the route most effective in bringing drug to the anterior portion of the eye. Although transport of hydrophilic and macromolecular drugs has been reported to occur by limbal or scleral routes, often this is at rates significantly reduced from those expected for transcorneal transport of conventional, modestly lipophilic agents of low molecular weight (19,26,32,210,223,224). Even here, transmembrane transport is a significant requirement for availability.

A Generalized Phenomenological Transport Model and Simple Consequences

One of the key parameters for correlating molecular structure and chemical properties with bioavailability has been transcorneal flux, or alternatively, the corneal permeability coefficient. The epithelium has been modeled as a lipid barrier (possibly, with a limited number of aqueous "pores" that, for this physical model, serve as the equivalent of the extracellular space in a more physiological description) and the stroma as an aqueous barrier (Fig. 11). The endothelium is very thin and porous compared with the epithelium (18) and often has been ignored in the analysis, although mathematically it can be included as part of the lipid barrier. Diffusion through bilayer membranes of various structures has been modeled for some time (225) and adapted to ophthalmic applications more recently (226,227). For a series of molecules of similar size, it was shown that the permeability increases with octanol-water distribution (or partition) coefficient until a plateau is reached. Modeling of this type of data has led to the earlier statement that drugs need to be both oil and water soluble. If pores are not included in the analysis, the steady-state corneal flux, J_S, can be approximated by

$$J_s = \frac{P\,C_w}{(P\,l_s\,/\,D_s) + (l_e\,/\,D_e)} \tag{3}$$

where C_w is the concentration of drug indoor phase, l_s and l_e are the stromal and epithelial thickness, respectively, D_s and D_e the corresponding diffusion coefficients, and P the distribution coefficients.

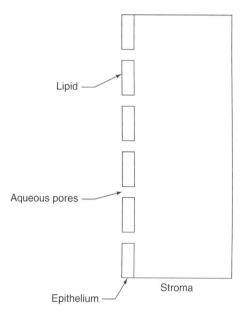

Figure 11 Schematic diagram of the physical model for transcorneal peremeation; features are not to scale.

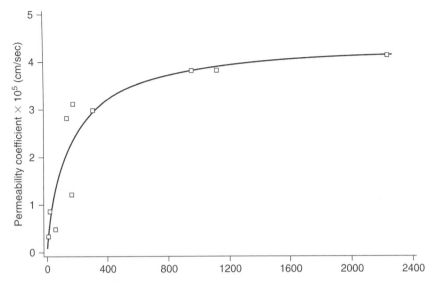

Figure 12 Predicted versus experimental values for corneal steroid permeability as a function of partition coefficient.

The permeability coefficient K_{per} is just the flux divided by C_w. It is apparent that the permeability coefficient is linear with P for small distribution coefficients and constant for large P. Thus, for small P the epithelium is the barrier, and for large P the stroma is the barrier. A fit for steroid permeability is shown in Figure 12, where the regression analysis gave $D_e = 1.4 \times 10^{-9}$ cm^2/sec and $D_s = 2.0 \times 10^{-6}$ cm^2/sec for $l_e = 4 \times 10^{-3}$ cm and $l_s = 3.6 \times 10^{-2}$ cm (228). These values for the diffusion coefficients are reasonable compared with those of aqueous gels and lipid membranes.

A simple estimate of the diffusion coefficients can be approximated from examining the effects of molecular size on transport through a continuum for which there is an energy cost of displacing solvent. Since the molecular weight dependence of the diffusion coefficients for polymers obeys a power law equation (229), a similar form was chosen for the corneal barriers. That is, the molecular weight (M) dependence of the diffusion coefficients was written as

$$D_e = D_e^{(0)} M^\alpha$$
$$D_s = D_s^{(0)} M^\delta$$

(4)

Using regression analysis on a data set of about 50 different molecules, it was found that $\alpha = -4.4$, $\delta = -0.5$, $D_e^{(0)} = 12$ cm^2/sec, and $D_s^{(0)} = 2.5 \times 10^{-5}$ cm^2/sec (19). A graphic representation of the effect of relative molecular mass (M_r) and distribution coefficient on corneal permeability is shown in Figure 13. One observes a rapid reduction in permeability coefficient with decreasing P and increasing M_r. The addition of pores to the model, a mathematical construct, is necessary to account for permeability of polar molecules such as mannitol and cromolyn. These would also be required for correlating effects of compounds, such as BAC, which may compromise the epithelial barrier by increasing the volume of the extracellular space.

Another perspective provided by this model is the effect of three physicochemical parameters: solubility, distribution coefficient, and molecular mass on transcorneal flux. All of these properties can be influenced by molecular design. The effects of these properties are illustrated in Figure 13 in which the logarithm of the flux is plotted as a

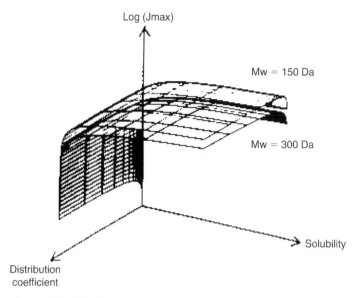

Figure 13 This figure illustrates the "mesa" response resulting for the diffusion model. Two plateau functions corresponding to different M_r are shown.

function of solubility and distribution coefficient for two different M_r values. Several features of the model are depicted, and these qualitative, or semiquantitative, aspects presumably encompass the principles of corneal permeation.

Inferred from this model is the relative independence of the effects of solubility and partitioning. For each property there is a characteristic threshold above which the log of the flux increases more slowly than below it, and the value of the threshold for one variable is not very dependent on the value of the other variable. This tabletop perspective has led to the name mesa model. The relative independence signifies that neither property can totally compensate for a deficiency in the other. This is not to say that these properties are independent of one another in a chemical sense, quite the contrary. However, in the hypothetical sense, if one property were varied independently of the other, then the consequences on flux are relatively independent. Clearly, dependence on molecular mass, even for relatively low-molecular-mass agents, can be significant.

Ex vivo studies of transcorneal transport in animal models have been used to establish the characteristics of passive diffusional motion, the conventional means by which drugs reach internal ocular tissues. Although such analysis neglects the complications of tear flow, tear drainage, nonproductive membrane absorption, elimination from the aqueous humor, and so forth, measurements of corneal transport measurements have been important in establishing correlations of model calculations with experimental measurements of transmembrane transport. Modifications (230) of the classical ex vivo experiments of transport across excised, but metabolizing, rabbit corneas (18,24,26,231) have provided information both about targeting of similar molecules from the same pharmacological class (19) and confirmation of the balance of different anatomical pathways for accession (32).

The rough brushstroke agreement between model and experiment is illustrated by the results shown in (Fig. 14), for which the correspondence of theoretical with experimental permeability coefficients for the compounds listed in Table 2 and β-adrenergic blockers studied by Lee (48,232) and Schoenwald (26) are plotted. The calculated values utilized

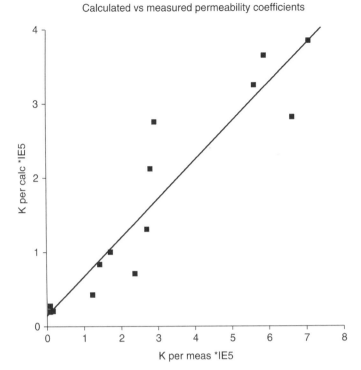

Figure 14 Plot of data in Table 2, the theoretically computed permeability coefficient versus that measured. The larger influence on flux is often the range of solubility, which can increase the range in flux by several orders of magnitude.

Table 2 Permeability of β-Adrenergic Blockers

Compound	Chemical formula	Molecular weight	Distribution coefficient	$K_{per}^{calc} \times IE5$ (cm/sec)	$K_{per}^{meas} \times IE5$ (cm/sec)
Acebutolol	$C_{18}H_{28}N_2O_4$	336.43	1.58	0.28	0.085
Alprenolol	$C_{15}H_{23}NO_2$	249.34	8.92	2.09	2.86
Atenolol	$C_{14}H_{22}N_2O_3$	266.34	0.03	0.20	0.068
Betaxolol	$C_{18}H_{29}NO_3$	307.44	60.3	2.72	3.02
Bevantolol	$C_{20}H_{27}NO_3$	345.44	154.8	2.78	6.76
Bufuralol	$C_{16}H_3NO_2$	261.36	204.2	3.82	7.24
Labetolol	$C_{19}H_{24}N_2O_3$	328.41	7.77	0.82	1.43
Levobunolol	$C_{17}H_{25}NO_3$	291.39	5.25	0.99	1.74
Metoprolol	$C_{15}H_{25}NO_3$	267.38	1.91	0.69	2.40
Nadolol	$C_{17}H_{27}NO_4$	309.42	0.15	0.17	0.10
Oxprenolol	$C_{15}H_{23}NO_3$	265.34	4.90	1.28	2.75
Penbutolol	$C_{18}H_{29}NO_2$	291.44	338.84	3.62	6.03
Propranolol	$C_{16}H_{21}NO_2$	259.34	41.69	3.22	5.75
Sotalol	$C_{12}H_{20}N_2O_3S$	272.36	0.06	0.20	0.16
Timolol	$C_{13}H_{24}N_4O_3S$	316.42	2.19	0.42	1.23

the physical model with pores (228). Characteristic of correlations of this type is the slope's value, less than 1. The origin of the smaller calculated values of permeability coefficients is unknown. A reasonable conjecture, however, is that the estimated diffusion coefficients, that is, the laws presented in equation (4), on which the permeability is based, are not quite correct for the drugs in different ocular environments. The predictability of the model is useful both for providing approximate values and distinguishing departure from simple diffusional transport. Also apparent from a comparison of the last two figures (Figs. 13 and 14) is the significance of solubility, since it is the value of C_w that controls flux by orders of magnitude.

A significant inference from the model is that if, as is the conventional behavior of a family of molecules, the solubility decreases with an increase in distribution coefficient, eventually this effect will profoundly reduce the transcorneal flux. Alternatively and conceptually, for any class of molecules with a desirable physiological response and without significant differences in potency or therapeutic index, the member of that family with the greatest promise for ophthalmic application is the one with lowest molecular weight, highest distribution coefficient, and highest aqueous solubility. However, since the last two requirements are in general inconsistent (the most soluble molecule is generally the one with lowest partition coefficient), the model helps select the molecular structure for which the flux is greatest.

Perhaps as more is learned about the molecular requirements for binding therapeutic agents to active sites of macromolecules as part of the intention to control physiological function, these simple transport requirements can be incorporated into the molecular design.

Role of Specialized Formulations

Many materials and specialized formulations have been devised with the intention of improving delivery of drugs to intraocular tissues by means of the transcorneal route. Carriers have been used both alone and in conjunction with viscosifying or responsive formulations to control concentration of the active therapeutic compound or sustain delivery. As calculations clearly demonstrate and experiments confirm, the impact on total drug availability for such systems is crucially dependent on the degree to which the vehicle is capable of sustaining residence time of the drug or drug carrier in the eye (183). The historical and current challenge remains to devise spontaneously responsive systems that are capable of being retained in the eye, sustaining the presence of the carrier without degrading its reservoir and delivery characteristics, and without producing such conventional side effects as blurring or undesirable residues.

In recent years a barrage of technologies has been developed for sustaining delivery of drug to the cornea. Corneal collagen shields and contact lenses loaded with drug have been placed directly on the cornea. But undesirable side effects including blurring, dumping of drug, packaging, and storage problems have prevented these technologies from being successful in the marketplace. Responsive polymeric systems have been more successful to date. Polymers whose solubilities and interactions are dominated by hydrogen bonding can be controlled with temperature, whose solubilities are dominated by coacervation-type interactions can be controlled by the concentration of the complementary polymer, whose solubilities are dominated by weak acid ionization can be controlled by pH, and whose solubilities are dominated by ion-pairing condensation can be controlled by ionic strength or even specific ion concentrations. Those systems utilizing mechanisms less impacted by the environment have proven more widely applicable.

Active Transport, a Potential Mechanism for Specific Structures

As more is learned about accession of drugs into the eye, it is becoming more obvious that passive diffusion through the cornea is not the only pathway likely to be exploited for future delivery of drugs. Many drugs are known either to bind to or to be taken up by and accumulated in epithelial cells. Interesting work is emerging in the areas of facilitated transport in which enhancers are used to diminish diffusional barriers temporarily (233,234) and in the areas of active transport in which drug carriers can be employed for transport of larger molecules (230).

As evermore potent therapeutic agents are developed, concentrations required diminish and importance of drug targeting, as a means of reducing systemic toxicity, increases. For biochemical and therapeutic agents included in specific classes of amino acids, dipeptides, polypeptides with resemblance to specific peptide sequences (e.g., the undecapeptide cyclosporin A), small cationic molecules, or monocarboxylates, and nucleosides, there are known transporters, antiports, cotransporters, etc., in conjunctiva and sometimes in cornea that at low concentrations of a drug may actively contribute to controlling flux into or out of specific tissues (235–239, 236, p. 1436). Carrier-mediated transport is not restricted to ocular conjunctiva and cornea, of course, but has been identified in other ocular tissues, specifically the RPE, as well as in numerous systemic tissues such as gastric, intestinal, hepatic, renal, and cardiac tissues, and in some ex vivo cell culture lines. As a consequence, information concerning structural and geometric specificity, co- or counterion requirements, proton and energy dependence, pump capacity (saturability), total ion flux and current, and directionality of mediated transport have been provided by biochemists, physiologists, and pharmacologists studying a variety of human and mammalian tissues.

For conventional therapeutic agents the presence of active drug transport is either nonexistent or obscured, since at high concentrations while both active and passive transport may occur concurrently, the passive component is the dominating and overwhelming fraction. However, as the concentration decreases, as it will for potent agents for which concentrations in the micromolar range may be adequate, some of these agents will experience facilitated, active, carrier-mediated transport. For example, the flux may be expected to have a complicated concentration dependence:

$$J = \frac{J_{\max}}{[K_{\mathrm{m}}/(C)] + 1} + K_{\mathrm{d}}(C) \tag{5}$$

where $J_{\max}$ is the maximum saturable flux from the active transport process, K_{m} the Michaelis–Menten constant, and K_{d} the passive diffusive permeation rate (236, p. 1436). Note both K_{m} and K_{d} are temperature dependent; however, the temperature dependence of K_{m} is much greater, so that the diagnostic for the presence of active transport is the essentially complete loss of the active component by the time the temperature is reduced to 4°C.

Some measure of the importance of active transport is the diversity of systems where it has been observed. For example, carrier-mediated transport of L-argenine, a substrate for nitric oxide (NO) synthase, can impact the concentrations of NO, a neurotransmitter. The same carrier, present in the conjunctiva, can be inhibited by competitive inhibitors such as nitro-L-argenine. This transporter appears to be coupled to the transport of Na^+ ions, and directionally transports the inhibitor preferentially into the tissues from the mucosal exterior surface. The utility of such a path might be to regulate production of NO in vivo and thereby control inflammation, a complication, for example, in Sjögren's syndrome. The potential for delivering a therapeutic agent to the uveal tract is also promising. Nucleoside transport for uridine has also been demonstrated to have similar directionality, preferential flow from mucosal to serosal, or apical to basolateral, sides of the conjunctival cells. Its role is presumably to salvage nucleosides from the tears and might be able to be exploited for compounds with antiviral activity.

Not all transporters, however, show the same preferential directions. Lee and coworkers also have discovered a pump glycoprotein in the conjunctiva with preferential flux directed toward the mucosal side of the tissue. This transporter has been shown to restrict conjunctival absorption of therapeutic agents, cyclosporin A, verapamil, and dexamethasone, for example. In some circumstances, transient inhibition of such xenobiotic transporters might be an effective means of increasing the efficacy of particular classes of therapeutic agents.

Delivery to the Vitreous and Posterior Segment

Intravitreal Administration

The most direct means of delivering drug to the vitreous humor and retina is by intravitreal injection. While this method of administration has been associated with serious side effects, such as endophthalmitis, cataract, hemorrhage, and retinal detachment (198), aggravated by the conventional need for serial injections further increasing the risk, intravitreal injection continues to be the mode of choice for treatment of acute intraocular therapy and has become the standard of care for providing treatment of several chronic ocular diseases, such as age-related macular degeneration (AMD) and associated retinal edema. For example, Lucentis (ranibizumab), injected monthly, can be highly effective in decreasing the thickness of the edematous retina in AMD patients.

In response to well-known risks of recurring intravitreal injections, intravitreal inserts have been, and are continuing to be, developed to deliver drug for protracted periods following implantation. The first was the Vitrasert® (Bausch & Lomb), delivering ganciclovir for treatment of cytomegalovirus (CMV) retinitis (240,241). Later, a similar device, the RETISERT™ (Fig. 15), was developed to deliver fluocinolone acetonide for

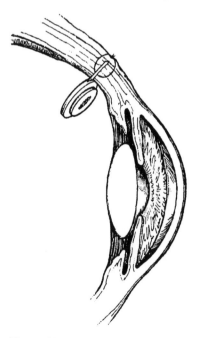

Figure 15 Drawing showing the optimum placement of an intravitreal sustained-release device in the eye. *Source*: From Ref. 240.

the treatment of uveitis (242). Surmodics' I-Vation™ device is a corkscrew-like thumbtack and has been used to incorporate triamcinolone acetonide for treatment of diabetic macular edema (DME) (243). Neurotech encapsulated cell technology is being investigated for delivery of ciliary neurotrophic factor (CNTF) for neurodegenerative retinal diseases (244). Because these devices must be surgically implanted and subsequently removed, biodegradable alternatives also are being evaluated. Two such devices under development are Allergan's Posurdex®, delivering dexamethasone (245), and Alimera Sciences Medidur™, delivering fluocinolone acetonide, both drugs used for the treatment of DME.

Owing to the nonstirred nature of the vitreal space, the kinetic behavior of intravitreally delivered drugs is governed by mechanisms of diffusion, hydrostatic and osmotic pressure, convective flow, and active transport (246). Diffusion is the predominant mechanism for transvitreal movement for small- to moderately sized molecules, such as fluorescein or dextran (18,246), with kinetics similar to that observed in water or saline. Although low-level convective flow has been observed within the vitreous, this flow has only a negligible effect on transvitreal movement in comparison with diffusion for drug molecules of low molecular weight (247,248). However, the change in viscoelasticity with age might increase the contribution of convective flow.

Two primary mechanisms of vitreal drug distribution and elimination are (*i*) diffusion from the lens region toward the retina with elimination via the retina-choroid-sclera and (*ii*) anterior diffusion with elimination via the hyaloid membrane and posterior chamber (18). Distribution to the retina from an intravitreal injection site is relatively slow, considering juxtaposition of the vitreous and retina, with the time for maximum drug concentration (t_{max}) in retina typically achieved at 4 to 12 hours, and reflects the inefficiency of diffusion over the distances encountered within the vitreous body. For example, ranibizumab, an ocular specific monoclonal VEGF antibody, distributes to the retina with t_{max} of 6 to 24 hours. While relatively rapid therapeutically, this is slow compared with the rate of redistribution in stirred compartments. (249).

The dominant path of distribution and elimination in the vitreous depends on a molecule's physicochemical properties and its substrate affinity. Lipophilic compounds, such as fluorescein (250) or dexamethasone (251), and compounds subject to active transport mechanisms, tend to be eliminated via the retina (Fig. 16). On the other hand, hydrophilic substances, such as fluorescein glucuronide, and compounds with poor retinal permeability, such as fluorescein dextran, tend to exit the vitreous anteriorly through the hyaloid membrane into the posterior chamber and subsequently into the anterior chamber, where they are subject to elimination pathways for aqueous humor (250). In general, shorter vitreal half-lives are associated with elimination through the retina, with its high surface area, whereas longer half-lives are indicative of elimination through the hyaloid membrane.

Volume and location of an intravitreal injection can impact the patterns of ocular distribution and elimination. Friedrich et al. demonstrated a substantial effect of both on vitreal distribution and elimination of fluorescein and fluorescein glucuronide (252), with evaluation of four extreme positions and two injection volumes, 15 or 100 μL. The mean drug concentration remaining in the vitreous 24 hours postdose varied up to 3.8-fold with injection position, and increasing injection volume reduced this effect.

Aphakia and retinal inflammation are common pathophysiological conditions that can alter vitreal retention and kinetics of elimination. Elimination is generally faster in aphakic eyes, especially for drugs with low retinal permeability and injected in the near vicinity of the lens capsule. For example, Wingard et al. showed that intravitreally injected amphotericin B progressively accumulated in the sclera-choroid-retina in control

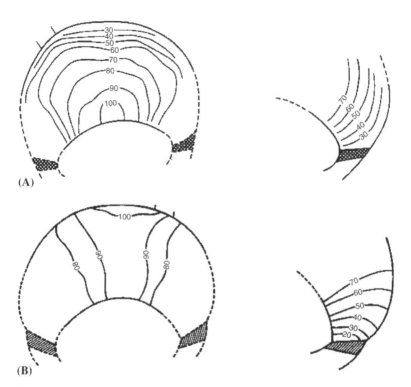

Figure 16 Contours of fluorescent intensity in frozen sections of the rabbit eye following 15 μL injection of marker solutions in the central vitreous cavity; injection was conducted through the superior rectus muscle. (**A**) Fifteen hours following injection of 0.2% sodium fluorescein. (**B**) Fourteen days following injection of 0.1% FITC-dextran, molecular weight 66,000. *Source*: From Ref. 250.

phakic eyes, a phenomenon not observed in aphakic eyes (253). Half-life in the whole phakic eye was 6.9 to 15.1 days, whereas that in the aphakic eye was only 1.8 days. Retinal inflammation is known to increase blood-retinal barrier permeability. Drug diffusivity and retinal permeability are important factors that determine elimination from the vitreous, particularly when the blood-retinal barrier is compromised (254).

In the case of infected eyes, Ben-Nun et al. demonstrated that the elimination rate of intravitreally injected gentamicin was greater in infected than normal eyes, attributed to alteration in blood-retinal barrier (255). The vitreal half-lives of ceftizoxime, ceftriaxone, ceftazidime, and cefepime in rabbits ranged from 5.7 to 20 hours in rabbits with uninflamed eyes and from 9.4 to 21.5 hours in rabbits with infected eyes (256).

As noted above, some compounds are actively and rapidly transported out of the vitreous through the blood-retinal barrier. The so-called efflux transporters of the blood-retinal barrier include P-glycoprotein (P-gp), multidrug resistance protein (MRP), and breast cancer–related protein (BRCP) (257). Evidence for active transport in the blood-retinal barrier has been provided by Mochizuki, who investigated the transport of indomethacin in the anterior uvea of the albino rabbit, both in vitro and in vivo, the latter following intravitreal injection (258). An energy-dependent carrier-mediated transport mechanism with low affinity was observed in the anterior uvea of the rabbit that could have accounted for the drug's rapid clearance (30%/hr) from the eye. In another example of active transport in the retina, Yoshida et al. characterized the active transport mechanism of the blood-retinal barrier by estimating its inward and outward permeability in monkey eyes using vitreous fluorophotometry following intravitreally injected fluorescein and fluorescein glucuronide (259). Outward permeability (P_{out}) was 7.7 and 1.7×10^{-4} cm/min, respectively, and P_{out}/P_{in} was 160 for fluorescein and 26 for fluorescein glucuronide. Moreover, intraperitoneal injection of probenecid caused a significant decrease in P_{out} for fluorescein but had no effect on fluorescein glucuronide P_{out}. Concomitant intraperitoneal injection of probenecid has been shown to prolong the vitreal half-life of the cephalosporins indicating a secretory mechanism. Barza et al. studied the ocular pharmacokinetics of carbenicillin, cefazolin, and gentamicin following intravitreal administration to rhesus monkeys (260).

The simplest model for exploring the kinetics of elimination assumes a well-stirred vitreous body; this applies almost exclusively to studies employing larger injection volumes, 100 μL or more, where the injection process itself can "stir" and alter the vitreal space. More relevant and sophisticated modeling explores diffusion through a relatively stagnant vitreous humor. For example, Ohtori and Tojo applied Fick's second law of diffusion to understand the process of elimination of dexamethasone sodium *m*-sulfobenzoate (DMSB) following injection in the rabbit vitreous body. They demonstrated that the rate of elimination was greater in vivo than in vitro (261). The model assumed a cylindrical vitreous body with three major elimination pathways: posterior aqueous chamber, retinal-choroidal-scleral membrane, and lens. The results showed that the retina, with its large surface area, is a major pathway for elimination. In a separate study, Tojo and Ohtori used the cylindrical model approach to demonstrate three potential pathways of elimination, including the annular gap, the lens, and the retina-choroid-sclera (262). The drug's site of injection or initial distribution profile affected retinal levels. Drug injected into the anterior segment of the vitreous was shown to exit rapidly through the annular gap into the posterior chamber. It follows that that drugs injected into the posterior vitreous can prolong therapeutic levels in the retina.

More precise modeling of vitreal pharmacokinetics employs the engineering technique of finite element analysis, which has now been conducted by a number of investigators (247,248,252,254,263–268). This approach accounts for the geometry and boundary conditions of the vitreous and predicts with relatively high resolution the concentration gradients. The power of these methods for accurately predicting the disposition of drug in the eye is illustrated in Figure 17, where finite element analysis was used to simulate the experiments of Ref. 250. When the retinal permeability is high, the contours resemble the experimental result for fluorescein, with the highest concentration immediately behind the lens. When the only pathway allowed is through the hyloid membrane, the contours resemble those obtained for the dextran polymer, with the highest concentration at the rear of the vitreous cavity. Other physiological details included in simulations have been the hydrodynamics of the aqueous humor (264), the influence of the directionality of release from an intravitreal device (247,265), dynamic partitioning of drug between various ocular tissues (266) (also simulated in Fig. 17), and IOP (247). Figure 18 demonstrates that IOP does not appreciably alter the concentration profile for small drug molecules. The very marked concentration gradients depicted have been confirmed by experimental measurements using nuclear magnetic resonance (NMR) imaging of a paramagnetic drug surrogate (269).

Periocular Administration

While intravitreal injection can be quite effective and has become the route of choice by retinal specialists, in spite of known risks, periocular drug administration, using

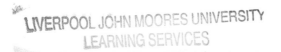

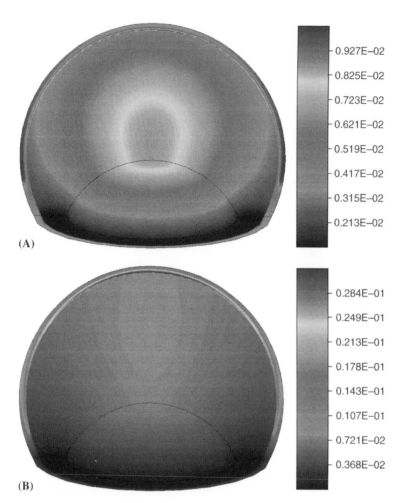

Figure 17 Finite element modeling of concentration profiles established after central intravitreal bolus injection, using FIDAP, 3D geometric model for the posterior rabbit eye, similar to Ref. 247, comprising the vitreous region, the retina, choroid, and sclera. At time zero, a spherical bolus of drug having unit concentration was placed in the center, behind the lens. (**A**) Contours of drug concentration simulated six hours after injection, assuming a reasonable value (250) for the diffusion coefficient (6×10^{-6} cm^2/sec) and efficient clearance by the choroid. Permeability across the lens and hyloid membrane is assumed to be negligible. (**B**) Simulated concentration profile two days after injection of FITC-dextran (diffusion coefficient 6×10^{-7} cm^2/sec), assuming zero retinal permeability and hyloid permeability 8×10^{-5} cm/sec. Drug partition coefficients in the vitreous, retina, choroid, and sclera were assumed to be roughly 1, 4, 4, and 2, respectively.

subconjunctival, sub-Tenon's, or retrobulbar injection, can be a reasonable alternative for delivering some drugs to the posterior segment (198).

Subconjunctival administration In addition to being less invasive compared with intravitreal injection, subconjunctival injection can be well suited to drug depots for prolonging the duration of drug therapy. Furthermore, subconjunctival administration may avoid much of the toxicity encountered with systemic administration, with drug concentrations in the eye typically substantially higher and systemic levels lower following subconjunctival versus systemic administration. For example, following

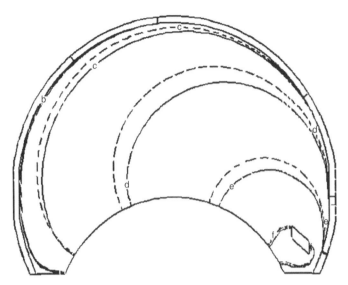

Figure 18 Finite element modeling of steady-state concentration profiles in the human eye (247) from a hypothetical device that releases drug toward the front of the eye, for a low-molecular-weight drug that is efficiently eliminated through the retina. Solid contours represent changes of 1 log unit with the eye under zero pressure. Dashed contours show the influence of the normotensive 5 mmHg intraocular pressure difference between the ocular interior and the episclera.

subconjunctival injection of 6-mercatopurine, mean peak concentrations in aqueous and vitreous were 15 and 10 times those following intravenous administration, while serum levels were about half (270). In another example, rabbits administered ^{14}C-5-fluoruracil either subconjunctivally or intravenously exhibited similar peak levels of parent in the serum and urine for the two routes; however, subconjunctival injection resulted in peak aqueous concentrations of 125 and 380 times that after intravenous injection (271).

The mechanism for ocular penetration following subconjunctival administration has been studied by Maurice and Mishima, who identify direct penetration into deeper tissues as the main absorption pathway (18), with the prerequisite condition that the sclera be saturated with drug. The consequential diffusion can occur by various routes: (*i*) laterally into corneal stroma and across the endothelium, (*ii*) across trabecular meshwork, (*iii*) through the iris stroma and across its anterior surface, (*iv*) into the ciliary body stroma and into newly generated aqueous humor, and (*v*) into the vitreous body via the pars plana and across its anterior hyaloid membrane (18). In addition to these pathways, direct transcorneal absorption can result from a mechanism dependent on the dose volume in which excess volume injected is squeezed out from the injection site with subsequent spillage onto the cornea. For example, Conrad and Robinson demonstrated that, at high injection volumes (>200 μL), the primary mechanism for uptake into the aqueous was reflux of the drug solution from the injection site followed by corneal absorption (272). At lower volumes, the mechanism involved reflux and transconjunctival penetration, permeation of the globe, and systemic absorption followed by redistribution.

Periocular injection (sub-Tenon's and retrobulbar) More posterior, sub-Tenon's or juxtascleral, injection involves periocular delivery of drug, usually forming a depot, between the sub-Tenon's capsule and sclera or episclera. This route conveniently places drug in very close proximity to, or in direct contact with, the sclera. Given that the sclera is quite permeable to a wide range of molecular weight compounds, most drugs easily diffuse through the sclera to underlying tissues (198,273). However, the diffusion of drug from the dose site can be highly localized, so the preferred location of dose is directly external to the target, for example, the macula. Freeman et al. injected corticosteroid sub-Tenon's and used echography to show drug within the sub-Tenon's space over the macula in 11 of 24 cases (274). They attributed the lack of therapeutic response to inaccurate placement relative to target.

Retrobulbar (or peribulbar) injection administers drug around the eyeball, usually posteriorly, but not necessarily juxtasclerally. With injection of a depot, drug delivery can be sustained, allowing for relatively infrequent injections. Hyndiuk and Reagan have demonstrated the penetration and persistence of retrobulbar depot corticosteroid in monkey ocular tissues (275). Concentrations of drug were high in posterior uvea and ultimately sustained at lower concentrations. Steroid concentrated in the optic nerve after retrobulbar but not after systemic administration. No drug was detected in other ocular tissues, with the exception of lens and vitreous, after two and nine days. Weijten et al. studied the penetration of dexamethasone into the human vitreous and its systemic uptake following peribulbar injection (276). Mean levels in the vitreous peaked at 13 ng/mL at 6 to 7 hours postdose, and maximal serum level was 60 ng/mL at 20 to 30 minutes postdose.

Systemic administration Systemic administration is generally not preferred for treatment of posterior-segment eye diseases because most drugs poorly penetrate the blood-retinal barrier, including both the inner (microvessel endothelial cells) and outer (RPE) layers (277). As a result, large doses must be administered orally or intravenously, thus increasing the probability of systemic side effects. On the other hand, local ocular delivery typically provides direct access to the site of action and, in most cases, substantially reduces systemic exposure and toxicity. However, for drug delivery to the posterior segment or vitreous body, systemic administration could be the best choice depending on the drug's ability to penetrate the blood-retinal barrier or blood-vitreous barrier and its systemic toxicity profile. For example, in a study by Ueno et al., concentrations of the anticancer drug BCNU (also known as carmustine) were measured in aqueous and vitreous of rabbits following intravenous, subconjunctival, and topical ocular administration (278). Distribution was dependent on dose route in that topical, followed by subconjunctival, was best for distribution into the iris, while intravenous was best for distribution into the choroid-retina. In another example, Liu et al. demonstrated that rifampin penetrated vitreous humor after an intravenous single dose (279).

Disruption of the blood-vitreous or blood-retinal barrier can augment ocular absorption following systemic administration. For example, in a study by Elliot et al., following intravenous injection of ganciclovir with and without the bradikynin analog RMP-7, a compound known to increase the permeability of the blood-brain barrier, RMP-7 enhanced retinal uptake through the blood-retinal barrier (280). In another example, Wilson et al. demonstrated increased intravitreal penetration of carboplatin in rabbit eyes treated with triple or single freeze-thaw cryotherapy at one or two locations, one day before intravenous carboplatin with or without cyclosporine (281). In general, however, if systemic exposure can be prevented, this is to be preferred.

Topical ocular distribution to the posterior segment Historically, ophthalmologist and vision scientists have accepted the dogma that drugs applied topically to the eye do not reach therapeutic levels in the posterior segment tissues, except perhaps by way of absorption from the precorneal area into the systemic circulation and redistribution to the posterior segment tissues (198). The local distribution pathway was considered therapeutically irrelevant. There are a growing number of studies, however, challenging this dogma. The history and more recent evidence of topical delivery to the posterior segment are summarized elsewhere (277,282).

Local distribution of an effectively administered topical ocular drug is exemplified in a study by Hollo et al., who estimated the contributions of local ocular versus systemic delivery to posterior-segment concentrations of betaxolol at steady state following multiple topical dosing of Betoptic S in monkeys and humans (283). Significant levels of betaxolol were found in the retina and optic nerve head. A comparison of concentrations of dosed versus nondosed ocular tissue in monkeys revealed that most of the drug in the posterior segment was from local delivery (absorption), with some contribution from the systemic plasma. High concentrations in the iris-ciliary body, choroid, and sclera suggested the presence of a depot that presumably facilitated transfer to the retina and optic nerve head. Further evidence of local distribution after topical administration was provided by Chien et al., who evaluated the ocular distribution of brimonidine in albino and pigmented rabbits following a single topical ocular dose of ^{14}C-labeled drug (284). The results indicated that drug was retained in choroid-retina and optic nerve head. Levels in the nondosed contralateral eyes were much lower than those in the treated eyes for both albino and pigmented rabbits, suggesting that the majority (>99%) of the intraocularly absorbed drug was due to local topical application and not to redistribution from plasma.

The mechanism by which drugs may be locally delivered to the posterior segment from the precorneal area is not fully understood, but the evidence seems to indicate a noncorneal route, possibly involving conjunctival/scleral absorption followed by distribution to choroid, vitreous, and retina. Hughes et al. have proposed four routes of entry and distribution: (*i*) diffusion into the posterior chamber via the iris root and subsequently into the posterior tissues; (*ii*) entry via the pars plana, followed by distribution posteriorly; (*iii*) lateral diffusion along the sclera with subsequent penetration of Bruch's membrane and the RPE; and (*iv*) absorption into the systemic circulation via the conjunctival blood vessels or via the nasolacrimal duct, followed by redistribution to the retina (277). This evidence suggests that topically applied drugs that are effective in reaching the retina achieve this target not by passing through the vitreous or anterior chamber but by a more efficient route through the conjunctiva and sclera.

DIETARY SUPPLEMENTATION FOR OCULAR HEALTH

One of the exciting pharmaceutical opportunities afforded when exploring formulations for ocular applications is the direct visual observation and measurement of the consequences of dosage design on therapeutic activity. The disadvantages of treating such an intricate organ are often outweighed by the advantages of its accessibility and the prospect of monitoring a pharmacological benefit of therapeutic intervention. With investigation of impacts of environment and nutrition on ocular health, short-term observations are now replaced by long-term monitoring of the gradual and progressive changes over many years. While pathological conditions are still observable, such as deposits in the retina known as drusen, or changes in gross physiological state measured by visual acuity, or tissue and cellular structure and function by novel technologies such as OCT (285–289) and electroretinograms (ERGs) (290,291), respectively, discovering underlying biochemical etiologies poses the same difficulties as that existing for internal organs and tissues. Conversely, observation of progressive structural and functional changes observed over years often provides a window into the state of not just ocular but systemic health.

Because the eye is unique in its demand for oxygen required to sustain its high rate of metabolism (214), and because whenever functioning its tissues are concurrently exposed to the stress of electromagnetic radiation, it should not be surprising that the retina is exquisitely sensitive to homeostatic balance, influenced by the state of systemic health (292). It had been suspected by physicians for some time and epidemiologists more recently that nutrition, and in particular certain essential nutrients, might retard progression of age-related disease, and in particular, age-related eye disease (293–295). However, it was not until a large trial [AREDS (Age-Related Eye Disease Study) trial] of extended duration was undertaken by the National Eye Institute (NEI), initiated about 1992 and extending beyond seven years, that there was clinical evidence for benefit of dietary modification through supplementation. The AREDS trial demonstrated unambiguous benefit of supplementation with five essential vitamins and minerals at high potency. The formulation consisted of β-carotene, vitamin C, vitamin E, zinc, and copper, either well-known antioxidants or enzyme cofactors of antioxidant enzymes.

In a series of papers in *Archives of Ophthalmology* and other journals, investigators described significant findings, perhaps the most noteworthy being that even with relatively late-stage intervention, individuals with the advanced dry form of AMD could delay progression of this insidious disease, which ultimately robs sight from a significant fraction of the elderly (296,297). In this segment of the population, physicians reported that over a five-year period there was about a 25% reduction in the rate of progression to advanced AMD, observed as neovascularization and hemorrhage or geographic atrophy. Because of the epidemiological significance from this recognized prophylaxis, as well as the sociological and economic implications for public policy, administration of high-potency nutrients has become the standard of care for subpopulations at risk of AMD (298). Because of extensive evaluations and dissections of the trial's statistics, numerous valuable observations have been made affecting prognosis and treatment (299,300). Safety of the formulation, an initial concern of some physicians based on the high potency of these nutrients relative to their dietary reference intakes (DRIs), has been allayed, though in a new trial, AREDS2, the required levels of those ingredients seemingly posing greatest risk, zinc and β-carotene, are being reevaluated. Genetic sampling has contributed to the understanding of the role of single nucleotide polymorphism (SNP) in complement factor H as a risk factor for AMD (301,302). While the AREDS trial did not support an effect on cognition or vascular function in the elderly, alternate studies of antioxidants have suggested the value of antioxidant nutrients that appear capable of influencing inflammatory states (300). Consequently, several ancillary studies have been incorporated into the AREDS2 trial. The rationale for these extensions of the study is supported by the observation that the decreased survival rates of AMD patients appears to be countered for those patients in particular arms of the AREDS trial, and that AMD patients' decrease in cognitive function appears correlated with the disease's visual impairment (303).

Because two essential carotenoids, the C_{40} xanthophylls lutein and zeaxanthin, are found concentrated in the retina with increased level in the macula (304), because these compounds are both antioxidants and absorbers of short-wavelength visible light (305), because of the risk engendered in exposure to blue light that can produce fluorescent excitation of A2E chromophores (a 2,4-bis retinoid pyridinyl ethanol salt) in lipofuscin (306,307), because epidemiological evidence suggesting reduced incidence of AMD for those individuals in the higher quintiles of these compounds in their diet, because of the protection observed from light damage by these two compounds in preclinical studies (304,308,309), because of demonstrable clinical benefit in delaying the effects of AMD on visual function from using xanthophyll supplementation (310,311), because of evidence for binding by specific retinal proteins of these xanthophylls (312), and because analysis of the AREDS population disclosed that there was a reduced likelihood of neovascular AMD, geographic atrophy, and large drusen for those individuals in the highest quintiles of lutein and zeaxanthin consumption (313), NEI has embarked on an extension of the AREDS trial, designated as AREDS2, in which the impact of these carotenoids on progression of AMD is being evaluated. Another class of lipid, the essential ω-3 fatty acids, eicosapentaenoic acid (EPA, 20:5, n-3) and docosahexaenoic acid (DHA, 22:6, n-3), also is of interest. Because these antioxidants are abundant in photoreceptor disk membranes, are significant enough to be reprocessed by the RPE so they can be reused by the photoreceptors, are incorporated in neural membranes contributing to controlling their growth and function, are known to influence inflammatory responses by influencing arachidonic acid metabolism, and in epidemiological investigations appear to reduce the incidence of AMD, they also are being evaluated in this new trial (300,313). As evermore information, both basic and clinical, about the subtle nutritional requirements of the eye and its age dependence emerges, benefit from more complex formulations can be anticipated (314–317).

The linkage of the impact of these studies on dosage form, the influence of nutrient administration on compliance, and ultimately the effect on the health of patients is appreciated by a review of the types and timing of the administrations available. In the AREDS trial, supplementation was provided by four tablets, taken twice a day with meals. Relatively large tablet volumes were needed because, in addition to the high potency of the actives, high loads of excipients were required to confine lipophilic materials and avoid "bleed-through" and discoloration of the tablets, or the need to satisfy other tableting requirements (297). Specifically, in the original trial, a daily dose of AREDS antioxidants provided along with 69.6 mg of zinc as zinc oxide and 1.6 mg of copper as cupric oxide, 400 mg of vitamin E as DL-α-tocopheryl acetate and 28,640 IU (about 17.2 mg) of vitamin A as β-carotene. Because the latter two need to be provided as free-flowing powders, they are incorporated into the tablet as beadlets, conventionally made from gelatin or starch, whose amounts can be in excess of the nutrient. Another nutrient, also present at high levels, more than seven times the DRI, is the water-soluble and effective antioxidant vitamin C, at 452 mg/day. While vitamin C can be provided as a free-flowing crystalline powder of nearly 100% active nutrient, it also is well known to be sensitive to oxidation on prolonged exposure to air. For example, many vitamin C tablets once exposed to the atmosphere have been observed to discolor. For that reason, one class of additional excipient required for extending the shelf life to two years is a protective antioxidant, an ingredient more readily oxidized than any of the other effective antioxidants in the formulation! In a tablet formulation, several additional classes of excipient may be required to provide the appropriate flow and mixing characteristics of the blend, hardness, and fracture properties under compression and disintegration attributes following ingestion (318). Tablet coatings serve to impart good barrier characteristics contributing to product stability, lubricity to facilitate swallowing, and color to assist in tablet identification, providing consumer recognition (319).

While compliance with this regimen of four tablets per day was very high during the AREDS trial, that is, found to be better than 75% for 71% of the participants with very few lost to follow-up (<2.4%), later analysis of compliance for a broader spectrum of AMD patients, for tablets available in the marketplace, appears to dwindle (297). It is not clear whether this loss of compliance was driven by inconvenience of the dosage form, their cost, or simple and conventional attrition accompanying normal loss of discipline to the regimen. The consequence, nonetheless, is obvious, since any regimen less than the design deprives the patients of the high potency found effective. In part these failings can be addressed through redesign of the dosage form, which has been provided for the second-tier evaluation occurring in AREDS2, to be a softgel dosed as two softgels per day. And the composition of the precise AREDS multivitamin mineral formulation was slightly readjusted so that it more nearly approached the design composition indicated in the original descriptions of the trial, 500 mg of vitamin C, 400 IU of vitamin E, 15 mg of β-carotene, 80 mg of zinc, and 2 mg of copper, a design intended to be compliant with USP requirements over the shelf life of the product. The new formulation provided for the AREDS2 trial, donated to the study by Alcon Research, Ltd., meets the current operative DSHEA legislation, as provided in the Federal Register and Code of Federal Regulations (CFR) (320). The softgel dosage form (321), with primary capsule fill excipient and carrier being oil in which the lipophilic vitamins are soluble, reduces posology by half. The oil barrier also serves to protect the ingredients from hydrolytic and oxidative instability. Because the new AREDS2 trial is so large, nominally 4000 participants, there is high probability that the results will be able to offer broad guidelines of essential nutrients, spanning vitamins, minerals, and lipids, capable of contributing to the reduction in rate of progression of AMD, and perhaps contributing to improved systemic health as measured by the impact of these nutrients on cardiovascular health and cognition. As the number, amounts, and diversity in properties of these nutrients increase to support good nutrition and maintenance of health, it is expected that new dosage forms will emerge to facilitate treatment and support compliance.

MANUFACTURING CONSIDERATIONS

Because the official compendia require all topically administered ophthalmic medications to be sterile, manufacturers of such medications must weigh numerous alternative approaches as they design manufacturing procedures. Ideally, as preferred by some regulators especially from Europe, all ophthalmic products would be terminally sterilized in the final packaging because it offers the best chance of assuring patients of their sterility. In effect, this would rule out any aseptic processing for the manufacture of ophthalmic products; however, the use of sterile filtration and/or aseptic assembly of ophthalmic products has been shown not to constitute a risk to public health.

It is quite rare that the composition or the packaging of an ophthalmic pharmaceutical will lend itself to terminal sterilization, the simplest form of manufacture of sterile products. Only a few ophthalmic drugs formulated in simple aqueous vehicles are stable to normal autoclaving temperatures and times (121°C for 20–30 minutes). Such heat-resistant drugs may be packaged in glass or other heat-deformation-resistant packaging and thus can be sterilized in this manner. The convenience of plastic dispensing bottles is possible today using modern polyolefins that resist heat deformation with proper sterilization cycles.

Most ophthalmic products, however, cannot be heat sterilized. In general, the active principle is not particularly stable to heat, either physically or chemically. Moreover, to impart viscosity, aqueous products are generally formulated with the inclusion of high-molecular-weight polymers, which may, similarly, be affected adversely by heat.

Because of these product sensitivities, most ophthalmic pharmaceutical products are aseptically manufactured and filled into previously sterilized containers in aseptic environments using aseptic filling and capping techniques. This is the case for ophthalmic solutions, suspensions, and ointments, and specialized technology is involved in their manufacture.

All pharmaceutical manufacturers are required to follow Current Good Manufacturing Practice (CGMP) Part 210—Current Good Manufacturing Practice in Manufacturing,

Processing, Packaging, or Holding of Drugs and General Part 211—Current Good Manufacturing Practice for Finished Pharmaceuticals. Readers can access more information from FDA's Web site at www.fda.gov. These guidelines cover all aspects of manufacture of pharmaceutical products.

Manufacturing Environment

Aside from drug safety, stability, and efficacy and shelf life considerations associated with tonicity, pH, and buffer capacity, the major design criteria of an ophthalmic pharmaceutical product are the additional safety criteria of sterility, preservative efficacy, and freedom from extraneous foreign particulate matter. Current U.S. standards for Good Manufacturing Practices (GMPs) (322) provide for the use of specially designed environmentally controlled areas for the manufacture of sterile large- and small-volume injections for terminal sterilization. These environmentally controlled areas must meet the requirements of class 100,000 space in all areas where open containers and closures are not exposed, or where product-filling and -capping operations are not taking place. The latter areas must meet the requirements of class 100 space (323). As defined in Federal Standard 209E, classes 100,000 and 100 spaces contain not more than 100,000 or 100 particles, respectively, per cubic foot of air of a diameter of 0.5 µm or larger. The readers are also referred to the *British Standard 5295: 1989* for classification of clean room environments. Often these design criteria are coupled with laminar airflow concepts (324,325). This specification deals with total particle counts and does not differentiate between viable and nonviable particles. Federal Standard 209 was promulgated as a "hardware" or mechanical specification for the aerospace industry and has found applications in the pharmaceutical industry as a tool for the design of aseptic and particle-free environments. Class 100,000 conditions can be achieved in the conventionally designed clean room where proper filtration of air supply and adequate turnover rates are provided. Class 100 conditions over open containers can be achieved with properly sized high-efficiency particulate air (HEPA)-filtered laminar airflow sources. Depending on the product need and funds available, some aseptic pharmaceutical environments have been designed to class 100 laminar-flow specifications throughout the manufacturing area. However, during actual product manufacture the generation of particulate matter by equipment, product, and (most importantly) people may cause these environments to demonstrate particulate matter levels two or more orders of magnitude greater than design. It is for this reason that specialists in the design of pharmaceutical manufacturing and hospital operating room environments are beginning to view these environments not only from the standpoint of total particles per cubic foot of space alone but also from that of the types of particles, for example, the ratio of disease-transmitting biocontaminants to inert particulates (326).

Such environmental concepts as mass air transfer may lead to meaningful specifications for the space in which a nonterminally sterilized product can be manufactured with a high level of confidence (327).

When dealing with the environment in which a sterile product is manufactured, the materials used for construction of the facility, as well as personnel attire, training, conduct in the space; the entrance and egress of personnel, equipment, and packaging; and the product, all bear heavily on the assurance of product sterility and minimization of extraneous particulate matter.

The importance of personnel training and behavior cannot be overemphasized in the maintenance of an acceptable environment for the manufacture of sterile ophthalmic products or sterile pharmaceutical agents in general. Personnel must be trained in the proper mode of gowning with sterile, nonshedding garments and also in the proper techniques and conduct for aseptic manufacturing. The Parenteral Drug Association can be contacted at their offices in Bethesda, Maryland, for a listing of training films on this subject. To maximize personnel comfort and to minimize sloughing of epidermal cells and hair, a cool working environment should be maintained, with relative humidity controlled to between 40% and 60%. Additional guidelines on pharmaceutical clean room classifications—which became effective on January 1, 1997, for Europe—are contained in a "Revision of the Annexes to the EU Guide to Good Manufacturing Practice— Manufacture of Sterile Medicinal Products" (328).

Manufacturing Techniques

In general, aqueous ophthalmic solutions are manufactured by methods that call for the dissolution of the active ingredient and all or a portion of the excipients into all or a portion of the water, and the sterilization of this solution by heat or by sterilizing filtration through sterile depth or membrane filter media into a sterile receptacle. If incomplete at this point, then this sterile solution is mixed with the additional required sterile components, such as previously sterilized solutions of viscosity-imparting agents, preservatives, and so on, and the batch is brought to final volume with additional sterile water.

Aqueous suspensions are prepared in much the same manner, except that before bringing the batch to final volume with additional sterile water, the solid that is to be suspended is previously rendered sterile by heat, by exposure to ethylene oxide, or ionizing radiation (γ or electrons), or by dissolution in an appropriate solvent, sterile filtration, and aseptic crystallization. The sterile solid is then added to the batch, either directly or by first dispersing the solid in a small portion of the batch. After adequate dispersion, the batch is brought to final volume with sterile water (329). Because the eye is sensitive to particles larger than 25 μm in diameter, proper raw material specifications for particle size of any dispersed solids must be established and verified on each lot of raw material and final product. The control of particle size of the final suspended material is very important, not only for comfort of the product but also for improving physical stability and resuspendability of the suspension throughout the shelf life and the in-use life by patients.

When an ophthalmic ointment is manufactured, all raw material components must be rendered sterile before compounding unless the ointment contains an aqueous fraction that can be sterilized by heat, filtration, or ionizing radiation. The ointment base is sterilized by heat, and appropriately filtered while molten to remove extraneous foreign particulate matter. It is then placed into a sterile steam-jacketed kettle to maintain the ointment in a molten state under aseptic conditions, and the previously sterilized active ingredient(s) and excipients are added aseptically. While still molten, the entire ointment may be passed through a previously sterilized colloid mill for adequate dispersion of the insoluble components.

After the product is compounded in an aseptic manner, it is filled into previously sterilized containers. Commonly employed methods of sterilization of packaging components include exposure to heat, ethylene oxide gas, and ^{60}Co (γ) irradiation. When a product is to be used in conjunction with ophthalmic surgical procedures and must enter the aseptic operating area, the exterior of the primary container must be rendered sterile by the manufacturer and maintained sterile with appropriate packaging. This may be accomplished by aseptic packaging or by exposure of the completely packaged product to ethylene oxide gas, ionizing radiation, or heat. Whenever ethylene oxide is used as a sterilant for either the raw material or packaging components, strict processing controls and validated aeration cycles are required to assure lower residual limits permitted by the regulatory agencies.

With the need of, and the preference for, unpreserved formulations of active drug(s) by ophthalmologists and patients, the blow/fill/seal concept, also termed the "form/fill/ seal method," has gained acceptance for manufacture of unpreserved ophthalmic products, especially for artificial tear products. In this process, the first step is to extrude polyethylene resin, at high temperature and pressure, and to form the container by blowing the resin into a mold with compressed air. The product is filled as air is vented out, and finally the container is sealed on the top. There are several published articles describing and validating this technology (330–335). Automatic Liquid Packaging, Incorporated, located in Woodstock, Illinois, U.S., designs and fabricates bow/fill/seal machines as well as provides contract manufacture in the U.S. Hollopack (BottlePack-6) and similar equipment in Europe.

Raw Materials

All raw materials used in the compounding of ophthalmic pharmaceutical products must be of the highest quality available. Complete raw material specifications for each component must be established and verified for each lot purchased. As many pharmaceutical companies improve efficiency and increase product distribution by qualifying a single plant to provide product globally, it becomes necessary to qualify excipients for global distribution. Excipients used in the product need to be tested for multiple pharmacopoeial specifications to meet global requirements (USP, Pharma Europe, Japanese Pharmacopoeia). When raw materials are rendered sterile before compounding, the reactivity of the raw material with the sterilizing medium must be completely evaluated, and the sterilization must be validated to demonstrate its capability to sterilize raw materials contaminated with large numbers (10^5–10^7) of microorganisms that have been demonstrated to be most resistant to the mode of sterilization appropriate for that raw material. As mentioned previously, for raw material components that will enter the eye as a suspension in an appropriate vehicle, particle size must be carefully controlled both before use in the product and as a finished product specification.

As for most sterile (and nonsterile) aqueous pharmaceuticals, the largest portion of the composition is water. At present, USP 31 allows the use of "purified water" as a pharmaceutical aid for all official aqueous products, with the exception of preparations intended for parenteral administration, inhalation administration, and hemodialysis (336). For preparations intended for parenteral administration, USP 31 requires the use of WFI, sterile water injection, or bacteriostatic WFI as a pharmaceutical aid. Because some pharmaceutical manufacturers produce a line of parenteral ophthalmic drugs and devices (large-volume and small-volume irrigating and "tissue-sparing" solutions) as well as topical ophthalmic drugs, the provision of WFI-manufacturing capability is being designed into new and existing facilities to meet this requirement. Some manufacturers have made the decision to compound all ophthalmic drugs from WFI, thus employing the highest grade of this raw material economically available to the pharmaceutical industry. In doing so, systems must be designed to meet all the requirements for WFI currently listed in the USP (336) and the guidelines listed for such systems by the FDA in their GMPs guidelines for large-volume and small-volume parenterals (337). Briefly, these proposals call for the generation of water by distillation or by reverse osmosis and its storage and circulation at relatively high temperatures of up to 80°C (or, alternatively, its disposal every 24 hours) in all stainless steel equipment of the highest attainable, corrosion-resistant quality.

Equipment

The design of equipment for use in controlled environment areas follows similar principles, whether for general injectable manufacturing or for the manufacturer of sterile ophthalmic pharmaceuticals. All tanks, valves, pumps, and piping must be of the best available grade of corrosion-resistant stainless steel. In general, stainless steel type 304 or 316 is preferable. All product-contact surfaces should be finished either mechanically or by electropolishing to provide a surface as free as possible from scratches or defects that could serve as a nidus for the commencement of corrosion (338). Care should be taken in the design of such equipment to provide adequate means of cleaning and sanitization. For equipment that will reside in aseptic-filling areas, such as filling and capping machines, care should be taken in their design to yield equipment as free as possible from particle-generating mechanisms. Wherever possible, belt or chain-drive concepts should be avoided in favor of sealed gear or hydraulic mechanisms. Additionally, equipment bulk located directly over open containers should be held to an absolute minimum during filling and capping operations to minimize introduction of equipment-generated particulate matter or creation of air turbulence. This precaution is particularly important when laminar flow is used to control the immediate environment around the filling-capping operation.

In the design of equipment for the manufacture of sterile ophthalmic (and nonophthalmic) pharmaceuticals, manufacturers and equipment suppliers are turning to the advanced technology in use in the dairy and aerospace industries, where such concepts as clean in place (CIP), clean out of place (COP), automatic heliarc welding, and electropolishing have been in use for several years. As a guide here, the reader is referred to the so-called 3A Standards of the dairy industry issued by the U.S. Public Health Service (339).

Some of the newer and more potent drugs, like the prostaglandins, which are produced at very low concentrations in the finished formulation, may require special precautions during compounding and processing to prevent loss of actives due to adsorption/absorption to the walls of fill lines and/or storage tanks.

Modern Risk-Based Approaches

In recent years, the concept of quality is transforming. Product quality and performance are achieved and assured through effective designing and efficient manufacturing processes. ICH guidelines provide the foundation to the modern risk-based approaches to pharmaceutical quality and manufacturing (340). Risk, quality, and uncertainty are very broad concepts and are not suitable for formal analysis until they are well defined within a specific concept (341). These approaches have influenced both industry and regulatory agencies worldwide (342).

CLASSES OF OPHTHALMIC PRODUCTS

Topical Eyedrops

Administration and Dosage

Although many alternate experimental methods have been tried, eyedrops remains the major method of administration for the topical ocular route. The usual method of self-administration is to place the eyedrop from a dropper or dropper bottle into the lower cul-de-sac by pulling down the eyelid, tilting the head backward, and looking at the ceiling after the tip is pointed close to the sac and applying a slight pressure to the rubber bulb or plastic bottle to allow a single drop to form and fall into the eye. Most people become quite adept at this method with some practice and may develop their own modifications. However, elderly, arthritic, low-vision, and glaucoma patients often have difficulty in self-administration and may require another person to instill the drops.

The pharmacist should instruct patients to keep in mind the following considerations in administering drops to help improve the accuracy and consistency of dosage and to prevent contamination: be sure that the hands are clean; do not touch the dropper tip to the eye, surrounding tissue, or any surface; prevent squeezing or fluttering of lids, which causes blinking; place the drop in the conjunctival sac, not on the globe; and close the lids for several moments after instillation. The administration of eyedrops to young children can be a difficult task. A way to simplify the task involves the parent's sitting on the floor or a flat surface and placing the child's head firmly between the parent's thighs and crossing legs over the child's lower trunk and legs. The parent's hands are then free to lower the eyelid and administer the drops.

In addition to the proper technique to administer eyedrops, the pharmacist may need to explain to the patient the correct technique for temporary punctal occlusion. Punctal occlusion is usually reserved for use with potent drugs, which can have adverse systemic effects from topical ocular administration such as with ocular β-blockers. Tear fluid drains into the nasolacrimal duct via the puncta located on the medial portion of the eyelid, and fluid is directed into the puncta by the blinking action of the lids. The nasal meatus is a highly vascular area within the nasal cavity, which receives the fluid of the nasolacrimal duct, and drugs contained in tears can be absorbed into the systemic circulation from this area as well as from gastrointestinal absorption. Punctal occlusion can be performed immediately after instillation of an eyedrop by closing the eye and placing a finger between the eyeball and the nose and applying pressure for several minutes.

Eyedrops are one of the few dosage forms that are not administered by exact volume or weight dosage, yet this seemingly imprecise method of dosing is quite well established and accepted by ophthalmologists. The volume of a drop is dependent on the physicochemical properties of the formulation, particularly surface tension, the design and geometry of the dispensing office, and the angle at which the dispenser is held in relation to the receiving surface. The manufacturer of ophthalmic products controls the tolerances necessary for the dosage form and dispensing container to provide a uniform drop size. How precise does the actual dose have to be? As noted earlier, the normal tear volume is about 7 μL, and with blinking about 10 μL can be retained in the eye. Approximately 1.2 μL of tear fluid is produced per minute, for about a 16% volume replacement per minute. Commercial ophthalmic droppers deliver drops from about 30 to 50 μL/drop. Therefore, the volumes delivered normally are more than threefold in excess of that that the eye can hold, and the fluid that does remain in the eye is continuously being removed until the normal tear volume is attained. It can be seen, then, that the use of more than one drop per dose must take into account the fluid volume and dynamics of the lacrimal system of the eye. If the effect of multiple drops is desired, they should be administered one drop at a time with a three- to five-minute interval in between dosings. Some doctors may prescribe more than one drop per dose to ensure that the patients retains at least one drop in the eye.

Dosage Forms

Solutions The two major physical forms of eyedrops are aqueous solutions and suspensions. Nearly all the major ophthalmic therapeutic agents are water soluble or

Table 3 Effects of Salt Form on Product Properties

Salt form	Discomfort reaction	pH range	Buffer capacity
Epinephrine hydrochloride	Mild to moderate stinging	2.5–4.5	Medium
Epinephrine bitartrate	Moderate to severe stinging	3–4	High
Epinephrine borate	Only occasional mild stinging	5.5–7.5	Low

can be formulated as water-soluble salts. A homogeneous solution offers the assurance of greater uniformity of dosage and bioavailability and simplifies large-scale manufacture. The selection of the appropriate salt form depends on its solubility, therapeutic concentrations required, ocular toxicity, the effect of pH, tonicity, buffer capacity, its compatibility with the total formulation, and the intensity of any possible stinging or burning sensations (i.e., discomfort reactions). The most common salt forms used are the hydrochloride, sulfate, nitrate, and phosphate. Salicylate, hydrobromide, and bitartrate salts are also used. For drugs that are acidic, such as the sulfonamides, sodium and diethanolamine salts are used. The effect that choice of salt form can have on resulting product properties is exemplified by the epinephrine solutions available, as shown in Table 3. The bitartrate form is a 1:1 salt and may cause considerable stinging, and the free carboxyl group acts as a strong buffer, resisting neutralization by the tears. The borate form results in a solution with lower buffer capacity, a more nearly physiological pH, and better patient tolerance; however, it is less stable than the other two salts. The hydrochloride salt combines better stability than the borate with acceptable patient tolerance.

Gel-forming solutions One disadvantage of solutions is their relatively short residence time in the eye. This has been overcome to some degree by the development of solutions that are liquid in the container and thus can be instilled as eyedrops but gel on contact with the tear fluid and provide increased contact time with the possibility of improved drug absorption and increased duration of therapeutic effect.

A number of liquid-gel phase transition-dependent delivery systems have been researched and patented. They vary according to the particular polymer(s) employed and their mechanism(s) for triggering the transition to a gel phase in the eye. The mechanisms that make them useful for the eye take advantage of changes in temperature, pH, ion sensitivity, or ionic strength upon contact with tear fluid or the presence of proteins such as lysozyme in the tear fluid. Thermally sensitive systems, which are transformed to a gel phase by the change in temperature associated with reaching body temperature, have the disadvantage of possibly gelling in the container when subjected to warmer climatic conditions. The pH-sensitive systems may have limited use for drugs that require a neutral to slightly alkaline environment for stability, solubility, etc.

Gel-forming ophthalmic solutions have been developed and approved by the FDA for timolol maleate, which is used to reduce elevated IOP in the management of glaucoma. Timolol maleate ophthalmic solutions, as initially developed, require twice-a-day dosage for most patients. With the gel-forming solutions, IOP-lowering efficacy was extended from 12 to 24 hours and thus required only once-a-day dosing. This extended duration of efficacy was demonstrated for both gel-forming products in controlled clinical trials. The first gel-forming product, Timolol®-XE, uses the polysaccharide gellan gum and is reported to gel in situ in response to the higher ionic strength of tear fluid (U.S. patent 4,861,760). Alternative ion-sensitive gelling systems have been patented (3–7). The second product, Alcon's timolol gel-forming solution (timolol maleate), uses the polysaccharide xanthan gum as the gelling agent and is reported to gel upon contact with the tear fluid, at least in part, due to the presence of tear protein lysozyme (PCT Application WO 99/51273). Another more recent application of a gel-forming product is the ocular lubricant eyedrop SYSTANE that contains hydroxypropyl guar (343).

Suspensions If the drug is not sufficiently soluble, it can be formulated as a suspension. A suspension may also be desired to improve stability, bioavailability, or efficacy. The major topical ophthalmic suspensions include but are not limited to steroid anti-inflammatory agents and IOP-lowering agents: prednisolone acetate, dexamethasone, fluorometholone, nepafenac, brinzolamide, betaxolol hydrochloride, and rimexolone. Water-soluble salts of prednisolone phosphate and dexamethasone phosphate are available; however, they have a lower steroid potency and are poorly absorbed.

An ophthalmic suspension should use the drug in a microfine form; usually 95% or more of the particles have a diameter of 10 μm or less. This is to ensure that the particles do not cause irritation of the sensitive ocular tissues and that a uniform dosage is delivered to the eye. Since a suspension is made up of solid particles, it is at least theoretically possible that they may provide a reservoir in the cul-de-sac for slightly prolonged activity. However, it appears that this is not so, since the drug particles are extremely small, and with the rapid tear turnover rate, they are washed out of the eye relatively quickly.

Pharmaceutical scientists have developed improved suspension dosage forms to overcome problems of poor physical stability and patient-perceived discomfort attributed to some active ingredients. An important development and compendial aspect of any suspension is the ability to resuspend easily any settled particles prior to instillation in the eye and ensure a uniform dose is delivered. It would be ideal to formulate a suspension that does not settle since the patient may not always follow the labeled instructions to shake well before using. However, this is usually not feasible or desirable since the viscosity required to retard settling of the insoluble particles completely would likely be excessive for a liquid eyedrop. The opposite extreme, of allowing complete settling between doses, usually leads to a dense layer of agglomerated particles that are difficult to resuspend.

An improved suspension has been developed, which controls the flocculation of the insoluble active ingredient particles, such that they will remain substantially resuspended (95%) for many months, and any settled particles can be easily resuspended with only a few seconds of gentle handshaking. This improved vehicle utilizes a charged water-soluble polymer and oppositely charged electrolyte such as negatively charged carbomer polymer of very high molecular weight and large dimension and a cation such as sodium or potassium. The negatively charged carboxy vinyl polymer is involved in controlling the flocculation of the insoluble particles, such as the steroid rimexolone, and the cation assists in controlling the viscosity of the vehicle such that the settling is substantially retarded, yet can be easily and uniformly resuspended and can be dispensed from a conventional plastic eyedrop container (U.S. patent 5,461,081).

In some cases it may be advantageous to convert a water-soluble active ingredient to an insoluble form for development as an ophthalmic suspension dosage form. This could be the case when it is beneficial to extend the practical shelf life of the water-soluble form to improve the compatibility with other necessary compositional ingredients or to improve its ocular tolerability. Such an example is the β-blocker betaxolol hydrochloride, which is an effective IOP-lowering agent with clinically significant safety advantages for many asthmatic patients. With the ophthalmic solution dosage form some patients experienced discomfort characterized as a transient stinging or burning upon instillation. Although, this did not interfere with the safety or efficacy of the product, it was desirable to improve the patient tolerability. Many solution-based formulations were tried but with limited success. It was discovered that an insoluble form of betaxolol (Betoptic® S) could be produced in situ with the use of a combination of a high-molecular-weight polyanionic polymer such as carbomer and a sulfonic acid cation exchange resin. The resultant optimized suspension increased the ocular bioavailability of betaxolol such that the drug concentration required to achieve equivalent efficacy to the solution dosage form was reduced by one-half and the ocular tolerance was improved significantly. It would appear that the sustained release of the active betaxolol occurs through exchange with cations such as sodium and potassium in tear fluid, resulting in prolonged tear levels of the drug and substantial increase in ocular bioavailability (U.S. patent 4,911,920).

Powders for reconstitution Drugs that have only limited stability in liquid form are prepared as sterile powders for reconstitution by the pharmacist prior to dispensing to the patient. In ophthalmology, these drugs include α-chymotrypsin, echothiophate iodide (Phospholine Iodide®), dapiprazole HCl (Rev-Eyes®), and acetylcholine (Miochol®). The sterile powder is usually manufactured by lyophilization in the individual glass vials. In powder form these drugs have a much longer shelf life than in solution. Mannitol is usually used as a bulking agent and lyophilization aid and is dissolved in the solution with the drug prior to drying. In the case of echothiophate iodide, it was found that potassium acetate used in place of mannitol as a drying aid produced a more stable product. Apparently the presence of potassium acetate with the drug allows freeze-drying to lower residual moisture content (U.S. patent 3,681,495). A stable echothiophate product has also been produced by freeze-drying from an alcoholic solution without a codrying or bulking agent, but the product is no longer marketed.

A separately packaged sterile diluent and sterile dropper assembly is provided with the sterile powder and requires aseptic technique to reconstitute. The pharmacist should only use the diluent supplied by the manufacturer since it has been developed to maintain the optimum potency and preservation of the reconstituted solution. The storage conditions and expiration dating for the final solution should be emphasized to the patient.

Inactive Ingredients in Topical Drops

The therapeutically inactive ingredients in ophthalmic solution and suspension dosage forms are necessary to perform one or more of the following functions: adjust concentration and tonicity, buffer and adjust pH, stabilize the active ingredients against decomposition, increase solubility, impart viscosity, and act as solvent. The use of unnecessary ingredients is to be avoided, and the use of ingredients solely to impart a color, odor, or flavor is prohibited.

The choice of a particular inactive ingredient and its concentration is based not only on physical and chemical compatibility but also on biocompatibility with the sensitive and delicate ocular tissues. Because of the latter requirement, the use of inactive ingredients is greatly restricted in ophthalmic dosage forms.

The possibility of systemic effects due to nasolacrimal drainage as previously discussed should also be kept in mind. FDA has cataloged all inactive ingredients in approved drug products and provides this information in a searchable database at http://www.accessdata.fda.gov/scripts/cder/iig/index.cfm. The FDA database provides route and dosage form, CAS number, UNII, and maximum potency for each listed inactive ingredient.

Tonicity and tonicity-adjusting agents In the past a great deal of emphasis was placed on teaching the pharmacist to adjust the tonicity of an ophthalmic solution correctly (i.e., exert an osmotic pressure equal to that of tear fluids, generally agreed to be equal to 0.9% NaCl). In compounding an eye solution, it is more important to consider the sterility, stability, and preservative aspects, and not jeopardize these aspects to obtain a precisely isotonic solution. A range of 0.5% to 2.0% NaCl equivalency does not cause a marked pain response, and a range of about 0.7% to 1.5% should be acceptable to most persons. Manufacturers are in a much better position to make a precise adjustment, and thus their products will be close to isotonic, since they are in a competitive situation and are interested in a high percentage of patient acceptance for their products. In certain instances, the therapeutic concentration of the drug will necessitate using what might otherwise be considered an unacceptable tonicity. This is the case for sodium sulfacetamide, for which the isotonic concentration is about 3.5%, but the drug is used in 10% to 30% concentrations. Fortunately, the eye seems to tolerate hypertonic solutions better than hypotonic ones. Various textbooks deal with the subject of precise tonicity calculations and determination. Several articles (344) have recommended practical methods of obtaining an acceptable tonicity in extemporaneous compounding. Common tonicity-adjusting ingredients include NaCl, KCl, buffer salts, dextrose, glycerin, propylene glycol, and mannitol.

pH adjustment and buffers The pH and buffering of an ophthalmic solution is probably of equal importance to proper preservation, since the stability of most commonly used ophthalmic drugs is largely controlled by the pH of their environment. Manufacturers place particular emphasis on this aspect, since economics indicates that they produce products with long shelf lives that will retain their labeled potency and product characteristics under the many and varied storage conditions outside the makers' control. The pharmacist and wholesaler must become familiar with labeled storage directions for each product and ensure that it is properly stored. Particular attention should be paid to products requiring refrigeration. The stability of nearly all products can be enhanced by refrigeration, except for those few in which a decrease in solubility and precipitation might occur. Freezing of ophthalmic products, particularly suspensions, should be avoided. A freeze-thaw cycle can induce particle growth or crystallization of a suspension and increase the chance of ocular irritation and loss of dosage uniformity. Glass-packaged liquid products may break owing to the volume expansion of the solution when it freezes. It is especially important that the pharmacist fully advise the patient on proper storage and use of ophthalmic products to ensure their integrity and safe and efficacious use.

In addition to stability effects, pH adjustment can influence comfort, safety, and activity of the product. Comfort can be described as the subjective response of the patient after instillation of the product in the cul-de-sac (i.e., whether it may cause a pain response such as stinging or burning). Eye irritation is normally accompanied by an increase in tear fluid secretion (a defense mechanism) to aid in the restoration of normal physiological conditions. Accordingly, in addition to the discomfort encountered, products that produce irritation will tend to be flushed from the eye, and hence a more rapid loss of medication may occur with a probable reduction in the therapeutic response (11).

Ideally, every product would be buffered to a pH of 7.4, considered the normal physiological pH of tear fluid. The argument for this concept is that the product would be comfortable and have optimum therapeutic activity. Various experiments, primarily in rabbits, have shown an enhanced effect when the pH was increased, owing to the solution containing a higher concentration of the nonionized lipid-soluble drug base, which is the species that can more rapidly penetrate the corneal epithelial barrier. This would not be true if the drug were an acidic moiety. The tears have some buffer capacity of their own, and it is believed that they can neutralize the pH of an instilled solution if the quantity of solutions is not excessive and if the solution does not have a strong resistance to neutralization. Pilocarpine activity is apparently the same whether applied from vehicles with nearly physiological pH values or from more acidic vehicles, provided the latter are not strongly buffered (345). A pH difference of 6.6 versus 4.2 produced a statistically insignificant difference in pilocarpine miosis (346). The pH values of ophthalmic solutions are adjusted within a range to provide an acceptable shelf life. When necessary, they are buffered adequately to maintain stability within this range for at least two years. If buffers are required, their capacity is controlled to be as low as possible, thus enabling the tears to bring the pH of the eye back to the physiological range. Since the buffer capacity is determined by buffer concentration, the effect of buffers on tonicity must also be taken into account and is another reason that ophthalmic products are usually only lightly buffered.

The pH value is not the sole contributing factor to discomfort of some ophthalmic solutions. It is possible to have a product with a low pH and little buffer capacity that is more comfortable than a similar product with a higher pH and a stronger buffer capacity. Epinephrine hydrochloride and dipivefrin hydrochloride solutions, used for treatment of glaucoma, have a pH of about 3, yet they have sufficiently acceptable comfort to have been used daily for many years. The same pH solution of epinephrine bitartrate has an intrinsically higher buffer capacity and will produce much more discomfort.

The acidic nonsteroidal anti-inflammatory agents produce significant stinging and burning upon topical ocular instillation, and this limits the concentration of drug that can be developed. Caffeine, a xanthine derivative, has been found to improve significantly the comfort of drugs such as suprofen (Profenal®) by forming in situ weak complexes with the NSAID (U.S. patent 4,559,343).

Stabilizers Stabilizers are ingredients added to a formula to decrease the rate of decomposition of the active ingredients. Antioxidants are the principal stabilizers added to some ophthalmic solutions, primarily those containing epinephrine and other oxidizable drugs. Sodium bisulfite or metabisulfite are used in concentration up to 0.3% in epinephrine hydrochloride and bitartrate solutions. Epinephrine borate solutions have a pH in the range 5.5 to 7.5 and offer a more difficult challenge to formulators who seek to prevent oxidation. Several patented antioxidant systems have been developed specifically for this compound. These consist of ascorbic acid and acetylcysteine and sodium bisulfite and 8-hydroxyquinoline. Isoascorbic acid is also an effective antioxidant for this drug. Sodium thiosulfate is used with sodium sulfacetamide solutions.

Surfactants The use of surfactants is greatly restricted in formulating ophthalmic solutions. The order of surfactant toxicity is anionic > cationic >> nonionic. Several nonionic surfactants are used in relatively low concentrations to aid in dispersing steroids in suspensions and to achieve or to improve solution clarity. Those principally used are the sorbitan ether esters of oleic acid (polysorbate or Tween 20 and 80), polymers of oxyethylated octyl phenol (tyloxapol), and polyoxyl 40 stearate. The lowest concentration possible is used to perform the desired function. Their effect on preservative efficacy and possible binding by macromolecules as well as effect on ocular irritation must be taken into account. The use of surfactants as cosolvents for an ophthalmic solution of chloramphenicol has been described (347). This composition includes polyoxyl 40 stearate and polyethylene glycol to solubilize 0.5% chloramphenicol. These surfactants-cosolvents provide a clear aqueous solution of chloramphenicol and a stabilization of the antibiotic in aqueous solution. Polyethoxylated ethers of castor oil are used reportedly for solubilization in Voltaren® (diclofenac sodium) ophthalmic solution (U.S. patent 4,960,799).

Viscosity-imparting agents Polyvinyl alcohol, methylcellulose, hydroxypropyl methyl-cellulose, hydroxyethylcellulose, and one of the several high-molecular-weight cross-lined polymers of acrylic acid, known as carbomers (346), are commonly used to increase the viscosity of ophthalmic solutions and suspensions. Although they reduce surface tension significantly, their primary benefit is to increase the ocular contact time, thereby decreasing the drainage rate and increasing drug bioavailability. A secondary benefit of the polymer solutions is a lubricating effect that is largely subjective, but noticeable to many patients. One disadvantage to the use of the polymers is their tendency to dry to a film on the eyelids and eyelashes; however, this can be easily removed by wiping with a damp tissue.

Numerous studies have shown that increasing the viscosity of ophthalmic products increases contact time and pharmacological effect, but there is a plateau reached after which further increases in viscosity produce only slight or no increases in effect. The location of the plateau is drug and formulation dependent. Blaugh and Canada (347) using methylcellulose solutions found increased contact time in rabbits up to 25 cP and a leveling off at 55 cP. Lynn and Jones (348) studied the rate of lacrimal excretion in humans using a dye solution in methylcellulose concentration from 0.25% to 2.5%, corresponding to viscosities of 6 to 30,000 cP, the latter being a thick gel.

Chrai and Robinson (42) conducted studies in rabbits and found that over a range of 1.0 to 12.5 cP viscosity there is a threefold decrease in the drainage rate constant and a further threefold decrease over the viscosity range of 12.5 to 100 cP. This decrease in drainage rate increased the concentration of drug in the precorneal tear film at zero time and subsequent time periods, which resulted in a higher aqueous humor drug concentration. The magnitude of the increase in drug concentration in the aqueous humor was smaller than the increase in viscosity, about 1.7 times, for the range 1.0 to 12.5 cP, and only a further 1.2-fold increase at 100 cP. Since direct determination of ophthalmic bioavailability in humans is not possible without endangering the eye, investigators have used fluorescein to study factors affecting bioavailability in the eye, because its penetration can be quantified in humans through the use of slit-lamp fluorophotometer. Adler (349), using this technology, found only small increases in dye penetration over a wide range of viscosities. The use of fluorescein data to extrapolate vehicle effects to ophthalmic drugs in general would be questionable owing to the large differences in chemical structure, properties, and permeability existing between fluorescein and most ophthalmic drugs.

The major commercial viscous vehicles are hydroxypropyl methylcellulose (Isopto®) and polyvinyl alcohol (Liquifilm®). Isopto products most often use 0.5% of the cellulosic and range from 10 to 30 cP in viscosity. Liquifilm products have viscosities of about 4 to 6 cP and use 1.4% polymer.

Although usually considered to be inactive ingredients in ophthalmic formulations added because they impart viscosity, many of these polymers function as ocular lubricants. They are marketed as the active ingredients in OTC ocular lubricants used to provide relief from dry eye conditions. The regulatory requirements for these OTC products are found in the FDA CFR (21 CFR 349 Ophthalmic Drug Products for Over-the-Counter Human Use), and their formulations are presented in the 15th edition of the *APhA Handbook of Nonprescription Drugs*.

In summary, there are numerous variables to be adjusted and many choices of excipients required when tailoring a formulation of a particular therapeutic agent for ophthalmic application. But ultimately the choice rests on finding an economically viable formulation, which clinically enhances the therapeutic index for that drug.

Vehicles Ophthalmic drops are, with few exceptions, aqueous fluids using purified water USP as the solvent. WFI is not required as it is in parenterals. Purified water meeting USP standards may be obtained by distillation, deionization, or reverse osmosis.

Oils have been used as vehicles for several topical eyedrop products that are extremely sensitive to moisture. Tetracycline HCl is an antibiotic that is stable for only a few days in aqueous solution. It is supplied as a 1% sterile suspension with Plastibase 50W and light liquid petrolatum. White petrolatum and its combination with liquid petrolatum to obtain a proper consistency is routinely used as the vehicle for ophthalmic ointments.

When oils are used as vehicles in ophthalmic fluids, they must be of the highest purity. Vegetable oils such as olive oil, castor oil, and sesame oil have been used for extemporaneous compounding. These oils are subject to rancidity and, therefore, must be used carefully. Some commercial oils, such as peanut oil, contain stabilizers that could be irritating. The purest grade of oil, such as that used for parenteral products would be advisable for ophthalmics.

Packaging

Eyedrops have been packaged almost entirely in plastic dropper bottles since the introduction of the Drop-Tainer® plastic dispenser in the 1950s. A few products still remain in glass dropper bottles because of special stability considerations. The main advantage of the Drop-Tainer and similarly designed plastic dropper bottles are convenience of use by the patient, decreased contamination potential, lower weight, and lower cost. The plastic bottle has the dispensing tips as an integral part of the package. The patient simply removes the cap and turns the bottle upside down and squeezes gently to form a single drop that falls into the eye. The dispensing tip will deliver only one drop or a stream of fluid for irrigation, depending on the tip design and pressure applied. When used properly, the solution remaining in the bottle is only minimally exposed to airborne contaminants during administration; thus, it will maintain very low to nonexistent microbial content compared with the old-style glass bottle with its separate dropper assembly.

The plastic bottle and dispensing tip are made of low-density polyethylene (LDPE) resin, medium-density polyethylene (MDPE), or a high-density polyethylene (HDPE) resin, which provides the necessary flexibility and inertness. Because these components are in contact with the product during its shelf life, they must be carefully chosen and tested for their suitability for ophthalmic use. In addition to stability studies on the product in the container over a range of normal and accelerated temperatures, the plastic resins must pass the USP biological and chemical tests for suitability. The LDPE resins are by far the most commonly used and are compatible with a very wide range of drugs and formulation components. Their one disadvantage is their sorption and permeability characteristics. Volatile ingredients, such as the preservatives chlorobutanol and phenylethyl alcohol, can migrate into the plastic and eventually permeate through the walls of the container. The sorption and permeation can be detected by stability studies if it is significant. If the permeating component is a preservative, a repeat test of the preservative effectiveness with time will determine if the loss is significant. If necessary, a safe and reasonable excess of the permeable component may be added to balance the loss during the product's shelf life. Another means of overcoming permeation effects is to employ a secondary package, such as a peel-apart blister or pouch composed of nonpermeable materials (e.g., aluminum foil or vinyl). The plastic dropper bottles are also permeable to water, but weight loss by water vapor transmission has a decreasing significance as the size of the bottle increases. The consequences of water vapor transmission must be taken into consideration when assessing the stability of a product.

The LDPE resins are translucent, and if the drug is light sensitive, additional package protection may be required. This can be achieved by using a resin containing an opacifying agent such as titanium dioxide, by placing an opaque sleeve over the exterior of the container, or by placing the bottle in a cardboard carton. Extremely light-sensitive drugs, such as epinephrine and proparacaine, may require a combination of these protective measures.

The MDPE and HDPE resins were developed to address formulator's needs when an LDPE resin was not adequate; on the basis of parameters such as weight loss, adsorption, or additional package rigidity is required. The MDPE resins provide intermediate properties between low- and high-density polyethylene, where more rigidity than LDPE and less rigidity than HDPE are required. The HDPE resins are of a natural milky color with much better barrier properties than LDPE and MDPE.

Colorants, other than titanium dioxide, are rarely used in plastic containers; however, the use of colorants is required for the cap. The American Academy of Ophthalmology (AAO) recommended to the FDA that a uniform color coding system be established for the caps and labels of all topical ocular medications. Industry new drug applicants are required to either follow this system or provide an adequate justification for any deviations from the system. The AAO color codes, as revised and approved by the AAO Board of Trustees in June 1996, are shown in Table 4. The FDA and AAO have extended the cap color scheme to differentiate different classes of newer Rx drugs for the benefit of the patient who may be using more than one product. The intent is to help prevent errors in medication and improve patient compliance. It is important for the pharmacist to explain this color coding to the patient and/or caregiver since it can be defeated if the cap is not returned to the proper container after each use.

The pharmacist should dispense the sterile ophthalmic product only in the original unopened container. A tamper-evident feature such as a cellulosic or metal band around

Table 4 AAO-Recommended Color Coding of Caps and Labels for Topical Ophthalmic Medications

Class	Color	Pantone® number
Anti-infectives	Tan	467
Anti-inflammatories/steroids	Pink	197, 212
Mydriatics and cycloplegics	Red	485C
Nonsteroidal anti-inflammatories	Gray	4C
Miotics	Green	374, 362, 348
β-Blockers	Yellow or blue[a]	
Yellow C	290, 281	
Adrenergic agonists (e.g., propine)	Purple	2583
Carbonic anhydrase inhibitors	Orange	1585
Prostaglandin analogs	Turquoise	326C

[a]The AAO notes that as new classes of drugs are developed, this coding system may be modified in the future by reassigning the blue color to a new class of drugs while keeping yellow for β-blockers.
Abbreviation: AAO, American Academy of Ophthalmology.

the cap and bottleneck is provided by the manufacturer, and the container should not be dispensed if these are missing or there is evidence of prior removal and reapplication. The LDPE, MDPE, and HDPE resins used for the bottles and the dispensing tips cannot be autoclaved, and they are sterilized either by ^{60}Co γ-irradiation or ethylene oxide. The cap is designed such that when it is screwed tightly onto the bottle, it mates with the dispensing tip and forms a seal. The cap is usually made of a harder resin than the bottle, such as polystyrene or polypropylene, and is also sterilized by γ-radiation or ethylene oxide gas exposure. A plastic ophthalmic package has been introduced that uses a special grade of polypropylene that is resistant to deformation at autoclave temperatures. With this specialized packaging, the bottle can be filled, the dispensing tip and cap applied, and the entire product sterilized by steam under pressure at 121°C.

The glass dropper bottle is still used for products that are extremely sensitive to oxygen or contain permeable components that are not sufficiently stable in plastic. Powders for reconstitution also use glass containers, owing to their heat-transfer characteristics, which are necessary during the freeze-drying process. The glass used should be USP type I for maximum compatibility with the sterilization process and the product. The glass container is made sterile by dry heat or steam autoclave. Amber glass is used for light resistance and is superior to green glass. A sterile dropper assembly is usually supplied separately. It is usually gas sterilized in a blister composed of vinyl and Tyvek, a fused, porous polypropylene material. The dropper assembly is made of a glass or LDPE plastic pipette and a rubber dropper bulb. The manufacturer carefully tests the appropriate plastic and rubber materials suitable for use with the product; therefore, they should be dispensed with the product. The pharmacist should place the dropper assembly aseptically into the product before dispensing and instruct the patient on precautions to be used to prevent contamination.

Multidose packaging of unpreserved topical drops In some cases it may be desirable to prescribe a product without an antimicrobial preservative for patients who exhibit sensitivity to various preservatives. This can be accomplished with the use of unit-dose containers but these usually contain more than that needed for a single use, so if the patient ignores the labeling and makes multiple use of the contents, there is increased risk for contamination. Recent product introductions of this type include the VISMED® multilubricant eyedrops from TRB CHEMMEDICA, who are marketing an innovative unpreserved multidose eye lubricant that contains a pump that needs to be primed prior to first use (http://www.trbchemedica.co.uk). The VISMED eyedrops contain a proprietary formulation of highly purified specific fraction of sodium hyaluronate. In this formulation, sodium hyaluronate due to its main physical characteristic, viscoelasticity, delivers a high viscosity between blinks and a low viscosity during blinking, ensuring efficient coating of the surface of the eye. In addition to being unpreserved, the pH of VISMED is adjusted to 7.3, similar to that of the natural tear film, for further potential patient comfort. The VISMED product is currently marketed in the European Union as a medical device under a CE mark, and a clinical trial sponsored by Lantibio Inc., Chapel Hill, North Carolina, U.S. is recruiting patients in the United States.

FDA regulations for ophthalmic liquids allow the use of unpreserved multidose packaging if the product is packaged and labeled in such a manner as to afford adequate protection and minimize the hazards resulting from contamination during use (21 CFR 200.50). Thus, the same unit-dose containers can be modified to use a resealable cap and the labeling modified to limit the usage to a minimum number of doses such as to discard after 12 hours from initial use and limit the content volume to the expected number of doses with only a small overfill if necessary. It may be necessary to use a secondary package to retard moisture vapor transmission significantly, depending on the surface to volume ratio of the primary package.

Semisolid Dosage Forms: Ophthalmic Ointments and Gels

Formulation
The principal semisolid dosage form used in ophthalmology is an anhydrous ointment with a petrolatum base. The ointment vehicle is usually a mixture of mineral oil and white petrolatum. The mineral oil is added to reduce the melting point and modify the consistency. The principal advantages of the petrolatum-based ointments are their blandness and anhydrous and inert nature, which make them suitable vehicles for moisture-sensitive drugs. Ophthalmic ointments containing antibiotics are used quite frequently following operative procedures, and their safety is supported by the experience of a noted eye surgeon Ramon Castroviejo (350), who, in over 20,000 postsurgical patients, saw no side effects secondary to ointment use. No impediment to epithelial or stromal wound healing was exhibited by currently used ophthalmic ointments tested by Hanna et al. (351). The same investigators have reported that, even if these ointments were entrapped in the anterior chamber and did not exceed 5% of the volume, little or no reaction was caused (352). Ganulomatous reactions requiring surgical excision have been reported secondary to therapeutic injection of ointment into the lacrimal sac (353).

The chief disadvantages of the use of ophthalmic ointments are their greasy nature and the blurring of vision produced. They are most often used as adjunctive nighttime therapy, with eyedrops administered during the day. The nighttime use obviates the difficulties produced by blurring of vision and is stated to prolong ocular retention when compared with drops. Ointments are used almost exclusively as vehicles for antibiotics, sulfonamides, antifungals, and anti-inflammatories. The petrolatum vehicle is also used as an ocular lubricant following surgery or to treat various dry eye syndromes. Anesthesiologists may prescribe the ointment vehicle for the nonophthalmic surgical patients to prevent severe and painful dry eye conditions that could develop during prolonged surgeries. A petrolatum ointment is recognized as a safe and effective OTC emollient (21 CFR 349.14), and marketed OTC emollient products are discussed in the 12th edition of the *APhA Handbook of Nonprescription Drugs*.

The anhydrous petrolatum base may be made more miscible with water through the use of an anhydrous liquid lanolin derivative. Drugs can be incorporated into such a base in aqueous solution if desired. Polyoxyl 40 stearate and polyethylene glycol 300 are used in an anti-infective ointment to solubilize the active principle in the base so that the ointment can be sterilized by aseptic filtration. The cosmetic-type bases, such as the oil-in-water (o/w) emulsion bases popular in dermatology, should not be used in the eye, nor should liquid emulsions, owing to the ocular irritation produced by the soaps and surfactants, used to form the emulsion.

In an attempt to formulate an anhydrous, but water-soluble, semisolid base for potential ophthalmic use, five bases were studied and reported on (354). The nonaqueous portion of the base was either glycerin or polyethylene glycols in high concentrations. The matrix used to form the phases included silica, Gantrez® AN-139, and Carbopol® 940. Eye irritation results were not reported, but the authors have studied representative bases from that research report and found them to be quite irritating in rabbit eyes. The irritation is believed to be primarily due to the high concentration of the polyols used as vehicles.

An aqueous semisolid gel base has been developed that provides significantly longer residence time in the cul-de-sac and increases drug bioavailability and, thereby, may prolong the therapeutic level in the eye. The gel contains a high-molecular-weight, cross-linked polymer to provide the high viscosity and optimum rheological properties for prolonged ocular retention. Only a relatively low concentration of polymer is required, so that the gel base is more than 95% water.

Schoenwald et al. (355) have demonstrated the unique ocular retention of this polymeric gel base in rabbits, in which the miotic effect of pilocarpine was significantly prolonged. The use of other polymers, such as cellulosic gums, polyvinyl alcohol, and polyacrylamides at comparable apparent viscosities, did not provide a significantly prolonged effect. The prolonged effect of pilocarpine has also been demonstrated in human clinical trials, in which a single application of 4% pilocarpine HCl-containing carbomer gel at bedtime provided a 24-hour reduced IOP, compared with the usually required q.i.d. dosing for pilocarpine solution (356). As a result, some glaucoma patients can now use pilocarpine in this aqueous gel base (Pilopine® HS Gel) dosing only once a day at bedtime to control their IOP without the significant vision disturbance experienced during the day for the use of conventional pilocarpine eyedrops. The gel is applied in a small strip in the lower conjunctival sac from an ophthalmic ointment tube.

The carbomer polymeric gel base itself has been used successfully to treat moderate to severe cases of dry eye (keratoconjunctivitis sicca) (357). The dry eye syndrome is usually characterized by deficiency of tear production and, therefore, requires frequent instillation of aqueous artificial tear eyedrops to keep the corneal epithelium moist. The gel base applied in a small amount provides a prolonged lubrication to the external ocular tissues, and some patients have reduced the frequency of dosing to control their symptoms to thrice a day or fewer.

Sterility and Preservation

Since October 1973, FDA regulations require that all U.S. ophthalmic ointments be sterile. This legal requirement was a result of several surveys on microbial contamination of ophthalmic ointments, and followed reports in Sweden and the United Kingdom of severe eye infections resulting from use of nonsterile ointments. In its survey published in 1973, the FDA found that of 82 batches of ophthalmic ointments tested from 27 manufacturers, 16 batches were contaminated, including 8 antibiotic-containing ointments. The contamination levels were low and were principally molds and yeasts (358). The time lag in imposition of a legal requirement for sterility of ointments compared with solutions and suspensions was due to the absence of a reliable sterility test for the petrolatum-based ointments until isopropyl myristate was employed to dissolve these ointments and allow improved recovery of viable microorganisms by membrane filtration. Manufacturers found that, in fact, many of their ointments were sterile, but revised their manufacturing procedures to increase the assurance of sterility.

A suitable substance or mixture of substances to prevent growth of, or destroy, microorganisms accidentally introduced during use must be added to ophthalmic ointments that are packaged in multiuse containers, regardless of the method of sterilization employed, unless otherwise directed in the individual monograph or unless the formula itself is bacteriostatic in accordance with the USP ⟨771⟩, Ophthalmic Ointments. Schwartz (359) has commented that a sterile ointment cannot become excessively contaminated by ordinary use because of its consistency and the fact that in a nonaqueous medium microorganisms merely survive, but do not multiply. Antimicrobial preservative effectiveness of ophthalmic ointments is evaluated by use of the USP ⟨51⟩.

Packaging

Historically, ophthalmic ointments were packaged in small tin collapsible tubes, usually holding 3.5 g. The tin tube was compatible with a wide range of drugs in petrolatum-based ointments; however, epoxy-phenolic-lined aluminum tubes are becoming more widespread. Plastic tubes made from flexible LDPE resins have also been considered as an alternative material, but do not collapse and tend to suck back the ointment. The various types of metal tubes are sealed using an adhesive coating covering only the inner edges of the bottom of the open tube to form the crimp, which does not contact the product. Laminated tubes are usually heat sealed. The crimp usually contains the lot code and expiration date. Filled tubes may be tested for leaks by storing them in a horizontal position in an oven at 60°C for at least 8 hours. No leakage should be evidenced except for a minute quantity that could only come from within the crimp of the tube or the end of the cap. The screw cap is made of polyethylene or polypropylene. Polypropylene must be used for autoclave sterilization, but either material may be used when the tubes are gas sterilized. A tamper-evident feature is required for sterile ophthalmic ointments, and may be accomplished by sealing the tube or the carton holding the tube such that the contents cannot be used without providing visible evidence of destruction of the seal.

The tube can be a source of metal particles and must be cleaned carefully before sterilization. The USP ⟨751⟩ metal particles in ophthalmic ointments is a test procedure that sets the limits of the level of metal particles in ophthalmic ointments. The total number of metal particles detected under 30 times magnification that are 50 μm or larger in any dimension is counted. The requirements are met if the total number of such particles counted in 10 tubes is not more than 50, and if not more than one tube is found to contain more than eight such particles.

Solid Dosage Forms: Ocular Inserts

In earlier times, it has been reported that lamella or disks of glycerinated gelatin were used to supply drugs to the eye by insertion beneath the eyelid. The aqueous tear fluids dissolved the lamella and released the drug for absorption. The medical literature also describes a sterile paper strip impregnated with drug for insertion in the eye. These appear to have been the first attempts at designing a sustained-release ocular dosage form.

Nonerodible Ocular Inserts

In 1975, the first controlled-release topical dosage form was marketed in the United States by the Alza Corporation. Zaffaroni (360) describes the Alza therapeutic system as a drug-containing device or dosage form that administers a drug or drugs at programed rates, at a specific body site, for a prescribed time period to provide continuous control of drug therapy and to maintain this control over extended periods. Therapeutic systems for uterine delivery of progesterone, transdermal delivery of scopolamine, and oral delivery of systemic drugs have also been developed.

The Ocusert® Pilo-20 and Pilo-40 Ocular Therapeutic System is an elliptical membrane that is soft and flexible and designed to be placed in the inferior cul-de-sac between the sclera and the eyelid and to release pilocarpine continuously at a steady rate for seven days. The design of the dosage form is described by Alza in terms of an open-looped therapeutic system, having three major components: (*i*) the drug, (*ii*) a drug delivery module, and (*iii*) a platform. In the Ocusert Pilo-20 and Pilo-40 systems, the drug

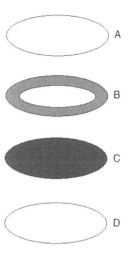

Figure 19 Exploded view of the pilocarpine Ocusert system (**A,D**) Transparent rate-controlling membranes. (**B**) Plastic ring, opaque white for visibility in handling and insertion. (**C**) Drug reservoir. Total thickness of the assembled system is 0.3 mm. Major and minor axes of the ellipsoidal device are 13.4 and 5.7 mm, respectively.

delivery module consists of (*i*) a drug reservoir, pilocarpine (free base), and a carrier material, alginic acid; (*ii*) a rate controller, ethylene-vinyl acetate (EVA) copolymer membrane; (*iii*) an energy source, the concentration of pilocarpine in the reservoir; and (*iv*) a delivery portal, the copolymer membrane. The platform component for the pilocarpine Ocusert consists of the EVA copolymer membranes, which serve as the housing, and an annular ring of the membrane impregnated with titanium dioxide that forms a white border for visibility. The laminate structure of the Ocusert is seen in (Fig. 19). The free-base form of pilocarpine is used, since it exhibits both hydrophilic and lipophilic characteristics. Use of the extremely water-soluble salts of pilocarpine would have necessitated the use of a hydrophilic membrane, which, if it osmotically imbibed an excessive amount of water, would cause a significant decline in the release rate with time. Use of the free base allowed a choice of more hydrophobic membranes that are relatively impermeable to water; accordingly, the release rate is independent of the environment in which it is placed. EVA, the hydrophobic copolymer chosen, was found to be very compatible with the sensitive ocular tissues (111, p. 1037), an important feature.

The pilocarpine Ocusert was seen by Alza to offer a number of theoretical advantages over drop therapy for the glaucoma patient. The Ocusert exposes a patient to only one-fourth to one-eighth the amount of pilocarpine, compared with drop therapy. This could lead to reduced local side effects and toxicity. It provides continuous round-the-clock control of IOP, whereas drops used four times a day can permit periods where the IOP might rise. Additionally, the Ocusert provides for more patient convenience and improved compliance, as the dose needs to be administered only once per week. However, clinical experience seems to indicate that the Ocusert has a compliance problem of its own (i.e., retention in the eye for the full seven days). The patient must check periodically to see that the unit is still in place, particularly in the morning on arising. Replacement of a contaminated unit with a fresh one can increase the price differential of the already expensive Ocusert therapy compared with the inexpensive drop or once-a-day gel therapy. In addition, some patients find positioning the Ocusert in the eye to be challenging.

Soft contact lenses, made of the same hydrophilic plastic materials used for vision correction, are also used as corneal bandages to protect the cornea during the healing process following surgery. They can be fitted to the eye and inserted and removed by the ophthalmologist. They are usually used without correction (plano lens) and removed by the ophthalmologist. Since they are used in a compromised cornea, great care must be taken to prevent microbial contamination.

A recent investigation of a nonerodible ocular insert was conducted by QLT Plug Delivery, Inc. and evaluated the safety and efficacy of its Latanoprost Punctal Plug Delivery System (L-PPDS) for the treatment of open angle glaucoma. The company released proof-of-concept phase II clinical data from their CORE study that suggest that this might be a novel drug delivery route for ocular compounds. The PPDS was designed to address the unmet medical need of poor compliance and adherence patterns to treatment regimens seen in glaucoma and ocular hypertensive patients. Additional confirmatory clinical trials will be necessary to enable market registration of this product for the lowering of IOP, and potentially other indications when the PPDS is loaded with different therapeutic agents.

Erodible Ocular Inserts

Since polymers have been added to solutions to increase viscosity and ocular retention, it is not surprising that similar solutions have been dried to form films of the polymer-drug system. These films inserted into the lower cul-de-sac of the eye have been reported to increase retention time and drug bioavailability and prolong therapeutic effect. Ocular inserts made with water-soluble polymers imbibe the tear fluid and slowly dissolve and erode, releasing their drug content. The erodible inserts have potential advantages of not having to be removed at the end of their useful dosing interval. They provide a more precise dosage to the eye from a unit dosage form, and no preservative is required, thus reducing the risk of sensitivity reactions. Also, it may be possible to reduce the applied dose compared with conventional eyedrops and reduce the risk of local or systemic adverse effects. Potential disadvantages include the difficulty of achieving constant zero-order drug delivery as the matrix is eroding, and in some cases they may be squeezed out of the eye due to movement of the eyelids before their delivery cycle is complete. They may require terminal sterilization, and this may adversely affect stability and could produce unwanted degradation products. Considerable drug delivery research has been conducted and reported for various erodible ocular inserts (361–365).

An erodible insert developed as a potential ocular drug delivery system is marketed as a prescription drug for the lubricant properties of the polymer base. Lacrisert® is a sterile ophthalmic insert that is used in the treatment of moderate-to-severe dry eye syndrome and is usually recommended for patients unable to obtain symptomatic relief with artificial tear solutions. The insert is composed of 5 mg of hydroxypropylcellulose in a rod-shaped form, about 1.27 mm in diameter and about 3.5 mm long. No preservative is used, since it is essentially anhydrous. The quite rigid cellulose rod is placed in the lower conjunctival sac and first imbibes water from the tears, and after several hours, forms a gel-like mass, which gradually erodes as the polymer dissolves. This action thickens the tear film and provides increased lubrication, which can provide symptomatic relief for dry eye states. It is usually used once or twice daily.

Corneal shields are medical devices that are used as a bandage for protection of the cornea and to allow healing following surgery. Initially, hydrophilic soft contact lenses used for vision correction were employed as corneal shields. Collagen was then introduced as a substitute for the plastic noneroding bandage lens. They are widely used today as temporary protective devices for healing corneas. In addition to their approved use of corneal bandages, they have been investigated as drug delivery vehicles to provide sustained delivery of drugs to the cornea by the ophthalmologist (366).

Collagen is widely used for biomedical applications. It makes up about 25% of the total body protein in mammals and is the major protein of connective tissue, cartilage, and bone. Importantly, the secondary and tertiary structures of humans, porcine and bovine collagen, are very similar, making it possible to use animal-sourced collagen in the human body. Collagen shields are designed to be sterile, disposable, temporary bandage lens, which conform to the shape of the eye and protect the cornea. They are not optically clear and reduce visual acuity to the 20/80 to 20/200 range. They differ mainly in the source of the collagen, usually bovine or porcine, and their dissolution time on the cornea ranging from 12 to 72 hours. The dissolution time is controlled during manufacture by varying the degree of cross-linking usually by exposure to ultraviolet light.

Intraocular Dosage Forms

Ophthalmic products, which are introduced into the interior structures of the eye either during ocular surgery or via an intravitreal injection, are a special class that requires the application of technology from parenteral dosage forms in their design, packaging, and manufacture. The development of cytomegalovirus (CMV) retinitis as a common opportunistic infection in patients with AIDS has resulted in the initial expansion of this class of ocular product to include solid inserts and injections of antiviral agents administered directly to the vitreous cavity. As discussed previously, topical and systemic administration often fail to achieve therapeutic concentrations in the vitreous cavity.

Ophthalmic surgery has rapidly advanced in the last three decades particularly with the ability of the surgeon to operate in back of the eye. The ophthalmologist can perform vitreoretinal surgery and restore significant visual function in patients with diabetic complications, endophthalmitis, and retinal tears and detachments. Also, significant advances have been made in anterior segment surgery, especially for cataract surgery where replacement of a cloudy or opaque natural crystalline lens with a plastic or silicone intraocular lens can restore visual acuity and allow the patient to achieve a significant improvement in his or her quality of life. These technological advances have placed greater emphasis on the development of products specifically formulated and packaged for intraocular use. This has led to the development of improved irrigating solutions, intraocular injections, viscoelastics, vitreous inserts, and intravitreal injections.

Intraocular Irrigating Solutions

An essential component of ocular surgery is the use of physiological solution to moisten and irrigate ocular tissue on the external surface as well as intraocular anterior and posterior segments of the eye. Externally, the solution maintains a moist surface, preventing cellular desiccation, which can inhibit the surgeon's ability to see inside the eye. The solution also acts as a substitute for the natural aqueous intraocular fluid and aids in the removal of blood and cellular debris. Normal saline and lactated Ringer's solution were used initially since they were available in parenteral dosage form; but they lacked key components of ocular fluids. In the 1960s, a balanced salt solution was developed specifically for ocular surgical use and became widely used. It contains the five essential ions: sodium, potassium, calcium, magnesium, and chloride. It also contains citrate and acetate ions, which provide some buffer capacity and a potential source of bicarbonate. It is formulated to be iso-osmotic with aqueous humor (about 305 mOsm) and has a neutral to slightly alkaline physiological pH (49,111,367).

Balanced salt solution (BSS®) provided an improved ocular irrigating solution; however, as the surgical techniques for cataract surgery evolved and new vitreoretinal surgical procedures were introduced, larger volumes of irrigating solutions have been used, and surgical operating times for the very delicate vitreoretinal procedures can exceed several hours. This put additional physiological demands on the irrigating solution, and an enriched BSS (BSS® Plus) was developed. The enriched product contains the essential electrolyte components of BSS with the addition of glutathione (oxidized) and dextrose as energy sources, bicarbonate as a physiological buffer, and a phosphate buffer system to maintain the products storage pH in the physiological range (112,368).

The enriched BSS formulation presented chemical and physical stability issues not present in the original BSS product. It was necessary to use a two-part formulation to develop a commercially viable product with several years of storage stability; the two parts are aseptically combined just prior to surgery. The two-part formulation consists of a large volume part containing sodium, potassium, chloride, phosphate, and bicarbonate components at physiological pH and osmolality. The second part contains the calcium and magnesium divalent ions and the oxidized glutathione and dextrose in an acidic environment for long-term storage stability. The smaller-volume second part has a minimal buffer capacity and when added to the larger-volume first part does not significantly change the final product's physiological pH. Once aseptically combined, it is stable for at least 24 hours, although it is labeled to be used within 6 hours as a sterility precaution.

Providing the product as a two-part system was necessary to overcome the physical and chemical incompatibilities inherent in the final composition. Bicarbonate is stable only in an alkaline environment while glutathione and dextrose are stable in a pH range of about 3 to 5. Consideration was also given to which of the two parts should be of the larger volume in the irrigation bottle since there could be inadvertent failure to mix the two parts prior to use. The large volume component contains a bicarbonate saline solution at physiological pH and osmolality and thus would be more tissue compatible than irrigating with a hypo-osmotic acidic pH solution.

The large volume part is packaged in type 1 glass IV bottle and as such can be autoclave sterilized. The quality of the glass is important to prevent leaching of silicates, which can increase pH during autoclaving and storage. IV parenteral grade rubber stoppers must be used to minimize coring and extraction. Type 1 glass is also used for the additive part vial with a parenteral grade rubber stoppers. With a small volume in the larger volume package, the additive part can be easily added through the stopper via a transfer needle.

Intraocular irrigating solutions are required to be preservative-free to prevent toxicity to the internal tissues of the eye, particularly the corneal endothelium, lens, and the retina (369,370). These products are intended for single use only to prevent intraocular infections, which can be difficult to treat and seriously threaten sight. In addition to being sterile, they must be nonpyrogenic, therefore requiring sterile WFI as the vehicle.

These irrigating solutions have been developed and are labeled to be used without the addition of any drugs, that is, not as a delivery vehicle. However, some drugs such as epinephrine are added to the irrigating solution prior to surgery and used extensively by cataract surgeons to achieve and maintain pupillary dilation, facilitating removal of the natural lens and insertion of the prosthetic intraocular lens. Use of some commercial epinephrine injections that contain sodium bisulfite in addition to their acidic pH as the source for the epinephrine additive have been reported to be the cause of intraocular toxicity, even though it is diluted as much as 500-fold before irrigation (113).

Intraocular Injections and Implants

Very few injectable dosage forms have been specifically developed and approved by the FDA for intraocular use. However, the ophthalmologist uses available parenteral dosage forms to deliver anti-infectives, corticosteriods, and anesthetic products to achieve higher therapeutic concentrations intraocularly than can ordinarily be achieved by topical or systemic administration. These unapproved or off-label uses have developed over time as part of the physician's practice of medicine and include subconjunctival, retrobulbar, sub-Tenon's, and intravitreal injections.

The FDA approved intraocular injections include miotics, triamcinolone acetonide, pegaptanib sodium, ranibizumab, formivirsen sodium, viscoelastics and viscoadherents, and an antiviral agent for intravitreal injection. There are many small and large molecules currently in clinical trials that are delivered via intravitreal injection for the treatment of a variety of retinal diseases with a large area of focus on the treatment of AMD and macular edema.

Antivirals are used to treat the ocular sequelae of AIDS such as CMV retinitis. They are treated with systemic administration; but with the need for higher localized ocular therapeutic concentrations, products have been developed and approved for direct administration into the vitreous cavity.

Intraocular implants for treatment of diseases of the posterior segment have been described in the section "Delivery to the Vitreous and Posterior Segment."

Viscoelastics

Highly purified fractions of sodium hyaluronate have become an important ocular surgical adjunct because of their lubricant and viscoelastic properties. They are injected into the anterior segment of the eye during surgery for removal of cataracts and implantation of an IOL, trabeculectomy, and corneal transplantation. They are also used as a surgical aid in the vitreous cavity during retinal surgery. Their viscoelasticity provides a mechanical barrier between tissues and allows the surgeon more space for manipulation with less trauma to surrounding tissues, particularly the corneal endothelium. It is also used to coat the IOL prior to insertion and lessen the potential for tissue damage upon implantation. In posterior segment surgery, it is used to separate tissue away from the retina and as a tamponade to maneuver tissue, such as a detached retina, back into place for reattachment. The viscoelastic material is usually removed at the end of the surgery since it may take several days to be cleared from the eye and has the potential to elevate IOP.

Sodium hyaluronate is a high-molecular-weight polysaccharide, which is widely distributed throughout the tissues of the body of animals and humans. The viscoelastic materials used as ocular surgical aids are specific fractions from animal tissue, which are highly purified to remove foreign proteins and are tested to be nonantigenic and noninflammatory in the eye. The purified fraction is formulated to yield a high viscoelasticity determined by the interplay of molecular weight and concentration. The solution is packaged in disposable glass syringes, which are terminally sterilized and aseptically packaged so that they can be used in the sterile surgical field (Healon®, ProVisc®, Amvisc®).

Chondroitin sulfate (Viscoat[®], DuoVisc[®], DisCoVisc[®]) also is used in combination with sodium hyaluronate as a viscoelastic surgical aid to provide higher viscosities, which may provide additional tissue protection during the irrigation and aspiration accompanying phacoemulsification, a common means of removing the cloudy crystalline lens prior to IOL implantation.

Nonpyrogenic solutions of sterile hydroxypropyl methylcellulose are also used as ocular surgical aids similar to the viscoelastics in cataract surgery (OcuCoat[®]). These lubricants are sometimes classified as viscoadherents because they are used to coat the IOL prior to implantation and the tips of surgical instruments prior to deployment inside the eye. This is the same cellulosic material, but in a highly purified form, serving as a viscosifying agent in topical eyedrops and as an OTC ocular lubricant. Since it is not a natural product, it does not have the antigenic potential of the other viscoelastics. It can be stored at room temperature, whereas the sodium hyaluronate solutions must be stored in the refrigerator.

CONTACT LENS CARE PRODUCTS

Contact lenses are optical devices that are either fabricated from preformed polymers or polymerized during lens manufacture. The main purpose of contact lenses is to correct defective vision, and they are generally referred as corrective lenses. However, due to the recent advances in material manufacturing, reduction in fabrication cost, and their availability in many colors, they are extensively used to change the appearance of the eye. For this application, they are called cosmetic lenses. Contact lenses used medically for the treatment of certain corneal diseases are called bandage lenses.

Evolution of Contact Lenses

In 1508, Leonardo da Vinci conceived the concept of the contact lens. It was not until 1887 that scleral contact lenses were fabricated by Dr. A. E. Fick, a physician in Zurich; F. A. Mueller, a maker of prosthetic eyes in Germany; and Dr. E. Kalt, a physician in France. Muller, Obrig, and Gyorry fabricated contact lenses made from polymethyl methacrylate (PMMA) in the late 1930s. K. Tuohy filed the patent for contact lens design in 1948, which were made of PMMA material (371). Although they were safe and effective, these lenses were uniformly uncomfortable, thus suppressing their potential growth for contact lens wear. Lenses made from polyhydroxyethyl methacrylate (HEMA), the so-called soft lenses or hydrophilic lenses were introduced in 1970. Since then, significant technological advances have been made in the lens materials, lens fabrication, and lens designs (372). Consequently, a phenomenal growth in lens wearers necessitated the need for, and development of, lens care products. Recent development in polymers has led to a broad acceptance of materials prepared by combining HEMA with silicone (silicone hydrogels) (373). Such materials are considered to improve oxygen permeability required to maintain healthy cornea.

Composition of Contact Lenses

Contact lenses are broadly classified as PMMA, RGP, and soft hydrogel (HEMA) lenses. Dyes may be added during polymerization or after fabrication to improve lens handling or to change the color of the lens wearer's eyes. Lenses made from numerous polymers are available today (374). In soft hydrogel lenses, HEMA is a commonly used monomer.

However, to avoid infringement of existing patents, many comonomers, as, for example, methyl methacrylic acid or a blend of comonomers, are used. Comonomers produce changes in the water content or ionic nature of lenses that is significantly different from HEMA lenses. For example, addition of acrylic acid in HEMA increases the water content and ionic nature of lenses. Some lenses are made from *n*-vinylpyrrolidone and have high water contents. Such lenses have pore sizes that are much larger than low water content lenses. Cross-linkers, such as ethyleneglycol dimethacrylate, and initiators as, for example, benzyl peroxide, in appropriate amounts are added for polymerization and to achieve desirable physical and chemical properties. Recently, contact lenses made from HEMA and silicone were made available. These lenses combine the properties of hydrogel and gas-permeable polymers (374). Table 5 gives a list of monomers, comonomers, and cross-linkers along with their effects on polymer properties. In 1985, the FDA published a classification for soft hydrophilic lenses based on their water content and ionic nature. Groupings for soft lenses and their generic names are listed in Table 6. Adequate levels of oxygen are necessary to maintain normal corneal metabolism (375). Lenses that are poorly designed and worn overnight deprive the cornea of oxygen, causing edema (376). Contact lenses made from PMMA materials are virtually impermeable to gases (377). The PMMA lenses are also inflexible, causing discomfort in a large percentage of individuals while the lens is worn. During the 1980s, lenses were made from either cellulose acetate butyrate (CAB) or silicone elastomer. Although comfortable and flexible, such lenses accumulated lipids, were nonwettable, and adhered to the cornea. Several reports detailing difficulty in removing CAB and silicone lenses appeared in the published literature (378). Lenses made from fluorocarbons and in various combinations of fluorocarbon, silicone, methyl methacrylate, and acrylic acid are currently available. Desired properties of these lenses include flexibility, wettability, and gas transmissibility. Grouping for RGP lenses was published by the FDA in 1989. The generic names and oxygen permeabilities of RGP lens materials are provided in Table 7 (379). The development of silicone hydrogels has initiated discussions among regulatory agencies worldwide to add additional groups. Recently, the International Standards Organization (ISO) has recognized that silicone hydrogels do not effectively "fit" within the existing FDA lens grouping and that a further "group V" category should be added for this class of high oxygen permeability hydrogel materials.

Table 5 Commonly Used Monomers, Comonomers, and Cross-Linkers in Contact Lens Polymers

Name	Abbreviation	Lens properties
Acrylic acid	AA	Flexibility Hydrophilicity pH sensitivity: acidic Reactivity: ionically interacts with positively charged tear components Wettability
Butyl methacrylate	BMA	Softness Flexibility Hydrophobicity: attracts lipids Wettability Gas transmissibility
Cellulose acetate butyrate	CAB	Clarity Wettability Gas transmissibility Physical stability

Table 5 Commonly Used Monomers, Comonomers, and Cross-Linkers in Contact Lens Polymers (*Continued*)

Name	Abbreviation	Lens properties
Dimethyl siloxane	DMS	Hydrophobicity Wettability Gas transmissibility Physical stability
Diphenyl siloxane	DPS	Hydrophobicity Wettability Gas transmissibility Physical stability
Ethonyethyl methacrylate	EOEMA	Flexibility Softness Hydrophobicity Wettability Gas transmissibility
Ethylene glycol dimethacrylate	EGDMA	Hydrophobicity Wettability
Glyceryl methacrylate	GMA	Wettability Gas transmissibility Hydrophilicity Machinability
Hydroxyethyl methacrylate	HEMA	Flexibility Wettability Gas transmissibility Softness Machinability
Methacrylic acid	MA	Hardness Machinability Wettability Gas transmissibility Hydrophobicity
Methyl methacrylate	MMA	Hardness Machinability Wettability Gas transmissibility Hydrophobicity
Methylphenyl siloxane	MPS	Hydrophobicity Gas transmissibility
Methyl vinyl siloxane	MVS	Hydrophobicity Gas transmissibility
N-Vinyl pyrrolidone	NVP	Hydrophilicity Wettability Machinability Color, clarity
Siloaxanyl methacrylate	SMA	Hardness Wettability Gas transmissibility

Table 6 FDA Grouping for Soft Hydrophilic Lenses and Generic Names

Group I	Group 2	Group 3	Group 4
Low water ($<$50% H_2O)	High water ($>$50% H_2O)	Low water ($<$50% H_2O)	High water ($>$50% H_2O)
Nonionic polymers	Nonionic polymers	Ionic polymers	Ionic polymers
Tefilcon (38%)	Lidofilcon (70%) Lidofilcon B (79%)	Etafilcon (43%)	Bufilcon A (55%)
Tetrafilcon A (43%) Grofilcon (39%) Dimefilcon A (38%) Hefilcon A (43%)	Surfilcon (74%) Vilifilcon A (55%) Scafilcon A (71%) Xylofilcon A (67%)	Bufilcon A (45%) Deltafilcon A (43%) Dronifilcon A (47%) Phenifilcon A (38%) Ocufilcon (44%)	Perfilcon (71%) Etafilcon A (58%) Ocufilcon C (55%) Phenfilcon A (55%) Tetrafilcon B (58%)
Hefilcon B (43%) Phenifilcon A (30%) Isofilcon (36%) Polymacon (38%) Mafilcon (33%)		Mafilcon (33%)	Methafilcon (55%) Vifilcon A (55%)

Table 7 FDA Grouping of Hydrophobic Hard and Rigid Gas-Permeable Lenses

Lens materials	Generic name	D_k
Cellulose acetate butyrate	Cabufocon A	$>$150
	Powfocon A	$>$150
	Powfocon B	$>$150
t-Butylstyrene	Aufocon A	$>$150
Silicone	Elastofilcon A	$>$150
	Dimofocon	$>$150
	Dilafilcon A	$>$150
t-Butylstyrene-silicon acrylate	Pentasilcon P	120
Fluoracrylate	Fluorofocon A	100
Fluoro silicone acrylate	Itafluorofocon A	60
	Porflufocon A	30–92
Silicone acrylate	Pasifocon A	14
	Pasifocon B	16
	Pasifocon C	45
	Itafocon A	14
	Itafocon B	26
	Nefocon A	20
	Telefocon A	15–45
	Amefocon A	40

Complications of Contact Lens Wear and the Need for Care Products

Lens design, user compliance with manufacturer's instructions, hygiene, environmental conditions, poor fit, lens materials, and tear chemistry are the major causes of lens wear complications. Complications owing to lens design, compliance, hygiene, environmental conditions, and poor fit are beyond the scope of this chapter and are not

Table 8 Major Proteins of the Tear Film

Name	Total protein (%)	Function
Lysozyme	30–40	Antimicrobial, collagenase regulator
Lactoferin	2–3	Bacteriostatic, anti-inflammatory
Albumin	30–440	Anti-inflammatory
Immunoglobulins	0.1	Immunological, anti-inflammatory

critical to an understanding of the concepts required for the development of care products. However, knowledge of tear chemistry is important in understanding the complex chemical interactions between tear components and contact lenses. The tear film can be broadly divided into three distinct layers: lipids, aqueous, and mucin (380). Each layer of the tear film performs a specific function. The mucin layer spreads and coats the hydrophobic corneal cells and extends into the aqueous layer. The aqueous layer contains 98% water and 2% solids. Dissolved solids in this layer are predominately the electrolytes (Na^+, K^+, C^{2+}, Mg^{2+}, Cl^-, and HCO_3^-), non-electrolytes (urea and glucose), and proteins. Major proteins in the tear film are presented in Table 8.

The lipid layer, which consists of cholesterol esters, phospholipids, and triglycerides, prevents and regulates aqueous evaporation from the tear film.

Components of the tear attach to contact lenses by electrostatic and van der Waals forces and build up to form deposits. Deposits on the surface and in the lens matrix may result in reduced visual acuity, irritation, and in some instances, serious ocular complications. The composition of deposits varies because of the complexity of an individual's ocular physiology-pathology. Lysozyme is a major component of soft lens deposits, especially found on high water content ionic lenses (381). Calcium (382) and lipids (383) are infrequent components of deposits, occurring as inorganic salts, organic salts, or as an element of mixed deposits, or as a combination thereof (384,385).

Lenses are exposed to a broad spectrum of microbes during normal wear and handling and become contaminated relatively quickly. Failure to remove microorganisms effectively from lenses can cause ocular infections. Ocular infections, particularly those caused by pathogenic microbes, such as *P. aeruginosa*, can lead to the loss of the infected eye if left untreated.

Types of Lens Care Products

Contact lens care products can be divided into three categories: cleaners, disinfectants, and lubricants. Improperly cleaned lenses can cause discomfort, irritation, decrease in visual acuity, and giant papillary conjunctivitis (GPC). This latter condition often requires discontinuation of lens wear, at least until the symptoms clear. Deposits can also accumulate preservatives from lens care products and produce toxicity and can act as a matrix for microorganism attachment to the lens (386). Thus, cleaning with the removal of surface debris, tear components, and contaminating microorganisms is one of the most important steps contributing to the safety and efficacy of successful lens wear (387).

Daily cleaners and weekly cleaners are employed to clean deposits that accumulate on lenses during normal wear. A list of cleaning agents commonly used in daily cleaners is provided in Table 9. Single-cleaning agents or combinations of cleaning agents may be used in a cleaner. Surfactant(s), surface-active polymer(s), solvent(s), and complexing agent(s) chosen for cleaner formulations must be capable of solubilizing lens deposits and

Table 9 Cleaning Agents Commonly Used in Daily Cleaners

Class	Trade name	Chemical name
Abrasive particles	Nylon 11	11-Aminoundecanoic acid
	Silica	Silicon dioxide
Complexing agents	Citric acid	2-Hydroxy-1,2,3-propane tricarboxylic acid
Solvents	Isopropyl alcohol	2-Propanol
	Propylene glycol	1,2-Propanediol
	Hexamethyene glycol	1,6-Hexanediol
Surfactants (nonionic)	Tween 21	Polysorbate 21
	Tween 80	Polysorbate 80
	Tyloxapol	4-(1,3,3-Tetramethylbutyl)-phenol polymer with formaldehyde and oxirane
	Pluronic	Poloxamer
	Tetronic	Poloxamine
Surfactants (ionic)	Miracare	Cocoamphocarboxyglycinate

must have low irritation potential. They must be rinsed easily, leaving very low or nondetectable residue levels on the lens. Many problems that contact lens wearers experience with their lenses are the results of incomplete removal of deposit(s) (388). Nonionic and amphoteric surfactants are commonly used in daily cleaner products. Because of their toxicity to the cornea and binding to the lenses, anionic and cationic surfactants are avoided. Solvents capable of solubilizing lens deposits without altering the lens polymer properties should be selected carefully. Complexing agents, such as citrates, are included in daily cleaner formulations (389). They retard the binding of positively charged proteins to the lenses, and by ion pairing or salt formation, render the proteins more soluble in the media.

Mechanical force is a key aspect in the cleaning process. For daily cleaning, mechanical force is generally provided through the rubbing action of the fingers over the lens during the actual cleaning process. Rubbing typically removes 1.7 ± 0.5 logs of microorganisms, rinsing the lens removes 1.9 ± 0.5 logs of microorganisms, and cleaning and rinsing the lens removes 3.7 ± 0.5 logs of microorganisms of a typical challenge by 10^6 colony-forming units (CFU)/mL (389). Abrasive particles are included in products to enhance the mechanical force applied to the lens during the cleaning process (390). The abrasive properties are evaluated by testing the hardness of the included abrasive particles. Typically, particles that have Rockwell hardness lower than the hardness of the lens polymers are used. If the hardness of abrasive particles is higher than the hardness of the lens polymer, it is possible that the lens would be damaged. Some contact lenses are reported to require special treatment. Abrasive particles may alter surface treatment effects even when their hardness is lower than that of the lens polymer.

Enzymatic cleaners contain enzymes derived from animals, plants, or microorganisms. Plant and microorganism-derived enzymes may cause sensitization in many lens wearers (391). A list of commonly used enzymes is provided in Table 10. All these enzymes are effective in removing deposits from the contact lens surface (392). They are biochemical catalysts that are specific for catalyzing certain chemical reactions. Those that aid in removing debris from contact lenses are protease (protein-specific enzyme), lipase (lipid-specific enzyme), and amylase (polysaccharide-specific enzyme). Such enzymes catalyze breakdown of substrate molecules—protein, lipid, and mucin—into smaller molecular units. This process yields fragments that are readily removed by mechanical force and rinsing.

Table 10 Enzymes Commonly Used in Weekly Cleaners

Name	Origin	Active against	Active at pH
Pancreatin	Animal (porcine)		
Proteases		Proteins	7.0
Lipase		Lipids	8.0
Amylase			6.7–7.2
		Carbohydrates	
Papain	Plant (papaya)	Proteins	5.0
Subtilisin A	Microorganisms	Proteins	8–10
Subtilisin B	Microorganisms	Proteins	8–10

In the past, only tablet dosage forms of enzymatic cleaners were available. They required soaking lenses in solutions prepared from a tablet for a period of 15 minutes to more than 2 hours before disinfecting the lenses. Although this process provided sufficient time for cleaning, it was a cumbersome process and required multiple steps. A complicated or cumbersome process inevitably leads to poor user compliance. Enzymes in aqueous liquid compositions are inherently unstable. New technological advances have led to the stabilization of enzymes in liquid vehicles, which are compatible with soft and RGP contact lenses (393). The newer products are either in a tablet or a solution product form. Simultaneous cleaning and disinfection can be achieved, which reduces care time and the need for multiple steps (394).

Contact lenses are contaminated with microorganisms during lens handling and lens wear. They must be disinfected to prevent ocular infections, especially from pathogenic microorganisms. The two disinfection methods used are thermal and chemical. In thermal disinfection systems, lenses are placed in preserved or unpreserved solution in a lens case and then heated sufficiently by a device to kill the microorganisms. The current FDA requirement for thermal disinfection requires heating at a minimum of 80°C for 10 minutes. The unpreserved salines are either packaged in a unit-dose or an aerosol container, and they do have some antimicrobial activity (395). Preservatives must be used in salines packaged in nonaerosol multidose containers. The type and names of preservatives and antimicrobial disinfectants commonly used in lens care products are listed in Table 11. Thimerosal and sorbic acid are commonly used preservatives in these products; however, concerns of sensitization potential and discoloration of lenses has led to the introduction of new and safer molecules like polyquad (a polymerically bound quaternary ammonium compound) and dymed. Specifically, polyquad is resistant to absorption into the lenses; thus, there is little to diffuse out of the lens into the eye, leading to corneal toxicity, an inherent problem associated with nonpolymerically bound quaternary ammonium compounds. The FDA and the USP have specific standards for preservative effectiveness that these products must meet. The FDA standards detailing the method were published in 1985 (396). Oxidizing agents and nonoxidizing chemical disinfectants that are nontoxic at product concentrations are used to disinfect lenses chemically. Primarily, hydrogen peroxide is used as an oxidizing agent (397). It is used in concentrations of 0.6% to 3.0%. Peroxides are very toxic to the cornea of the eye. After the disinfection cycle, and before placing the lens in the eye, hydrogen peroxide must be completely neutralized by reducing agents, catalase, or transition metals, such as platinum.

An ideal chemical-disinfecting agent would have the following properties: (*i*) it should be nonirritating, nonsensitizing, and nontoxic in tests for cytotoxicity; (*ii*) it should have an adequate antimicrobial spectrum and be able to kill ocular pathogens during a

Table 11 Antimicrobial Agents Commonly Used in Lens Care Products

Class	Generic	Molecularweight	Soft	RGP, PMMA
Acids	Benzoic acid	122	No	Yes
	Boric acid	62	Yes	Yes
	Sorbic acid	112	Yes	Yes
Alcohols	Benzyl alcohol	108	No	Yes
	Phenyl ethyl alcohol	122	No	Yes
Biguanide	Chlorhexidine	505	Yes	Yes
	Polyaminopropyl biguanide	~1200	Yes	Yes
Mercurial	Thimerosal	404	Yes	Yes
	Phenylmercuric nitrate	634	Yes	Yes
Oxidizing	Hydrogen peroxide	34	Yes	No
	Sodium dichloroisocyanurate	220	Yes	No
Quaternary	Tris(2-hydroxyethyl) tallow ammonium chloride	≈424	Yes	No
	Benzalkonium chloride	≈363	No	Yes
	Benzethonium chloride	448	No	Yes
	Polyquaternium-1	≈6000	Yes	Yes

Abbreviations: RGP, rigid gas permeable; PMMA, polymethyl methacrylate.

short lens-soaking period; (*iii*) it should not bind to the lens surface; and (*iv*) it should be compatible with the lens and not cause lens discoloration or alter the tint of colored contact lenses. Polyquad and dymed have most of these characteristics. They have been introduced recently into the marketplace and are performing to expectations (398,399).

Contact lens wearers may experience increasing awareness of their lenses during the day owing to ocular dryness (400). With some lens materials, this increase in awareness may arise from a decrease in the wettability of the lens surface. Dehydration of the lens or accumulation of debris on the lens surface can cause similar symptoms (401). The lens wearer may achieve relief from these symptoms with periodic administration of lubrication of rewetting drops (402). These solutions contain polymers or surfactants that enhance the wettability of the surface, facilitate the spreading of tears, and improve the stability of the tear film. They may also provide cushioning and lubrication actions, thereby reducing the frictional force between the eyelids and the lens. Some products are specifically designed to rehydrate the lens. These products are unpreserved and packaged in a unit-dose container. However, a preservative is required for a multidose product.

The emphasis that patients place on convenience has led to the development of single-bottle care products referred to as "multipurpose solutions". Such products do not require a separate cleaner and in some instances can be used as a rewetting drop. However, they require rubbing and rinsing of lenses to achieve adequate cleaning. Recent advances in technology along with careful selection of formulation components have resulted in products that do not require a rubbing step (403). These products have met all the microbiological and cleaning efficacy requirements, including those proposed in the ISO Guidelines. However, some newer products, although meeting the regulatory requirements during development, were found to cause microbial infection (404). FDA/ CDRH issued advice to patients wearing soft contact lenses, alerting them regarding an increase in incidence of reports of fungal infection in the United States. This fungal keratitis caused by *Fusarium* fungus can result in permanent loss of vision. Several patients with this infection required corneal transplants to save their vision.

Summary

Generally, contact lens products are sterile solutions or suspensions. Formulators for these products must have training in technologies practiced during development of sterile pharmaceutical products, such as injectable and large-volume IV fluids. The products must be effective and compatible with a wide range of lens materials. Components of the formulations should not accumulate in the lens or change the lens properties. They must be preserved adequately and be well tolerated by the sensitive ocular tissues. The products should also be simple to use to assure good compliance on the part of lens wearers. Additionally, they should be developed following the guidelines enumerated in Table 12.

Table 12 Types of Tests and Requirements Proposed by the FDA for Product Development

Chemistry/manufacturing
Solution/container descriptions
Solution stability testing
Lens group selection for solution testing
Toxicology
Solution testing
Acute oral toxicity assessment
Acute systemic toxicity assessment
Acute ocular irritation and cytotoxicity assessment
Sensitization/allergic response assessment
Preservative uptake and release test
Guinea pig maximization testing
Container/accessory testing
In vitro testing
Systemic toxicity testing
Primary ocular irritation testing
Microbiology
Sterilization of the solution by the manufacturer
Validation of the sterilization cycle
USP sterility tests
USP-type preservative effectiveness test
USP microbial limits test
Shelf life–testing requirements
Shelf life sterility
Shelf life preservative effectiveness
Extension of shelf life protocol
Disinfection of the lens
Chemical disinfection systems
Contribution of elements test
D-value determinations
Multi-item microbial challenge test
Clinical
Patient characteristics
Number of eyes duration and number of investigators
Initial patient visit parameters

Abbreviation: USP, United States Pharmacopoeia.

REFERENCES

1. Joeres S, Tsong JW, Updike PG, et al. Invest Ophthalmol Vis Sci 2007; 49:4300–4307.
2. The United States Pharmacopeia 31 (USP)/The National Formulary 26. Sections ⟨771⟩ Ophthalmic Ointments and ⟨1151⟩ Pharmaceutical Dosage Forms. Rockville, MD: U.S. Pharmacopeial Convention; 2008.
3. Rozier A, Mazuel C, Grove J, et al. Int J Pharm 1997; 153:191.
4. Lang JC, Keister JC, Missel PJT, et al. U.S. patent 5,403,841. 1995.
5. Missel PJT, Lang JC, Jani R. U.S. patent 5, 212,162. 1993.
6. Bawa R, Hall R, Kabra B, et al. U.S. patent 6,174,524. 2001.
7. Asgharian B. U.S. patent 7,169,767. 2007.
8. Majno G. The Healing Hand-Man and Wound in the Ancient World. Cambridge, MA: Harvard University Press, 1975; 43–45, 112–114, 154, 216,359, 348,377.
9. Deardorf DL. Remington's Pharmaceutical Sciences. 14th ed. Easton, PA: Mack Publishing, 1970:1545–1548.
10. Riegleman S, Sorby DL. Dispensing of Medication. 7th ed. Easton, PA: Mack Publishing, 1971:880–884.
11. Lang JC, Stiemke MM. "Biological Barriers to Ocular Delivery" in Ocular Therapeutics and Drug Delivery, A Multidisciplinary Approach. In: Reddy IK, ed. Technomic Publishing Company, 1996:51–132.
12. Chiou GCY. Toxicol Methods 1992; 2:139.
13. Tuft SJ, Costner DJ. Eye 1990; 4:389.
14. Cheng JW, Matsumoto SS, Anger CB. J Toxicol Cutan Ocul Toxicol 1995; 14:287.
15. Burstein NL, Anderson JA. J Ocul Pharmacol 1985; 1:309.
16. Lee VHL, Robinson JR. J Ocul Pharmacol 1986; 2:67.
17. Mishima S. Invest Ophthalmol Vis Sci 1981; 21:504.
18. Maurice DM, Mishima S. "Ocular pharmacokinetics". In: Sears ML, ed. Pharmacology of the Eye. Berlin: Springer-Verlag, 1984:19–116.
19. Schoenwald RD. Clin Pharmacokinet 1990; 18:255.
20. Davies NM. Clin Exp Pharmacol Physiol 2000; 27:558.
21. Schoenwald RD. "Ocular pharmacokinetics/pharmacodynamics". In: Mitra AK, ed. Ophthalmic Drug Delivery Systems. New York: Marcel Dekker, Inc., 1993:83–110.
22. Worakul N, Robinson JR. J Pharm Biopharm 1997; 44:71.
23. Chastain JE. "General considerations in ocular drug delivery". In: Mitra AK, ed. Ophthalmic Drug Delivery Systems. 2nd ed. New York: Marcel Dekker, Inc., 2003:59–107.
24. Schoenwald RD, Ward RL. Pharm Sci 1978; 67:786.
25. Cox WV, Kupferman A, Leibowitz HM. Arch Ophthal 1972; 88:549.
26. Schoenwald RD, Huang HS. J Pharm Sci 1983; 72:1266.
27. Huang HS, Schoenwald RD, Lach JL. J Pharm Sci 1983; 72:1272.
28. Madhu C, Rix PJ, Shackleton MJ, et al. J Pharm Sci 1996; 85:415.
29. Ahmed I, Patton TF. Invest Ophthalmol Vis Sci 1985; 26:584–587.
30. Ahmed I, Patton TF. Int Pharmaceutics J 1987; 38:9.
31. Ahmed I, Gokhale RD, Shah MV, et al. J Pharm Sci 1987; 76:583.
32. Chien DS, Homsy JJ, Gluchowske C, et al. Curr Eye Res 1990; 9:1051.
33. Schoenwald RD, Deshpande GS, Rethwisch DG, et al. Ocul Pharmacol Ther 1997; 13:41.
34. Romanelli L, Valeri P, Morrone LA, et al. Science 1994; 54:877.
35. Ling TL, Combs DL, J Pharm Sci 1987; 76:289.
36. Tang-Liu DDS, Liu S, Neff J, et al. J Pharm Sci 1987; 76:780.
37. Chrai SS, Patton TF, Mehta A, et al. J Pharm Sci 1973; 62:1112.
38. Chrai SS, Makoid M, Eriksen SP, et al. Pharm Sci 1974; 63:333.
39. Keister JC, Cooper ER, Missel PJ, et al. Pharm Sci 1991; 80:50.
40. Zaki I, Fitzgerald P, Hardy JG, et al. J Pharm Pharmacol 1986; 38:463.
41. Patton TF, Robinson JR. J Pharm Sci 1975; 64:1312.
42. Chrai SS, Robinson JR, J Pharm Sci 1974; 63:1218.

43. Kaila T, Huupponen R, Salminen L. J Ocul Pharmacol 1986; 2:365.
44. Zimmerman TJ, Kooner KS, Kandarakis AS, et al. Arch Ophthalmol 1984; 102:551.
45. Linden C, Alm A. Acta Ophthalmol 1990; 68:633.
46. Lee Y-H, Kompella UB, Lee VHL. Exp Eye Res 1993; 57:341.
47. Hitoshe S, Bungaard H, Lee VHL. Invest Ophthalmol Vis Sci 1989; 30(suppl):25.
48. Ashton P, Podder SK, Lee VHL. Pharm Res 1991; 8:1166.
49. Havener WH. Ocular Pharmacology. 2nd ed. St. Louis, MO: Mosby CV, 1970.
50. Smith B. Handbook of Ocular Pharmacology. Acton, MA: Publication Sciences Group, 1974.
51. Ellis P, Smith DL. Ocular Therapeutics and Pharmacology. 3rd ed. St. Louis, MO: Mosby CV, 1969.
52. Grayston JT, Wang SP, Woolridge RL, et al. JAMA 1962; 172:602.
53. Bartlett JD, Jaanus SD. Clinical Ocular Pharmacology. Boston, MA: Butterworth-Heinemann, 1995:275.
54. Byers JL, Holland MG, Allen JH. Am J Ophthalmol 1960; 49:267.
55. Gingrich WD. JAMA 1962; 179:602.
56. Mishima S, Maurice DM. Invest Ophthalmol 1962; 1:794.
57. Maurice DM. Invest Ophthalmol 1967; 6:464.
58. Kimura SJ. Am J Ophthalmol 1951; 34:446.
59. Wessing A. Fluorescein Angiography of the Retina (trans. by von Noorden GK). St. Louis, MO: Mosby CV, 1969.
60. Koller K. Arch Ophthalmol 1884; 13:404.
61. Council on Drugs, New drugs and developments in therapeutics, JAMA 1963; 183:178.
62. Lemp MA, Dohlman CH, Holly FJ. Ann Ophthalmol 1970; 2:258
63. Lemp MA. Szymanski ES. Arch Ophthalmol 1975; 93:134.
64. Lemp MA. Scientific Exhibit. Dallas: American Academy of Ophthalmology and Otolaryngology, September 1975.
65. The United States Pharmacopeia 31 (USP)/The National Formulary 26. Section ⟨71⟩ Sterility Tests. Rockville, MD: U.S. Pharmacopeial Convention, 2008.
66. British Pharmacopoeia 2000. Department of Health. London: The Stationery Office, 2000.
67. The United States Pharmacopeia 31 (USP)/The National Formulary 26. ⟨1211⟩ Sterilization and Sterility Assurance of Compendial Aritcles. Rockville, MD: U.S. Pharmacopeia, 2008.
68. The Japanese Pharmacopoeia. English Version JP XIV, 5 – 15, 87, 1304–1305, April 2001.
69. The European Pharmacopoeia. 6th ed., 2008; 6.2, 07 Dosage Forms.
70. Marzulli FN, Simon ME. Am J Optom 1971; 48:61.
71. Hackett RB, McDonald TO. Eye Irritation. In: Marzulli FN, Maibach HL, eds. Dermatoxicology. 5th ed. Washington D.C.: Hemisphere Publishing, 1996:299–305, 557–566.
72. Basu PK, Toxicol J. Cutan Ocul Toxicol 1984; 2:205–227.
73. Seifried HE. J Toxicol Cutan Ocul Toxicol 1986; 5:89–114.
74. Friedenwald JS, Hughes WF Jr., Hermann H. Arch Ophthalmol 1944; 31:379.
75. Carpenter C, Symth H. Am J Ophthalmol 1946; 29:1363.
76. Hazelton LW. Proc Sci Sect Toilet Goods Assoc 1973; 17:490.
77. Carter LM, Duncan G, Rennie GK. Exp Eye Res 1952; 17:5.
78. Kay JH, Calandra JC. J Soc Cosmet Chem 1962; 13:281.
79. Russell KL, Hoch SG. Pro Sci Sect Toilet Goods Assoc 1962; 37:27.
80. Gaunt I, Harper KH. J Soc Cosmet Shem 1964; 15:290.
81. Battista SP, McSweeney ES. J Soc Cosmet Chem 1965; 16:119.
82. Becklet JH. Am Perum Cosmet 1965; 80:51.
83. Bonfield CT, Scala RA. Proc Sci Sect Toilet Goods Assoc 1965; 43:34.
84. Buehler EV, Newmann EA. Toxicol Appl Pharmacol 1964; 6:701.
85. Dohlman CH, Invest Ophthalmol 1971; 10:376.
86. Hogan MJ, Zimmerman LE. Ophthalmic Pathology: An Atlas and Textbook. 2nd ed. Philadelphia: W.B. Saunders, 1962.
87. Phister RR. Invest Ophthalmol 1973; 12:654.
88. Maurice DM. In: Davson H, ed. The Eye. Vol 1. New York: Academic Press, 1969:489–600.

89. Prince JH, Diesen CD, Eglitis I, et al. Anatomy and Histology of the Eye and Orbit in Domestic Animals. Springfield, IL: Charles C Thomas, 1960.
90. Davson H. In: Davson H, ed. The Eye. Vol 1. New York: Academic Press, 1969:217–218.
91. Fine BS, Yanoff M. Ocular Histology: A Text and Atlas. New York: Harper & Row, 1972.
92. Green WR, Sullivan JB, Hehir RM, et al. A Systemic Comparison of Chemically Induced Eye Injury in the Albino Rabbit and Rhesus Monkey. New York: Soap and Detergent Association, 1978:405–415.
93. Committee for the Revision of NAS Publication 1138, National Research Council, Principles and Procedures for Evaluating the Toxicity of Household Substances. Washington, D.C.: National Academy of Sciences, 1977:41–56.
94. Interagency Regulatory Liaison Group, Testing Standards and Guidelines Work Group, Recommended Guidelines for Acute Eye Irritation Testing, 1981.
95. Ophthalmic optics—Contact lenses and contact lens care products—Determination of biocompatibility by ocular study with rabbit eyes. ISO 9394:1998(E), 1998.
96. Draize JH. Food Drug Cosmet Law J 1955; 10:722.
97. Draize JH, Kelley EA. Proc Sci Sect Toilet Goods Assoc 1959; 17:1.
98. Draize JH. J Pharmacol Exp Ther 1944; 82:377.
99. Food Drug Cosmet Law Rep. 233:8311; 440:8313; 476:8310.
100. Bruner LH, Parker RD, Bruce RD. Fund Appl Toxicol 1992; 19:330–335.
101. York M, Steiling W. J Appl Toxicol 1998; 18:233.
102. Nussenblatt RB, Bron A, Chambers W. et al. J Toxicol Cut Ocul Toxicol 1998; 17:103.
103. Balls M, Botham PA, Bruner LH, et al. Toxic in Vitro 1995; 9:871.
104. ICCVAM Test Method Evaluation Report: In Vitro Ocular Toxicity Test Methods for Identifying Severe Irritants and Corrosives. National Institute of Environmental Health Sciences. National Institutes of Health Publication 07–4517, 2007.
105. Guidance on Nonclinical Safety Studies for the Conduct of Human Clinical trials for Pharmaceuticals. FDA Docket No 97D-0147. Fed Regist 1997; 62(227):62922.
106. Timing of Non-Clinical Safety Studies for the Conduct of Human Clinical trials for Pharmaceuticals. Fourth International Conference on Harmonization. Brussels; International Conference on Harmonization, 1997.
107. Hackett RB. Lens Eye Toxic Res 1990; 7:181.
108. Hayes AW. Principles and Methods of Toxicology. 3rd ed. New York: Raven Press, 1994.
109. Guidance for Industry: Premarket Notification (510(k)) Guidance Document for Contact Lens Care Products. Rockville, MD: Center for Devices and Radiologic Health, FDA, 1997
110. Biological evaluation of medical devices – Part 5: Tests for cytotoxicity: in vitro methods. ISO 10993–5:1992(E). International Standards Organization, 1992.
111. Shell JW, Baker RW. Ann Ophthalmol 1975; 7:1637.
112. Grant WM. Toxicology of the Eye. Springfield, IL: Charles C Thomas, 1974:259.
113. Edelhauser HF, Van Horn DL, Scholtz RW, et al. Am J Ophthalmol 1976; 81:473.
114. Herrell SE, Heilman D. Am J Med Sci 1943; 206:221.
115. Baldwin HA, McDonald TO, Beasley CH. J Soc Cosmet Chem 1973; 25:181.
116. Shopsis C, Borenfreund E, Walberg J, et al. In: Goldberg AM, ed. Alternative Methods in Toxicology. Vol 2. New York: Mary Ann Liebert, 1984:103–114.
117. Borenfreund E, Borrero O. Cell Biol Toxicol 1984; 1:55–65.
118. Shopsis C, Sathe S. Toxicology 1984; 29:195–206.
119. Neville R, Dennis P, Sens D, et al. Curr Eye Res 1986; 5:367.
120. Stern ME, Edelhauser HF, Hiddemen JW. Methods of Evaluation of Corneal Epithelial and Endothelial Toxicity of Soft Contact Lens Preservatives. Presented at Contact Lens International Congress; Las Vegas, Nevada; March 1985.
121. Edelhauser HF, Antione ME, Pederson HJ, et al. J Toxicol Cutan Ocul Toxicol 1983; 2(1):7.
122. Krebs SJ, Stern ME, Hiddemen JW, et al. CLAO J 1984; 10(1):35.
123. Stark DM, Shopsis C, Borenfreund E, et al. Alternative Methods of Toxicology. Vol 1. Product Safety Evaluation. New York: Mary Ann Liebert, 1983:127–204.

124. Frazier JM. Dermatotoxicology. 4th ed. In: Marzulli FN, Maibach HL, eds. Washington, DC: Hemisphere Publishing, 1991:817.
125. Burstein NL. Invest Ophthalmol Vis Sci 1984; 25:1453–1457.
126. Maurice D, Singh T. A permeability test for acute corneal toxicity. Toxicol Lett 1986; 31: 125–130.
127. Burstein NL. Invest Ophthalmol Vis Sci 1980; 7:308–313.
128. Pfister RR, Burstein N. Invest Ophthalmol Vis Sci 1976; 15:246–249.
129. Tonjum AM. Acta Ophthalmol 1975; 53:358–366.
130. Ichijima H, Petroll WM, Jester JV, et al. Cornea 1992; 11:221–225.
131. Imperia PS, Lazarus HM, Botti RE Jr., et al. J Toxicol Cutan Ocul Toxicol 1986; 5:309–317.
132. Collins HB, Grabsch BE. Am J Optom Physiol Opt 1982; 59:215–222.
133. Ubels J. J Toxicol Cutan Ocul Toxicol 1982; 1:133–145.
134. Tripathi BJ, Tripathi RC. Lens Eye Toxicol Res 1987; 6:395–403.
135. Federal Register. 1953; 18:351.
136. Furrer P, Mayer JM. Eur J Pharm Biopharm 2002; 53:263–280.
137. Yee RW. Curr Opin Ophthalmol 2007; 18:134–139.
138. Lewis RA. J Glaucoma 2007; 16:98–103.
139. Diestelhorst M, Grunthal S, Suverkrup R. Graefes Arch Clin Exp Ophthalmol 1999; 237:394.
140. Levrat F, Pisella PJ, Baudouin C. J Fr Ophtalmol 1999; 22:186.
141. Becquet F, Goldschild M, Moldovan MS, et al. Curr Eye Res 1998; 17:419.
142. Weiner ML, Kotkoskie LA. eds. Excipient Toxicity and Safety. New York: Marcel Dekker, 2000.
143. Green K, Chapman JM. J Toxicol Cutan Ocul Toxicol 1986; 5:133.
144. Green K, Chapman J, Cheeks L, et al. Conc Toxicol 1987; 4:126.
145. Thode C, Kilp H. Fortschr Ophthalmol 1982; 79:125.
146. Gassett AR, Ishii Y, Kaufman HE, et al. Am J Ophthalmol 1975; 78:98.
147. Sasaki H, Nagano T, Yamamura K, et al. J Pharm Pharmacol 1995; 47:703.
148. Sasaki H, Tei C, Yamamura K, et al. J Pharm Pharmacol 1994; 46:871–875.
149. Richards RME. Aust J Pharm Sci 1967; 55:S86, S96.
150. Mullen W, Shephard W, Labovitz J. Surv Ophthalmol 1973; 17:469.
151. J Am Coll Toxicol 1989; 8:589–625.
152. Baudouin C, Pisella PJ, Fillacier K, et al. Ophthalmol 1999; 106:556.
153. De-Saint-Jean M, Brignole F, Bringuier AF, et al. Invest Ophthalmol Vis Sci 1999; 40:619.
154. Debbasch C, De-Saint-Jean M, Pisella PJ, et al. J Toxicol Cutaneous Ocul Toxicol 2000; 19:79.
155. Miller MJ. In:Ascenzi JM, ed. Handbook of Disinfectants and Antiseptics. New York: Marcel Dekker, 1996:83–110.
156. Binder PS, Rasmussen D, Gordon M. Arch Ophthalmol 1981; 99:87.
157. Tosti A, Tosti G. Contact Dermatitis 1988; 18:268–273.
158. Shaw E. Contact Intraocul Lens Med J 1980; 6:273.
159. Molinari J, Nash R, Badham D. Int Contact Lens Clin 1982; 9:323.
160. Gual EL. J Invest Dermatol 1958; 31:91.
161. Ellis FA, Robinson HM. Arch Fermatol Syphilol 1941; 46:425.
162. Reisman RE. Allergy J 1969; 43:245.
163. Mackeen D. Contact Lens J 1978; 7:14.
164. Meyer RC, Cohn LB. J Pharm Sci 1978; 67:1636.
165. Baily WR. Contact Lens Soc Am J 1972; 6:33.
166. Grant WM, Toxicology of the Eye. 4th Ed. Springfield, IL: Charles C Thomas, 1993:365.
167. Salonen EM, Vaheri A, Tervo T, et al. J Toxicol Cutan Ocul Toxicol 1991; 10:157–166.
168. Doughty MJ. Optom Vis Sci 1994; 71:562.
169. Tripathi BJ, Tripathi RC, Susmitha PK. Lens Eye Toxicol Res 1992; 9:361–375.
170. Rudnick DE, Edelhauser HF, Hendrix CL, et al. ARVO, 1997.
171. Chang JH, Ren H, Petroll WM, et al. Curr Eye Res 1999; 19:171.

172. Chowhan MA, Helton DO, Harris RG, et al. To Alcon Laboratories, Inc. U.S. patent 5,037,647.
173. Burstein NL. Invest Ophthalmol 1975; 53:358.
174. Tonjum AM. Acta Ophthalmol Vis Sci 1980; 19:308.
175. Dormans JA, Van Logten JJ. Toxicol Appl Pharmacol 1982; 62:251.
176. Gassett AR, Ishii Y. Can J Ophthalmol 1975; 10:98.
177. Green K, Livingston V, Bowman K, et al. Arch Ophthalmol 1980; 19:1273.
178. Begley CG, Waggoner PJ, Hafner GS, et al. Opt Vis Sci 1991; 68:189–197.
179. Green K, Johnson RE, Chapman JM, et al. Lens Eye Toxicol Res 1989; 6:37–41.
180. Bron AJ, Daubas P, Siou-Mermet R, et al. Eye 1998; 12:839.
181. Noecker R. Effects of common ophthalmic preservatives on ocular health. Adv Ther 2001; 18:205–215.
182. Noecker RJ. Corneal and conjunctival changes caused by commonly used glaucoma medications. Cornea 2004; 23:490–496.
183. Rozen S. IOVS 1998; 39:2486–B2343.
184. Katz LJ. J Glaucoma 2002; 11:119–126.
185. Kahook MY. Comparison of corneal and conjunctival changes after dosing of travoprost preserved with sofZia, latanoprost with 0.02% benzalkonium chloride, and preservative-free artificial tears. Cornea 2008; 27:339–343.
186. Kahook MY. Expert Rev Ophthalmol 2007; 2:363–368.
187. Gross RL. J Glaucoma 2008; 17:217–22.
188. Neuwelt EA, ed. Implications of the Blood-Brain Barrier and Its Manipulation. Vol 1. Basic Science Aspects. New York: Plenum Medical Book Company, 1989.
189. Segal MB, ed. Barriers and Fluids of the Eye and Brain. Cleveland, OH: CRC Press, 1992.
190. Kaufman HE, Barron BA, McDonald MB, et al., eds. The Cornea. New York: Churchill Livingstone, 1988.
191. Mitra AK, ed., Ocular Drug Delivery Systems. New York: Marcel Dekker, 1993.
192. Fine BS, Yanoff M. Ocular Histology. New York: Harper and Row, 1979.
193. Robinson JR, ed., Ophthalmic Drug Delivery Systems, Academy of Pharmaceutical Sciences. Washington, D.C.: American Pharmaceutical Association, 1980.
194. Conroy CW, Maren TH. J Ocul Pharm Ther 1999; 15:179.
195. Conroy CW, Maren TH. J Ocul Pharm Ther 1998; 14:565.
196. Olsen TW, Edelhauser HF, Lim JI, et al. Invest Ophthalmol Vis Sci 1995; 36:1893.
197. Olsen TW, Aaberg SY, Geroski DH, et al. Am J Ophthalmol 1998; 125:237.
198. Geroski DH, Edelhauser HF. Invest Ophthalmol Vis Sci, 2000; 41:961.
199. Rudnick DE, Noonan JS, Geroski DH, et al. Invest Ophthal Vis Sci 1999; 40:3054.
200. Weiss DI, Schaffer RD. Arch Ophthalmol 1962; 68:727.
201. Fraunfelder FT, Meyer SM. Drug-Induced Ocular Side Effects and Drug Interactions. Philadelphia: Les & Febiger, 1989:442–487.
202. Polak BCP. Drugs used in ocular treatment. In: Dukes MNG, ed. Meyler's Side Effects of Drugs. New York: Elsevier, 1988:988–998.
203. Patton TF. In: Robison JR, ed. Ophthalmic Drug Delivery Systems. Washington, D.C.: Academy of Pharmaceutical Sciences, American Pharmaceutical Association, 1980:23–54.
204. Rozier A, Mazuel C, Grove J, et al. Int J Pharm 1989; 57:163.
205. Zimmerman TJ, Sharir M, Nardin GF et al. Am J Ophthalmol 1992; 114:1.
206. Stevens LE, Missel PJ, Lang JC. Anal Chem 1992; 64:715.
207. Perry RH, Chilton CH. Chemical Engineer's Handbook. 5th ed. New York: McGraw-Hill, 1973:Sec. 4.
208. Smith JM. Chemical Engineering Kinetics. 3rd ed. New York: McGraw-Hill, 1981.
209. Hill CG. An Introduction to Chemical Engineering Kinetics and Reactor Design. New York: John Wiley & Sons, 1977.
210. Narawane N. Oxidative and Hormonal Control of Horseradish Peroxidase Transytosis Across the Pigmented Rabbit Conjunctiva [master's thesis]. University of Southern California, 1993.
211. Veng-Pedersen P, Gillespie WR. J Pharm Sci 1988; 77:39.

212. Gillespie WR, Veng-Pedersen P, Antal EJ, et al. J Pharm Sci 1988; 77:48.
213. Maurice DM, Riley MV. The cornea. In: Graymore CN, ed. Biochemistry of the Eye. New York: Academic Press, 1970.
214. Berman ER. Biochemistry of the Eye. New York: Plenum Press, 1991.
215. Edwards A, Prausnitz MR. AICHE J 1998; 44:214.
216. Edwards A, Prausnitz MR. Pharm Res 2001; 18:1497–1508.
217. Alberts B, Bray D, Lewis J, et al. Molecular Biology of the Cell. New York: Garland Publishing, Inc., 1983.
218. Stryer L. Biochemistry. New York: WH. Freeman and Company, 1981.
219. Lodish H, Baltimore D, Berk A, et al., Molecular Cell Biology. New York: W. H. Freeman and Company, 1995.
220. Mullins JD, Hecht G. Ophthalmic preparations. In: Genaro AR, ed. Remington's Pharmaceutical Sciences. Vol 18. Easton, PA: Mack Publishing, 1990:1581–1595.
221. Moses RA. Adler's Physiology of the Eye. 5th ed. St. Louis, MO: Mosby CV, 1970:49.
222. Durward A. The skin and the sensory organs. In: Romanes GJ, ed. Cunningham's Testbook of Anatomy. London: Oxford University Press, 1964:796.
223. Candia OA. Invest Ophthalmol Vis Sci 1992; 33:2575.
224. Huang AJ, Tseng SC, Kenyon KR. Invest Ophthalmol Vis Sci 1989; 30:684.
225. Flynn GL, Yalkowsky SH, Roseman TJ. J Pharm Sci 1974; 63:479.
226. Cooper ER, Kasting G. J Control Release 1987; 6:23.
227. Hecht G, Roehrs RE, Cooper ER, et al. Design and evaluation of ophthalmic pharmaceutical products. In: Banker GS, Rhodes CT, eds. Modern Pharmaceutics. 2nd ed. New York: Marcel Dekker, 1990.
228. Cooper ER. Optimization of Transport and Biological Response with Epithelial Barriers in Biological and Synthetic Membranes. New York: Alan Liss R, 1989:249–260.
229. Baker RW, Lonsdale HK. Controlled release: mechanisms and rates. In: TanquaryAC, RE Lacy, eds. Controlled Release of Biologically Active Agents. New York: Plenum Press, 1974:15–71.
230. Hayakawa E, Chien D-S, Ingagaki K, et al. Pharm Res 1992; 9:769.
231. Edelhauser HF, Hoffert JR, Fromm PO. Invest Ophthalmol 1965; 4:290.
232. Wang W, Sasaki H, Chien DS, Lee VH. Curr Eye Res 1991; 10:57.
233. Liaw J, Robinson JR. Ocular penetration enchancers. In: Mitra AK, ed. Ophthalmic Drug Delivery Systems. New York: Marcel Dekker, 1993:369–381.
234. Rojanaskul Y, Liaw J, Robinson JR. Int J Pharm 1990; 66:133.
235. Hosoya K-I, Horibe Y, Kim K-J, et al. J Pharm Exp Therap 1998; 285:223.
236. Hosoya KI, Horibe Y, Kim K-J, et al. Invest Ophthamol Vis Sci 1998; 39:372.
237. Saha P, Yang JJ, Lee VHL. Invest Ophthamol Vis Sci 1998; 39:1221.
238. Basu SK, Haworth IS, Bolger MB, et al. Invest Ophthamol Vis Sci 1998; 39:2365.
239. Ueda H, Horibe Y, Kim K-J, et al. Invest Ophthamol Vis Sci 2000; 41:870.
240. Smith TJ, Pearson PA, Blandford DL, et al. Arch Ophthalmol 1992; 110:255.
241. Sanborn GE, Anand R, Torti RE. Arch Ophthalmol 1992; 110:188–195.
242. Driot JY, Novack GD, Rittenhouse KD, et al. J Ocul Pharmacol Ther 2004; 20:269–275.
243. Dugel PU, Cantrill HL, Eliott D, et al. Invest Ophthalmol Vis Sci 2007; 48:ARVO E-Abstract 1413.
244. Bush RA, Weng Tao BL, Raz D, et al. Invest Ophthalmol Vis Sci 2004; 45:2420–2430.
245. Kuppermann BD, Blumenkranz MS, Haller JA, et al. Invest Ophthalmol Vis Sci 2003; 44:E-Abstract 4289.
246. Sebag J. The Vitreous. In: Hart WM Jr., ed. Adler's Physiology of the Eye: Clinical Applications. St. Louis: Mosby Year Book, 1992:305–308.
247. Missel PJ. Pharm Res 2002; 19:1636–1647.
248. Stay MS, Xu J, Randolph TW, et al. Pharm Res 2003; 20:96–102.
249. Gaudreault J, Fei D, Rusit J, et al. Invest Ophthalmol Vis Sci 2005; 46:726.
250. Araie M, Maurice DM. Exp Eye Res 1991; 52:27–39.
251. Graham RO, Peyman GA. Arch Ophthalmol 1974; 92:149.

252. Friedrich S, Cheng Y–L, Saville B. Curr Eye Res 1997; 16:663.
253. Wingard LB, Zuravleff JJ, Doft BH, et al. Invest Ophthalmol Vis Sci 1989; 30:2184–9.
254. Friedrich S, Saville B, Cheng Y-L. J Ocul Pharmacol Ther 1997; 13:445.
255. Ben-Nun J, Joyce DA, Cooper RL, et al. Invest Ophthalmol Vis Sci 1989; 30:1055.
256. Barza M, Lynch E, Baum JL. Arch Ophthalmol 1993; 111:121.
257. Mannermaa E, Vellonen K-S, Urtti A. Adv Drug Deliv Rev 2006; 58:1136.
258. Mochizuki M. Jpn Ophthalmol J 1980; 24:363.
259. Yoshida A, Ishiko S, Kojima M. Graefe's Arch Clin Exp Ophthalmol 1992; 230:78.
260. Barza M, Kane A, Baum J. Invest Ophthalmol Vis Sci 1983; 24:1602.
261. Ohtori A, Tojo K. Biol Pharm Bull 1994; 17:283.
262. Tojo KJ, Ohtori A. Math Biosci 1994; 123:59.
263. Pinsky PM, Maurice DM, Datye DV. Invest Ophthalmol Vis Sci 1996; 37(Suppl):S700.
264. Friedrich S, Cheng YL, Saville B. Ann Biomed Eng 1997; 25:303.
265. Friedrich S. Thesis, University of Toronto, Department of Chemical Engineering and Applied Chemistry, 1996.
266. Missel PJ. Annals Biomed Eng 2000; 28:1311–1321.
267. Missel PJ. Annals Biomed Eng 2002; 30:1128–1139.
268. Park J, Bungay PM, Lutz RJ, et al. J Control Release 2005; 105:279–295.
269. Kim H, Robinson MR, Lizak MJ, et al. Invest Ophthalmol Vis Sci 2004; 45:2722–2731.
270. Gudauskas G, Kumi C, Dedhar C, et al. Can J Ophthalmol 1985; 20:110.
271. Rootman J, Ostry A. Gudauskas G. Can J Ophthalmol 1984; 19:187.
272. Conrad JM, Robinson JR. J Pharm Sci 1980; 69:875.
273. Maurice DM, Polgar J. Exp Eye Res 1977; 25:577.
274. Freeman WR, Green RL, Smith RE. Am J Ophthalmol 1987; 103:281.
275. Hyndiuk RA, Reagan MG. Arch Ophthalmol 1968; 80:499.
276. Weijten O, van der Sluijs FA, Schoemaker RC, et al. Am J Ophthalmol 1997; 123:358.
277. Hughes PM, Olejnik O, Chang-Lin J-E, et al. Adv Drug Deliv Rev 2005; 57:2010.
278. Ueno N, Refojo MF, Liu LHS. Invest Ophthalmol Vis Sci 1982; 23:199.
279. Liu QF, Dharia N, Mayers M, et al. Invest Ophthalmol Vis Sci 1995; 36:S1018.
280. Elliot PJ, Bartus RT, Mackic JB, et al. Pharm Res 1997; 14:80.
281. Wilson TW, Chan HSL, Moselhy GM, et al. Arch Ophthalmol 1996; 114:1390.
282. Maurice DM. Surv Ophthalmol 2002; 47(suppl 1):S41.
283. Hollo G, Whitson JT, Faulkner R, et al. Invest Ophthalmol Vis Sci 2006; 47:235.
284. Chien D-S, Richman J, Zolezio H, et al. Pharm Res 1992; 9:S336.
285. Schuman JS, Puliafito CA, Fujimoto JG. Optical Coherence Tomography of Ocular Diseases. 2nd ed. NJ: Slack, Inc, 2004.
286. Schmitt JM. IEEE J Select Topics Quantum Electron 1999; 5:1205–1215.
287. Rollins AM, Izatt JA. Opt Lett 1999; 24:1484–1486.
288. Izatt JA, Hee MR, Swanson EA, et al. Arch Ophthalmol 1994; 112:1584–1589.
289. Hee MR, Izatt JA, Swanson EA, et al. Arch Ophthalmol 1995; 113:325–332.
290. Biersdorf WR. Doc Ophthalmol 2004; 73:313–325.
291. Palmowski AM, Sutter EE, Bearse MA Jr., et al. Invest Ophthalmol Vis Sci 1997; 38: 2586–2596.
292. Eperjesi F, Beatty S. Nutrition and the Eye. New York: Elsevier, 2006.
293. Seddon JM, Ajani UA, Sperduto RD, et al. For the Eye Disease Case-Control Study Group. JAMA 1994; 272:1413–1420.
294. Cho E, Hung S, Willett WC, et al. Am J Clin Nutr 2001; 73:209–218.
295. Mares-Perlman JA, Fisher A, Klein R, et al. Am J Epidemiol 2001; 153:424–432.
296. Age-related disease study research group. J Nutr 2002; 132:697–702.
297. Age-related disease study research group. Arch Ophthalmol 2001; 119:1417–1436.
298. Age-related disease study research group. Arch Ophthalmol 2003; 121:1621–1624.
299. Age-related disease study research group. Arch Ophthalmol 2007; 125:671–679.
300. Age-related disease study research group. Arch Ophthalmol 2007; 125:1225–1232.

301. Zareparsi S, Branham KEH, Li M, et al. Abecasis and Swaroop A. Am J Hum Genet 2005; 77:149–153.
302. Klein RJ, Zeiss C, Chew EY, et al. Science 2005; 308:385–389.
303. Johnson EJ, Schaefer EJ. Am J Clin Nutr 2006; 93(suppl):1494S–1498S.
304. Snodderly DM. Am J Clin Nutr 1995; 62(suppl):1448s–1461s.
305. Krinsky NI, Landrum JT, Bone RA. Annu Rev Nutr 2003; 23:171–201.
306. Sprarrow JR, Parish CA, Hashimoto M, et al. Invest Ophthalmol Vis Sci 1999; 40:2988–2995.
307. Shaban H, Richter C. Biol Chem 2002; 383:537–545.
308. Neuringer M, Sandstrom MM, Johnson EJ, et al. Invest Ophthalmol Vis Sci 2004; 45: 3234–3243.
309. Leung IYF, Sandstrom MM, Zucker CL, et al. Invest Ophthalmol Vis Sci 2004; 45: 3244–3256.
310. Richer S, Stiles W, Statkute L, et al. Optometry 2004; 75:216–230.
311. Falsini B, Piccardi M, Iarossi G, et al. Ophthalmology 2003; 110:51–61.
312. Bhosale P, Larson AJ, Frederick JM, et al. J Biol Chem 2004; 279:49446–49454.
313. National Eye Institute, Age-related eye disease study 2 (AREDS2). Available at: http// clinicaltrials.gov/ct/show/NCT00345176.
314. Miles EA, Calder PC. Proc Nutr Soc 1998; 57:277–292.
315. Bazan NG. Invest Ophthalmol Vis Sci 2007; 48:4866–4881.
316. Doucet JP, Squinto SP, Bazan NG. Mol Neurobiol 1990; 4:27–55.
317. Yang H, Yang X, Lang JC, et al. J Cell Biochem 2006; 98:1560–1569.
318. Kottke MK, Rudnic EM. Tablet dosage forms. In: Banker GS, Rhodes CT, eds. Modern Pharmaceutics. 4th ed. New York: Marcel Dekker, 2002:287–333.
319. Brotherman DP, Bayraktaroglu TO, Garofalo RJ. J Am Pharm Assoc 2004; 44:587–593.
320. 21 Code of Federal Regulations, Part 111.
321. Augsberger LL. Hard and soft shell capsules. In: Banker GS, Rhodes CT, eds. Modern Pharmaceutics. 4th ed. New York: Marcel Dekker, 2002:335–380.
322. Code of Federal Regulations, 21, § 210–211.
323. Clean Room and Work Station Requirements, Controlled Environment, Sec. 1–5 Federal Standard 209, Office of Technical Services, U. S. Department of Commerce, Washington, D.C., December 16, 1963.
324. Austin PR, Timmerman SW. Design and Operation of Clean Rooms. Detroit, MI: Business News Publishers, 1965.
325. Austin PR. Clean Rooms of the World. Ann Arbor, MI: Ann Arbor Science Publishers, 1967.
326. Goddard KR. Air filtration of microbial particles, Publication 953, U. S. Public Health Service, Washington, D.C., 1967.
327. Goddard KR. Bull Parenter Drug Assoc 1969; 23:699.
328. The Rules Governing Medicinal Products in the European Union, Vol 4. "Good Manufacturing Practices – Medicinal Products for Human and Vetrinary Use", Annex 1 "Manufacture of Sterile Medicinal Products", Commission Directive 91/356/EEC of 13 June 1991.
329. Alcon Laboratories, Inc. U.S. patent 6,071,904. June 6, 2000.
330. Jones D. Environmental microbial challenges to an aseptic blow-fill-seal process- a practical study. PDA J Pharm Sci Technol 1995; 49(5):226–234.
331. Sharp JR. Manufacture of sterile pharmaceutical products using 'blow-fill-seal' technology. Pharm J 1987; 239:106.
332. Sharp JR. Validation of a new form-fill-seal installation. Manuf Chem 1988:22–27, 55.
333. Leo F. Blow/Fill/Seal Aseptic Packaging Technology in Aseptic Pharmaceutical Technology for the 1990s. Prairie View, IL: Interpharm Press, 1989:195–218.
334. Sharp JR. Aseptic validation of a form/fill/seal installation: principles and practice. J Parenter Sci Technol. 1990; 44(5):289–292.
335. Bradely A, Probert SP, Sinclaire CS, et al. Airborne microbial challenges of blow/fill/seal equipment: a case study" J Prenter Sci Technol 45(4):187–192.
336. The United States Pharmacopeia 31 (USP)/The National Formulary 26. Rockville, MD: United States Pharmacopeia, 2008:3523–3525.

337. Federal Register, 41, 106, June 1, 1976.
338. Grimes TL, Fonner DE, Griffin JC, et al. Bull Parenter Drug Assoc 1975; 29:64.
339. E-3A Accepted Practices for Permanently Installed Sanitary Product Pipeline and Cleaning Systems, Serial E-60500, U. S. Public Health Service, Washington, D.C.
340. Zu Y, Luo Y, Ahmed SU. J PAT 2007; 10:7.
341. Claycamp HG. J PAT 2006; 2:8.
342. Joshi Y, LoBrutto R, Serajuddin ATM. J PAT 2006; 4:6.
343. Christensen MT, Cohen S, Rinehart J, et al. Curr Eye Res 2004; 28:55–62.
344. Cadwallader DE. Am J Hosp Pharm 1967; 24:33.
345. Kronfeld FG, McDonald JE. J Am Pharm Assoc (Sci Ed) 1951; 42:333.
346. Riegelman S, Vaughn DG. J Am Pharm Assoc (Pract Pharm Ed) 1958; 19:474.
347. Blaugh SM, Canada AT. Am J Hosp Pharm 1965; 22:662.
348. Linn ML, Jones LT. Am J Ophthalmol 1968; 65:76.
349. Adler CA, Maurice DM, Patterson ME. Exp Eye Res 1971; 11:34.
350. Castroviejo R. Arch Ophthalmol 1965; 74:143.
351. Hanna C, Fraunfelder FT, Cable M, et al. Am J Ophthalmol 1973; 76:193.
352. Fraunfelder FT, Hanna C, Cable M, et al. Am J Ophthalmol 1973; 76:475.
353. Mouly R. Ann Chir Plast 1972; 17:61.
354. Newton DW, Becker CH, Torosian G. J Pharm Sci 1973; 62:1538.
355. Schoenwald RL, Ward RL, DeSantis LM, Roehrs RE. JPharm Sci 1978; 67:1280.
356. March WF, Stewart RM, Mandell AI, Bruce L. Arch Ophthalmol 1982; 100:1270.
357. Liebowitz HM, Chang RK, Mandell AI. Ophthalmology 1984; 91:1199.
358. Bowman FW, Knoll EW, White M, Mislivic P. J Pharm Sci 1972; 61:532.
359. Schwartz TW. Am Perum Cosmet 1971; 86:39.
360. Zaffaroni A. Proc. 31st International Congress on Pharmaceutical Science, Washington, D.C., 1971.
361. Lerman S, Reininger B. Can J Ophthalmol 1971; 6:14.
362. Maichuk YF. Invest Ophthalmol 1975; 14:87.
363. Loucas SP, Haddad HM. J Pharm Sci 1972; 61:985.
364. Hiller J, Baker RW. To Alza Corporation. U.S. patent 3,811,444, 1974.
365. Michaels A. To Alza Corporation. U. S. patent 3,867,519. 1975.
366. Keller N, Longwell AM, Biros SA. Arch Ophthalmol 1976; 94:644.
367. Edelhauser HF. Arch Ophthalmol 1975; 93:649.
368. McCarey BE, Edelhauser HF, Van Horn DL. Invest Ophthalmol 1973; 12:410.
369. Merrill DL, Fleming TC, Girard LJ. Am J Ophthalmol 1960; 49:895.
370. Girard LJ. Proceedings International Congress on Ophthalmology; Brussels; September 1958.
371. Jaffee NS. Bull Parenter Drug Assoc 1970; 24:218.
372. Baily NJ. Contact Lens Spectrum 1987; 2(7):6–31.
373. Randeri KJ, Quintana RP, Chowhan MA. Lens care products. In: Swarbrick J, Boylan JC, eds. Encyclopedia of Pharmaceutical Technology. Vol 8. New York: Marcel Dekker, 1993: 361–402.
374. Tan J, Keay L, Sweeney D. Contact Lens Spectrum 2000:42–44.
375. Kastl PR, Refojo MJ, Dabezies OH Jr., Review of polymerization for the contact lens fitter. In: Dabezies OH Jr., ed. Contact Lenses: The CLAO Guide to Basic Science and Clinical Practice. 2nd ed., Vol 1. Boston: Little, Brown & Co., 1989:6.21–6.24.
376. Polse KA, Mandell RB. Arch Ophthalmol 1970; 84:505–508.
377. Binder PS. Ophthalmology 1978; 86:1093.
378. Fatt I, Hill RM. Am J Optom Arch Am Acad Optom 1970; 47:50.
379. Fatt I. Contacto 1978; 23(1):6.
380. Food and Drug Administration, Guidance Document for Class III Contact Lenses, United States Food and Drug Administration; Silver Springs, MD; 1989.
381. Van Haeringen NJ. Clinical biochemistry of tear, Surv. Opthalmol 1981; 26(2):84–96.
382. Castillo EJ, Koenintg JL, Anderson JM. Biomaterials 1986; 7:89–96.
383. Ruben M. Br J Ophthalmol 1975; 59:141.

384. Hart DE. Int Contact Lens Clin 1984; 11:358–360.
385. Begley CG, Waggoner PJ. J Am Optom Assoc 1991; 62:208–214.
386. Tripathi RC, Tripathi BJ, Millard CB. CLAO J. 1988; 14:23–32.
387. Miller MJ, Wilson LA, Ahrean DG. J Clin Microbiol 1988; 16:513–517.
388. Chowhan M, Bilbault T, Quintana RP, et al. Contactologia 1993; 15:190–195.
389. Jacob R. Int Contact Lens Clin 1988; 15:317–325.
390. Holsky D. J Am Optom Assoc 1993; 55:205–211.
391. Hom MM, Pickford M. Int Eyecare 1986; 2:325–326.
392. Davis RL. Int Contact Lens Clin 1983; 10:277–284.
393. Chowhan MA, Quintana RP, Hong BS, et al. To Alcon Laboratories, Inc. U.S. patent 5,948,738.
394. Begley CG, Paraguia S, Sporm C. An analysis of contact lens enzyme cleaner. J Am Optom Assoc 1990; 61:190–193.
395. Tarrantino N, Courtney RC, Lesswell LA. et al. Int Contact Lens Clin 1988; 15:25–32.
396. Houlsby RD, Ghajar M, Chavez G. J Am Optom Assoc 1988; 59:184–188.
397. Anger CB, Ambrus K, Stocker J, et al. Spectrum 1990; 9:46–51.
398. Chowhan M, Bilbault, T, Quintana RP. To Alcon Laboratories, Inc. U.S. patent 5,370,744.
399. Chowhan M, Keith D, Chen H, Stone R. Poster at Annual Meeting. Las Vegas: CLAO, 1998.
400. Food and Drug Administration, Draft Testing Guidelines for Class III Soft (Hydrophilic) Contact Lens Solutions, U. S. Food and Drug Administration; Silver Springs, MD; 1985.
401. Brennan NA, Efron N. Optom Vis Sci 1989; 66:834–838.
402. Efron N, Goldwig TR, Brennan NA. CLAO J 1991; 17:114–119.
403. Chowhan M, Stone R, Rosenthal RA, et al. Alcon Laboratories, Inc, Technical Reports, XXXX.
404. Gorscak JJ, Ayres BA, Bhagat N, et al. Cornea 2007; 26:10.

5

Delivery of Drugs by the Pulmonary Route

Anthony J. Hickey
*Dispersed Systems Laboratory, Division of Molecular Pharmaceutics,
University of North Carolina at Chapel Hill, School of Pharmacy,
Chapel Hill, North Carolina, U.S.A.*

Heidi M. Mansour
*Department of Pharmaceutical Sciences-Drug Development, College of
Pharmacy, University of Kentucky, Lexington, Kentucky, U.S.A.*

INTRODUCTION

Background and Historical Perspective

Inhaled therapies have existed for at least 5000 years (1). Modern drug therapy can be traced to the propellant-driven (also known as "pressurized") metered-dose inhaler (pMDI) of the 1950s (2). The surge in interest that has arisen in the last decade relates to the chlorofluorocarbon (CFC) propellant ban and the development of biotechnology products. The observation that CFC propellants play a significant role in ozone depletion in the upper atmosphere (3), which in turn results in greater surface ultraviolet (UV) radiation and impact on public health, particularly the incidence of skin cancer, led to regulation in the late 1980s (4). In addition, the burgeoning biotechnology industry of the late 1980s and early 1990s actively sought alternative methods of delivering macromolecular drugs, which were difficult to deliver in therapeutic doses by the oral or parenteral route (5). The urgent need for alternative methods explains the diversity of devices that have been described in the patent literature, many of which are currently on the market, and the others are under development.

The factors governing lung deposition may be divided into those related to the physicochemical properties of the droplets or particles being delivered, the mechanical aspects of aerosol dispersion usually associated with the delivery device, and the physiological and anatomical considerations associated with the biology of the lungs.

Physicochemical Factors Governing Lung Deposition

A number of physicochemical properties are associated with aerosol droplets of particles, which impact on their characteristics as aerosols. The most important of these may be related to the aerodynamic properties of aerosols (6).

The size of any particle may be related to a characteristic dimension (7). As examples, visual examination allows determination of projected area diameter, surface area measurement allows determination of equivalent surface diameter, and volume displacement allows determination of equivalent volume diameter. A full discussion of particle size measurement is beyond the scope of this chapter. It is sufficient to acknowledge that the method of describing particle size most relevant to describing aerosol particles is based on the aerodynamic behavior of the particle being studied. The size may then be described in terms of the equivalent diameter of a unit-density sphere with the same terminal settling velocity as the particle being studied. The terms of an expression relating different particle diameters in terms of terminal settling velocity take the following form (8):

$$V_{\mathrm{T}} = \frac{\rho_{\mathrm{p}} g D_{\mathrm{e}}^2 C(D_{\mathrm{e}})}{\kappa_{\mathrm{p}} 18\eta} = \frac{\rho_0 g D_{\mathrm{ae}}^2 C(D_{\mathrm{ae}})}{\kappa_0 18\eta} \tag{1}$$

where κ_{p} and κ_0 are the shape factors for the particle (>1) and an equivalent sphere (1), respectively; ρ_{p} and ρ_0 are the densities of the particle and a unit-density (1 g/cm^3) sphere, respectively; $C(D_{\mathrm{e}})$ and $C(D_{\mathrm{ae}})$ are the slip correction factors for an equivalent volume and an aerodynamically equivalent sphere, respectively; D_{e} and D_{ae} are the equivalent volume diameter and aerodynamically equivalent (aerodynamic) diameter, respectively; and g is the acceleration due to gravity.

Equation (1) points to a number of important particle properties. Clearly, the particle diameter, by any definition, plays a role in the behavior of the particle. The particle properties of density and shape are also of significance in aerosol behavior. The shape becomes important if particles deviate significantly from sphericity. The majority of pharmaceutical aerosol particles exhibit a high level of rotational symmetry and consequently do not deviate substantially from spherical behavior. The notable exception is that of elongated particles, fibers, or needles, which exhibit shape factor κ_{p} substantially greater than 1. Density will frequently deviate from unity and must be considered in comparing aerodynamic and equivalent volume diameters.

The slip correction factors are important for particles smaller than 1 μm in diameter, which is rarely the case for pharmaceutical aerosols. Slip correction is required for the Stokes' equation to remain predictive of particle behavior for these small particles. Therefore, assuming the absence of shape effects for particles in the Stokes' regime of flow, equation (1) collapses into the following expression:

$$D_{\mathrm{ae}} = (\rho_{\mathrm{p}})^{0.5} D_{\mathrm{e}} \tag{2}$$

The capacity for aerosols to take on moisture by hygroscopicity gives rise to a kinetic phenomenon of change in particle size as a function of residence time at a particular ambient relative humidity (RH). This phenomenon can best be described in terms of the relationship between saturation ratio and particle size according to the following expression (9):

$$\frac{p}{p_{\mathrm{s}}} = \left[1 + \left(\frac{6imM_{\mathrm{w}}}{M_{\mathrm{s}}\rho\pi d_{\mathrm{p}}^3} \right) \right]^{-1} \exp\left(\frac{4\gamma M_{\mathrm{w}}}{RT d_{\mathrm{p}}} \right) \tag{3}$$

where p and p_{s} are the partial and saturation vapor pressures of water in the atmosphere, respectively; M_{s} and M_{w} are the molecular weights of the solute and water, respectively; ρ and γ are the density and surface tension of the solution, respectively; i is the number of ions into which the solute dissociates; and d_{p} is the particle diameter. This phenomenon is of significance, since a change in the size of particles in transit through the high-humidity environment of the lungs (99.5% RH at 37°C) will give rise to altered deposition characteristics (10,11).

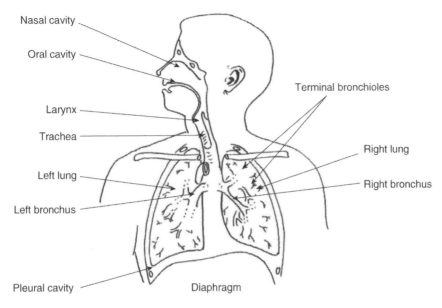

Nasal cavity

Oral cavity

Larynx

Trachea

Left lung

Left bronchus

Pleural cavity

Terminal bronchioles

Right lung

Right bronchus

Diaphragm

Figure 1   The anatomy of the lungs showing the major airway subdivisions.

Physiological and Anatomical Features Governing Lung Deposition

Anatomically, the lung is a series of bifurcating tubes, which begin at the trachea, divide into the main bronchii, the conducting bronchioles, and conclude in the terminal bronchioles and the alveoli, as shown in Figure 1. Casts of the upper airways have been constructed in an attempt to predict aerosol deposition in the lungs. From these casts, a number of anatomical models have been constructed, the most notable assuming symmetrical (12) and asymmetrical (13) branching. Figure 2 illustrates the Weibel symmetrical branching model of the lung. The average lengths, cross-sectional areas, and linear velocities achieved at various locations in the lungs were estimated early in the last century (14), and some examples are shown in Table 1.

Most lung deposition models are based on the influence of particle size on aerosol deposition. Breathing parameters, such as breathing frequency and tidal volume, play a key role in lung deposition (15). Table 2 shows the breathing parameters for healthy male volunteers subjected to various levels of exercise on a bicycle ergometer (16). There are known differences in these parameters based on gender, age, and disease state, all of which should be considered in evaluating aerosol therapies.

A variety of species of laboratory animal are employed to study aerosol deposition for both efficacy and toxicity. It is important to recognize that the breathing parameters (17), not to mention the anatomy (18), of these animals differ substantially from that of humans. Table 3 shows a range of breathing parameters for several species of laboratory animal. Clearly, there is a matter of scale involved in that small animals cannot generate the same airflow volumes as humans and, to some extent, compensate by increasing their respiratory rate.

The physicochemical properties of particles influence their behavior in transit through the airways of the lungs according to three mechanisms: impaction, sedimentation, and diffusion.

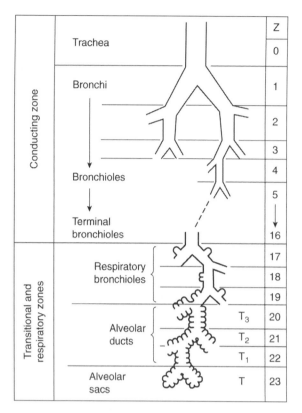

Figure 2 The Weibel symmetrical branching model of the lung. *Source*: From Ref. 12.

Table 1 Estimates of the Length, Cross-Sectional Areas, and Linear Velocities of Airways Indicating the Geometry and Dynamics of Discrete Regions of the Lungs

Lung region	Length (cm)	Cross-sectional area (cm^2)	Linear velocity (cm/sec)
Trachea	11.0	1.3	150
Main bronchi	6.5	1.1	180
Second-order bronchi	1.5	3.1	65
Terminal bronchiole	0.3	150	1.3
Alveolar duct	0.02	8200	0.025

Table 2 Respiratory Rates and Tidal and Minute Volumes for Healthy Young Men at Rest and Under Two Levels (Light, 622 kg.m/min; Heavy, 1660 kg.m/min)

Degree of exertion	Respiratory rate[a] (breaths/min)	Tidal volume[b] (L)	Minute volume[a] (L)
Sedentary	14.6	0.705	10.3
Light	23.0	1.622	37.3
Heavy	47.6	2.391	113.8

[a]Measured
[b]Calculated

Table 3 Resting Respiratory Rates and Tidal and Minute Volumes in Laboratory Animals[a]

Species	Respiratory rate (breaths/min)	Tidal volume (mL)	Minute volume (L)
Dog	18	320.0	5.2
Cat	25	12.4	0.32
Rat	85	1.5	0.1
Mouse	163	0.15	0.023
Guinea pig	90	1.8	0.16
Rabbit	46	21.0	1.07

[a]Measured
Source: Modified from Ref. 17.

The principle of inertial impaction is employed to sample aerosols aerodynamically for characterization of particle size and will be dealt with theoretically later in this chapter.

Sedimentation of particles follows the principle outlined above in equation (1) in which particles in the Stokes' regime of flow have attained terminal settling velocity. In the airways, this phenomenon occurs under the influence of gravity. The angle of inclination, ψ, of the tube of radius R, on which particles might impact, must be considered in any theoretical assessment of sedimentation (14,19), Landahl's expression for the probability, S, of deposition by sedimentation took the form

$$S = 1 - \exp\left[\frac{-(0.8V_T \cdot .t \cdot .\cos\psi)}{R}\right] \qquad (4)$$

where $V_T \cdot .t \cdot .\cos\psi/R$ has been designated the deposition parameter.

From equation (1), V_T includes a term for the particle size and gravitational acceleration. Landahl's expression adds terms describing the geometry of the tube and the residence time of the particle to allow a probability of deposition to be derived. As an example of the manner in which this expression is applied, assuming a deposition parameter of one and a probability of deposition of 55% for 2-μm particles, 1-μm and 0.5-μm particles would be expected to deposit with 29% and 10% efficiency, respectively. The probabilities of particle deposition, by the U.S. Atomic Energy Commission and American Conference of Governmental and Industrial Hygienists, have been used to designate the fraction of an aerosol that is respirable, as shown in Table 4. This considers deposition in all of the airways of the lungs. Thorough descriptions of theoretical and experimental studies of lung deposition have been collated and may be found in the literature (20).

Particulate diffusion does not play a significant role in the deposition of pharmaceutical aerosols. However, it is worth noting the mechanism by which diffusion of particles occurs in the lungs. The principle of Brownian motion is responsible for particle deposition under the influence of impaction with gas molecules in the airways. The amplitude of particle displacement, Λ, is given by the following equation:

$$\Lambda = \left[\left(\frac{RT}{N}\right)\left(\frac{Ct}{3\pi\eta d}\right)\right]^{0.5} \qquad (5)$$

where R is the universal gas constant, T is absolute temperature (Kelvin), N is Avogadro's number, C is the slip correction factor, t is time, η is the air viscosity, and d is the particle diameter.

Table 4 Respirable Fractions as Designated by the American Conference of Governmental and Industrial Hygienist (ACGIH) and the U.S. Atomic Energy Commission (USAEC)

Aerodynamic diameter (μm)	Respirable fraction[a] (%)	Respirable fraction[b] (%)
10	1	0
8	5	—
5	30	25
4	50	—
2	91	100
1	97	—

[a]ACGIH (1997)
[b]USAEC (1961)

Diffusion plays an important role in one of the most efficient aerosol delivery devices, the cigarette, because of the submicron size of the particles produced by combustion (21). It is conceivable that the next generation of inhalers may take greater advantage of this mechanism of delivery. However, the major limitation to this approach is that an aerosol with a significant submicron fraction tends to be exhaled without depositing. The closer the particle size approaches the mean free path of the conducting gas, the more likely it is that deposition will not occur within usual lung residence times.

Mechanism of Drug Clearance and Pharmacokinetics of Disposition

The first purified and characterized drug substances were administered as aerosols as a topical treatment for asthma approximately 50 years ago. More recently, drugs have been evaluated for systemic delivery by this route. For each category of drug, the mechanism of clearance from the airways must be considered. These mechanisms may be listed as mucociliary transport, absorption, and cell-mediated translocation. The composition and residence time of the particle will influence the mechanism of clearance.

The importance of clearance mechanisms from the lungs relates to the action of the drug. For drugs that act in the lungs, such as bronchodilators or anti-inflammatory agents, an extended residence time in the lungs might be beneficial. For drugs intended to act systemically, such as ergotamine alkaloids for migraine or insulin for the treatment of *diabetes mellitus*, rapid absorption may be desirable. This is not to imply that all systemically acting agents must be delivered rapidly, but this allows a contrast in rates of delivery.

The nature of the mechanisms involved and the interaction with the aerosol particles complicate the pharmacokinetics of drug clearance from the lungs. Figure 3 illustrates the sites of deposition in the lungs and the nasal, oropharyngeal, tracheobronchial, and pulmonary regions. Also shown in this figure are the routes for clearance by absorption into the blood circulation, by mucociliary transport to the gastrointestinal tract, and cell-mediated transport to the lymphatics and from there to the blood circulation.

Mucociliary transport in the conducting airways takes approximately 24 hours from the lung periphery to the epiglottis. Absorption takes place at a rate dictated by the physicochemical properties of the drug (hydrophobic, hydrophilic, strong or weak electrolyte, molecular weight). These properties impact on the paracellular and transcellular mechanisms of transport across the alveolar or bronchiolar epithelium. Studies of fluorescent dextrans of a range of molecular weights have shown that paracellular transport occurs more rapidly for small-molecular-weight molecules than for

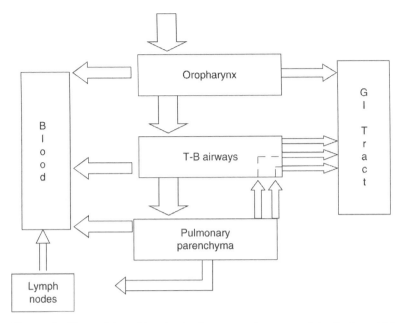

Figure 3 Sites of deposition in the lungs, oropharynx, and tracheobronchial and pulmonary regions.

large molecular weight ones (22). A plot of log clearance (min^{-1}) against log molecular weight (D) appears to be linear in the range of clearances of $10^{-1}-10^{-4}$ for molecular weights of 10^2-10^5 Da, respectively (22). The data were collected for a number of different species (rat, rabbit, dog, sheep, lamb, dog, and human).

Particles that exhibit long residence times in the periphery of the lungs, beyond the mucociliary escalator, are subject to uptake by alveolar macrophages, phagocytic cells responsible for clearing debris from the pulmonary region of the lungs. These cells are also the primary immunological defense, presenting the initial response to antigenic materials, usually foreign material of biological origin including infectious micro-organisms (bacteria, viruses, and fungi). Cellular clearance may take weeks or months depending on the nature of the particles.

Mathematical models for drug disposition have been proposed (23) and elaborated upon (24). The latter model proposed dividing the airways into tracheobronchial and two pulmonary regions, long and short residence time regions, also considering the availability of drug that enters the gastrointestinal tract. A series of equations were derived for the fraction remaining in each of the regions under steady-state conditions. These models examine thoroughly the influence of the physicochemical properties on drug disposition from the lungs. More subtle models have also been evaluated on the basis of receptor occupancy of glucocorticoids (25).

CATEGORIES OF AEROSOL DELIVERY DEVICE

Before discussing the three categories of delivery device, the nature of the emitted aerosol will be considered. Droplet formation may be characterized in terms of the nature of the propulsive force and the liquid being dispersed, and this topic is dealt with for specific situations in the following sections. However, dry particles, which are delivered from suspension in pMDIs or from dry powder inhalers (DPIs) alone or from a blend, must be prepared in respirable sizes. The production of respirable aerosol particles has traditionally been achieved by micronization of the drug (26). This is commonly achieved through air-jet milling (27,28). This involves the introduction of bulk particles on a gas stream into the path of an opposing gas stream under high pressure. Particles impact on each other and are thereby ground into small particles, which ultimately pass through a cyclone separator and are collected in a vessel or a bag filter. These particles can be produced in size ranges less than 5 μm, which is suitable for lung deposition.

A variety of technologies (27,29) exist for creating respirable colloidal particles in the solid state. In recent years, spray drying has been employed as an alternative method of production (27,30–33). This method has the advantage that particles produced are frequently spherical. In addition, it may be the case that the particles are not subject to such high-energy input as in the case of jet milling, and consequently, this may be more suitable for thermolabile materials. As more sophisticated techniques are being developed for the production of particles, they are finding applications in the production of aerosol particles. One of the more successful of these approaches is the supercritical fluid method of manufacture, which involves controlled crystallization of drugs from dispersion in supercritical fluids, notably carbon dioxide (27,32,34,35). Many supercritical fluid technologies exist and have found demonstrated utility in generating respirable solid-state particles for a variety of pulmonary materials and emulsion systems (27,33,35–43).

Propellant-Driven Metered-Dose Inhalers

The formulation for a pMDI consists of several key components: propellant(s), drug, cosolvents, and surfactants.

Propellants may be of a number of different types: CFCs, hydrofluoroalkanes (HFAs), or alkanes. The composition impacts on performance. A numerical system is employed to identify fluorinated propellants. The rules governing this numbering system allow the molecular structure to be derived from the numerical descriptor. The rules may be listed as follows:

- The digit on the extreme right, e.g., propellant 114, represents the number of chlorine atoms.
- The second digit from the right, e.g., propellant 114, represents one more than the number of hydrogen atoms.
- The third digit from the right, e.g., propellant 114, represents one less than the number of carbon atoms.
- A subscripted lowercase letter represents the symmetry of the molecule: the earlier in the alphabet, the more symmetrical the molecule being described, e.g., propellant 134a.

Two additional rules have not been required for pharmaceutical purposes but may be included for completeness.

- A fourth number from the right indicates the number of double bonds in the molecule.
- A prefixed lowercase c indicates that the molecule is cyclic.

The vapor pressure and density of propellants are employed to assist in formulation. The vapor pressure dictates the force of emission of the droplets from the metering valve of the inhaler. The force of emission is derived from the difference between the product vapor pressure and atmospheric pressure. The density of the propellant may be matched to

Table 5 Physicochemical Properties of Chlorofluorocarbon and Alternative Hydrofluoroalkane Propellants such as Hydrofluorocarbons

Propellant (chemical formula)	Molecular weight (g/mol)	Vapor pressure (psia at 25°C)	Boiling point (°C at 1 atm)	Density (g/cm³ at 25°C)
011 (CCl_3F)	137.4	13.4	23.8	1.48
012 (CCl_2F_2)	120.9	94.5	−29.8	1.31
114 ($C_2Cl_2F_4$)	170.9	27.6	3.8	1.46
134a (CH_2FCF_3)	102.0	96.0	−26.5	1.20
227 ($CHF_2C_2F_5$)	170.0	72.6	17.3	1.42

the drug particles to assist in the suspension formulation stability. Table 5 shows the characteristic physicochemical properties of the common propellants.

Hydrocarbons have also been considered as potential propellants for pharmaceutical aerosols. To date, concerns regarding flammability seem to have precluded significant developments with propane, isobutane, butane, and mixtures of these alkanes (44).

A cosolvent, typically ethanol, may be used to bring drug into solution. A small number of insoluble surfactants (sorbitan trioleate, oleic acid, and lecithin) may be dispersed in propellant systems and can aid in suspension stability and in valve lubrication.

The significance of a propellant is its ability to generate high-velocity emission as it vaporizes upon equilibrium with atmospheric pressure. Raoult's and Dalton's laws may be applied to estimate the vapor pressure of propellant blends.

Raoult's law states that the partial pressure (P') is equal to the product of the pure vapor pressure (P^0) and the mole fraction (X) of the component being considered as follows (45,46):

$$P' = P^0 X \tag{6}$$

where for a two-component system (a and b)

$$X_a = \frac{n_a}{(n_a + n_b)}$$

and

$$X_b = \frac{n_b}{(n_a + n_b)}$$

where n_a and n_b are the number of moles of components a and b, respectively, present in the product.

Dalton's law states that the total vapor pressure (P_T) over a solution is equal to the sum of partial vapor pressures attributable to each component ($a, b, \ldots n$).

$$P_T = P'_a + P'_b + \cdots + P'_n \tag{7}$$

An empirical relationship between median droplet diameter, D_i, and atomizer conditions has been demonstrated (47). The relationship is described in the following expression.

$$D_i = \frac{C_s}{Q_e^m[(P_e - P_A)/P_A]^n} \tag{8}$$

where C_s is a constant, relating pressure and quality to droplet size, Q_e the mass fraction of vapor phase in the expansion chamber, m a constant relating quality of flow to droplet

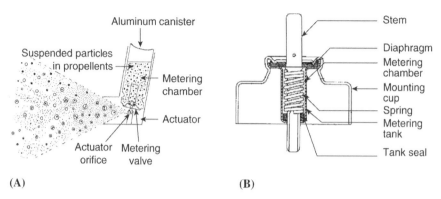

Figure 4 (**A**) Propellant-driven metered-dose inhaler. (**B**) Metering valve.

size, n a constant relating pressure to droplet size, P_e and P_A are the pressure downstream of discharge orifice and atmospheric pressure, respectively.

A theoretical approach was also taken to predicting the droplet formation from a pMDI, and this was followed by experimental validation studies (48,49).

The container components include a canister, valve, and actuator. Each of these components should be considered in the preparation of a pMDI product. The majority of products marketed are in plastic-coated glass or aluminum containers of various sizes.

Figure 4A shows the assembled components of a pMDI in operation. The therapeutic usefulness of this device stems from the accurate metering of small doses of drug, which is achieved by a small but complex metering valve. The components of a metering valve are shown in Figure 4B.

The performance should be evaluated in terms of drug and component physical and chemical compatibilities. Particle size and emitted dose determinations are required. Through-life performance should be evaluated as this is a multidosing reservoir system. The influence of temperature and humidity on stability and performance of the product should also be considered.

Filling may be conducted at low temperature or high pressure and requires specialized equipment. Low-temperature filling is carried out at a temperature substantially lower than the boiling point of the propellant to allow manipulation at room temperature in an open vessel. Pressure filling is conducted in a sealed system from which the propellant is dispensed at its equilibrium vapor pressure at room temperature through the valve of the container (50).

Dry Powder Inhalers

The 1987 Montreal protocol (4) initially limited the use of CFC propellants and then banned them by 2009 in the United States (51). In addition, degradation kinetics of therapeutic biomolecules is slower in the solid state than in the liquid state. Combined with bypassing the "first-pass effect" of hepatic metabolism and drug degradation in the gastrointestinal tract, the lungs have been an attractive route of administration of sensitive biomacromolecules in the solid state. The forces of interaction between particles present barriers to their flow and dispersion. The major forces of interaction are van der Waals, electrostatic, and capillary forces (52).

Van der Waals forces are derived from the energy of interaction between two molecules, V_{ss}. These can be derived from London's theory as follows:

$$V_{ss} = -\frac{3}{4}h v_0 \frac{\alpha^2}{\alpha^6} \tag{9}$$

where α is the polarizability, h is Planck's constant, and v_0, the characteristic frequency. Because v is found in the UV region of the absorption spectra and plays a key role in optical dispersion, the intermolecular London–van der Waals forces are also called dispersion forces. These forces operate at short ranges but when integrated over all molecules give rise to large interparticulate forces.

The dipole-induced dipole interactions are summed over all atoms and expressed as the Hamaker constant (A). The total molecular potential, U_m, for two perfectly spherical particles with diameters d_1 and d_2 for particles 1 and 2, respectively, is

$$U_m = \frac{A d_1 d_2}{12z(d_1 + d_2)} \tag{10}$$

where z is the shortest interparticulate distance. The Hamaker constant is given by

$$A = \pi^2 n_1 n_2 C_{ss} \tag{11}$$

where n_1 and n_2 are molecular densities and C_{ss} is the London–van der Waals constant.

Two dissimilar materials, with Hamaker constants A_{11} and A_{22}, interact as follows:

$$A_{12} = (A_{11} \cdot A_{22})^{0.5} \tag{12}$$

Equation (10) may be applied when $z \ll D = d_1 d_2 /(d_1 + d_2)$. This is not a practical limitation, but an applicable equation can be obtained by differentiating equation (10) with respect to z.

$$F = \frac{\delta}{\delta z}(U_m) = \frac{AD}{12z^2} \tag{13}$$

The attractive force (F) is dependent on the Hamaker constant and the shortest distance between the particles, z. F may be decreased by decreasing A or increasing z. Theoretically, the Hamaker constant can be decreased by decreasing the densities of the two interacting particles. Since the separation distance plays a significant role in van der Waals attraction, any means to increase this distance will reduce the attractive force and increase the ease of dispersion. Surface roughening and the use of spacers can increase interparticulate separation with the improved particle dispersion.

Electrostatic forces are smaller than van der Waals forces for conducting particles, but most pharmaceutical products are poor conductors. Therefore, electrostatic charge must be considered. Two adjacent solid surfaces give rise to a contact potential and, in turn, interfacial electrostatic attractive forces that increase interparticulate interfacial interactions (52,53) and, consequently, powder aggregation. Surface electrostatic charge phenomena play an important role in aerosol dispersion and delivery of respirable particles in the solid state (53). Particle collisions and surface contacts give rise to contact charging and additional surface electrostatic interactions. Triboelectric (frictional) charging, a potential difference between two interacting particles in motion having different work functions, further contributes to electrostatic interactions. The potential difference causes electrons to migrate from the body that has a smaller work function to that with a larger work function until equilibrium is achieved. A reduction in charge does not always occur on contact with another particle whether the latter is charged or

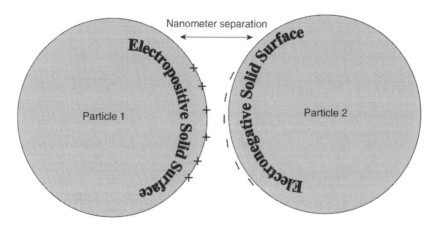

Figure 5 Illustration of interfacial electrostatic attraction between two particles.

uncharged. A persistent charge will induce an equal and opposite charge on neighboring particles or surfaces, as depicted in Figure 5. This induced electrical force on a particle may be expressed as follows:

$$F_1 = \frac{\varepsilon q^2}{h^2} \tag{14}$$

where q is the charge on the particle and h is the separation distance between the adhering particles in a dielectric medium, ε.

The Coulomb equation describes triboelectric charging (F_c) between a spherical particle and an adjacent uncharged particle.

$$F_c = q^2 \left[1 - \frac{h}{(R^2 + h^2)^{0.5}} \right] \times \frac{1}{16\pi\varepsilon_0 h^2} \tag{15}$$

where R is the particle radius, q the charge, h the separation distance, and ε_0 the permittivity of vacuum. This Coulomb attraction between two solid-state particles, illustrated in Figure 5, reduces to zero in a humid environment because of decharging of the system, but attractive forces then become complicated by capillary forces of interaction.

In the presence of a potential difference, particles of different work functions are brought into contact by a force of attraction defined as follows:

$$F_w = \pi\varepsilon_0 \frac{R(\Delta U)^2}{h} \tag{16}$$

Capillary condensation, illustrated in Figure 6, results from capillary force and changes in partial vapor pressures as a result of increased curvature, as defined by the Kelvin equation. Capillary forces increase in relationship to the RH of the ambient air and the presence of porous structures, where the high curvature of the pore in the solid results in the lowering of the vapor pressure of water. This vapor pressure–lowering effect results in small amounts of water vapor to condense to liquid water at lower relative humidities of 10% to 50% RH. When nonporous solid particles are exposed to a RH greater than 65% RH, fluid condenses in the space between the adjacent nonporous solid particles. This leads to liquid bridges as a consequence of the interfacial attractive forces due to the intrinsically high surface tension of water.

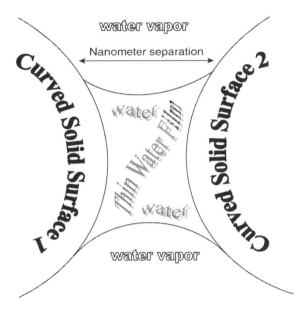

water vapor

Nanometer separation

water

Thin Water Film

water

water vapor

Curved Solid Surface 1

Curved Solid Surface 2

Figure 6 Illustration of capillary condensation of water vapor to a thin film of water at the interfacial space between two curved surfaces.

For a smooth spherical particle with radius R, the force, F_H, experienced is

$$F_H = 2\pi\gamma R \qquad (17)$$

where γ is the surface tension.

A thin film of liquid confined at the interface of two solid bodies gives rise to boundary forces. A pressure difference, P_c, arises and is known as the capillary pressure. This can be calculated from the Laplace equation.

$$P_c = \gamma\left(\frac{1}{R_1} + \frac{1}{R_2}\right) \qquad (18)$$

where γ is the surface tension at the liquid-gas interface and R_1 and R_2 are the principal radii of curvature of the interface. The pulmonary mechanics of alveolar function and the work of breathing is often described by the Laplace equation, in the context of the process of exhalation/inhalation and the modulation of lung surface tension to decrease the work of breathing by normally maintaining a constantly low P_c. The Laplace equation describes the interrelationship and the elegant balance between the surface tension of the nanofilm of lung surfactant lining the alveolus and alveolar diameter. In respiratory distress syndrome (i.e., the absence or dysfunction of alveolar lung surfactant) present in premature babies and adults with pulmonary disease, the work of breathing increases significantly because of an increase in P_c as a result of an abnormal increase in the surface tension of the aqueous nanofilm lining the interior of the alveoli. Consequently, the rise in alveolar capillary forces leads to alveolar collapse and a severe decrease in alveolar gas exchange. It should also be remembered that surface asperities might increase the potential for mechanical interlocking (structural cohesion) of particles, which will influence the aggregation state and ease of dispersion of particles.

The formulation of DPIs is dependent on the nature of particles employed in the formulation. The delivery of dry powder products is dependent on effective dispersion of particles in respirable size ranges. This has been brought about by blending with carrier particles, most notably α-lactose monohydrate (28,53,54). Other approaches include developing particles to overcome the forces of interaction, which include van der Waals forces, capillary forces, electrostatic forces, and mechanical interlocking (53,54). Spherical porous particles that exhibit unique properties of dispersion and aerodynamic behavior have been produced. These particles disperse readily since their van der Waals forces are smaller. However, capillary forces are enhanced in porous structures, hence, capillary condensation can occur at relatively lower relative humidities (10–50% RH), which can adversely affect particle deaggregation and enhance agglomeration. This is especially true for respirable aerosol particles in the solid state. Irregularly shaped porous particles can experience decreased or increased structural cohesion (mechanical interlocking) and surface electrostatics depending on whether the number of contact points between particles is decreased or increased and on the extent of surface asperities (52,53). Once airborne, these particles, which may be geometrically large, behave as aerodynamically small particles, following equation (2).

The metering of DPIs is closely linked to the device itself and may be divided into three common systems (27): capsules, multidose blister packs, and powder reservoir systems. The considerations that go into these metering systems include convenience to the patients, stability on storage, compatibility with product, and ease of filling.

The components of a DPI are the formulation, the metering system, and the device. The device may involve various dispersion mechanisms, pressure drops/shear stress/ resistance levels. The performance of a DPI involves evaluation of component compatibility and influence on device performance. The performance of commercial passive inhaler devices is influenced by the pressure drop (i.e., shear stress or resistance) (55) generated by a patient during an inspiratory flow cycle (56). Recently, it has been suggested that particle size and emitted dose determinations should be conducted as a function of pressure drop/shear stress/device resistance. For powder reservoir devices (27), such as the Turbuhaler (57), evaluation throughout the life of the device is required as part of a stability program. For unit-dose systems (27), such as the Spinhaler (58), barrier integrity must be evaluated for the unit-dose packaging.

Several successful DPI products are currently on the U.S. market (27). Figure 7 shows examples of two DPIs, the Turbuhaler and the Diskus, currently marketed in the United States for the delivery of the steroids budesonide and fluticasone, respectively. Table 6 shows the major elements of a number of passive DPIs. In addition to the

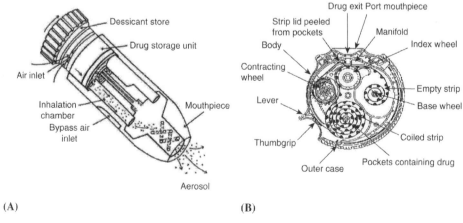

(A)   (B)

Figure 7 Examples of two dry powder inhalers: (**A**) the Turbuhaler™ and (**B**) the Diskus™.

Table 6 Characteristics of Select Passive Dry Powder Inhalers

Inhaler	Carrier	Doses	Powder supply	Passive fluidization	Dispersion
Inhalator Ingelheim™	Glucose	6	Capsule	Capillary	Shear force
Diskhaler™	Lactose monohydrate	4, 8	Blister	Shear force	Turbulence
Diskus™	Lactose monohydrate	60	Blister	Shear force	Turbulence
Turbuhaler™	—	200	Reservoir	Shear force, capillary	Shear force
Easyhaler™	Lactose monohydrate	200	Reservoir	Shear force	Turbulence
MAGhaler™	Lactose monohydrate	200–500	Tablet	Mechanical	Mechanical

Source: Modified from Ref. 28.

Table 7 Characteristics of Select Active Dispersion Dry Powder Inhalers

Inhaler	Carrier	Doses	Powder supply	Active fluidization	Dispersion
Spiros™	n/a[a]	1, 16, or 30	Unit-dose blister or cassette	Mechanical	Turbulence, impaction, shear force
Prohaler™	Mannitol	—	—	Gas assist	Turbulence, shear force
Dynamic Powder Disperser™	Lactose monohydrate	12	Cartridge	Gas assist	Turbulence, shear force
Inhaler Device™	Lactose monohydrate	1	Blister	Gas assist	Turbulence, shear force

[a]n/a denotes information not available.
Source: Modified from Ref. 28.

commercially available passive inhalation products, a number of active dispersion systems are under development; the key characteristics of selected devices are shown in Table 7.

The DPI insulin, lactose carrier-free DPI product, is the only FDA-approved DPI product utilizing an active dispersion system, thereby independent of the patient's inspiratory flow cycle (27).

Nebulizers

Nebulizer formulation conforms to sterile product preparation, which means that drug stability in solution in the presence of additives must be evaluated. Historically, it was sufficient to use antimicrobial agents in the formulation, notably benzalkonium chloride. Adding antimicrobials is not considered now an acceptable approach to the formulation of nebulizer solutions. The solubility of the drug is important since it may impact on the performance of the solution in a selected nebulizer. Additives may form complexes with the drug.

Components include an energy source (gaseous, electrical), a site of energy input to solution (capillary tubes, piezoelectric plate), a means of removing large droplets (baffle plate), and tubing and a face mask to deliver aerosol.

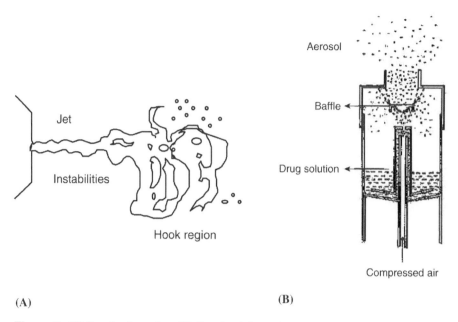

Figure 8 (A) Droplet formation. (B) Droplet delivery from an air-blast nebulizer.

The mechanisms of delivery are either air-blast or air-jet and ultrasonic systems. The theory for each of these mechanisms has been elucidated to the same degree.

Droplet delivery from an air-blast nebulizer is governed by the surface tension, density, and viscosity of the fluid, and the applied pressure, which can be passive or forced. Droplet breakup is illustrated in Figure 8. Droplets form during this breakup at a critical Weber number (We).

$$We_{crit} = \frac{8}{C_D} \tag{19}$$

where C_D is the coefficient of discharge, and

$$We = \rho_A \frac{U_R^2}{\eta} D \tag{20}$$

where ρ_A is the air density, U_R the velocity, D the diameter of the nozzle, and η the liquid viscosity.

Droplets are dispersed from nebulizer nozzles by one of five basic mechanisms based on Bernoulli (Venturi) effect. There are two categories of arrangement of liquid feed supply with respect to the driving gas supply: separate liquid and air feed nozzles and coaxial nozzles. The latter coaxial arrangement has four potential orientations: central gas with internal mixing, central gas with external mixing, central liquid with internal mixing, and central liquid with external mixing. The high-pressure airstream passes over or around the liquid feed nozzle, inducing a low-pressure region, which draws solution through a capillary. The liquid is subsequently dispersed in the air.

Performance of nebulizers is not measured in the same manner as pMDIs and DPIs. Since the drug solution is not supplied with the device, the time scale of compatibility is much smaller. Droplet size and distribution and dose delivery are, however, very important.

The manifestation of through-life evaluation, which is important to these devices, is the delivery of a single dose. The emitted dose and droplet size may vary from the beginning to the end of the delivery period.

CHARACTERIZATION OF PHARMACEUTICAL AEROSOLS

Emitted Dose

The therapeutic effect of aerosols is dependent on their delivery to the lungs. Clearly, the first measure of the potential to deliver drug to the lungs is the dose delivered from the device. A number of methods have been suggested for this purpose. Two unit-dose samplers are popular and are shown in Figure 9. A sampler, consisting of a tube and an absolute filter, through which air is drawn, enables the collection of bolus aerosols delivered by metered-dose inhalers (MDIs) and DPIs, as shown in Figure 9A. These airborne particulates are sampled at a fixed flow rate of 60 L/min. Nebulizer output is more difficult to collect as it is delivered over an extended period of time and often saturates filters, compromising their collection efficiency. These devices may more easily be evaluated by passing them through an immersed sintered glass or steel frit, as shown in Figure 9B.

Particle Size Characterization

In Vitro Characterization
Inertial impaction is the method of choice for evaluating particle or droplet size delivery from pharmaceutical aerosol systems. This method lends itself readily to theoretical analysis. It has been evaluated in general terms (59) and for specific impactors (60). Inertial impaction employs Stokes' law to determine the aerodynamic diameter of particles being evaluated. This has the advantage of incorporating shape and density effects into a single term.

The collection efficiency of particles at a stage of an impactor is based on curvilinear motion and assumes Reynolds' numbers for flow greater than 500 but less than

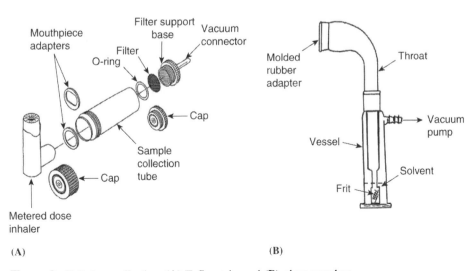

(A)   (B)

Figure 9   Unit-dose collection. (**A**) Teflon tube and (**B**) glass samplers.

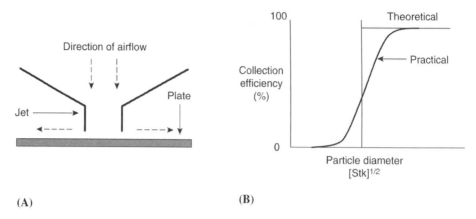

Figure 10 (**A**) General principle of inertial sampling through a jet onto a collection plate. (**B**) Generalized collection efficiency curve.

3000. Figure 10A illustrates the principle of inertial sampling in which particles with high momentum travel in the initial direction of flow of an airstream impacting on an obstructing surface and those with low momentum adjust to the new direction of flow and pass around the obstruction. The efficiency of this phenomenon can be described as follows:

$$d_{50}[C(D)]^{0.5} = \left\{ \frac{9[D_{\mathrm{j}}(\mathrm{Stk}_{50})]}{\rho_{\mathrm{p}}U} \right\}^{0.5} \tag{21}$$

where d_{50} is the 50% collection efficiency cutoff diameter for the stage, D_{j} and U are the jet diameter and linear velocity, respectively, Stk_{50} is the Stokes' number for 50% efficiency, which by definition for circular orifices is 0.22, and ρ_{p} is the particle density usually taken as unity (1 g/cm^3) for aerodynamic purposes. The linear velocity can be derived from the ratio of the volumetric flow rate through the impactor divided by the cross-sectional area of the orifice(s). Figure 10B shows the characteristic theoretical and practical collection efficiency curve. The x-axis may be plotted as particle diameter, in which case a series of curves at ever-decreasing sizes representing different stages of the impactor would exist. Converting the data to the square root of Stokes' number overlays each of the particle size curves. The characteristic Stokes' number for circular jets is 0.22.

Theoretical approximations of deposition on impactor collection plates can be validated by calibration of the instrument using monodisperse aerosol particles. A number of methods exist for the preparation of monodisperse aerosols, including vibrating orifice aerosol generation (61) and spinning-disk aerosol generation (62). Schematic diagrams of the key elements of these devices are shown in Figure 11. Each of these methods lends itself to theoretical prediction of particle size output, which is important to the calibration process.

The droplet size delivered from a vibrating orifice monodisperse aerosol generator can be derived from the following expressions:

$$d_{\mathrm{d}} = \left(\frac{6Q}{\pi f} \right)^{0.33} \tag{22}$$

where Q is the volumetric flow rate and f is the frequency of the piezoelectric ceramic.

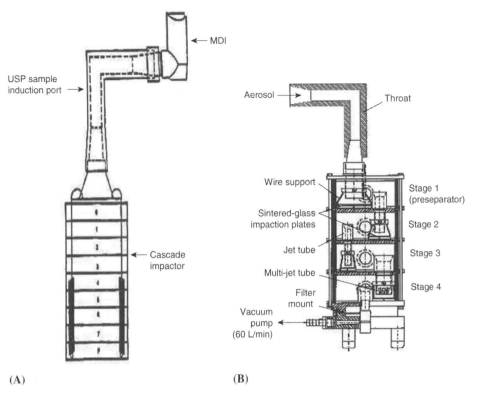

(A)   **(B)**

Figure 11 Magnified diagrams of monodisperse aerosol–generating devices. **(A)** Spinning-disk aerosol generator. **(B)** Vibrating orifice aerosol generator.

When a nonvolatile solute is incorporated in a volatile solvent droplet, the dry particle diameter can be derived from the following expression:

$$d_p = C^{0.33} d_d \tag{23}$$

where C is the volumetric concentration of the nonvolatile solute.

The droplet size delivered from a spinning-disk monodisperse aerosol generator can be derived from the following expression:

$$d = \left(\frac{k}{\omega}\right) \left[\frac{\gamma}{(D\rho_1)}\right]^{0.5} \tag{24}$$

where ω is the angular disk velocity, γ the surface tension, D the disk diameter, and ρ_1 the liquid density.

When the liquid fed to the disk contains solids in a concentration C and the droplets are dried slowly in air, the diameter of the resultant spherical particles, d_p, is given by

$$d_p = \left[\frac{C}{\rho}\right]^{0.33} d \tag{25}$$

An alternative method of calibration involves the dispersion of monodisperse polystyrene microparticles. This has recently been made an efficient process by the incorporation of these particles in pMDI suspensions to allow for metering of small well-dispersed boluses sufficient for use as aerosol calibration standards (63).

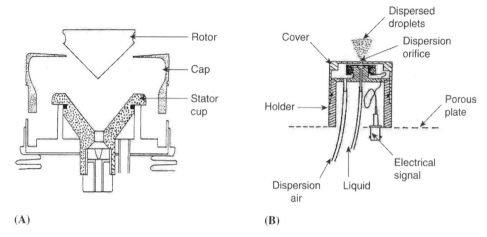

Figure 12 Aerodynamic particle size characterization techniques using (**A**) Andersen eight-stage nonviable cascade impactor and (**B**) four-stage liquid impinger.

Figure 12A depicts a stacked Andersen eight-stage nonviable impactor with calibrated cutoff diameters of 9.0, 5.8, 4.7, 3.3, 2.1, 1.1, 0.7, and 0.4 µm and a lower absolute filter (0.22 µm) when operated at 28.3 L/min. Figure 12B depicts a four-stage liquid impinger with calibrated cutoff diameters of 13.3, 6.7, 3.2, and 1.7 µm at 60 L/min.

Inertial impactors are calibrated at designated flow rates. This may vary depending on the instrument (28). The range of flow rates selected for early impactors was based on passive inhalation of environmental and occupational particulates. Thus, the Delron, Batelle type, six-stage impactor operates at 12.5 L/min, and the Andersen eight-stage nonviable impactor operates at 28.3 L/min [1 ACFM (actual cubic feet per minute)]. The sampling of pharmaceutical aerosols has proven more difficult than ambient particulates. After a period of debate regarding suitable inlets for the device, the USP adopted a right-angled tube as the standard for sampling pMDI output (64). When used with the Andersen impactor, the inlet is arranged immediately above the first stage of the impactor.

The next-generation pharmaceutical impactor (NGPI or NGI), is the most recent type of inertial impactor that is becoming a part of routine aerosol research because of its increased efficiency and ease of use. It has been characterized extensively, including comparison with the Andersen cascade impactor (65–71). This can be attributed to its many advantageous properties including minimal aerosol material loss and is much less labor intensive. Hence, it possesses high-throughput capability, since the solvent used for chemical analysis can be easily incorporated into the impactor prior to the experiment.

Dry powder aerosols are more complicated to sample as the commercially available devices disperse the aerosol on the patient's inspiratory flow, as described above. To challenge the efficiency of these devices, it is important to sample at multiple flow rates. The standard flow rate has become 60 L/min. Additional flow rates of 30 (28.3) and 90 L/min have also been used. Each impactor must be calibrated at the different flow rates employed. In recent compendial specifications, the duration of sampling (four seconds) and pressure drop across the device (4 kPa) have also been suggested. This corrects for the effort on the part of a patient in a single breath.

There have been attempts to conduct in vitro experiments in a manner that gives more meaningful data with regard to lung deposition. These methods, which are loosely based on inertial impaction, utilize inspiratory flow cycles rather than fixed flow rates for sampling the aerosol. These "electronic lung" approaches give interesting results, which may prove useful in the development of aerosol products. Their suitability as quality control tools is influenced by the effect of variable flow rates on impactor calibration.

A viable bio-impactor enables experimental evaluation of aerosol particulate interactions with viable cells placed as cell cultures (specific to different lung regions and different lung disease states) (27) on each stage of the impactor. A number of excellent reviews exist, which discuss suitable pulmonary cell culture models (72–75). Immortalized (continuous) pulmonary cell lines representing distinct regions of the respiratory tract used include A549 (76–79), Calu-3 (78,80–85), and HBE14o (86–88). Primary cultures at an air-liquid interface of normal (noncontinuous) human pulmonary cells have been successful for normal human alveolar epithelial cells (77,78,84,89–92) and normal human bronchial epithelial cells (93). Recognizing the vital importance of pulmonary dendritic cells in pulmonary defense, a triple coculture (94) of dendritic cells, macrophages, and A549 cells is possible to decipher cellular-cross talk between different respiratory cells in particle uptake behavior.

General Sizing Methods

A number of alternative sizing methods are available, and these are described in Table 8. The American Association of Pharmaceutical Scientists, Inhalation Focus Group conducted a comprehensive review of available methods, which was published in a series of articles identified in the last column of the table. All of the methods described either have been or are currently employed in the development of aerosol products. However, at this time, only the inertial samplers, cascade impactors, and impingers appear in compendial standards and in regulatory guidelines (64,95–97). Other methods, such as thermal imaging, are also under development and may give complementary size information to the current methods.

Table 8 General Particle Sizing Methods

Sizing technique (Refs)	Description	Size range (μm)	Limitations
Microscopy with image analysis (98)	Scanning electron microscopy (SEM)	1–300	Sampling shape effects
Inertial sampling methods (99,100)	Impactors, impingers	0.2–20	Number of data points for a distribution; re-entrainment
Right-angle light scattering (101)	Population measure	0.5–40	Sampling refractive index
Phase Doppler anemometry (102)	Cumulative with time	>0.5[a]	Limited to droplets, sampling
Laser diffraction (103)	Population measure	0.1–800	Coincidence errors, sampling
Time of flight (104)	Cumulative with time	0.4–100	Obscuration, coincidence, sampling
Holography (105)	Population measure	3–1000	Obscuration, coincidence, sampling
Direct imaging (106)	Photography	5–1000	Obscuration, coincidence, sampling

[a]Depends on optical configuration.
Source: From Ref. 107.

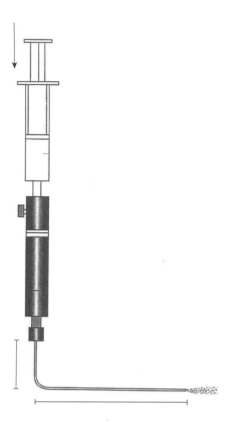

Figure 13 Diagram of the PennCentury powder insufflator.

In Vivo Characterization (Animals and Humans)

The use of animals to evaluate aerosol performance has certain limitations. Toxicological studies have been conducted utilizing whole-body or nose-only exposure chambers (108). However, since pharmaceutical aerosols are not administered as standing clouds, dose estimation by this method would be difficult. Certain species are good pharmacological or immunological models for humans. Only large animals are capable of inhaling or receiving a propelled bolus dose equivalent to a human one. Consequently, instillation and insufflation have been employed to deliver drugs to the lungs of various rodent species. Figure 13 shows an insufflator (PennCentury, Philadelphia, U.S.) and illustrates the dimensions of the device, which is suitable for delivery of powders to rats or guinea pigs (109). Similar devices are available for delivery of drugs to mice and for the delivery of aqueous solutions. Solution volumes are limited to several hundred microliters. Considerable progress is being made in reported aerosol studies involving animals, humans, and in vitro/in vivo correlations, as described recently in depth by these authors (27).

γ-Scintigraphic and single-positron-emission computer-aided tomography imaging methods have been used to evaluate the site of deposition of drugs administered as aerosols. γ-Scintigraphy has become a routine method for the comparison of the performance of various products and for in vivo/in vitro correlation (110–123). It has been proposed that comparison of lung deposition might be employed as a surrogate bioequivalence measure for drugs that act in the lung. This seems a reasonable proposition as the receptors being targeted are located in the airways. It is not clear whether the site of deposition translates into bioequivalence for systemically acting agents.

Efficacy

In the years since the first pMDI asthma therapy was introduced, a host of new products have been developed. The major therapeutic categories are β_2-adrenergic agonists, anticholinergics, glucocorticosteroids, and other anti-inflammatory agents (cromolyn, nedocromil) (27,124). The β_2-adrenergic agonists and anticholinergics act on the parasympathetic and sympathetic nervous system to induce bronchodilation, which relieves bronchoconstriction, a symptom of asthma. Since the underlying cause of asthma is small-airways inflammation, glucocorticoids act as anti-inflammatories. Cromolyn blocks the production of histamine, an inflammatory mediator, by stabilizing mast cells, among other actions, which are not fully understood.

Long-acting agents, such as salmeterol and formoterol, have superseded short-duration bronchodilators such as albuterol and fenoterol. In addition, more potent, site-specific, rapid-onset, and long-acting glucocorticoids, such as fluticasone and budesonide, have superseded the delayed onset of action of less specific molecules such as beclomethasone.

As greater control of the disease state is achieved with aerosol therapy, manufacturers are considering combining some of their most successful products to achieve bronchodilation and anti-inflammatory effect in a single dose. These combinations may increase interest in the use of anticholinergics in addition to β_2-adrenergic agonists.

The systemic delivery of drugs was pioneered with a pMDI product, leuprolide acetate, for the treatment of prostate cancer. A considerable amount of work was conducted to demonstrate feasibility of delivery of this nonapeptide (125). Insulin aerosol development has followed closely behind leuprolide, with a number of companies now looking at various formulations of insulin (126) from pMDI, DPI, and aqueous delivery systems. Exubera® was approved as the first inhaled insulin DPI product (lactose sugar carrier free) delivering a macromolecule and by use of an active dispersion (27,127,128). Despite similar therapeutic blood levels of insulin (compared with injection), Exubera was voluntarily withdrawn from the U.S. market in late 2007 by the manufacturer (Pfizer, Inc., New York, U.S.) because of low patience acceptance of the large indiscrete inhaler device. A range of polypeptide molecules have been studied for their potential, as shown in Table 9. It is now accepted that as a general guide, the window of opportunity for acceptable rates of delivery of such molecules range from 5 to 20 kDa (129,130).

Table 9 Examples of Polypeptides and Their Residence Times in the Lungs

Polypeptide	Molecular weight (g/mol)	t_{max} (hr)
Leuteinizing hormone–releasing hormone (LHRH)	1,067	1
1-Deamino-8-D-arginine vasopressin	1,209	0.5
Calcitonin	3,418	0.25
Parathyroid hormone (PTH)	4,109	0.25
Insulin	5,700	0.25
Granulocyte colony-stimulating factor (GCSF)	18,600	1.5
Interferon-α	19,000	6
Human growth hormone (HGH)	22,000	0.75
α-1-Antitrypsin	45,000	12
Albumin	68,000	20
Immunoglobulin G (IgG)	150,000	16

Source: From Refs. 129 and 130.

CONCLUSION

Drug delivery to the respiratory tract has been characterized in the past decade by an increase in knowledge of drug droplet or particle manufacture, behavior aerosol dispersion, lung deposition, and clearance. The number of diseases for which aerosol therapy may be applicable has increased dramatically. The pharmaceutical scientist is no longer limited to pulmonary diseases as therapeutic targets. Substantial progress has been made in every area of pharmaceutical aerosol science, and it is anticipated that this will ultimately lead to many new therapies.

BIBLIOGRAPHY

Adjei AL, Gupta PK. Inhalation Delivery of Therapeutic Peptides and Proteins. New York: Marcel Dekker, 1997.

Byron PR. Respiratory Drug Delivery. Boca Raton: CRC Press, 1990.

Derendorf H, Hochhaus G. Handbook of Pharmacokinetic/Pharmacodynamic Correlation. Boca Raton: CRC Press, 1995.

Fuchs NA. Mechanics of Aerosols. Minneola: Dover Press, 1964.

Ganderton D, Jones T. Drug Delivery to the Respiratory Tract. New York: VCH/Ellis Horwood, 1987.

Gehr P, Heyder J. Particle-Lung Interactions. New York: Marcel Dekker, 2000.

Hickey AJ. Pharmaceutical Inhalation Aerosol Technology. 2nd ed. New York: Marcel Dekker, 2004.

Hickey AJ. Inhalation Aerosols. 2nd ed. New York: Informa Healthcare, 2007.

Lefebvre AH. Atomization and Sprays. New York: Hemisphere Publishing Corporation, 1989.

Newman SP. Deposition and Effects of Inhalation Aerosols. Lund, Sweden: AB DRACO (subsidiary to ASTRA), 1983.

Purewal TS, Grant DJW. Metered Dose Inhaler Technology. Buffalo Grove: Interpharm Press, Inc., 1998.

Reist P. Aerosol Science and Technology. 2nd ed. New York: McGraw-Hill, 1993.

REFERENCES

1. Sciarra JJ. Pharmaceutical aerosols. In: Lachman L, Lieberman HA, Kanig JL, eds. The Theory and Practice of Industrial Pharmacy. Philadelphia: Lea and Febiger, 1970:605–638.
2. Thiel CG. From Susie's Question to CFC Free: An Inventor's Perspective on Forty Years of MDI Development and Regulation. Respiratory Drug Delivery V. Phoenix, AZ: Davis Healthcare International Publishing, LLC, 1996:115–123.
3. Molina MJ, Rowland FS. Stratospheric sink for chlorofluoromethanes: chlorine atom catalyzed destruction of ozone. Nature 1974; 249:1810.
4. Montreal Protocol 1987. Montreal protocol on substances that deplete the ozone layers, 1987.
5. Hickey AJ, Dunbar CA. A new millenium for inhaler technology. Pharm Technol 1997; 21:116–125.
6. Gonda I. Targeting by deposition. In: Hickey AJ, ed. Pharmaceutical Inhalation Aerosol Technology. New York: Marcel Dekker, Inc., 1992:61–82.
7. Allen T. Particle Size Measurement. 4th ed. London: Chapman and Hall, 1993.
8. Raabe OG. Aerosol aerodynamic size conventions for inertial sampler calibration. J Air Pollut Control Assoc 1976; 26:856–860.
9. Hinds WC. Aerosol Technology: Properties, Behavior, and Measurement of Airborne Particles. 2nd ed. New York: John Wiley and Sons, Inc, 1999.
10. Ferron GA, Oberdorster G, Henneberg R. Estimation of the deposition of aerosolized drugs in the human respiratory tract due to hygroscopic growth. J Aerosol Med 1989; 2:271–283.

11. Hickey AJ, Martonen TB. Behavior of hygroscopic pharmaceutical aerosols and the influence of hydrophobic additives. Pharm Res 1993; 10:1–7.

12. Weibel ER. Morphometry of the Human Lung. Berlin: Springer Verlag, 1963.

13. Horsfield K, Woldenberg MJ. Branching ratio and growth of tree-like structures. Respir Physiol 1986; 63:97–107.

14. Findeisen W. Über das Absetzen kleiner, in der Luft suspendierten Teilchen in der menschlichen Lunge bei der Atmung. Arch Ges Physiol 1935; 236:367.

15. Martonen TB, Katz I, Fults K, et al. Use of analytically defined estimates of aerosol respirable fraction to predict lung deposition patterns. Pharm Res 1992; 9:1634–1639.

16. Hatch TF, Gross P. Physical Factors in Respiratory Deposition of Aerosols. Pulmonary Deposition and Retention of Inhaled Aerosols. New York: Academic Press, 1964:27–43.

17. Chaffee VW. Surgery of laboratory animals. In: Melby EC, Altman NH, eds. Handbook of Laboratory Animal Science. Cleveland: CRC Press, Inc., 1974:233–273.

18. Phalen RF, Oldham MJ. Tracheobronchial airway structure as revealed by casting techniques. Am Rev Respir Dis 1983; 128:S1–S4.

19. Landahl HD. On the removal of air-borne droplets by the human respiratory tract. I. The Lung. Bull Math Biophys 1950; 12:43.

20. ICRP P. Human respiratory tract model for radiological protection. Ann ICRP 1994; 24:1–3.

21. McCusker K, Hiller FC, Wilson JD, et al. Aerodynamic sizing of tobacco smoke particulate from commercial cigarettes. Arch Environ Health 1983; 38:215–218.

22. Effros RM, Mason GR. Measurements of pulmonary epithelial permeability in vivo. Am Rev Respir Dis 1983; 125:S59–S65.

23. Byron PR. Prediction of drug residence times in regions of the human respiratory tract following aerosol inhalation. J Pharm Sci 1986; 75:433–438.

24. Gonda I. Drugs administered directly into the respiratory tract: modeling of the duration of effective drug levels. J Pharm Sci 1988; 77:340–348.

25. Hochhaus G, Suarez S, Gonzalez-Rothi RJ, et al. Pulmonary Targeting of Inhaled Glucocorticoids: How Is it Influenced by Formulation. Respiratory Drug Delivery VI. . Hilton Head, SC: Interpharm Press, Inc., 1998:45–52.

26. Hickey AJ. Lung deposition and clearance of pharmaceutical aerosols: what can be learned from inhalation toxicology and industrial hygiene? Aerosol Sci Technol 1993; 18:290–304.

27. Hickey AJ, Mansour HM. Formulation challenges of powders for the delivery of small molecular weight molecules as aerosols. In: Rathbone MJ, Hadgraft J, Roberts MS, et al. (eds.), Modified-Release Drug Delivery Technology, Vol 2, Drugs and the Pharmaceutical Sciences Series, 2nd ed. New York: Informa Healthcare, 2008: 573–602.

28. Dunbar C, Hickey AJ, Holzner P. Dispersion and characterization of pharmaceutical dry powder aerosols. KONA Powder Part 1998; 16:7–45.

29. Chow AHL, Tong HHY, Chattopadhyay P, et al. Particle engineering for pulmonary drug delivery. Pharm Res 2007; 24:411–437.

30. Mosen K, Backstrom K, Thalberg K, et al. Particle formation and capture during spray-drying of inhalable particles. Pharm Dev Technol 2004; 9:409–417.

31. Vidgrén MT, Vidgren PA, Paronen TP. Comparison of physical and inhalation properties of spray-dried and mechanically micronized disodium cromoglycate. Int J Pharm 1987; 35:139–144.

32. Van Oort MM, Sacchetti M. Spray-drying and supercritical fluid particle generation techniques. In: Hickey AJ, ed. Inhalation Aerosols: Physical and Biological Basis for Therapy. 2nd ed. New York: Informa Healthcare, 2007:307–346.

33. Tong HHY, Chow AHL. Control of physical forms of drug particles for pulmonary delivery by spray drying and supercritical fluid processing. KONA Powder Part 2006; 24:27–40.

34. Tom JW, Debendetti PG. Particle formation with supercritical fluids—a review. J Aerosol Sci 1991; 22:555–584.

35. York P, Kompella UB, Shekunov BY. Supercritical Fluid Technology for Drug Product Development. 1st ed. New York: CRC Press, 2004.

36. Rehman M, Shekunov BY, York P, et al. Optimisation of powders for pulmonary delivery using supercritical fluid technology. Eur J Pharm Sci 2004; 22:1–17.

37. Shekunov BY. Production of powders for respiratory drug delivery. In: York P, Kompella UB, Shekunov BY, eds. Supercritical Fluid Technology for Drug Product Development. New York: Marcel Dekkar, 2004:247–282.

38. Shekunov BY, Chattopadhyay P, Seitzinger J, et al. Nanoparticles of poorly water-soluble drugs prepared by supercritical fluid extraction of emulsions. Pharm Res 2006; 23:196–204.

39. Shekunov BY, Feeley JC, Chow AHL, et al. Physical properties of supercritically-processed and micronised powders for respiratory drug delivery. KONA Powder Part 2002; 20:178–187.

40. Shekunov BY, Feeley JC, Chow AHL, et al. Aerosolisation behaviour of micronised and supercritically processed powders. J Aerosol Sci 2003; 34:553–568.

41. Schiavone H, Palakodaty S, Clark A, et al. Evaluation of SCF-engineered particle-based lactose blends in passive dry powder inhalers. Int J Pharm 2004; 281:55–66.

42. Velaga SP, Bergh S, Carlfors J. Stability and aerodynamic behaviour of glucocorticoid particles prepared by a supercritical fluids process. Eur J Pharm Sci 2004; 21:501–509.

43. Lobo JM, Schiavone H, Palakodaty S, et al. SCF-engineered powders for delivery of budesonide from passive DPI devices. J Pharm Sci 2005; 94:2276–2288.

44. Dalby RN. Halohydrocarbons, pharmaceutical usesIn: Swarbrick J, Boylan JC, eds. Encyclopedia of Pharmaceutical Technology. New York: Marcel Dekker, Inc., 1993:161–180.

45. Atkins P. Physical Chemistry. 5th ed. New York: W.H. Freeman and Company, 1994.

46. Sinko PJ. Martin's Physical Pharmacy and Pharmaceutical Sciences. 5th ed. Philadelphia: Lippincott Williams & Wilkins, 2006.

47. Clark AR. Metered Atomisation for Respiratory Drug Delivery [PhD thesis]. Loughborough University of Technology, U.K., 1991.

48. Dunbar CA, Watkins AP, Miller JF. An experimental investigation of the spray issued from a pMDI using laser diagnostic techniques. J Aerosol Med 1997; 10:351–368.

49. Dunbar CA, Watkins AP, Miller JF. A theoretical investigation of the spray issued from a pMDI. Atomization Sprays 1997; 7:417–436.

50. Sirand C, Varlet JP, Hickey AJ. Aerosol-filling equipment for the preparation of pressurized pack pharmaceutical formulations. In: Hickey AJ, ed. Pharmaceutical Inhalation Aerosol Technology. New York: Marcel Dekker, Inc, 2004:311–343.

51. U.S. Food and Drug Administration. Use of ozone-depleting substances; removal of essential-use designation. U.S. Food and Drug Administration, 2005.

52. Hickey AJ, Concessio NM, Van Oort MM, et al. Factors influencing the dispersion of dry powders as aerosols. Pharm Technol 1994; 18:58–64, 82.

53. Hickey AJ, Mansour HM, Telko MJ, et al. Physical characterization of component particles included in dry powder inhalers. I. Strategy review and static characteristics. J Pharm Sci 2007; 96:1282–1301.

54. Hickey AJ, Mansour HM, Telko MJ, et al. Physical characterization of component particles included in dry powder inhalers. II. Dynamic characteristics. J Pharm Sci 2007; 96:1302–1319.

55. Louey MD, Van Oort M, Hickey AJ. Standardized entrainment tubes for the evaluation of pharmaceutical dry powder dispersion. J Aerosol Sci 2006; 37:1520–1531.

56. Clark AR, Hollingworth AM. The relationship between powder inhaler resistance and peak inspiratory conditions in healthy volunteers—implications for in vitro testing. J Aerosol Med 1993; 6:99–110.

57. Wetterlin K. Turbuhaler: a new powder inhaler for administration of drugs to the airways. Pharm Res 1988; 5:506–508.

58. Rubin LD. Intal (Cromolyn Sodium) A Monograph. 1st ed. Bedford, MA: Fisons Corporation, 1973.

59. Marple VA. Simulation of respirable penetration characteristics by inertial impaction. J Aerosol Sci 1978; 9:125–134.

60. Vaughan NP. The Andersen impactor: calibration, wall losses and numerical simulation. J Aerosol Sci 1989; 20:67–90.

61. Berglund RN, Liu BYH. Generation of monodisperse aerosol standards. Environ Sci Technol 1973; 7:147–152.

62. Byron PR, Hickey AJ. Spinning-disk generation and drying of monodisperse solid aerosols with output concentrations sufficient for single-breath inhalation studies. J Pharm Sci 1987; 76:60–64.

63. Vervaet C, Byron PR. Polystyrene microsphere spray standards based on CFC-free inhaler technology. J Aerosol Med 2000; 13:105–115.

64. Aerosols, Nasal Sprays, Metered-Dose Inhalers, and Dry Powder Inhalers Monograph. USP 29-NF 24 The United States Pharmacopoeia and The National Formulary: The Official Compendia of Standards. Rockville, MD: The United States Pharmacopeial Convention, Inc, 2006:2617–2636.

65. Kamiya A, Sakagami M, Hindle M, et al. Aerodynamic sizing of metered dose inhalers: an evaluation of the Andersen and next generation pharmaceutical impactors and their USP methods. J Pharm Sci 2004; 93:1828–1837.

66. Marple VA, Olson BA, Santhanakrishnan K, et al. Next generation pharmaceutical impactor: a new impactor for pharmaceutical inhaler testing. Part III. Extension of archival calibration to 15 L/min. J Aerosol Med 2004; 17:335–343.

67. Leung K, Louca E, Gray M, et al. Use of the next generation pharmaceutical impactor for particle size distribution measurements of live viral aerosol vaccines. J Aerosol Med 2005; 18:414–426.

68. Myrdal PB, Mogalian E, Mitchell J, et al. Application of heated inlet extensions to the TSI 3306/3321 system: comparison with the Andersen cascade impactor and next generation impactor. J Aerosol Med 2006; 19:543–554.

69. Berg E, Svensson JO, Asking L. Determination of nebulizer droplet size distribution: a method based on impactor refrigeration. J Aerosol Med 2007; 20:97–104.

70. Mitchell JP, Nagel MW, Wiersema KJ, et al. Aerodynamic particle size analysis of aerosols from pressurized metered-dose inhalers: comparison of Andersen 8-stage cascade impactor, next generation pharmaceutical impactor, and model 3321 aerodynamic particle sizer aerosol spectrometer. AAPS PharmSciTech 2003; 4:E54.

71. Guo C, Gillespie SR, Kauffman J, et al. Comparison of delivery characteristics from a combination metered-dose inhaler using the Andersen cascade impactor and the next generation pharmaceutical impactor. J Pharm Sci 2007; 97(8):3321–3334.

72. Mathias NR, Yamashita F, Lee VHL. Respiratory epithelial cell culture models for evaluation of ion and drug transport. Adv Drug Deliv Rev 1996; 22:215–249.

73. Mobley C, Hochhaus G. Methods used to assess pulmonary deposition and absorption of drugs. Drug Discov Today 2001; 6:367–375.

74. Steimer A, Haltner E, Lehr CM. Cell culture models of the respiratory tract relevant to pulmonary drug delivery. J Aerosol Med 2005; 18:137–182.

75. Sakagami M. In vivo, in vitro and ex vivo models to assess pulmonary absorption and disposition of inhaled therapeutics for systemic delivery. Adv Drug Deliv Rev 2006; 58:1030–1060.

76. Foster KA, Oster CG, Mayer MM, et al. Characterization of the A549 cell line as a type II pulmonary epithelial cell model for drug metabolism. Exp Cell Res 1998; 243:359–366.

77. Bruck A, Abu-Dahab R, Borchard G, et al. Lectin-functionalized liposomes for pulmonary drug delivery: interaction with human alveolar epithelial cells. J Drug Target 2001; 9:241.

78. Ehrhardt C, Fiegel J, Fuchs S, et al. Drug absorption by the respiratory mucosa: cell culture models and particulate drug carriers. J Aerosol Med 2002; 15:131–139.

79. Hermanns MI, Unger RE, Kehe K, et al. Lung epithelial cell lines in coculture with human microvascular endothelial cells: development of an alveolo-capillary barrier *in vitro*. Lab Invest 2004; 84:736–752.

80. Foster KA, Avery ML, Yazdanian M, et al. Characterization of the Calu-3 cell line as a tool to screen pulmonary drug delivery. Int J Pharm 2000; 208:1–11.

81. Florea BI, van der Sandt ICJ, Schrier SM, et al. Evidence of p-glycoprotein mediated apical to basolateral transport of flunisolide in human broncho-tracheal epithelial cells (Calu-3). Br J Pharm 2001; 134:1555–1563.

82. Borchard G, Cassara ML, Roemele PE, et al. Transport and local metabolism of budesonide and fluticasone propionate in a human bronchial epithelial cell line (Calu-3). J Pharm Sci 2002; 91:1561–1567.

83. Florea BI, Cassara ML, Junginger HE, et al. Drug transport and metabolism characteristics of the human airway epithelial cell line Calu-3. J Control Release 2003; 87:131–138.

84. Forbes B, Ehrhardt C. Human respiratory epithelial cell culture for drug delivery applications. Eur J Pharm Biopharm 2005; 60:193–205.

85. Grainger CI, Greenwell LL, Lockley DJ, et al. Culture of Calu-3 Cells at the air-water interface provides a representative model of the airway epithelial barrier. Pharm Res 2006; 23:1482–1490.

86. Ehrhardt C, Kneuer C, Bies C, et al. Salbutamol is actively absorbed across human bronchial epithelial cell layers. Pulm Pharmacol Ther 2005; 18:165–170.

87. Ehrhardt C, Kneuer C, Laue M, et al. 16HBE14o-human bronchial epithelial cell layers express P-glycoprotein, lung resistance-related protein, and caveolin-1. Pharm Res 2003; 20:545–551.

88. Manford F, Tronde A, Jeppsson AB, et al. Drug permeability in 16HBE14o-airway cell layers correlates with absorption from the isolated perfused rat lung. Eur J Pharm Sci 2005; 26:414–420.

89. Robinson PC, Voelker DR, Mason RJ. Isolation and culture of human alveolar type-II epithelial cells. Characterization of their phospholipid secretion. Am Rev Respir Dis 1984; 130:1156–1160.

90. Elbert KJ, Shafer UF, Shafers HJ, et al. Monolayers of human alveolar epithelial cells in primary culture for pulmonary absorption and transport studies. Pharm Res 1999; 16:601–608.

91. Fuchs S, Hollins AJ, Laue M, et al. Differentiation of human alveolar epithelial cells in primary culture: morphological characterization and synthesis of caveolin-1 and surfactant protein-C. Cell Tissue Res 2003; 311:31–45.

92. Bur M, Huwer H, Lehr CM, et al. Assessment of transport rates of proteins and peptides across primary human alveolar epithelial cell monolayers. Eur J Pharm Sci 2006; 28:196–203.

93. Lin HC, Li H, Cho HJ, et al. Air-liquid interface (ALI) culture of human bronchial epithelial cell monolayers as an *in vitro* model for airway drug transport studies. J Pharm Sci 2007; 96:341–350.

94. Rothen-Rutishauser BM, Kiama SG, Gehr P. A three-dimensional cellular model of the human respiratory tract to study the interaction with particles. Am J Respir Cell Mol Biol 2005; 32:281–289.

95. U.S. Department of Health and Human Services, Food and Drug Administration, Center for Drug Evaluation and Research. Guidance for Industry: Nasal Spray and Inhalation Solution, Suspension, and Spray Drug Products-Chemistry, Manufacturing, and Controls Documentation. Washington, D.C.: U.S. FDA, CDR, 2002:45.

96. U.S. Food and Drug Administration. Draft Guidance for Industry–Metered Dose Inhaler (MDI) and Dry Powder Inhaler (DPI) Drug Products Chemistry, Manufacturing, and Controls Documentation. Washington, D.C.: FDA, 1998.

97. European Pharmacopeia. Preparations for Inhalation. European Pharmacopeia, 2001.

98. Evans R. Determination of drug particle size and morphology using optical microscopy. Pharm Technol 1993; 17:146–152.

99. Milosovich SM. Particle-size determination via cascade impaction. Pharm Technol 1992; 16:82–86.

100. Atkins PJ. Aerodynamic particle-size testing–impinger methods. Pharm Technol 1992; 16:26–32.

101. Jager PD, DeStefano GA, McNamara DP. Particle-size measurement using right-angle light scattering. Pharm Technol 1993; 17:102–120.

102. Ranucci JA, Chen F-C. Phase Doppler anemometry: a technique for determining aerosol plume-particle size and velocity. Pharm Technol 1993; 17:62–74.

103. Ranucci J. Dynamic plume-particle size analysis using laser diffraction. Pharm Technol 1992; 16:109–114.

104. Niven RW. Aerodynamic particle size testing using a time-of-flight aerosol beam spectrometer. Pharm Technol 1993; 72–78.

105. Gorman WG, Carroll FA. Aerosol particle-size determination using laser holography. Pharm Technol 1993; 17:34–37.

106. Hickey AJ, Evans RM. Aerosol generation from propellant-driven metered dose inhalers. In: Hickey AJ, ed. Inhalation Aerosols: Physical and Biological Basis for Therapy. New York: Marcel Dekker, Inc., 1996:417–439.

107. Dunbar CA, Hickey AJ. Selected parameters affecting characterization of nebulized aqueous solutions by inertial impaction and comparison with phase-Doppler analysis. Eur J Pharm Biopharm 1999; 48:171–177.

108. Leong BKJ, ed. Inhalation Toxicology and Technology. Ann Arbor: Ann Arbor Science, 1981.

109. Concessio NM, Oort MMV, Knowles M, et al. Pharmaceutical dry powder aerosols: correlation of powder properties with dose delivery and implications for pharmacodynamic effect. Pharm Res 1999; 16:828–834.

110. Newman S, Wilding IR, Hirst P. Human lung deposition data: the bridge between in vitro and clinical evaluations for inhaled drug products? Int J Pharm 2000; 208:49–60.

111. Meyer T, Brand P, Ehlich H, et al. Deposition of Foradil P in human lungs: comparison of in vitro and in vivo data. J Aerosol Med Deposition Clear Eff Lung 2004; 17:43–49.

112. Bondesson E, Asking L, Borgstrom L, et al. In vitro and in vivo aspects of quantifying intrapulmonary deposition of a dry powder radioaerosol. Int J Pharm 2002; 232:149–156.

113. Sebti T, Pilcer G, Van Gansbeke B, et al. Pharmacoscintigraphic evaluation of lipid dry powder budesonide formulations for inhalation. Eur J Pharm Biopharm 2006; 64:26–32.

114. Eberl S, Chan HK, Daviskas E. SPECT imaging for radioaerosol deposition and clearance studies. J Aerosol Med Deposition Clear Eff Lung 2006; 19:8–20.

115. Dolovich M. Lung dose, distribution, and clinical response to therapeutic aerosols. Aerosol Sci Technol 1993; 18:230–240.

116. Vidgren M, Arppe J, Vidgren P, et al. Pulmonary deposition and clinical response of 99mTc-labelled salbutamol particles in healthy volunteers after inhalation from a metered-dose inhaler and from a novel multiple-dose powder inhaler. Pharm Res 1994; 11:1320–1324.

117. Vidgren M, Waldrep JC, Arppe J, et al. Study of 99mTechnetium-labeled beclomethasone dipropionate dilauroylphosphatidylcholine liposome aerosol in normal volunteers. Int J Pharm 1995; 115:209–216.

118. Vidgren MT, Karkkainen A, Paronen P, et al. Respiratory tract deposition of 99mTc-labelled drug particles administered via a dry powder inhaler. Int J Pharm 1987; 39:101–105.

119. Vidgren M, Arppe J, Vidgren P, et al. Pulmonary deposition of 99mTc-labelled salbutamol particles in healthy volunteers after inhalation from a metered-dose inhaler and from a novel multiple-dose powder inhaler. STP Pharm Sci 1994; 4:29–32.

120. Pitcairn GR, Hooper G, Luria X, et al. A scintigraphic study to evaluate the deposition patterns of a novel anti-asthma drug inhaled from the Cyclohaler dry powder inhaler. Adv Drug Deliv Rev 1997; 26:59–67.

121. Pitcairn GR, Lim J, Hollingworth A, et al. Scintigraphic assessment of drug delivery from the ultrahaler dry powder inhaler. J Aerosol Med 1997; 10:295–306.

122. Newman SP, Pitcairn GR, Hirst PH, et al. Scintigraphic comparison of budesonide deposition from two dry powder inhalers. Eur Respir J 2000; 16:178–183.

123. Newman SP, Pitcairn GR, Hirst PH, et al. Radionuclide imaging technologies and their use in evaluating asthma drug deposition in the lungs. Adv Drug Deliv Rev 2003; 55:851–867.

124. Kaliner MA, Barnes PJ, Persson CGA. Asthma, Its Pathology and Treatment. New York: Marcel Dekker, 1991.

125. Adjei A, Garren J. Pulmonary delivery of peptide drugs: effect of particle size on bioavailability of leuprolide acetate in healthy male volunteers. Pharm Res 1990; 7:565–569.

126. Patton JS, Bukar J, Nagarajan S. Inhaled insulin. Adv Drug Deliv Rev 1999; 35:235–247.

127. White S, Bennett DB, Cheu S, et al. EXUBERA: pharmaceutical development of a novel product for pulmonary delivery of insulin. Diabetes Technol Ther 2005; 7:896–906.

128. NDA 21-868/Exubera US Package Insert. New York, NY: Pfizer Labs, 2006:1–24.

129. Byron PR, Patton JS. Drug delivery via the respiratory tract. J Aerosol Med 1994; 7:49–75.

130. Patton JS, Byron PR. Inhaling medicines: delivering drugs to the body through the lungs. Nat Rev Drug Discov 2007; 6:67–74.

6

Pediatric and Geriatric Pharmaceutics and Formulation

Jörg Breitkreutz
Institute of Pharmaceutics and Biopharmaceutics, Heinrich-Heine University, Düsseldorf, Germany

Catherine Tuleu
Department of Pharmaceutics and Centre for Paediatric Pharmacy Research, The School of Pharmacy, University of London, London, U.K.

INTRODUCTION

Age-appropriate drug formulations are a challenge in drug development. A critical review of available drugs shows that a number of marketed products cannot be easily used for pediatric or geriatric patients who differ in many aspects from the "adult standard patient" (1). It is well known that the human body undergoes fundamental changes from birth to death. In childhood the maturation of organs and consciousness is the predominant factor that influences drug therapy. In the advanced life the diminution of organs' capacity and functions and additionally the reduced cognitive abilities of some elderly limit the effective and safe treatment with drugs. Although the pediatric and geriatric subpopulations show fundamental differences to be considered, there are a number of similarities not only concerning the drug delivery, the devices, and the drug formulations but also special demands of the patients. Recent technological developments are promising. The present chapter includes well-established methods and future trends for drug delivery to both subpopulations.

Definition of Pediatric Age Groups

The rapid physical maturation that occurs between birth and adulthood is well known. Logically, it would be anticipated that these changes would result in altered responses to

Adapted from
Michele Danish
St. Joseph Health Services, Providence, Rhode Island

Mary Kathryn Kottke
Cubist Pharmaceuticals, Inc., Lexington, Massachusetts

Table 1 Classification by Age of the Pediatric Population

Age group	FDA classification	ICH classification
Intrauterine	Conception to birth	
Preterm newborn infants		<37 wk of gestational age
Neonate or term newborn infant	Birth to 1 mo	0–27 day
Infant and toddlers	1 mo–2 yr	28 day–23 mo
Children	2 yr to onset of puberty	2–11 yr
Adolescent	Onset of puberty to adult	12–16 or 18 yr (depending on regions)

xenobiotics. Within the first five years of life 95% of children have been prescribed medications. Yet only few new molecular entities that have potential usefulness in pediatric patients have pediatric labeling at the time of approval.

In its continuing effort to improve the safety and efficacy of drugs in the pediatric population, the U.S. Food and Drug Administration (FDA) has defined five subgroups of this population based on age. Each subgroup is not homogeneous but does contain similar characteristics that are considered milestones in drug safety development. The International Conference of Harmonization (ICH) approach uses similar age groups in relation to developmental stages in children (ICH Topic E11 Clinical Investigation of Medicinal Products in the Paediatric Population). The FDA and ICH classifications are listed in Table 1.

Age classifications do not provide an all-inclusive method for establishing pediatric doses because it assumes that the body weight is appropriate for the child's age and do not take into account developmental differences, disease state, etc. On the basis of current knowledge, the most accurate pediatric doses are determined utilizing both age and weight. Most formulary will normalize children doses by body weight; occasionally body surface area (calculated from height and weight in square meter) is used as it correlates better with many physiological phenomena. It should be reserved for potent drugs as it limits the risk of overdosing. Apart from very young infants who show dramatic age-related differences in drug disposition, allometric scaling can also be used. In this dosing system, clearance and volume of distribution are scaled to body weight, which relates morphology and physiological function to body size (2).

The classification listed in Table 1 will be utilized throughout this chapter. Caution must be exercised when referring to observations in the neonatal period, however, since premature and/or very low birth weight neonates often have drug responses and disposition significantly different from those of full-term neonates. These differences will be clearly identified in the text.

Definitions of Elderly

Although there are commonly used definitions of "old age", there is no general agreement on the age at which a person becomes old. Most developed world countries have fixed the age of 65 years as a definition of "elderly" or older persons. Conventionally, the subgroups "young old" (65–74 years), "middle old" (75–84 years), and "old old" (>85 years) have been derived (3). This chronological concept obviously does not reflect the health situation in poorly developed countries, for example, in Africa, where the life expectation is quite short. Moreover, in some countries the date of birth is not even known because of lack of birth registers, and, thereby, the age of an individual has to be estimated. The chronological categorization does not reflect the continuous increase of life expectation achieved in the most recent years and most probably continuing in the near future.

While the chronological definition is somewhat arbitrary, the old age is often associated with the retirement from job or profession for an average individual receiving pension benefits. People aged between 18 and 64 years are regarded as the working population, and both the pediatric and geriatric population are distinguished from that age group. Nevertheless there are many people still working beyond 65 years, often in key roles as senior manager or consultant. At the moment, there is no accepted international numerical criterion for this age, but the United Nations agreed a cutoff of 60 years to refer to the older population as per the definition of an older or elderly person given by the World Health Organization. Again, this classification is mainly attributed to the developed countries in the world where the job or profession determines the personal income and the social status. In contrast, in many parts of the developing world time has little or no importance for the type of income of an individual (4). Elderly often own the highest social status in the community like tribal elders or medicine men.

From a medicinal point of view the aging process, however, is a dynamic process that is mostly beyond human control. The human body undergoes various changes and develops different illnesses causing reduced capabilities. Many geriatric patients suffer from various diseases with multiple-drug treatment. Some of these patients are addicted to alcohol, nicotine, and pharmaceuticals. Reduced kidney and liver functions as well as dehydration may dramatically alter the pharmacokinetic (PK) parameters. Limited audiovisual and ergonomic abilities must be considered. In rare diseases like progeria (Hutchinson–Gilford syndrome) a child may look, feel, and be realized as an elderly person. Considering all the different factors, it is very difficult to define a general cutoff for aging (Table 2). The "Clinical Assessment Scales for the Elderly (CASE^{TM})" have been developed mainly for typical mental disorders in the geriatric population like cognitive competence, fear of aging, obsessive compulsiveness, and others. The test allows assessing patients from 55 to 90 years. In the developing countries, patients from 50 years and more are often recruited for clinical studies in the geriatric population (5). An interesting approach is to use a "functional age" that is independent from chronological and socioeconomic scales (6,7), but so far no functional age scale has been adopted as a general approach (8). The variables in the different diseases are too complex for a single scale.

THE PEDIATRIC POPULATION

The Effects of Maturational Changes on Drug Disposition

Traditionally, drug dosing in infants and children has been based on age or weight ratio reduction of the adult dose. Data compiled in the past 40 years on maturational changes in

Table 2 Mostly Accepted Classifications for Defining Elder Subpopulations

Criterion	Method	Cutoff
Time	Chronological	65 yr (65–74 yr: young old, 75–84 yr: middle old, >85 yr: old old)
Social role	Socioeconomic	60 yr
Capabilities	Biological, medicinal	50–55 yr

organ function have allowed gaining a much greater appreciation of the differences in drug disposition in pediatrics when compared with adults. Numerous recent review articles have addressed in detail clinical PK in infants and children (2,9–11).

In this chapter some changes that are pertinent in the development of pediatric dosage forms will be highlighted.

Absorption

Age affects the capacity of all the physiological functions of the gastrointestinal (GI) tract (gastric acidity, gastric emptying, intestinal motility, activity of GI enzymes, biliary function, surface area, and maturation of the mucosal membrane), which can affect the rate and extent of absorption of drugs depending on the physicochemical properties of the drug and its dosage form. Except for the first hours or days, neonates have neutral gastric pH, which slowly falls to reach adult values. Acid output on a kilogram basis is similar to adult levels by age 24 months (12). Premature babies have little or no free acid during the first fortnight of life (2). Enteral feedings influence gastric acid secretion (13). This suggests that hospitalized neonates receiving only parenteral nutrition will be relatively achlorhydric. This hypothesis is supported by reports of increased absorption of acid-labile drugs in the newborn period (14).

Gastric-emptying time and intestinal transit time are reduced and erratic in neonates. Gastric-emptying time is influenced by gestational and postnatal age and the type and frequency of feeding (15). Although there is some controversy over the postnatal age at which adult patterns are attained, it is generally accepted that the rate at which most drugs are absorbed may be expected to be slower in neonates and young infants and that adult values are reached by ages six to eight months. There have been reports of erratic absorption of sustained-release products in children up to age six years (16), but the possible role of gastric emptying on this clinical finding is unknown.

Pancreatic enzyme activity is very low in premature neonates. Lipase activity increases 10-fold in the first nine months of life, whereas amylase activity increases 200-fold. Since concentration of bile salts is also low in neonate and infants, it is anticipated that lipid-soluble vitamins and drugs would be poorly absorbed in early infancy (9).

The first-pass effect has not been extensively evaluated in infants and children. The maturational rate of metabolic pathways would be directly related to the oral bioavailability of a drug subject to first-pass effect. Drugs that undergo glucuronidation during enterohepatic recirculation may have altered systemic availability in children up to approximately age three years because of delayed maturation of conjugation.

Colonization and metabolic activity of GI bacterial flora do not approach adult values until ages two to four years (17). This has resulted in increased bioavailability of digoxin in infants and young children (18). The absorption of vitamin K depends, to some extent, on the development of intestinal flora as it synthesizes large amounts of menaquinones, which are potentially available as a source of vitamin K.

Drugs absorbed by active transport mechanisms appear to have a delayed rate, but not extent of absorption, in the neonatal period (17). Drug absorption is highly variable and unpredictable in neonates and infants (19,20). Older children appear to have absorption patterns similar to adults unless chronic illness or surgical procedures alter absorption. Differences in bile excretion, bowel length, and surface area probably contribute to the reduced bioavailability of cyclosporine seen in pediatric liver transplant patients (21). Impaired absorption has also been observed in severely malnourished children (22). A rapid GI transit time may contribute to the malabsorption of carbamazepine tablets, which has been reported in a child (23).

Distribution

Significant changes occur in amount of body water, fat, and protein from the neonatal period through adulthood (24). The most rapid changes of relative percentage of total body water and extracellular water occur in early life (25,26), with values decreasing to approach adult levels by age 12 years (24). Water-soluble substances such as aminoglycosides will then have a greater volume of distribution and would require a larger dose in neonates; inversely a decrease in volume of distribution could be expected from a lipid-soluble drug such as diazepam (27). Adult levels of total body water and fat content are reached in adolescence (24). Plasma protein binding is altered in neonates and young infant due to a decrease of total protein, albumin, and α-1 acid glycoprotein and the presence of fetal albumin and competing substances such as bilirubin, resulting in relatively high levels of circulating free drug (26). This is especially important for highly bound drugs (e.g., phenytoin, phenobarbital, furosemide), which may require a lower total plasma concentration to achieve therapeutic effects. Malnourished children, who represent 40% of the pediatric population living in developing countries, have significantly reduced concentrations of albumin and α-1 acid glycoprotein (22).

As the blood-brain barrier (BBB) is less formed in neonate, the drug is more likely to penetrate the central nervous system (CNS).

Metabolism

The most noticeable changes occur in the first year of life and again at puberty. Parental exposure to inducing agents, nutritional status, and hormonal changes all play a role in metabolic activity. An added consideration is the fact that neonates requiring medications are often subject to other medical and surgical interventions that may influence drug disposition by liver (28). The underlying genetic pattern of enzymatic activity must also be considered in the assessment of dose-related effects (29).

In general, phase I reactions, such as oxidation and *n*-demethylation, are delayed in the neonate but mature after birth and are fully operational at or above adult levels by age six months in the full-term neonate (29–32). Cytochrome P450 (CYP) enzymes are mainly responsible for phase I reactions. Apart from CYP3A, which is already abundant in fetuses, all other CYPs develop postnatally in an enzyme-dependent fashion (9).

Phase II reactions or conjugation pathways, such as glucuronidation, do not approach adult values until ages three or four years, but there is no consistent pattern of expression. Sulfation activity does appear to reach adult levels in early infancy. For drugs that are subject to metabolism by both pathways, such as acetaminophen, the efficient activity of the sulfation pathway allows infants and children to compensate for low glucuronidation ability (33). Other compounds in which sulfation (e.g., chloramphenicol) is not an alternative pathway are subject to prolonged elimination half-lives and potential toxicity (34).

Infants and children older than one year are considered to be very efficient metabolizers of drugs and may actually require larger doses than those predicted by weight adjustment of adult doses or shorter dosing intervals (35). On the basis of metabolic activity, sustained-release formulations would appear to be ideal for children of 1 to 10 years if bioavailability issues would prove not to be problematic. The ability to clear drugs in critically ill children may be severely compromised; therefore, dosing in this subgroup of patients requires careful titration (36).

Metabolic activity declines with the onset of adolescence. After puberty, adolescents metabolize drugs at a rate similar to adults (29,37). Nevertheless, recent studies have shown that puberty, genetic polymorphism, and disease states such as cystic fibrosis also influence expression of CYP enzymes.

Renal Excretion

The renal excretion of drugs depends on glomerular filtration rate (GFR), tubular secretion, and tubular absorption. GFR is linked to the renal blood flow, which increases with age to reach adults' values at age six months. In preterm, GRF may be as low as 0.6 to 0.8 mL/min/1.73 m^2, but 2 to 4 mL/min/1.73 m^2 in term neonates (11). A twofold increase in GFR occurs in the first 14 days of life (38). The GFR continues to increase rapidly in the neonatal period and reaches a rate of about 86 mL/min/1.73 m^2 by age three months. Children aged 3 to 13 years showed an average clearance of 134 mL/min/1.73 m^2 (39). It is assumed that GFR reaches adult levels by age six months in most full-term infants (9). Tubular secretion matures at a slower rate (1 year) than glomerular function, and there is more variability observed in maturation of tubular reabsorption capacity. This is likely linked to fluctuations in lower urinary pH in the neonatal period (40).

These physiological differences lead to longer half-life in renally cleared drugs in neonates.

Summary

Differences exist in physiology and diseases, which may affect PK/pharmacodynamics (PD) in children (41). These differences are often associated with developmental growth and maturation processes. It is evident from the foregoing discussion that the greatest effects of maturation on drug disposition are observed in the first six months of life. However, individual variation in maturation in the first three years necessitates individual monitoring in the ill neonate, the infant, and the young child. Pediatric formulations that readily provide flexible doses would greatly facilitate dosing in this age group.

Drug Delivery System and Compliance Issues

Inactive Ingredients

Hundreds of excipients have been approved by FDA for use as "inactive ingredients" in drug products. The FDA Division of Drug Information Resources compiles a list of all inactive ingredients in approved prescription drug products in the *Inactive Ingredient Guide* (available at: http://www.fda.gov/cder/drug/iig/default.htm). The FDA requires the listing of excipients in pharmaceuticals other than oral. The labeling of inactive ingredients in oral drug products is voluntary. The reported incidence of adverse drug reactions to excipients is much lower than the incidence reported with active drug. This may be due to several factors, including the generally safe nature of the excipients, the low concentration found in single doses, or lack of identification of an excipient as a causative agent.

Selecting excipients for incorporation into a drug product for human consumption is complex. In selecting excipients for drug products intended for use in the pediatric population, additional cautions must be taken. Several subgroups of the pediatric population who are likely to be hospitalized and receive both oral and parenteral drug products have been identified as being particularly susceptible to excipient reactions. Serious events have been reported in low birth weight neonates and infants, asthmatics, and diabetics. Reactions have ranged from dermatitis to seizures and death (42–46). Table 3 lists some of the excipients that have been reported to cause adverse events in the pediatric and geriatric population.

Many of these reactions are related to the quantity of excipient found in a dosage form in relation to acute toxicity and repeated cumulative exposure in relation to chronic toxicity. Benzyl alcohol benzalkonium chloride, propylene glycol, lactose, and polysorbates are all associated with dose-related toxic reactions (44,45,47). Large-volume parenterals containing 1.5% benzyl alcohol as a preservative have caused

Table 3 Excipients with Elevated Toxicological Risk for Subpopulations of the Pediatric and Geriatric Patients

Excipient	Administration	Adverse reaction
Preterm and term neonates, infants < 6 mo		
Benzyl alcohol	Oral, parenteral	Neurotoxicity, metabolic acidosis
Ethanol	Oral, parenteral	Neurotoxicity
Polyethylene glycol	Parenteral	Metabolic acidosis
Polysorbate 20 and 80	Parenteral	Liver and kidney failure
Propylene glycol	Oral, parenteral	Seizures, neurotoxicity, hyperosmolarity
Patients with reduced kidney function		
Aluminium salts	Oral, parenteral	Encephalopathy, microcytic anemia, osteodystrophy
Polyethylene glycol	Parenteral	Metabolic acidosis
Propylene glycol	Oral, parenteral	Neurotoxicity, hyperosmolarity
Hypersensitive patients		
Azo dyes	Oral	Urticaria, bronchoconstriction, angioedema
Benzalkonium chloride	Oral, nasal, ocular	Bronchoconstriction
Chlorocresol	Parenteral	Anaphylactic reactions
Dextran	Parenteral	Anaphylactic reactions
Macrogolglycerol-ricinoleate (Cremophor EL)	Parenteral	Anaphylactic reactions
Parabens	Oral, parenteral, ocular, topical	Allergies, contact dermatitis
Sorbic acid	Topical	Contact dermatitis (rarely)
Starches	Oral	Gluten-induced celiac disease
Sulfites, bisulfites	Oral, parenteral	Asthma attacks, rashes, abdominal upset
Wool wax	Topical	Contact dermatitis, urticaria
Patients with metabolic disorders		
Aspartame	Oral	Phenylketonuria
Fructose	Oral, parenteral	Hereditary fructose intolerance
Lactose	Oral	Lactose intolerance, diarrhea
Sorbitol	Oral	Hereditary fructose intolerance
Sucrose	Oral, parenteral	Hereditary fructose intolerance

Source: From Ref. 1.

metabolic acidosis, cardiovascular collapse, and death in low birth weight premature neonates and infants. The cumulative dose of benzyl alcohol ranged from 99 to 234 mg/kg/day in these patients (48,49). Dose-related adverse effects to excipients are of particular concern in the preterm, low birth weight infant because of the known immaturity of hepatic and renal function in this population. Dose-related reversible CNS effects have also been reported in children receiving long-term therapy in which propylene glycol was a cosolvent (50).

Dyes Dose does not appear to be a factor in patient reaction to dyes. The mandatory labeling of the azo dye tartrazine (FD&C Yellow No. 5) in over-the-counter (OTC) and prescription medications (51) has focused the attention of pharmaceutical manufacturers and the consumer on the potential danger of dyes in susceptible individuals. Hypersensitivity reactions have been reported with several azo dyes, particularly FD&C Yellow No. 5 and No. 6. Tartrazine-induced bronchoconstriction is commonly considered a cross-reaction to aspirin in sensitive asthmatics, although urticaria has been reported in other patient populations (52). In a double-blind challenge involving aspirin-sensitive asthmatics, hypersensitivity to dyes was only 2% (53); however, numerous case reports involving azo dyes suggest caution when using a drug containing an azo dye in asthmatics (54). Non-azo dyes are considered to be weak sensitizers.

In a recent study (55), two combinations of Tartrazine (E102), Quinoline Yellow (E104), Sunset Yellow FCF (E110), Ponceau 4R (E124), Allura Red AC (E129), Carmoisine (E122), and the preservative, sodium benzoate (E211), contained in drinks, were studied on the behavior of 153 three-year old and 144 eight- to nine-year old children. (All synthetic azo dyes except for Quinoline Yellow (E104), which is a quinophthalone.) In 2008, The European Food Safety Agency reported that the study carried considerable uncertainties, such as the lack of consistency and relative weakness of the effect and the absence of information on the clinical significance of the behavioral changes observed. The association of dye content (especially in medicines) with hyperactivity in children remains controversial and unproved.

Sweeteners Sweeteners are commonly included in pediatric formulations to increase palatability.

Sucrose is the most popular sweetener due to its combination of sweetness, solubility, viscosity-enhancing, texture, and preservation properties. Chewable tablets may contain 20% to 60% sucrose, and liquid preparations may contain up to 85% sucrose. In a survey of sweetener content of 107 pediatric antibiotic liquid preparations in 1988, only 4 were sucrose free (56). Nevertheless sugar-free formulations have been largely promoted and are more readily available these days. In a recent review (57), only 14 of the 32 pediatric oral liquids (e.g., solutions, suspensions, or syrups) commercially available in the United States were not sugar free, although five of the eight syrups did contained sucrose. The sucrose content of oral liquids may cause significant problems when these products are prescribed for long-term therapy (e.g., asthma, seizure control, recurrent infections). Oral liquid preparations can represent a substantial carbohydrate load to children with labile diabetes, particularly if a child is ingesting more than one liquid medication with a high sugar content or/and have a parallel poor controlled diet. Nevertheless a wider problem exists with the possible role of these liquid medications in dental caries formation (58). The extent of acid production from sucrose by the buccal bacteria in the oral cavity is closely related to caries formation. In a study of liquid medication, investigators have observed that medications with sucrose concentrations higher than 15% were able to significantly lower pH; there was an inverse relation between sucrose content and a decrease in oral cavity pH (59). In a comparison of sorbitol and sucrose-sweetened liquid iron preparations, only sucrose-containing products produced a significant decrease in oral cavity pH (60). Viscous formulations with high sucrose content are especially prone to contribute to caries formation because of their prolonged contact time in the oral cavity. This can be improved by rinsing the mouth after intake of such formulations.

To achieve sugar-free preparations, polyols (sugar alcohol) are replacing sucrose as bulk sugar substitutes. They are not fermented by oral bacteria, hence noncariogenic. However, they are slowly hydrolyzed by the enzymes of the small intestine into their constituent monomers, which are only slowly and incompletely absorbed compared with

Table 4 A Brief Summary of the Characteristics of Common Polyols

Polyols	E number	Carbons	MW	Solubility in water at 25°C (% w/w)	Relative sweetness	Digestive tolerance (g/kg)[a]	Caloric value (kcal/g)
Mannitol	E421	4	182	22	0.5	0.3	1.6
Erythritol	E968	4	122	37	0.6–0.7	0.73	0.2
Sorbitol	E420	4	182	235	0.6	0.205	2.6
Xylitol	E967	5	152	200	1	0.3	2.4
Maltitol	E965	12	344	175	0.8–0.9	0.3	2.1
Isomalt	E953	12	344	28	0.5–0.6	0.3	2
Sucrose		12	342	211.5	1	–	4

[a]Maximum bolus dose not causing laxation—data for adults.
All the polyols presented are considered as food additive or GRAS in the United States.
Source: Adapted from Ref. 61.

glucose and thus provide less energy per unit mass to the consumer and have lower glycemic and insulinemic indices. Sugar alcohols reaching the large intestine are almost completely digested by the colonic flora, which can cause certain side effects as fermentation of unabsorbed sugar leads to flatulence. In addition, as they are osmotically active, diarrhea may occur when the fermentation capacity is exceeded. Their main characteristics are resumed in Table 4, adapted from (61). In a survey of 129 oral liquid dosage forms stocked at a large university teaching hospital, 42% contained sorbitol (62). The sorbitol concentration in the identified products varied from 3.5% to 72% w/v (0.175–3.6 g/mL). In a recent review of pediatric oral formulations commercially available in the United States, 44% of the liquids contained sorbitol (57). The other polyols found were xylitol, mannitol, maltitol, and, in many, glycerol.

Artificial or intense sweeteners are often used not only to restrict the sugar intake in food and beverages but also to boost the degree of sweetness to mask bitter notes. Only few are approved for use in over 80 countries (e.g., saccharin, aspartame, sucralose, and acesulfame potassium). There is some ongoing controversy over whether artificial sweeteners are health risks despite lack of scientifically controlled peer-reviewed studies in general consistently to produce clear evidence. It is to be noted that if an acceptable daily intake (ADI) value is available, most of the time it is for a general adult population and not specifically for pediatric and geriatric population.

Both solid and liquid dosage forms may contain saccharin. Saccharin (E954) is a nonnutritive sweetening agent, which is 250 to 500 times as sweet as sucrose. In a survey of sweetener content of pediatric medications, seven of nine chewable tablets contained saccharin (0.45–8.0 mg/tablet) and sucrose or mannitol. Of 150 liquid preparations investigated, 74 contained saccharin (1.25–33 mg/5 mL) (56). Saccharin is a sulfanamide derivative that should be avoided in children with sulfa allergies (47). It is recommended that daily saccharin intake be maintained below 1 g because of a risk of bladder cancer. A lifetime daily diet containing 5% to 7.5% saccharin has induced bladder tumors in rats (63). However, it is probable that saccharin is only a very weak carcinogen in humans. The amount contained in pharmaceutical preparations is well below the recommended maximum human daily intake. It is not approved in Canada but is in the United States and in Europe, only for children older than three years. It was found in combination or alone in 10 of the 12 commercially available liquids containing intense sweeteners in a recent American review of the commercially available pediatric dosage forms (57).

Aspartame (E951), a phenylalanine derivative, is incorporated in many chewable tablets and sugar-free dosage forms. Aspartame-containing products should be avoided in children with autosomal recessive phenylketonuria (47). Neotame is a derivative of aspartame but is 7000 to 13,000 times sweeter than sucrose, with greater stability at higher and neutral pH as well as higher temperatures than aspartame. It has a clean sweet taste (no off-tastes) and is not metabolized into phenylalanine. It is generally recognized as safe (GRAS) listed and approved as a food in over 25 countries but is not yet widely used.

Acesulfam K (E950) is an oxathiazinone sweetener; it is widely used, as it is stable during typical manufacturing and storage conditions of many pharmaceutical dosage forms. It can be used on its own (~200 times sweeter than sucrose) but has interesting synergistic properties with other intense sweeteners as well as bulk sweeteners such as sugar alcohols. It is similar to sucralose (E955), which is the only intense sweetener made from sugar (chlorination). It is approximately 600 times sweeter than sugar, with a clean sugar-like taste with just a sweet aftertaste. Presently 1 of 32 oral liquid formulations on the American market contains sucralose (57).

Vehicle Selection

Ethanol has long been employed as a solvent in pharmaceuticals and is still prevalent; in a recent survey in America, it was found that 5 of the 32 pediatric liquids commercially available still contain alcohol (57). Since it also acts as a preservative, it is second only to water in its use in liquid preparations. It has also been suggested that it may enhance the oral absorption of some active ingredients (64).

There are severe acute and chronic concerns around pediatric medicines containing ethanol. Hepatic metabolism of ethanol involves a nonlinear saturable pathway. Young children have a limited ability to metabolize and thereby detoxify ethanol. Ethanol intoxication has been recorded in children with blood levels as low as 25 mg/dL. Alcohol has a volume of distribution of approximately 0.65 L/kg. Ingestion of 20 mL of a 10% alcohol solution will produce a blood level of 25 mg/dL in a 30-lb. child. The American Academy of Pediatrics (AAP) Committee on Drugs recommends that pharmaceutical formulations intended for use in children should not produce ethanol blood levels of >25 mg/dL after a single dose. In general, manufacturers have voluntarily complied with the recommendations. In 1992 the Nonprescription Drug Manufacturers Association established voluntary limits for alcohol content of nonprescription products (65).

1. A maximum of 10% alcohol in products for adults and teens, 12 years and older
2. A maximum of 5% alcohol in products intended for children aged 6 to 12 years
3. Less than 0.5% alcohol content for products intended for children less than 6 years

Extemporaneous production of pediatric dosage forms is commonly undertaken in hospitals. Without the sophisticated formulation capabilities of pharmaceutical manufacturers, alcohol-based vehicles have been recommended for extemporaneous preparation of liquid dosage forms (66). There is a critical need to conduct research studies to assist the pharmacist in replacing current formulations with stable, alcohol-free preparations.

Propylene glycol is used as solvents in many formulations (e.g., oral, topical, and parenteral routes) for poorly soluble compounds such as phenobarbital, phenytoin, diazepam, and multivitamin concentrates. Because of the limited metabolic pathways in children younger than four years, number of adverse events has been described (laxative effects per os, contact dermatitis) but mainly serious systemic CNS depression. Seven of the thirty-two liquids (solution, suspension, syrup) commercially available for children in America contained propylene glycol (57).

Administration Considerations in Dosage Form Development

Limited evidence-based information around acceptability and preference of dosage forms in children are available, despite the fact that the therapeutic outcomes are closely linked to it (67).

An ideal formulation should suit all subsets of the pediatric population, have minimum administration frequency, be palatable, contain nontoxic excipients, provide easy and accurate dose administration, and have minimal impact on lifestyle (68,69).

Oral administration Oral administration is the preferred route of administration. There is a general consensus among pediatricians and parents that children younger that five years have great difficulty with, or are unable to swallow, a solid oral dosage form. Manufacturers, therefore, tend to favor liquid formulations. It allows dosing flexibility for the heterogenous pediatric population (varying weight, PK/PD, physical abilities, and developmental capacity). Liquid dosage forms, however, are not free of problems. They are often less stable and have shorter expiration dates; accurate measurement depends on device used, and administration of the prescribed dose can also be a problem, especially in infants. Dose volumes are critical, and it is considered that children younger than five years should not receive more than 5 mL and that older children should not be dosed with more than 10 mL. It is evident that the less palatable the drug is, the smaller should this volume be. Appropriate administration devices have to be used (70). They should also be easy to use even with an uncooperative child. To achieve satisfactory dispensing of drops, usually concentrated liquids, carers should hold the dropper vertically (71). Formulating liquids can be more challenging, as they require a greater quantity and type of excipients, which are limited in choice and concentration for pediatric patients (43,72).

To overcome insufficient stability in liquid state, dispersible tablets and effervescent dosage forms provide a "dry" alternative to liquid but are not without inherent issues (large volume of diluent, bicarbonate ingestion, sodium and/or potassium content not suitable for renally impaired patients, difficult taste masking).

In adults, tablets and capsules are the most popular dosage forms because of the accuracy of dose, taste maskability, stability, portability, low-cost production, and modifiable drug delivery release. Nevertheless, their main disadvantage for children is the nonflexibility of dose and the difficulty or inability to be swallowed by the very young. This is frequently often overcome by crushing tablets or opening capsules and adding the powder to water or soft food or beverages despite proof of accurate dose and bioequivalence (73). In some instance the resulting powder is further diluted with powder excipients and repackaged in sachets or capsules for extemporaneous dispensing with few, if any, compatibility/stability consideration.

When tablets are not scored but yet cut to obtain the appropriate dose or to facilitate swallowing, dose accuracy cannot always be ensured: the weight of a split tablet can range from 50% to 150% of the actual half-tablet weight (74). Splitting tablets into segments is not recommended with narrow therapeutic index drugs, potent or cytotoxics drugs, or small tablets. Some tablets (e.g., coated, multilayered, modified release) cannot be manipulated without affecting taste, release properties, and possible therapeutic effects, unless especially stated by the manufacturer (75). A potentially very fruitful area for future research and development is sprinkle multiparticulates formulations as they offer a solution to many of the limitations highlighted above and have been very well received by both patients and their parents. They can be dosed intraorally or in a vehicle the child likes, from a bottle (dosing scoop), or from individual sachets or capsules.

Chewable tablets are considered to be safe for use in children with full dentition (2–3 years) (76–78) and under supervision. Orodispersible preparations in the oral cavity (e.g., tablets, films, wafers) stand also on the periphery of solids and liquids, with the extra challenge that the quantity of excipients available to improve the palatability is limited.

It is to be noted that few studies have been performed to assess age, development, and oral dosage forms of choice (i.e., applicability, acceptability, preference).

Buccal and sublingual administration Oromucosal drug administration is possible, although mainly limited by ability and compliance concerns in the younger age group. It might be difficult in babies due to feeding patterns. Safety needs to be established in children.

Rectal administration The administration of drugs by a solid rectal dosage form (i.e., suppositories) can result in a wide variability in the rate and extent of absorption in children (79). Rectal administration of a drug is not favored by adolescents, carers, and various ethnic groups and can sometime be difficult (premature loss of the dose) in the very young. These facts, coupled with the inflexibility of a dose, make this a route difficult to promote for pediatric patients with chronic conditions. Nevertheless it can be an alternative route if the oral route is not available or local effects or immediate systemic effects (epileptic seizures) are required.

Transdermal administration The development of the stratum corneum is complete at birth but is more perfused and hydrated than in adults. It is considered to have permeability similar to that of adults, except in preterm infants (80). Preterm neonates and infants have an underdeveloped epidermal barrier and are subject to excessive absorption of potentially toxic ingredients from topically applied products. Once matured (3–5 months after birth), infant skin presents less variability, but the ratio of surface area to weight is higher in children, when compared with that of adults.

Only few transdermal products (e.g., steroidal hormone, caffeine, theophylline, fentanyl, scopolamine, nicotine, methylphenidate) have been tested or marketed for use in the pediatric population. The development of transdermal products in pediatric doses could be very beneficial for children who are unable to tolerate oral medications. The need for several sizes of patches to cover different doses needed by different subsets of the pediatric population and to avoid accidents with cutting adult patches can be a limitation. The younger, the better permeation. Hence a compromise between topical versus transdermal efficacy and safety should be sought.

Parenteral administration Absorption of medication following an intramuscular (IM) injection is often erratic in neonates owing to their small muscle mass and an inadequate perfusion of the IM site (81,82). In a study of infants and children aged 28 days to 6 years, the IM administration of chloramphenicol succinate produced serum levels that were not significantly different from those produced in intravenous (IV) administration (83). However, the bioavailability of most drugs administered intramuscularly has not been evaluated in the pediatric population. In addition to bioavailability issues, there are other concerns specific to pediatrics with the IM administration of drugs. The volume of solution injected is directly related to the degree of pain and discomfort associated with an IM injection. Manufacturers' recommendations for reconstitution of IM products often result in a final volume that is excessive for a single injection site in a child's smaller muscle mass, thereby requiring multiple injections and a significant degree of discomfort for the patient. If a smaller volume is used for reconstitution, the problems of drug solubility and high osmotic load at the site of injection must be addressed (84,85). The inclusion of a local anesthetic, such as lidocaine, as part of the reconstituted product is often necessary (84–86).

In a report from the Boston Collaborative Drug Surveillance Program, pediatric nurses have reported a much higher frequency of complications from IM injections than that observed in the adult population. Twenty-three percent of pediatric nurses surveyed had observed complications (e.g., local pain, abscess, hematoma) versus a rate of 0.4% reported in adult patients (87). Serious complications, such as paralysis from infiltration of the sciatic nerve, quadriceps myofibrosis, and accidental intra-arterial injection, are usually the result of the difficulty in placement of an IM injection in children.

In hospital, many patients have a venous cannula, and systemic drugs not given orally are usually given intravenously rather than subcutaneously or intramuscularly.

The major problem with the IV route in children is dosing errors. Because of the unavailability of stock solutions prepared for pediatric doses, errors in dilution of an adult stock solution have resulted in 10- to 20-fold errors in administered doses (88,89). A secondary problem is the maintenance of patient IV lines in infants and nonsedated children.

Intranasal drug delivery This drug delivery provides fast and direct access to systemic circulation without first-pass metabolism. Administration is not easy especially with uncooperative children, but small volumes involved, rapidity of execution, feasibility at home has made it more attractive, particularly for no-needle approach to acute illnesses. Aerosols with an appropriate device can avoid swallowing and is more precise in terms of dose. Drugs such as benzodiazepines, fentanyl, diamorphine, and ketamine have been used successfully via this route (90).

Pulmonary drug delivery Endotracheal drug delivery is a very effective method of administering emergency medications (i.e., epinephrine, atropine, lidocaine, naloxone) to children when an IV line is not available. To optimize drug delivery to the distal portions of the airway, the drug must be administered rapidly, using an adequate volume of diluent: 5 to 10 mL in young children; 10 to 20 mL for adolescents (91).

Pressurized inhalation products have also been very successfully employed in the pediatric population to provide a drug directly to the desired site of action, the lung. These products are designed to deliver a unit dose at high velocity with small particle size, the ideal conditions for drug delivery to distal airways (92). Self-administration is difficult for younger patients without coordination.

The choice of inhalation devices is crucial and is made in relation to age. Pressured metered-dose inhaler (pMDI) can only be used by older children. Environmentally friendly chlorofluorocarbon (CFC)-free formulations, using hydrofluoroalkane (HFA) as the propellant, are now replacing CFCs, except for formulaic exemptions. To decrease oropharyngeal impaction and optimize and widen pMDI utilization, spacers can be used (93). With a face mask, it even enables pMDI for very young infants. Dry-powder inhaler (DPI) is for children with enough inspiratory flow to trigger particles' release and transport the particles deep in the lung. Nebulizers are applicable for all ages but very few are portable yet. Guidance for use of different inhaler types (i.e., nebulizers, pMDI, and DPI) has been established by the Global Initiative on Asthma (GINA), a panel of clinical experts who look at the various inhaler types, their features, and patient experience. Their guidance has been incorporated in national regulatory guidance throughout the world. The most appropriate device should be selected for each child.

- Children younger than four years should use a pMDI plus a spacer with face mask or a nebulizer with face mask.
- Children aged four to six years should use a pMDI plus a spacer with mouthpiece, a DPI, or, if necessary, a nebulizer with face mask.
- For children using spacers, the spacer must fit the inhaler, and attention should be paid to ensure that the spacer fits the child's face.
- Children of any age older than six years who have difficulty using pMDIs should use a pMDI with a spacer, breath-actuated inhaler, DPI, or nebulizer. DPIs require an inspiratory effort that may be difficult to achieve during severe attacks.
- Children having severe attacks should use a pMDI with a spacer or a nebulizer.
- Particularly among children younger than five years, inhaler techniques may be poor and should be monitored closely.

The use of the aerosol route for delivery of antibiotics for pulmonary infections remains controversial. The majority of pediatric studies have been conducted in children with cystic fibrosis. In these patients distribution of the antibiotic to the desired tissue site is impeded because of the viscosity of the sputum in patients with acute exacerbations of their pulmonary infections (94,95). Long-term studies have demonstrated preventive benefits of aerosolized antibiotics in children with cystic fibrosis who are colonizing *Pseudomonas aeruginosa* in their lungs but are not acutely ill (96,97). Cyclic administration of tobramycin administered by nebulizer has received FDA approval (98).

Systemic treatment via the respiratory tract needs further study to determine its usefulness.

Compliance Issues: Taste Preference and Palatability

Compliance and concordance issues have multivariate complex origins but an acceptable taste especially with pediatric patients (99). Two factors make taste preference and palatability critical considerations in pediatric adherence. The dosage forms most commonly employed for pediatric formulations are liquids and chewable tablets. A perceived unpleasant taste is much more evident with these dosage forms than when a drug is administered as a conventional solid oral dosage form. It is widely believed that children younger than six years have more acute taste perception than older children and adults. Taste buds and olfactory receptors are fully developed in early infancy. Different taste acuity and preferences occur between teenagers and infants, as well as between boys and girls (100–102). Loss of taste perception accompanies the aging process. Children's adherence to therapy is affected by their cognitive skills, their acceptability or ability to swallow, and their own taste perception, affected or not by their disease.

Smell, taste, texture, and aftertaste, therefore, are important factors in the development of pediatric dosage forms. In a study of six brands of OTC chewable vitamins, flavor type and intensity, soft texture, and short aftertaste were critical factors in product preference. The flavor and texture attributes of the best-selling product were significantly different from that of the other brands (103).

Flavoring standardization would be an ideal global development of formulation but is complex as it depends on many factors such as the geographical and sociocultural background and the health condition of the target population. There are at least 26 different flavorings used in pediatric antimicrobial preparations (104). In America, cherry is a very common flavoring, although a blind taste comparison found that other flavorings, such as orange, strawberry, and bubble gum, were well accepted in pediatric antimicrobial suspensions (105). In many circumstances it may be difficult to mask the unpleasant taste of the active ingredient. Regardless of the flavoring used, parents consistently report that children prefer cephalosporin products to penicillin suspensions (105).

Future Directions

Effective and safe drug therapy for newborns, infants, and children depends on knowledge of pediatric PK and PD and knowledge of the drug formulation and delivery issues specific to this population.

In the United States, there have been several attempts to stimulate the pharmaceutical industry to generate more data in children. The first successful attempt was the creation of the voluntary Pediatric Exclusivity (PE) within the FDA Modernization Act (FDAMA) 1997, re-authorized as Best Pharmaceuticals for Children Act (BPCA) in 2002. In 1997, PE was accompanied by the Pediatric Rule, which gave the FDA authority to mandate pediatric clinical development in drugs where the authority saw a high clinical need. When the Pediatric Rule was struck down by a U.S. federal court in 2002, both houses of the government rapidly agreed with the new legislation: the Pediatric Research Equity Act (PREA). The rule reestablished the FDA's authority to mandate pediatric drug development. PREA makes a pediatric assessment mandatory at the pre-IND meeting with the FDA. Through the link between PREA and BPCA both reauthorized in September 2007, pharmaceutical companies and the FDA are encouraged to negotiate a pediatric development plan that will at the end of the patent life result in a six-month prolonged exclusivity that protects drugs from generic erosion.

Similarly, a new piece of legislation—Regulation (EC) No. 1901/2006 governing the development and authorization of medicines for use in children aged 0 to 17 years was introduced in the European Union in January 2007. The objectives of the new regulation are to facilitate development and availability of medicines for children aged 0 to 17 years, to ensure that medicines for use in children are of high quality, ethically researched, and authorized appropriately, to improve the availability of information on use of medicines for children, without subjecting children to unnecessary trials or delaying the authorization of medicinal products for use in adults. Paediatric Committee (PDCO) is a new committee at EMEA, and its main responsibility will be to evaluate and agree upon a Paediatric Investigational Plan (PIP) presented by the company. The new regulation includes rewards, incentives, and obligations for both on-patent and off-patent medicines. Pharmaceutical companies are obliged to develop medicines for children. A six-month extension of the market exclusivity is given if studies are performed according to the PIP—no matter whether the studies lead to pediatric indication or not. The results of all the studies have to be submitted prior to a new market authorization for new medicines; if not, PDCO has decided on a deferral or waiver. With a deferral, studies on children are postponed until more knowledge on the use of medicine in adults is collected. With a waiver, studies on children are deemed not necessary because of safety concerns or lack of indication in children.

There has been tremendous progress in the identification of PK and PD parameters in chronically ill infants and children. Nevertheless issues in the acutely ill child deserve further evaluation. The critical void in pediatric drug therapy now lies in effective drug delivery systems. Some inroads have been made in the manufacturing of pediatric dosing systems, particularly OTC preparations. There needs to be a redirection of the focus in nonparenteral drug formulations toward pediatric dosage forms with proven stability and bioavailability that can be easily and accurately administered to infants and children.

THE ELDERLY POPULATION

Diminution of Physical Function and Its Effects on Drug Disposition

Within the medical community it has been acknowledged that elderly patients often respond to drug therapy differently from their younger counterparts. Aside from alteration of various PK and PD processes, elderly patients tend to suffer from a number of diseases and, thus, have more complex dosage regimens. Additionally, a variety of physical limitations prevalent among the elderly may hinder their ability to self-administer medication.

Elderly patients are the primary consumers of drug products today. As the geriatric population is rapidly growing in the developed countries, the impact of the elderly in the medical and pharmaceutical context will increase further. The effect of aging on drug disposition, efficacy, and safety has been rarely investigated in geriatrics. Before discussing the actual changes that occur with aging, four points must be stressed. First, because of wide variation among older individuals, it is very difficult to quantify the extent of changes that occur within this population. Second, most of these changes are related to the fact that, with increasing age, there is an overall decrease in the capacity of homeostatic mechanisms to respond to physiological changes. Moreover, with increasing age most patients suffer from numerous diseases that potentially affect the efficacy and safety of drugs administered for another illness. Physical impairments and the reduced cognitive ability may also affect the compliance of the elder patients.

Pharmacokinetics

During the past decade, numerous articles reviewing the effects of aging on drug delivery and PK processes according to the LADME model (i.e., liberation, absorption, distribution, metabolism, and elimination) have been published (106–123). An outline of the observations made in these reports is supplied in Table 5. The liberation and absorption are the predominant processes that will be covered in depth in this chapter as these can most easily be manipulated through formulation techniques.

Peroral administration/intestinal absorption First of all, there is a decrease in gastric secretion that causes the elevated pH that has been noted in elderly patients (106–126). This condition is commonly referred to as hypochlorhydria or, in severe cases, achlorhydria and may be the result of atrophic gastritis (115,125–127). It may result in drug degradation in the stomach and, hence, incomplete bioavailability. Drugs that are degraded in the acidic environment of the stomach (e.g., penicillin), however, may actually have an increased extent of absorption in elderly patients because less acid is available (107,108,115,125–127).

There appears to be an ongoing dispute over whether or not gastric-emptying rate (GER) and GI motility are affected by the aging process (107,108,116,125,128–134). Most studies tend to suggest that there is, indeed, a decrease in GER as the body ages. As GER is the primary physiological determinant of the rate of absorption of solid oral dosage forms, one can see that a decrease in GER may result in a subsequent decreased rate of absorption, particularly when coupled with the compromised blood flow to the GI track is also noted in elderly patients. Additionally, unpredictable GER has a significant influence on extended-release formulations, as it becomes difficult to predict whether or not acceptable blood levels will be obtained (115). To circumvent the possible problems that may arise from a decrease in GER, a liquid or readily disintegrating formulation may be used. In most instances, this decrease in the rate of absorption does not necessarily

Table 5 Changes in Pharmacokinetic Processes Observed with Aging

Process	Changes	Effects
Liberation	Gastric pH	Drug dissolution, drug stability, mucosal irritation
	Gastric emptying	Drug dissolution, onset of action
	Fluid volume	Drug dissolution, onset of action
Absorption	GI transit time	Onset of action, rate of absorption
	Intestinal blood flow	Rate of absorption
	Intestinal mucosa surface	Rate of absorption
	Active drug carriers	Rate of absorption; drug-drug, drug-excipient, and food-drug interactions
	Efflux pumps	Rate of absorption; drug-drug, drug-excipient, and food-drug interactions
Distribution	Cardiac output	V_d water-soluble drugs
	Water content	V_d water-soluble drugs
	Fat/lean body mass	V_d lipid-soluble drugs
	Serum albumin concentration	V_d protein-bound drugs
Metabolism	Hepatic blood flow	Hepatical extraction and metabolism
	Bile dysfunctions	Capacity of hepatical clearance, impaired enterohepatic circulation
	Liver size	Metabolism, clearance of hepatically extracted molecules
	Liver dysfunction	Metabolism (phases I and II), clearance of hepatically extracted molecules
Elimination	Renal blood flow	Clearance of renally excreted drugs
	GFR	Clearance of renally excreted drugs
	ARTS	Clearance of renally excreted drugs, drug-drug, and drug-excipient interactions
	Renal dysfunction	Clearance of renally excreted drugs, toxicity by increased drug levels

Abbreviations: GER, gastric-emptying rate; V_d, volume of distribution; GFR, glomerular filtration rate; ARTS, active renal tubular secretion; GI, gastrointestinal.

cause a decrease in the extent of absorption. In fact, only those compounds that are actively absorbed (e.g., riboflavin) have a decreased rate of absorption (125,127).

Absorption Within the Oral Cavity

When dealing with oral dosage forms, it is important to study the various changes occurring within the oral cavity, particularly if a buccal or sublingual formulation is being considered (Table 6). Table 6 lists the changes within the oral cavity that have thus far been elucidated (116,126,135–141). It is very important to note that there is a decrease in the capillary blood supply to the oral mucosa. This may make it difficult to predict accurately the absorption rates that will occur when using sublingual and buccal formulations in the elderly age group. Additional changes occurring in and about the oral cavity will be discussed at length later in this chapter.

Percutaneous Absorption

With the increasing acceptance of transdermal formulations by the pharmaceutical industry and the trend toward an aging population that is occurring in our nation, it is vital

Table 6 Changes in and About the Oral Cavity
Observed with Aging

Mucosa	Drier
Muscle	Increase susceptibility to injury
	Decrease capillary blood supply
	Decrease bulk and tone
	Decrease masticatory efficiency
Salivary glands	Decrease resting secretory rate
	Increase viscosity of saliva
	Decrease enzyme activity of saliva
Miscellaneous	Decrease number of taste buds
	Increase dysfunction and cancer

that the effects of aging on percutaneous absorption be evaluated. Elderly patients are one of the main target groups of such drug delivery systems (e.g., with glycerol trinitrate, isosorbidinitrate, testosterone, fentanyl, or buprenorphine as the drug substances). In light of this, it is surprising to find that there have been relatively few studies published that specifically address percutaneous absorption in the elderly (142,143). Table 7 provides an outline of changes in characteristics of the skin that occur with aging (142–145).

Researchers assessing the various factors surrounding percutaneous absorption (e.g., permeation and clearance) have theorized that although there is an increase in the rate of permeation through aging skin, substances that permeate through the skin have a slower rate of removal into the general circulation and, thus, distribution may be incomplete (142,143). Unfortunately there appear to be few published reports addressing this phenomenon. Studies that do specifically evaluate percutaneous absorption in the elderly have used only one compound, testosterone, in their analyses (142,143). Before formulating drugs for transdermal delivery in the elderly, changes in percutaneous absorption that occur on aging should be assessed furthering detail.

Physical Capabilities

Many of the most often diagnosed conditions prevail in the elderly population (137). Many of these conditions severely limit the range of activities that one can perform (Fig. 1) (137,146). Indeed, researchers have studied, in depth, the extent to which age limits one's activities of daily living (ADL) (146–150). Moreover, some of these conditions, such as arthritis and impaired vision, impair the patient's ability to accurately self-administer medication (Table 8).

Table 7 Changes in Skin Characteristics Observed with
Aging

Drier skin
Loss of elasticity
Impaired wound healing
Deletion and derangement of small blood vessels
Increased permeation to water and some chemicals
Decreased clearance into blood stream
Decreased absorption

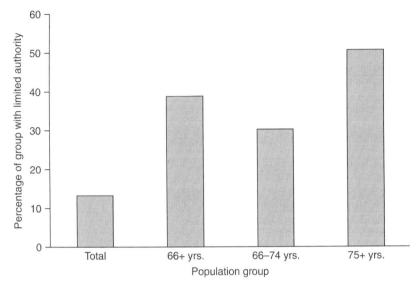

Figure 1 Limitation of activity by chronic conditions: United States, 1997. *Source*: From Ref. 150.

Table 8 Physical Impairments and Conditions with Impact on Drug Delivery

Capability	Disease	Affected formulations/drug handling
Dexterity	Arthritis	Bottle/blister opening
	Parkinson's disease	Tablet splitting
	Frailty	Subcutaneous injections
		Inhalers
		Eye drops
		Sublingual sprays
Vision	Diabetes	Subcutaneous injections
	Macula degeneration	Measuring liquids
	Glaucoma	Read instructions
Hearing	Amblyacousia	Clicking noise (e.g., inhalers, pens)
Swallowing	Dehydration	Tablets
	Mucosa degeneration	Capsules
	Reduced saliva production	
Consciousness	Alzheimer's disease	Medication instructions
	Obliviousness	Differentiate medication
		Time of dosing

Dexterity Dexterity may be impaired in the elderly for a variety of reasons, such as the following: (*i*) Over 43% of the elderly suffer from some form of arthritis (137); (*ii*) Many elderly experience tremors associated with Parkinsonism or other neurological disorders; and (*iii*) Frailty and weakness are prevalent in many elderly patients. The U.S. National Institute on Aging has been conducting a comprehensive study to assess all of the characteristics common among the elderly. This study reveals that at least 13% of the elderly have some difficulty in handling small objects (e.g., tablets) (149). Another government study reports that more than 4% of the elderly experience difficulty preparing their own meals and, therefore, are likely to encounter problems when self-administering

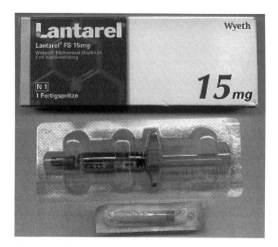

Figure 2 Syringe for single use for patients with reduced dexterity (Wyeth, Collegeville, Pennsylvania, U.S.).

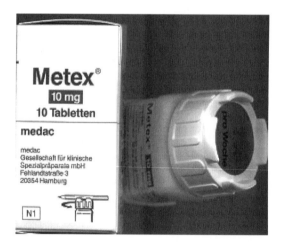

Figure 3 Multiple-dose container with special closure for patients with reduced dexterity (medac, Hamburg, Germany). The patient may apply a pencil, drawing the closure if he is not able to do it manually.

medication (148). Reduced motor capabilities have a direct impact on the drug dosing from numerous devices such as MDIs; powder inhalers; insulin pens; subcutaneous (SC) syringes; eye or nose spray containers, bottles, and tubes. Typical insulin pens need a force between 10 and 30 N for delivering the dose. When applying a lower force to the device, a lower dose might be released. The activation of inhalers or pressing eye drop containers also requires up to 30 N, which might be too much for a geriatric patient. In those cases the treatment will fail. For diseases that affect dexterity, e.g., arthritis, special delivery systems, and packaging materials have been developed. The syringes for SC injections in arthritis patients have been equipped with a broad mount to handle (Fig. 2). The multiple-dose containers have been improved (Fig. 3). The patient may use a pen applied to the closure, which is much easier than drawing the closure in the hand. Further, various devices are available for facilitating the application of eye drops. Some are

(A)

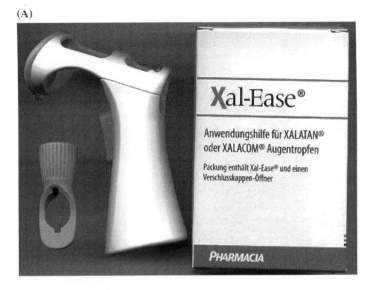

(B)

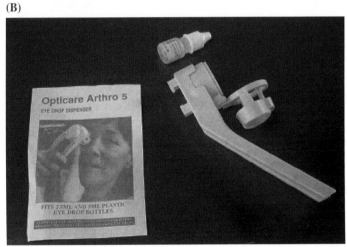

Figure 4 Devices for enabling arthritis patients to apply eye drops (**A**): Pfizer, Sandwich, Kent, U.K.; (**B**): Opticare Arthro 5, International Glaucoma Association, Ashford, Kent, U.K.

activated by using a pistol-like button to deliver a drop of the drug solution, others use the law of the lever to decrease the required force (Fig. 4). There are other devices available that help to target the conjunctiva, such as the Autodrop^{TM} or Easydrop^{TM} devices.

Vision Many people experience visual decline as they age (Fig. 5) (137,146). Moreover, there are typical diseases in the geriatric populations that affect the application of medicines. Macula degeneration and glaucoma diseases reduce the visual capabilities and may lead to blindness. A number of diabetic patients also show reduced visual potency. A special insulin pen has been developed, which is easy to handle and where the graduations are enlarged to facilitate the adjustment of the correct dose (Fig. 6). Impaired vision hinders one's ability to self-administer medication and to read instructions for the

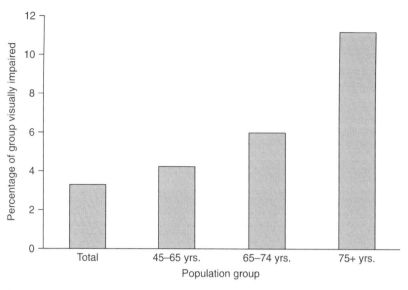

Figure 5 Incidence of visual impairment by age: United States, 1992. *Source*: From Ref. 137.

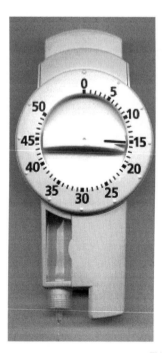

Figure 6 Insulin pen (Innolet™, Novo Nordisk, Denmark) with large graduations and numbers for diabetic patients with minor visual capabilities. Moreover, it requires only 6 N for activation, which is far below the average.

administration. Impaired vision may affect (*i*) the ability to accurately measure liquids, (*ii*) the ability to correctly read instructions, and (*iii*) the ability to differentiate between various types of medications (both the labeling of these drugs and their physical characteristics) (148,151–153).

Hearing The frequencies that are noticed by human beings range from 500 to 4000 Hz. In amblyacousia caused by degeneration of sensoric cells, the highest frequencies (>2000 Hz) vanish first followed by the lower ones. There are several drug delivery devices that need audiological capabilities (154–156). For instance, some powder inhalers are activated by moving a ring until it stops giving a clear "click" noise. If a patient does not hear the audio signal, he cannot be sure to have obtained the correct dose. The rotating of powder-releasing capsules in inhalers is quite loud and still recognizable by geriatric patients. However, connecting of a catheter to an insulin pump or perforating the capsule in an inhaler before administering is indicated by a more silent noise that cannot be registered by patients with amblyacousia (156).

Swallowing and chewing In addition to those changes occurring in the oral cavity (Table 6), there are other factors that may inhibit an elderly patient's ability to both swallow and chew. For instance, xerostomia, or dry mouth, is a condition that is prevalent among older people. Xerostomia may be caused by any one of the following conditions: (*i*) Elderly patients often do not consume adequate amounts of liquid and are thus dehydrated; (*ii*) Many elderly patients "mouth breathe" because of asthma or other respiratory diseases; and (*iii*) Elderly patients often take medications having anticholinergic side effects (e.g., antidepressants and neuroleptics) (136,157–160). Patients experiencing xerostomia often have difficulty swallowing tablets or capsules because they tend to adhere to the esophageal mucosa when it is dry (116,126,161–164). In addition, esophageal lesions are common among the elderly and may affect a patient's ability to swallow; this is compounded by the inhibition of peristalsis by the weakened esophageal musculature (126,128). The ability of elderly patients to chew is also compromised (126,135,139,141), perhaps as a result of the decreased bulk and tone of the oral musculature as one ages (135). Additionally, it has been estimated that 50% of all elderly persons in the United States are fully edentulous (i.e., toothless) (126,141). The absence of teeth not only hinders one's ability to chew, it also changes the bacterial flora within the oral cavity from predominantly anaerobic to aerobic (126).

Consciousness Many geriatric patients suffer from a reduced consciousness. Special diseases like Morbus Alzheimer as well as the "normal" obliviousness of elderly patients and headiness may affect the drug therapy. There are a number of aids to remind the patients of dosing the medicine, like alarm clocks (Fig. 7), calendar paks (C-paks), and medication boxes (dosage trays) with or without sealed doses.

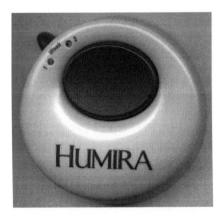

Figure 7 Alarm clock for reminding the patient of dosing by subcutaneous injection once a week (Humira, Abbott Laboratories, North Chicago, Illinois, U.S.).

Dosing Considerations Determined by Alterations in Physiology with Aging

The PK of each compound should be determined when one is deciding which drug candidates to use in designing formulations for the elderly. For instance, some medications have an increased half-life in older adults, either because these drugs undergo extensive hepatic metabolism (e.g., diazepam, verapamil, and pentazocine) or because they are excreted primarily by the kidneys (e.g., lithium, aminoglycosides, and digoxin) (106–112,122,150). In addition, drugs that are highly protein bound (e.g., warfarin) may be the cause of serious adverse reactions among elderly patients because of the decreased concentration of serum albumin in these patients and the subsequent rise in circulating "free" drug (106–112,118,122,150). So, if the PK behavior of the drug is known to change in elderly patients, it may be wise to avoid such drugs or to adjust the dosage accordingly. A guide has been recently published that lists a number of suggestions for dosing regimens in the geriatric patient (139).

Drug Delivery Systems and Compliance Issues

The changes experienced in aging may affect a patient's ability to use some of the drug delivery systems existing today. It should be kept in mind, however, that within the context of this chapter, a drug delivery system is not merely a novel dosage form: It is the dosage form with its container, labeling, *and* any other information supplied with the medication to the user.

Dosage Form Preferences

Solid oral dosage forms, particularly tablets, are the preferred type of formulation worldwide. Not only are these products widely accepted by consumers, but they are also relatively cheaper to develop and manufacture than oral liquids or suspensions, parenterals, or suppositories. Figure 4 shows, quite clearly, that the elderly primarily make use of solid oral dosage forms (165).

Oral Dosage Forms

Chewable tablets It has already been noted that most elderly patients experience a decrease in their ability to chew efficiently (124,136,139,148). Therefore, by virtue of their design, chewable tablets are not often recommended for use by elderly patients (particularly those who are edentulous) (159–167). Most chewable formulations also rely on an adequate amount of chewing action to obtain full release of their ingredients (e.g., chewing promotes the foaming action provided by some chewable antacid products). So, aside from being difficult for the elderly patient to use, full benefit of a chewable dosage form may not be achieved by these patients. Additionally, the use of chewable tablets by denture wearers may cause local irritation in the oral cavity (159).

Sublingual and buccal tablets Although sublingual and buccal tablets (e.g., nitroglycerin or isosorbide) are used by many elderly patients, few, if any, researchers have determined the effects that aging may have on the bioavailability of these dosage forms (137–141,148,157). Patient acceptance of these types of formulations must also be considered. Elderly patients who suffer from dry mouth conditions may find sublingual or buccal tablets irritating and may refuse to use such medications. Another problem may involve demented or contrary patients who may feel foreign objects inside their mouths and pull the tablets out before the active ingredients have been released from the formulation.

Capsules A number of scientists have investigated the effect of formulation on esophageal transit and have found that capsules tend to adhere to the esophageal mucosa more often than any other type of oral dosage form (161,163,164). Moreover, because of the conditions of xerostomia and hindered swallowing that are prevalent among the elderly, mucosal adherence of capsules in these patients may be more pronounced (124,126,138,151,158,159). In light of these observations, the use of capsules by older patients may not be advisable. This is an extremely important consideration if the drug to be delivered is one that is known to cause esophageal ulceration (e.g., tetracycline or aspirin) (161).

Liquids and suspensions Most liquid formulations are not packaged in unit-dosage forms. Therefore, before administration, the proper amount of medication to be taken for each dose must be measured. This additional requirement may compound any difficulties a patient may have in following a prescribed schedule. Patients suffering from visual impairment, arthritis, or tremors associated with neurological disorders are particularly likely to become frustrated with this type of formulation. Visual impairments make it difficult, if not impossible, for many elderly patients to measure the prescribed amounts of medication accurately. Impaired dexterity, owing to tremors or arthritis, may have effects on a patient's ability to hold both a spoon and a bottle at the same time while pouring out the desired amount of liquid.

Additional difficulties are encountered by elderly patients if a medication is in the form of a suspension. Problems may occur because a patient cannot see, or disregards, the words "Shake Well" on the label or is not able to exert the amount of agitation necessary to provide a uniform suspension. Certainly, unevenly distributed amounts of active ingredients throughout a suspension may result in serious consequences for a patient in terms of either under- or overdosing.

Transdermal delivery systems Although transdermal drug delivery may offer a means of increasing compliance among elderly patients, it is yet to be determined whether or not changes exist between the bioavailability of such products when administered to elderly patients versus young adults. Indeed, there may be a decrease in the absorption of compounds that are transdermally delivered to elderly patients (135,136,142,143). Still, some may prefer the transdermal design and may opt to perform all the preliminary investigations necessary to quantify percutaneous bioavailability in older patients. If this route is chosen, one should keep in mind that transdermal products formulated around these changes may be applicable to only the older patients for whom the product has been designed. Such products may have differing release characteristics in the rest of the population. Therefore, it is possible that these products, which will probably require lengthy preliminary studies, might be used effectively by only a limited portion of the population.

Parenteral dosage forms and invasive devices Parenteral and invasive devices provide the distinct advantage of the delivery of medication directly into the bloodstream or at the site of action. Additionally, these methods result in assuring patient compliance because, in most cases, an individual other than the patient is responsible for the administration of medication by these means. Unfortunately, this attribute is counteracted by numerous problems that are illustrated in Table 9.

In this table, it can be recognized that there are problems inherent in these types of formulations from both the patient's and the manufacturer's point of view. This is why most pharmaceutical companies make attempts to avoid these types of dosage forms, if at

Table 9 Possible Problems Associated with Parenteral Delivery

Cost to patient and manufacturer
Patient discomfort
Risk of infection
Administration by trained personnel required
Limitations on particle size
Sterilization necessary
Prone to chemical, mechanical, and microbial instability
Complex manufacturing processes
Cumbersome and fragile packaging

all possible. However, with the advent of biotechnological products, which often do not lend themselves to "conventional" dosage formulations, parenteral and invasive measures may be the only answer.

Alternative Delivery Systems   Although elderly patients seem to experience difficulties with the above-mentioned drug delivery systems, other systems are currently available that may be more suited to the needs of these patients. Although most of these systems are not specifically designed for the geriatric community, they may offer aid to this group of patients. This may be accomplished through the use of dosage formulations or packaging designs that are easier to handle or by supplying patients with devices or information that will enable them to better follow their prescribed dosing regimen.

Compliance aids   Many pharmacists and physicians have recognized that most elderly patients have complicated dosing schedules and need some sort of reminder that will help them keep track of their prescribed regimens (106,158,159,164,166,168–175). This can be achieved through several methods. First, various types of packages, such as dosett trays, C-paks, and patient med paks, can be prepared by pharmacists (171,172,176–178). These packages are usually devised so that all of the medications that have been prescribed to be taken at a specified time are packed together. For instance, all the medications that are to be taken before breakfast are placed in the same container, and all those to be taken one hour after breakfast are placed in another container. Labeling for each container should specify the time at which its contents are to be taken as well as a list of each individual medication it holds. In an effort to promote this type of packaging, the United States Pharmacopeia (USP) has set guidelines for pharmacists to follow when preparing patient med paks (178). In this manner, the USP has provided the pharmacist with a means to help out those patients with complex-dosing schedules and still comply with official-labeling criteria (i.e., it is not standard practice to supply more than one drug in a single container). Another way in which pharmacists and physicians can help patients regulate their dosing schedules is by supplying them with drug reminder cards (106,169,172,173). The concept for the cards is essentially the same as that for the labels on the packaging just described (i.e., time of day and all medications to be taken at that time). Various modifications of this design can be made, such as including the physical characteristics of each medication or providing stickers to be placed on the card and on its corresponding container (i.e., one sticker is placed on the prescription bottle and the other sticker is placed next to the medication's name on the reminder card) (169,173).

Unfortunately, both the drug reminder cards and packaging methods described here must be made for each patient on an individual basis, and some people are not willing to take the extra time needed to prepare these systems.

Oral dosage forms The advantages of oral dosage formulations have already been discussed. It appears that this route of delivery is preferred by physician, patients, and manufacturers alike. The relatively low cost of oral dosage forms makes them a particularly attractive means of drug delivery for those patients, such as the elderly, who may be economically depressed (179). These dosage forms are also comparatively easier to formulate, package, and ship than other types of dosage forms (180). Moreover, changes in PK parameters among the elderly have been assessed only in those formulations that are oral or parenteral in nature (106–124). Therefore, it is appropriate to focus on oral dosage formulations for drug delivery in the elderly.

Granules Granules are a type of oral formulation whose use among the elderly is warranted (166,167). This type of dosage form not only circumvents the difficulty in swallowing that may be encountered by older patients, but it also provides the patient with a certain amount of rehydration. As the elderly are often dehydrated, this is a feature that should not be overlooked. More importantly, medications that have been dispersed in a liquid are not likely to be affected by changes in GER that may occur in older patients.

Problems may still arise because granules may be supplied in either unit-dose packages or in bulk containers. If unit-dose packages are used, patients with impaired manual dexterity may have difficulty opening the packets. With bulk containers, most of the handling problems associated with administering liquid formulations that have been discussed can occur. However, bulk containers do offer the advantage of dosage flexibility that cannot be realized with other solid dosage formulations.

Coated tablets Investigators studying the effects of dosage formulation on esophageal transit have concluded that coated tablets are less likely to adhere to the esophageal mucosa than other solid dosage forms (e.g., uncoated tablets or capsules) (159,161,163,164). In addition, this effect may be complemented by the use of oval-shaped tablets, commonly referred to as "caplets" (161,162,164). This type of tablet offers advantages over uncoated tablets and capsules, especially in those patients who have difficulty swallowing. Still, it is imperative that physicians and pharmacists instruct patients to take their medications with a full glass of water because esophageal adherence is still possible in those patients who are dehydrated.

Effervescent tablets Effervescent tablets are another means of supplying medications to the elderly. This type of formulation provides the patient with an easy-to-swallow product that is aesthetically pleasing (i.e., forms a clear solution, rather than a cloudy suspension). However, pharmaceutical chemists are well aware of the problems that exist when preparing effervescent formulations. These problems may be partly solved by certain advances in pharmaceutical technology that allow direct compression of all excipients necessary to form such tablets (181–183). Although this makes the manufacture of such products easier, stability problems still exist because these formulations must be adequately protected against moisture. As with granules, the type of packaging required for effervescent tablets can be a problem for those patients with impaired manual dexterity. Moreover, and perhaps more importantly, the high sodium content necessary to manufacture effervescent products may have serious implications when used by patients with hypertension or congestive heart failure.

Dispersion or soluble tablets The trend toward formulation of dispersible tablets is evident in Europe (184,185) and is becoming more commonplace in the United States with OTC preparations available in the form of the following technologies: Zydis®

(Scherer DDS, Swindon, Wiltshire, U.K.); Lyoc® (Farmalyoc, Maisons-Alfort, France); WOW® Tab (Yamanouchi, Tokyo, Japan); FlashDose® (Fuisz Technologies, Chantilly, Virginia); OraSolv® (CIMA); and DuraSolv® (CIMA). These tablets are either placed in the mouth, where they quickly dissolve, or placed in a glass of water prior to ingestion. As with granules and effervescent tablets, dispersible tablets offer the patient a dosage form that is both portable and easy to swallow.

A challenge faced by formulators designing dispersible tablets is the ability to develop a formulation that rapidly disintegrates and is able to withstand shipping processes. In addition, this type of tablet should form a uniform and somewhat stable suspension when dispersed in water. An interesting answer to this challenge is the design of a "porous table" (186–188), in which a volatilizable solid (e.g., urethane or ammonium bicarbonate) is added to a standard, directly compressible formulation. After the tablets have been compressed, the volatilizable solid is removed by a freeze-drying or heating process. Water easily penetrates through the pores and promotes rapid disintegration of the tablets produced in this manner. Thus, these tablets are able to both maintain their mechanical strength and provide rapid disintegration or dispersion of product. Lyoc and Zydis tablets both use freeze-drying technologies.

Gel preparations Some Japanese investigators are promoting the use of jellylike preparations to help elderly patients overcome their difficulty in swallowing conventional tablets and capsules (189–191). These dosage forms rely on gelation of materials such as sodium casseinate, glycerogelatin, dried gelatin gel powder, and silk fibroin.

Tiltabs® Tiltab tablets represent one of the few dosage formulations that has been developed expressly to meet the needs of patients with impaired dexterity (192). Marketed by Smith, Kline & French Laboratories, Ltd. in several European countries, the novelty of the Tiltab design is its irregular shape that prevents it from lying fiat. Apparently, tablets manufactured in this fashion are easier to handle by those with impaired dexterity. Moreover, these tablets are readily identifiable by patients so that differentiation from other medication is facilitated. Other innovations like this are needed for drug delivery systems with the particular needs of the geriatric patient in mind.

Concentrated oral solutions Presentation of a drug may be made in the form of a concentrated solution that allows the entire dose to be held within a volume of less than 5 mL (e.g., Intensol® Concentrated Oral Solutions, Boehringer Ingelheim Roxanne Inc., Columbus, Ohio). This opens up another means of providing medication to the aged, infants, or any other patients experiencing difficulties in swallowing. Such preparations can be mixed with food or drink. Taste and poor solubility are problems that may set limits on the number of successful formulations that can be prepared in this way. Also, small errors in the measurement of such preparations represent large errors in dosing.

Taste Preferences in Oral Dosage Forms

Changes in elderly patients' abilities to taste various substances do not necessarily affect the ease or difficulty of administration of medications, but these changes do have an effect on the patients' acceptance of a product. For instance, although it may be easier for patients to swallow liquid medications, they may find the taste or smell of the product so objectionable that they will refuse to take any medication prepared in this manner. Indeed, even some solid dosage forms carry with them objectionable tastes or odors that result in limitation of patient acceptance. Although there have been few studies assessing elderly patients' taste preferences, these reports have indicated that differences in taste preference and perception do exist between elderly and young adult populations (126,133,139,193,194). It has been determined that although the number of taste buds declines with age, thresholds for certain tastes are affected, whereas others are not. Unfortunately, reports of taste threshold changes among the elderly are contradictory, and it is difficult to ascertain what changes really do occur (126,133,139,193,194). Current reports claim that these changes in taste thresholds are not due to the aging process, per se, but to medications that the patient may be taking (140,195). For example, it appears that an increased concentration of sour compounds must exist to be detected by patients taking medications (194).

Package and Label Design

One of the most important aspects of drug delivery design for the elderly is the presentation of the package and its label. If the patient is unable to open a package or cannot read a label properly, even the best dosage formulation design will be unsuccessful (178). For prescription medications the package design is difficult to control, because the container supplied by the manufacturer is not necessarily the container in which the medicine will be dispensed by the pharmacist. But pharmacist's selection of special packaging is a prospect open to most drugs whenever elderly-friendly packaging is in hand. The OTC products, in partial contrast, provide a manufacturer with the opportunity to make substantial changes in the design of packages and their labels. When developing a design, it is important to always keep in mind that impaired dexterity and visual decline are prevalent among the elderly. Listed in Table 10 are some suggestions that may be useful when designing a product's label (151,152,168,175,195,196).

In terms of the package itself, it is difficult to devise a package that is both childproof and tamperproof and still able to be opened easily by someone with impaired dexterity. It has been suggested that packaging a medication in unit-dose C-paks may increase patient compliance (197). The problem is that other studies have shown that most elderly patients encounter difficulties when attempting to open this type of packaging (blister packaging) (172,177). Additionally, this type of packaging (i.e., C-paks and the like) for OTC products may be unacceptable to the Federal Trade Commission and FDA as it promotes the daily use of the product. So, it is apparent that different types of packaging are needed, depending on whether a drug is for OTC or prescription-only use.

Table 10 Suggestions for Labels Designed to be Used by Elderly Patients

Use clear wording
Avoid too many information
Emphasize important handling advice (e.g., "shake before use") by color and font size
Avoid pastels
Use matte surfaces to minimize glare
Light colors on dark background are more visible than dark colors on light background
Use distinct spacing between letters
Increase height and thickness of letters
Use additional labels that clearly explain purpose of medication[a]

[a]This type of label is required on drugs dispensed in Denmark.

Conclusions

It is evident that numerous conditions exist that separate the elderly from young adults. Moreover, some of these conditions have a substantial impact on the use of drug delivery systems by elderly patients. With the ever-increasing proportion of elderly patients in our population, it is surprising that relatively few special products are marketed to accommodate the needs of these patients in terms of drug delivery design.

REFERENCES

1. Breitkreutz J, Boos J. Paediatric and geriatric drug delivery. Expert Opin Drug Deliv 2007; 4: 37–45.
2. Bartelink IH, Rademaker CM, Schobben AF, et al. Guidelines on paediatric dosing on the basis of developmental physiology and pharmacokinetic considerations. Clin Pharmacokinet 2006; 45:1077–1097.
3. Maddox GL. The Encyclopedia of Aging. 3rd ed. New York: Springer, 1987.
4. Gorman M. Development and the rights of older people. In: Randel J, German T, Ewing D, eds. The Ageing and Development Report: Poverty, Independence and the World's Older People. London: Earthscan Publications, 1993:3–21.
5. World Health Organization (WHO). Definition of an older or elderly person. 2008. Accessed January 2008. Available at: http://www.who.int/healthinfo/survey/ageingdefnolder/en/index.html
6. Costa PT, McCrae RR. Functional Age: A Conceptual and Empirical Critique. Washington, DC: U.S. Government Printing Office, 1977:23–32.
7. Graham JE, Mitnitski AB, Mogilner AJ, et al. Dynamics of cognitive aging: distinguishing functional age and disease from chronologic age in a population. Am J Epidemiol 1999; 150:1045–1054.
8. Orimo H, Ito H, Susuki T, et al. Reviewing the definition of "elderly". Geriatr Gerontol Int 2006; 6:149–158.
9. de Zwart LL, Haenen HE, Versantvoort CH, et al. Role of biokinetics in risk assessment of drugs and chemicals in children. Regul Toxicol Pharmacol 2004; 39:282–309.
10. Ginsberg G, Hattis D, Sonawane B. Incorporating pharmacokinetic differences between children and adults in assessing children's risks to environmental toxicants. Toxicol Appl Pharmacol 2004; 198:164–183.
11. Kearns GL, Abdel-Rahman SM, Alander SW, et al. Developmental pharmacology—drug disposition, action, and therapy in infants and children. N Engl J Med 2003; 349:1157–1167.
12. Deren JS. Development of structure and function in the fetal and newborn stomach. Am J Clin Nutr 1971; 24:144–159.
13. Hyman PE, Feldman EJ, Ament ME, et al. Effect of enteral feeding on the maintenance of gastric acid secretory function. Gastroenterology 1983; 84:341–345.
14. Assael BM. Pharmacokinetics and drug distribution during postnatal development. Pharmacol Ther 1982; 18:159–197.
15. Gupta M, Brans YW. Gastric retention in neonates. Pediatrics 1978; 62:26–29.
16. Hendeles L, Iafrate RP, Weinberger M. A clinical and pharmacokinetic basis for the selection and use of slow release theophylline products. Clin Pharmacokinet 1984; 9:95–135.
17. Jusko WJ, Levy G, Yaffe SJ. Effect of age on intestinal absorption of riboflavin in humans. J Pharm Sci 1970; 59:487–490.
18. Linday L, Dobkin JF, Wang TC, et al. Digoxin inactivation by the gut flora in infancy and childhood. Pediatrics 1987; 79:544–548.
19. Heimann G. Enteral absorption and bioavailability in children in relation to age. Eur J Clin Pharmacol 1980; 18:43–50.
20. Pedersen-Bjergaard L, Petersen KE. Oral absorption of pivampicillin and ampicillin in young children: cross-over study using equimolar doses of a suspension. Clin Pharmacokinet 1977; 2: 451–456.

21. Cooney GF, Habucky K, Hoppu K. Cyclosporin pharmacokinetics in paediatric transplant recipients. Clin Pharmacokinet 1997; 32:481–495.

22. Murry DJ, Riva L, Poplack D. Impact of nutrition on pharmacokinetics of anti-neoplastic agents. Int J Cancer 1998; 78(S11):48–51.

23. Gilman JT, Duchowny MS, Resnick TJ, et al. Carbamazepine malabsorption: a case report. Pediatrics 1988; 82:518–519.

24. Friss-Hansen B. Body water compartments in children: changes during growth and related changes in body composition. Pediatrics 1961; 28:169–181.

25. Heimler R, Doumas BT, Jendrzejczak BM, et al. Relationship between nutrition, weight change, and fluid compartments in preterm infants during the first week of life. J Pediatr 1993; 122(1):110–114.

26. Notarianni LJ. Plasma protein binding of drugs in pregnancy and in neonates. Clin Pharmacokinet 1990; 18:20–36.

27. Milsap RL, Jusko WJ. Pharmacokinetics in the infant. Environ Health Perspect 1994; 102 (suppl 11):107–110.

28. Gauntlett IS, Fisher DM, Hertzka RE, et al. Pharmacokinetics of fentanyl in neonatal humans and lambs: effects of age. Anesthesiology 1988; 69:683–687.

29. Leeder JS, Kearns GL. Pharmacogenetics in pediatrics. Implications for practice. Pediatr Clin North Am 1997; 44:55–77.

30. Aranda JV, MacLeod SM, Renton KW, et al. Hepatic microsomal drug oxidation and electron transport in newborn infants. J Pediatr 1974; 85:534–542.

31. Rosen JP, Danish M, Ragni MC, et al. Theophylline pharmacokinetics in the young infant. Pediatrics 1979; 64:248–251.

32. Carrier O, Pons G, Rey E, et al. Maturation of caffeine metabolic pathways in infancy. Clin Pharmacol Ther 1988; 44:145–151.

33. Miller RP, Roberts RJ, Fischer LJ. Acetaminophen elimination kinetics in neonates, children, and adults. Clin Pharmacol Ther 1976; 19:284–294.

34. Glazer JP, Danish MA, Plotkin SA, et al. Disposition of chloramphenicol in low birth weight infants. Pediatrics 1980; 66:573–578.

35. Thompson JA, Bloedow DC, Leffert FH. Pharmacokinetics of intravenous chlorpheniramine in children. J Pharm Sci 1981; 70:1284–1286.

36. Fisher DG, Schwartz PH, Davis AL. Pharmacokinetics of exogenous epinephrine in critically ill children. Crit Care Med 1993; 21:111–117.

37. Matsuda I, Higashi A, Inotsume N. Physiologic and metabolic aspects of anticonvulsants. Pediatr Clin North Am 1989; 36:1099–1111.

38. Guignard JP, Torrado A, Da CO, et al. Glomerular filtration rate in the first three weeks of life. J Pediatr 1975; 87:268–272.

39. Schwartz GJ, Feld LG, Langford DJ. A simple estimate of glomerular filtration rate in full-term infants during the first year of life. J Pediatr 1984; 104:849–854.

40. McCance RA. Renal function in early life. Physiol Rev 1948; 28:331–348.

41. Stephenson T. How children's responses to drugs differ from adults. Br J Clin Pharmacol 2005; 59:670–673.

42. American Academy of Pediatrics: committee on drugs. "Inactive" ingredients in pharmaceutical products: update (Subject Review). Pediatrics 1997; 99:268–278.

43. Ernest TB, Elder DP, Martini LG, et al. Developing paediatric medicines: identifying the needs and recognizing the challenges. J Pharm Pharmacol 2007; 59:1043–1055.

44. Golightly LK, Smolinske SS, Bennett ML, et al. Pharmaceutical excipients. Adverse effects associated with inactive ingredients in drug products (Part I). Med Toxicol Adverse Drug Exp 1988; 3:128–165.

45. Golightly LK, Smolinske SS, Bennett ML, et al. Pharmaceutical excipients. Adverse effects associated with 'inactive' ingredients in drug products (Part II). Med Toxicol Adverse Drug Exp 1988; 3:209–240.

46. Pawar S, Kumar A. Issues in the formulation of drugs for oral use in children: role of excipients. Paediatr Drugs 2002; 4:371–379.

47. Committee on Drugs. "Inactive" ingredients in pharmaceutical products: update (subject review). Pediatrics 1997; 99:268–278.
48. Menon PA, Thach BT, Smith CH, et al. Benzyl alcohol toxicity in a neonatal intensive care unit. Incidence, symptomatology, and mortality. Am J Perinatol 1984; 1:288–292.
49. Committee on Fetus and Newborn, Committee on Drugs. Benzyl alcohol: toxic agent in neonatal units. Pediatrics 1983; 72:356–358.
50. Arulanantham K, Genel M. Central nervous system toxicity associated with ingestion of propylene glycol. J Pediatr 1978; 93:515–516.
51. Anonymous. Yellow No 5. (tartrazine) labeling on drugs to be required. FDA Drug Bull 1979; 9(3):18.
52. Pohl R, Balon R, Berchou R, et al. Allergy to tartrazine in antidepressants. Am J Psychiatry 1987; 144:237–238.
53. Weber RW, Hoffman M, Raine DA Jr., et al. Incidence of bronchoconstriction due to aspirin, azo dyes, non-azo dyes, and preservatives in a population of perennial asthmatics. J Allergy Clin Immunol 1979; 64:32–37.
54. Buswell RS, Lefkowitz MS. Oral bronchodilators containing tartrazine. JAMA 1976; 235:1111.
55. McCann D, Barrett A, Cooper A, et al. Food additives and hyperactive behaviour in 3-year-old and 8/9-year-old children in the community: a randomised, double-blinded, placebo-controlled trial. Lancet 2007; 370:1560–1567.
56. Hill EM, Flaitz CM, Frost GR. Sweetener content of common pediatric oral liquid medications. Am J Hosp Pharm 1988; 45:135–142.
57. Strickley RG, Iwata Q, Wu S, et al. Pediatric drugs—a review of commercially available oral formulations. J Pharm Sci 2008; 97:1731–1774.
58. Shaw L, Glenwright HD. The role of medications in dental caries formation: need for sugar-free medication for children. Pediatrician 1989; 16:153–155.
59. Feigal RJ, Jensen ME, Mensing CA. Dental caries potential of liquid medications. Pediatrics 1981; 68(3):416–419.
60. Lokken P, Birkeland JM, Sannes E. pH changes in dental plaque caused by sweetened, iron-containing liquid medicine. Scand J Dent Res 1975; 83(5):279–283.
61. Mitchell H. Sweeteners and Sugar alternatives in food technology. London: Blackwell Publishing, 2007.
62. Lutomski DM, Gora ML, Wright SM, et al. Sorbitol content of selected oral liquids. Ann Pharmacother 1993; 27:269–274.
63. Arnold DL, Moodie CA, Grice HC, et al. Long-term toxicity of ortho-touenesulfonamide and sodium saccharin in the rat. Toxicol Appl Pharmacol 1980; 52:113–152.
64. Koysooko R, Levy G. Effect of ethanol on intestinal absorption of theophylline. J Pharm Sci 1974; 63:829–834.
65. Panel recommends limits on alcohol content of nonprescription products. FDA Over-The-Counter Drugs Advisory Committee. Am J Hosp Pharm 1993; 50:400.
66. Rappaport PL. Extemporaneous dosage preparations for pediatrics. Can J Hosp Pharm 1983; 36:66–70, 74.
67. Standing JF, Khaki ZF, Wong IC. Poor formulation information in published pediatric drug trials. Pediatrics 2005; 116:e559–e562.
68. Nunn T, Williams J. Formulation of medicines for children. Br J Clin Pharmacol 2005; 59:674–676.
69. Krause J, Breikreutz J. Improving drug delivery in paediatric medicines. Pharm Med 2008; 22:41–50.
70. Griessmann K, Breitkreutz J, Schubert-Zsilavecz M, et al. Dosing accuracy of measuring devices provided with antibiotic oral suspensions. Paediatr Perinat Drug Ther 2007; 10:61–70.
71. Brown D, Ford JL, Nunn AJ, et al. An assessment of dose-uniformity of samples delivered from paediatric oral droppers. J Clin Pharm Ther 2004; 29:521–529.
72. Standing JF, Tuleu C. Paediatric formulations—getting to the heart of the problem. Int J Pharm 2005; 300:56–66.

73. Blumer JL. Fundamental basis for rational therapeutics in acute otitis media. Pediatr Infect Dis J 1999; 18:1130–1140.

74. Teng J, Song CK, Williams RL, et al. Lack of medication dose uniformity in commonly split tablets. J Am Pharm Assoc 2002; 42:195–199.

75. Tuleu C, Grangé J, Seurin S. The need of paediatric formulation: administration of nifedipine in children, a proof of concept. J Drug Del Sci Tech 2005; 15:319–324.

76. Abdel-Rahman SM, Blowey DL, Kauffmann RE, et al. Comparative bioavailability of loracarbef chewable tablet vs. oral suspension in children. Pediatr Infect Dis J 1998; 17: 1171–1173.

77. Cornaggia C, Gianetti S, Battino D, et al. Comparative pharmacokinetic study of chewable and conventional carbamazepine in children. Epilepsia 1993; 34:158–160.

78. Cloyd JC, Kriel RL, Jones-Saete CM, et al. Comparison of sprinkle versus syrup formulations of valproate for bioavailability, tolerance, and preference. J Pediatr 1992; 120:634–638.

79. Nowak MM, Brundhofer B, Gibaldi M. Rectal absorption from aspirin suppositories in children and adults. Pediatrics 1974; 54:23–26.

80. Ghadially R, Shear N. Topical therapy and percutaneous absorption. In: Yaffe SJ, Aranda JV, eds. Pediatric Pharmacology: Therapeutic Principles in Practice. 2nd ed. Philadelphia: WB Saunders, 1992:72–77.

81. Loebstein R, Koren G. Clinical pharmacology and therapeutic drug monitoring in neonates and children. Pediatr Rev 1998; 19:423–428.

82. Paisley JW, Smith AL, Smith DH. Gentamicin in newborn infants. Comparison of intramuscular and intravenous administration. Am J Dis Child 1973; 126:473–477.

83. Shann F, Linnemann V, Mackenzie A, et al. Absorption of chloramphenicol sodium succinate after intramuscular administration in children. N Engl J Med 1985; 313:410–414.

84. Bradley JS, Compogiannis LS, Murray WE, et al. Pharmacokinetics and safety of intramuscular injection of concentrated certriaxone in children. Clin Pharm 1992; 11:961–964.

85. Suarez EC, Grippi JR. Comparative bioavailability and safety of two intramuscular ceftriaxone formulations. Ann Pharmacother 1996; 30:1223–1226.

86. Seay RE. Comment: bioavailability and safety of two ceftriaxone formulations - exposure to lidocaine questioned. Ann Pharmacother 1997; 31:501–502.

87. McIvor A, Paluzzi M, Meguid MM. Intramuscular injection abscess—past lessons relearned. N Engl J Med 1991; 324:1897–1898.

88. Hard R. Pharmacists work on pediatric dosage problems. Hospitals 1992; 66:46–48.

89. Koren G, Barzilay Z, Greenwald M. Tenfold errors in administration of drug doses: a neglected Iatrogenic disease in pediatrics. Pediatrics 1986; 77:848–849.

90. Goldman RD. Intranasal drug delivery for children with acute illness. Curr Drug Ther 2006; 1: 127–130.

91. Johnston C. Endotracheal drug delivery. Pediatr Emerg Care 1992; 8:94–97.

92. Hickey AJ. Factors influencing aerosol desposition in inertial impactors and their effect on particle size characterization. Pharm Technol 1990; 14:118–130.

93. Abrolat ML, Nguyen LP, Saca LF. Hold it! Correct use of inhalers in children with asthma. West J Med 2001; 175:303–304.

94. Saggers BA, Lawson D. Some observations on the penetration of antibiotics through mucus in vitro. J Clin Pathol 1966; 19:313–317.

95. Saggers BA, Lawson D. In vivo penetration of antibiotics into sputum in cystic fibrosis. Arch Dis Child 1968; 43:404–409.

96. Gibaldi M. Understanding and treating some genetic diseases. Ann Pharmacother 1992; 26: 1589–1594.

97. Jew LL, Hart LL. Inhaled aminoglycosides in cystic fibrosis. DICP 1990; 24:711–712.

98. Ross B, Ramsey L, Shepherd J. Delivery of aerosol therapy in the management of pulmonary disorders. Hosp Pharm Rep 2000; 14:3.

99. Matsui D. Assessing the palatability of medication in children. Paediatr Perinat Drug Ther 2007; 8:55–60.

100. Mennella JA, Pepino MY, Reed DR. Genetic and environmental determinants of bitter perception and sweet preferences. Pediatrics 2005; 115:e216–e222.

101. James CE, Laing DG, Oram N. A comparison of the ability of 8-9-year-old children and adults to detect taste stimuli. Physiol Behav 1997; 62:193–197.

102. James CE, Laing DG, Oram N, et al. Perception of sweetness in simple and complex taste stimuli by adults and children. Chem Senses 1999; 24:281–287.

103. Mantick N, Jantz C. Children's OTC pharmaceuticals: sensory directed flavor formulation. Profile Attribute Analysis. Cambridge, MA: Arthur D Little, 1991.

104. Kumar A, Weatherly MR, Beaman DC. Sweeteners, flavorings, and dyes in antibiotic preparations. Pediatrics 1991; 87:352–360.

105. Ruff ME, Schotik DA, Bass JW, et al. Antimicrobial drug suspensions: a blind comparison of taste of fourteen common pediatric drugs. Pediatr Infect Dis J 1991; 10:30–33.

106. Roberts J, Tumer N. Pharmacodynamic basis for altered drug action in the elderly. Clin Geriatr Med 1988; 4:127–149.

107. Vestal RE. Drug use in the elderly: a review of problems and special considerations. Drugs 1978; 16:358–382.

108. Rocci ML Jr., Vlasses PH, Abrams WB. Geriatric clinical pharmacology. Cardiol Clin 1986; 4:213–225.

109. Cromarty JA. Medicines for the elderly. Pharm J 1985; 235:511.

110. Pucino F, Beck CL, Seifert RL, et al. Pharmacogeriatrics. Pharmacotherapy 1985; 5:314–326.

111. Miura T, Kojima R, Sugiura Y, et al. Effect of aging on the incidence of digoxin toxicity. Ann Pharmacother 2000; 34:427–432.

112. Crooks J, O'Malley K, Stevenson IH. Pharmacokinetics in the elderly. Clin Pharmacokinet 1976; 1:280–296.

113. Kean WF, Buchanan WW. Pharmacokinetics of NSAID with special reference to the elderly. Singapore Med J 1987; 28:383–389.

114. A report of Royal College of Physicians. Medications for the elderly. J Royal Coll of Physicians of Lond 1984; 18:1–7.

115. Mayersohn M. Drug disposition in the elderly. In: Penta FB, ed. Pharmacy Practice for the Geriatric Patient. Alexandria, VA: American Association of Colleges of Pharmacy, 1986:9.5–9.11.

116. Shepherd AMM. Physiological changes with aging–relevance to drug study design. In: Cutler NR, Narang PK, eds. Drug Studies in the Elderly: Methodological Concerns. New York: Plenum Publishing, 1986:50–54.

117. Dilger K, Hofmann U, Klotz U. Enzyme induction in the elderly: effect of rifampin on the pharmacokinetics and pharmacodynamics of propafenone. Clin Pharmacol Ther 2000; 67: 512–520.

118. Grandison MK, Boudinot FD. Age-related changes in protein binding of drugs: implications for therapy. Clin Pharmacokinet 2000; 38:271–290.

119. Bachmann KA, Belloto RJ Jr. Differential kinetics of phenytoin in elderly patients. Drugs Aging 1999; 15:235–250.

120. Dresser GK, Spence JD, Bailey DG. Pharmacokinetic-pharmacodynamic consequences and clinical relevance of cytochrome P450 3A4 inhibition. Clin Pharmacokinet 2000; 38:41–57.

121. Dresser GK, Bailey DG, Carruthers SG. Grapefruit juice-felodipine interaction in the elderly. Clin Pharmacol Ther 2000; 68:28–34.

122. Sproule BA, Hardy BG, Shulman KI. Differential pharmacokinetics of lithium in elderly patients. Drugs Aging 2000; 16:165–177.

123. Cohen JS. Avoiding adverse reactions. Effective lower-dose drug therapies for older patients. Geriatrics 2000; 55:54–60, 63.

124. Castleden CM, Volans CN, Raymond K. The effect of ageing on drug absorption from the gut. Age Ageing 1977; 6:138–143.

125. Gerbino PP, Wordell CJ. Gastrointestinal disorder. In: Penta FB, ed. Pharmacy Practice for the Geriatric Patient. Alexandria, VA: American Association of Colleges of Pharmacy, 1986:20.1–20.24.

126. Sheely TW. The gastrointestinal system and the elderly. In: Gambert SR, ed. Contemporary Geriatric Medicine. 2nd ed. New York: Plenum Publishing, 1986.

127. Geokas MC, Haverback BJ. The aging gastrointestinal tract. Am J Surg 1969; 117:881–892.

128. Holt PR. Gastrointestinal drugs in the elderly. Am J Gastroenterol 1986; 81:403–411.

129. Anuras S, Loening-Baucke V. Gastrointestinal motility in the elderly. J Am Geriatr Soc 1984; 32: 386–390.

130. Moore JG, Tweedy C, Christian PE, et al. Effect of age on gastric emptying of liquid–solid meals in man. Dig Dis Sci 1983; 28:340–344.

131. Evans MA, Triggs EJ, Cheung M, et al. Gastric emptying rate in the elderly: implications for drug therapy. J Am Geriatr Soc 1981; 29:201–205.

132. Evans MA, Broe GA, Triggs EJ, et al. Gastric emptying rate and the systemic availability of levodopa in the elderly parkinsonian patient. Neurology 1981; 31:1288–1294.

133. Mojaverian P, Vlasses PH, Kellner PE, et al. Effects of gender, posture, and age on gastric residence time of an indigestible solid: pharmaceutical considerations. Pharm Res 1988; 5: 639–644.

134. Gryback P, Hermansson G, Lyrenas E, et al. Nationwide standardisation and evaluation of scintigraphic gastric emptying: reference values and comparisons between subgroups in a multicentre trial. Eur J Nucl Med 2000; 27:647–555.

135. Baum BJ, Bodner L. Aging and oral motor function: evidence for altered performance among older persons. J Dent Res 1983; 62:2–6.

136. Ben-Aryeh H, Miron D, Berdicevsky I, et al. Xerostomia in the elderly: prevalence, diagnosis, complications and treatment. Gerodontology 1985; 4:77–82.

137. Collins JG. Prevalence of selected chronic conditions: United States, 1990–1992. Vital National Health 1997; 10(194):1–89.

138. Exton-Smith AN, Weksler ME. Practical Geriatric Medicine. New York: Churchill Livingstone, 1985.

139. Ferguson BD. The Aging Mouth (Frontiers of Oral Physiology). 2nd ed. New York: S. Karger 1988.

140. Kamen S, Kamen LB. Contemporary Geriatric Medicine. In: Gambert SR,ed. New York: Plenum Publishing, 1986.

141. National Center for Health Statistics (NCHS). Health, United States, 1999, with Health and Aging Chartbook. Hyattsville, MD: DHSS eds. (US department of Health and Human Services), 1999. Available at: http://www.cdc.gov/nchs/data/hus/hus99ncb.pdf.

142. Christophers E, Kligman AM. Percutaneous adsorption in aged skin. In: Montagna W, ed. Advances in Biology of the Skin. New York: Permagon Press, 1964:163–175.

143. Behl CG, Bellantone NH, Flynn GL. Influence of age on percutaneous absorption of drug substance. In: Kyodonieus AF, Berner B, eds. Transdermal Delivery of Drugs. Boca Raton, FL: CRC Press, 1998:109–132.

144. Kligman AM. Perspectives and problems in cutaneous gerontology. J Invest Dermatol 1979; 73: 39–46.

145. Daly CH, Odland GF. Age-related changes in the mechanical properties of human skin. J Invest Dermatol 1979; 73:83–87.

146. Adams PF, Benson V. Current estimates from the National Health Interview Survey. Vital Health Stat 1990; 10(181):1–212.

147. Branch LG, Katz S, Kniepmann K, et al. A prospective study of functional status among community elders. Am J Public Health 1984; 74:266–268.

148. Cornoni-Huntley J, Brock DB, Ostfeld AM, et al. Established Populations for Epidemiologic Studies for the Elderly. Washington, DC: U.S. Government Printing Office, 1986.

149. Katz S, Downs TD, Cash HR, et al. Progress in development of the index of ADL. Gerontologist 1970; 10:20–30.

150. National Center for Health Statistics. Health, United States, 2000, Adolescent Health Chartbook. Hyattsville, MD: DHSS eds., 2000. Available at: http://www.cdc.gov/nchs/data/hus/hus00.pdf.

151. Cerella J. Age-related decline in extrafoveal letter perception. J Gerontol 1985; 40:727–736.

152. Kosnik W, Winslow L, Kline D, et al. Visual changes in daily life throughout adulthood. J Gerontol 1988; 43:63–70.

153. Maloney CC. Identifying and treating the client with sensory loss. Phys Occup Ther Geriatr 1987; 5:31.

154. Clarke A, Spollett G. Dose accuracy and injection force dynamics of a novel disposable insulin pen. Expert Opin Drug Deliv 2007; 4:165–174.

155. Kircher V. Ergonomische Probleme individuell lösen. Pharm Ztg 2005; 150:4570–4577.

156. Kircher V. Wie sich ergonomische und audiologische Probleme lösen lassen. Pharm Ztg 2007; 152: 2404–2413.

157. Heeneman H, Brown DH. Senescent changes in and about the oral cavity and pharynx. J Otolaryngol 1986; 15:214–216.

158. Lamy PP. Over-the-counter medication: the drug interactions we overlook. J Am Geriatr Soc 1982; 30(11 suppl):S69–S75.

159. Lamy PP. Appropriate and inappropriate drug use. In: Penta FB, ed. Pharmacy Practice for the Geriatric Patient. Alexandria, VA: American Association of Colleges of Pharmacy, 1985:13.1–13.27.

160. Fuselier CC. General principles of drug prescribing. In: Penta FB, ed. Pharmacy Practice for the Geriatric Patient. Alexandria, VA: American Association of Colleges of Pharmacy, 1985:8.1–8.28.

161. Channer KS, Virjee JP. The effect of formulation on oesophageal transit. J Pharm Pharmacol 1985; 37:126–129.

162. Hey H, Jorgensen F, Sorensen K, et al. Oesophageal transit of six commonly used tablets and capsules. Br Med J (Clin Res Ed) 1982; 285:1717–1719.

163. Kottke MK, Stetsko G, Rosenbaum SR, et al. Problems encountered by the elderly in the use of conventional dosage forms. J Geriatr Drug Ther 1990; 5:77–91.

164. Marvola M, Rajaniemi M, Marttila E, et al. Effect of dosage form and formulation factors on the adherence of drugs to the esophagus. J Pharm Sci 1983; 72:1034–1036.

165. Semla T, Breizer J, Higbee M. Geriatric Dosage Handbook. Washington, DC: American Pharmaceutical Association, 2000.

166. Hollenbeck RG, Lamy PP. Dosage form considerations in clinical trials involving elderly patients. In: Cutler NR, Narang PK, eds. Drug Studies in the Elderly. Methodological Concerns. New York: Plenum Publishing, 1986:335–353.

167. Wallace RB. Drug utilization in the rural elderly: Perspectives from a population study. In: Moore SR, Teal RW, eds. Geriatric Drug Use-Clinical and Social Perspectives. New York: Permagon Press, 1985:78–85.

168. Finchman JB. Over-the-counter drug use and misuse by the ambulatory elderly: a review of the literature. J Geriatr Drug Ther 1986; 1:3.

169. Hallworth RB, Goldberg LA. Geriatric patients' understanding of labelling of medicines. Br J Pharm Pract 1984; 6:6–14.

170. Lamy PP. The future is not what it used to be. Mol Pharm 1987; 63:10.

171. Richardson JL. Perspectives on compliance with drug regimens among the elderly. J Compliance Health Care 1986; 1:33.

172. Simonson W. Compliance to drug therapy. Medications and the Elderly. A Guide to Promoting Proper Use. Baltimore: Aspen Publishers, 1984:70–79.

173. Sumner BD. Compliance with drug therapy. Handbook of Geriatric Drug Therapy for Health Care Professionals. Philadelphia: Lea & Febiger, 1983:43–52.

174. Wade B, Bowling A. Appropriate use of drugs by elderly people. J Adv Nurs 1986; 11:47–55.

175. Williamson JR, Smith RG, Burley LE. Primary Care of the Elderly. A Practical Approach. London: IOP Publishing, 1987.

176. Wong BS, Norman DC. Evaluation of a novel medication aid, the calendar blister-pak, and its effect on drug compliance in a geriatric outpatient clinic. J Am Geriatr Soc 1987; 35:21–26.

177. Keram S, Williams ME. Quantifying the ease or difficulty older persons experience in opening medication containers. J Am Geriatr Soc 1988; 36:198–201.

178. Davidson JR. Presentation and packaging of drugs for the elderly. J Hosp Pharm 1973; 31:180.

179. United States Pharmacopeial Convention. Fourth Supplement of the United States Pharmacopeia National Formulary. Rockville, MD, 1988.
180. Banker GS, Anderson NR. Tablets. In: Lachman L, Lieberman HA, Kanig JL, eds. The Theory and Practice of Industrial Pharmacy. 3rd ed. Philadelphia, PA: Lea & Febiger, 1986.
181. Tsumara J, inventor; Process for the preparation of water-soluble tablets. US patent 3,692, 896. 1972.
182. Crivellaro G, Oldani F, inventors; Soluble tablet. US patent 3,819,824 1974.
183. Daunora LG, inventor; Water soluble tablet. US patent 4,347,235 1982.
184. Martini T. Tablet dispersion as alternative to mixtures. NZ Pharm 1987; 7:34.
185. Norris E, Guttadauria M. Piroxicam: new dosage forms. Eur J Rheumatol Inflamm 1987; 8: 94–104.
186. Heinemann H, Rothe W. Preparation of porous tablets. US patent 3,885,026 1975.
187. Corveleyn S, Remon JP. Stability of freeze-dried tablets at different relative humidities. Drug Dev Ind Pharm 1999; 25:1005–1013.
188. Seager H. Drug-delivery products and the Zydis fast-dissolving dosage form. J Pharm Pharmacol 1998; 50:375–382.
189. Hanawa T, Watanabe A, Tsuchiya T, et al. New oral dosage form for elderly patients: preparation and characterization of silk fibroin gel. Chem Pharm Bull (Tokyo) 1995; 43:284–288.
190. Hanawa T, Maeda R, Muramatsu E, et al. New oral dosage form for elderly patients. III. Stability of trichlormethiazide in silk fibroin gel and various sugar solutions. Drug Dev Ind Pharm 2000; 26:1091–1097.
191. Watanabe A, Hanawa T, Sugihara M, et al. Release profiles of phenytoin from new oral dosage form for the elderly. Chem Pharm Bull (Tokyo) 1994; 42:1642–1645.
192. Tovey GD. The development of the Tiltab tablets. Pharm J 1987; 239:363.
193. Murphy C. Aging and chemosensory perception. Front Oral Physiol 1987; 6:135.
194. Spitzer ME. Taste acuity in institutionalized and noninstitutionalized elderly men. J Gerontol 1988; 43:71–74.
195. Cooper BA. A model for implementing color contrast in the environment of the elderly. Am J Occup Ther 1985; 39:253–258.
196. Zuccollo G, Liddell H. The elderly and the medication label: doing it better. Age Ageing 1985; 14: 371–376.
197. Sumner BD. General considerations. Handbook of Geriatric Drug Therapy for Health Care Professionals. Philadelphia: Lea & Febiger, 1983:1–9.

7

Biotechnology-Based Pharmaceuticals

Lene Jorgensen, Hanne Moerck Nielsen, and Sven Frokjaer
*Department of Pharmaceutics and Analytical Chemistry, Faculty of
Pharmaceutical Sciences, University of Copenhagen, Copenhagen, Denmark*

INTRODUCTION/BACKGROUND

The area of biotechnology-based pharmaceuticals such as proteins and nucleic acid–based therapeutics has developed significantly during the last decade. The rapid advances in molecular biology, genetics, and recombinant DNA technology will continuously contribute to the development due to the greater understanding of the mechanisms behind the cause and progress of diseases, new methods for target identification, advances in production of biopharmaceuticals, and the development of innovative technologies for formulation and delivery of biopharmaceuticals. This development will expand the list of biotechnology-based pharmaceuticals and open for more and better treatments to the benefit of patients. As an example, the recent discovery of small-interfering RNA (siRNA) operating in mammalian cells has initiated a tremendous research activity to uncover new mechanisms of gene silencing, and to use this fundamentally new way to treat diseases by addressing molecular targets otherwise difficult to reach with existing medicines.

For the pharmaceutical scientists who formulate biopharmaceuticals as products with ideal therapeutic effects and storage characteristics, these products are highly challenging. Because of the unique physicochemical characteristics related to the biomacromolecular structure of biotechnology-based drugs, the formulation of biopharmaceuticals is in many ways different from conventional low-molecular drug formulation.

Recent reviews list more than 400 biotechnology-based pharmaceutical formulations either registered in clinical trials or undergoing review by the regulatory agencies for the treatment of nearly 150 diseases including cancer, infectious diseases, autoimmune diseases, and AIDS/HIV (1,2). Biotechnology-based pharmaceuticals already on the markets include: recombinant blood factors, recombinant hormones, cytokines, vaccines, monoclonal antibody-based products, and therapeutic enzymes.

This chapter focuses on the general formulation including aspects of production, delivery, stability, and analysis of biotechnology-based pharmaceuticals. Pharmaceutical formulation is, however, an interdisciplinary science, and a successful formulation of a biotechnology-based drug depends on a thorough understanding of, for example, recombinant DNA technology, purification technology, physicochemical and biological characteristics of the biomacromolecule including pharmacokinetic properties and immunogenicity.

PRODUCTION AND PURIFICATION

Typically, the biotechnology-based pharmaceuticals are proteins. Therapeutic proteins are available from a number of different sources, for example, animal tissues, plants, microorganisms, and cell culture systems. However, most commercially available therapeutic proteins are produced by large-scale fermentation using either recombinant microorganisms or mammalian cells as sources. In contrast to extraction from, for example, animal material, one of the advantages of recombinant technology is the possibility of producing pure substances in large quantities. In addition, recombinant technology makes it possible to produce substances that previously were impossible to produce in sufficient quantities. Another advantage of recombinant technology is the possibility to introduce chemical modifications to alter the physicochemical or pharmacokinetic characteristics of a protein to improve the stability or the therapeutic effect. This will be exemplified later. To clone a DNA molecule, it must be introduced into a host cell, where it is allowed to be replicated. This amplification of the original DNA sequence enables the production of proteins by large-scale fermentation.

The proteins obtained by fermentation are either secreted by the host cells into the culture medium or maintained intracellularly. In the subsequent downstream processing, extracellular proteins are normally much simpler to purify than intracellular proteins, as there is no requirement to disrupt the cells to harvest the protein. The protein product is present—often in low concentrations—in a crude, very complex mixture of cell fragments including subcellular components as well as a vast number of other cellular proteins. Compared to microbial sources, mammalian cell cultures; for example, Chinese hamster ovary (CHO) cells are generally more complex production systems, since various supplements, such as serum, often have to be added to the culture media in addition to the nutritional requirements. Addition of serum increases the risk of contamination of the final bulk protein with blood-borne pathogens. However, for a number of therapeutic proteins, mammalian cells are the cell system of choice since mammalian cells, unlike microorganisms, are capable of conducting important posttranslational reactions such as glycosylation.

The challenge for the bulk production of pharmaceutical proteins lies in the development of a purification process to isolate the protein of interest to obtain a highly purified and properly folded protein, which is a prerequisite for making a safe and therapeutic efficient medicine of optimal quality. A typical overall purification process is outlined in Figure 1.

DELIVERY CHALLENGES

The therapeutic application of biotechnology-based drug substances poses several problems, such as the low permeability across biological membranes due to the inherent physicochemical instability of biomacromolecules as well as their high molecular weight and polar surface characteristics. This implies that biotechnology-based pharmaceuticals for systemic treatment are administered parentally, although efforts are made to improve bioavailability via alternative routes of administration as for instance the nasal, pulmonary, and oral route (3–5). A crucial issue to consider is how to overcome these biological barriers, whether the drug delivery system is administered to a patient by

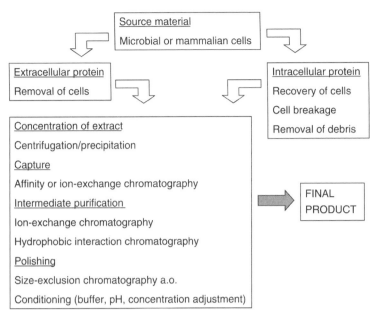

Figure 1 Schematic overview of protein purification from microbial and mammalian sources.

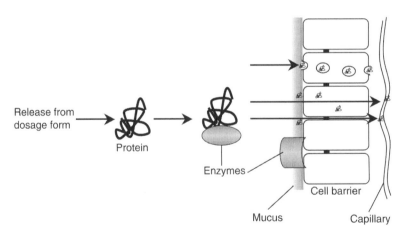

Figure 2 Major biological barriers for transmembrane delivery of biotechnology-based pharmaceuticals.

parenteral or nonparenteral route of delivery or aimed for local or systemic effects. Ways to overcome biological barriers are illustrated in Figure 2.

Briefly, upon release of the macromolecular drug from the delivery system, the drug should withstand hydrolysis and enzymatic activity in the extracellular milieu at the site of absorption. In the case of nonparenteral delivery, the unstirred water layer and especially the viscous mucin layer in particular, both present at the surface of epithelia constitute a barrier for absorption of biotechnology-based pharmaceuticals and must be permeated for the biomacromolecule to reach the surface of the epithelial membrane. A barrier of mucus cell layer does not cover endothelia. Irrespective of the delivery route, the cell layer must be permeated to reach the underlying capillaries. Permeation occurs sporadically by different mechanisms, for example, passive para- or transcellular diffusion or endocytotic transport mechanisms such as macropinocytosis. For macromolecular drugs such as proteins, the mechanism is believed to be dependent on the size, as its uptake and transport are expected to occur mainly by endocytosis (3,5). During the permeation of the epithelial or endothelial cell layer, the stability of the biomacromolecule is further challenged by the intra- and extracellular enzyme activity before the site of action is reached. The general principles of drug absorption and different routes of administration are discussed elsewhere in this book.

Both parenteral and nonparenteral local administration of macromolecular drugs are obviously advantageous for treatment of diseases such as cystic fibrosis and bone regeneration, and the primary biological barriers to overcome upon administration are thus elimination, that is, avoiding washout and enzymatic degradation.

However, when aiming at nonparenteral administration of biotechnology-based pharmaceuticals for systemic delivery, the barrier characteristics of the biological barrier to be permeated should also be taken into account. In Table 1, the properties of different barriers are compared, and the ranges of expected bioavailability are listed.

The formulation strategies ought to ensure that the drug is applied appropriately and released sufficiently from the formulation. Also, the formulation strategy ought to ensure

Table 1 Properties of Nonparenteral Routes of Administration with Respect to Systemic Delivery of Biotechnology-Based Pharmaceuticals

Route	Surface area and accessibility[a]	Physical barrier properties[a]	Enzymatic barrier properties[a]	Bioavailability
Oral	>200 m^2 fairly accessible, site-specific location difficult	Thick mucus layer, columnar epithelial monolayer (10 μm), pH variations	+++++ (and hepatic first pass metabolism)	0–1%
Oromucosal	~0.02 m^2 easily accessible	Mucus, stratified, partly keratinized epithelium (500–600 μm), hydrated	+++	0–5%
Nasal	~0.015 m^2 fairly accessible	Mucus, ciliated, columnar pseudostratified epithelium (10 μm)	+++	2–20%
Pulmonary	~80–140 m^2 not easily accessible	Bronchi and bronchioles: mucus, ciliated columnar pseudostratified epithelium (10–60 μm) Alveoli: squamous epithelial monolayer (<1μm)	++	20–80%
Cutaneous	~1.8 m^2 easily accessible	Keratinized stratified epithelium (100–200 μm)	+	0–1%

[a]Relative properties ranged at a level of + to +++++.
Source: Merged from Refs. 5–7.

that the drug is solubilized in the microenvironment where absorption should occur, and that the drug exists in an absorbable form avoiding complexation and ionization, and further that the drug is as stable as possible against hydrolysis and enzymatic degradation. Ensuring appropriate deposition at the site of absorption often require specific formulation strategies such as a proper aerodynamic diameter of particles for inhalation (8), or enterocoating and also mucoadhesiveness of drug delivery systems for oral and mucosal delivery (9–11). Protection against enzymatic degradation by particulate encapsulation (4) and/or coadministration of competitive enzyme inhibitors will, for most routes of delivery, be advantageous despite the differences in proteolytic activities. Also, for some routes of delivery it might be necessary to apply chemical enhancers or enhancing techniques to achieve a therapeutic level in the systemic circulation (12–15). However, this approach is often likely to compromise the barrier properties increasing the risk of unwanted side effects. Structural modifications of the biomacromolecule and use of drug delivery systems (16) are other approaches to optimize stability and/or membrane permeability.

PROTEIN STRUCTURE

Proteins are complex polymers of the naturally occurring L-amino acids. The amino acids are shown in Table 2, and divided into three classes according to the characteristics of the side chain: (*i*) hydrophobic, (*ii*) ionizable, or (*iii*) hydrophilic but nonionizable. For example, the more hydrophilic groups are those containing atoms or functional groups, which potentially are able to form hydrogen bonds (17).

The molecular weight of a protein is typically in the range of 10 to 100 kDa. Proteins are often discriminated from the smaller peptides due to their size; structures that are larger than 5 kDa are considered to be proteins whereas smaller structures are mostly referred to as peptides (18). The structure of proteins is classically divided into the primary, secondary, tertiary, and quaternary, all comprising different characteristics of the overall protein structure, cf. Figure 3. *The primary structure* is the sequence of amino acid residues, which fold in a certain predetermined manner into *the secondary structure* assisted by the formation of hydrogen bonds (19,20). The hydrogen bond is a strong dipol-dipol attraction either between covalently bonded hydrogen atoms and other electronegative atoms, such as (*i*) oxygen, (*ii*) nitrogen, (*iii*) or between the peptide amide and the carbonyl group (18,20,21). The hydrogen bond between the amide hydrogen and the carbonyl oxygen constitutes the major part, approximately 68%, of the total of hydrogen bonds formed in a globular protein (22). The secondary structural elements, the α-helix or the β-sheet are two of the more commonly observed structures. These structures are also stabilized by the interactions between adjacent side groups or helices (20,21,23). *The tertiary structure* is the overall distribution of the secondary structure into a three-dimensional structure, including the arrangement of the side chains in space. The tertiary structure is also stabilized by hydrophobic and electrostatic interactions. These interactions are caused by charge repulsion and ion pairing, salt bridges, van der Waals forces, and the formation of covalent bonds between the cystine residues, that is, the formation of disulphide bridges (18,20,23–25). In this regard, a distinction between peptides and proteins is also rational, since peptides do not contain a three-dimensional structure. Finally, the *quaternary structure* is the noncovalent assembly, oligomerization of two or more independent protein units into well-defined complexes (25,26). An example is given in Figure 3, where the dimer formation of two insulin monomers as well as the hexamer formation of six insulin monomers are shown (27,28).

Table 2 The Naturally Occurring Amino Acid Residues and Their Characteristics as Well as Commonly Used Abbreviations

Amino acids with side groups which are entirely hydrophobic

Alanine, Ala, A Glycine, Gly, G Valine, Val, V Cysteine, Cys*, C

Leucine, Leu, L Isoleucine, Ile, I Tryptophan, Trp, W

Proline, Pro, P Methinonine, Met, M Phenylalanine, Phe, F

Amino acids with ionisable side groups

Tyrosine, Tyr, Y Cysteine, Cys-H*, C pKa=8.35 Glutamine, Gln, Q

Arginine, Arg, N Lysine, Lys, K pKa=10.79

Aspartic acid, Asp, D pKa=3.9 Glutamic acid, Glu, E pka=4.07 Histidine, His, H pKa= 6.04

Amino acid with hydrophilic but non-ionisable side groups

Serine, Ser, S pKa=16 Threonine, Thr, T pKa=16 Asparagine, Asn, N

*Cystine is shown with two conformations: the single cystine (Cys-H) and the cystine involved in the formation of the disulphide bridge (Cys-).

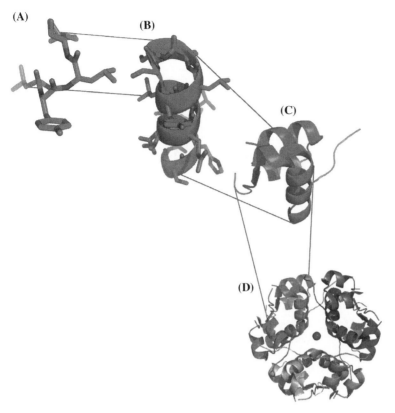

Figure 3 The structural levels of proteins, exemplified by human insulin in the T6 form. (**A**) Primary structure: residues 15–18 of human insulin B-chain, shown as sticks. (**B**) Secondary structure: residues 8–20 of the B-chain form an α-helix, here depicted as a superposition of sticks, and a cartoon-representation. (**C**) Tertiary structure: insulin A- and B-chains fold up to a monomer, which is assumed to be the active form, binding to the insulin receptor. Insulin can exist in different oligomeric forms, depending on formulation and protein concentration. (**D**): The Zn^{2+}-stabilized hexamer form is shown. 2 Zn^{2+} ions are bound per insulin hexamer (only one $Zn2^{+}$-ion is visible in this view). The hexamer is a trimer of dimmers. Figure based on pdb-file 1MSO, produced in Pymol. *Source*: Bente Vestergaard, Biostructural Research, Faculty of Pharmaceutical Sciences, University of Copenhagen.

PROTEIN STABILITY

As previously described, the physical as well as the chemical stability of biopharmaceuticals are critical and need to be optimized when formulating to optimize the outcome after production, processing, formulation, and storage. Specific approaches are addressed in this section.

Maintenance of the structural integrity of the therapeutic proteins is essential with respect to the biological activity, sustaining the release kinetics from a controlled-release formulation and avoiding unwelcome immunological reactions (18,29–31). Hence, the major challenge in the development of pharmaceutical formulations is to avoid unwanted changes in the structure and also to understand the processes and formulation parameters that affect the stability. In Table 3, the major degradation pathways are listed.

Table 3 Major Degradation Pathways for Peptides and Proteins

Physical degradation	Chemical degradation
Denaturation	Hydrolysis
Aggregation	Oxidation
Fibrillation	Racemization
Precipitation	Isomerization
Adsorption	β-elimination
	Deamidation
	Disulfide exchange
	Photodegradation

The physical degradation involves denaturation, precipitation, aggregation, changes in or unfolding of the secondary, tertiary, and quaternary structure of proteins (32–34), and also changes in the primary structure; for example, chemical degradation can lead to perturbation of the protein structure (33,35). However, some changes do not lead to any alteration in protein activity and might occur in areas of the protein that are not directly involved in its functional properties (23).

From a drug delivery aspect, the chemical degradation and the biological activity are, nevertheless, major points to consider, and a drug delivery system with a protein drug cannot be applied fully until the effects on the protein stability are studied. Whether the changes (physical or chemical) are reversible or not depends on the nature of the changes (25).

Physical Stability

In solution, the structure is not infinitely stable in the folded state (18,36), and therefore the structure is affected by production conditions, stress during preparation of the formulation, etc.

Denaturation

The term "denaturation" is used to denote *"a process (or sequence of processes) in which the spatial arrangement of the polypeptide chains within the molecule is changed from that typical of the native protein to a more disordered arrangement"* (33), where *"spatial arrangement"* can be replaced by configuration, conformation, or state of folding. The effect from denaturation can be alterations of specific parameters, such as solubility, loss of activity, or unfolding. In the following sections, denaturation and unfolding are used interchangeably.

One way to describe the unfolding process is the two-state model shown in Figure 4. It is an equilibrium, a single-transition step between the folded native (N) and the disordered, unfolded or denatured (D) species (36–38). An intermediate step, the formation of possible intermediates (I), can be present between the transformation from N to D. The intermediate state (I) has often been described as the molten globule, for example, for growth hormone (39). It is a stable compact, partly denatured species, which retains some ordered secondary structure but not the tertiary structure of the native protein (35,36,40,41). The aggregate (A) formed may occur from irreversible changes to the unfolded species (18,42–44).

Reversible denaturation also occurs, but the resulting structure formed may not always regain the biological activity (40). Many conditions lead to denaturation and not

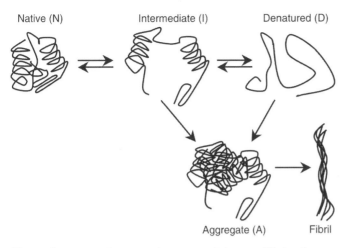

Native (N)   Intermediate (I)   Denatured (D)

Aggregate (A)   Fibril

Figure 4 The protein aggregation process. It is an equilibrium between the folded native (N) and the disordered, unfolded or denatured (D) species. An intermediate step, the formation of possible intermediates (I), can be present between the transformation from N to D. The aggregate (A) formed may occur from irreversible changes to the unfolded species and can result in formations of fibrils (F).

all proteins respond to these conditions in a similar manner. During production for example, proteins do undergo denaturation-renaturation cycles during extraction and purification, and proteins can be unfolded by various factors such as temperature, pH, and pressure. In addition, the characteristics of the denatured state can vary significantly (25). Some of the frequently applied denaturing conditions include denaturants such as, urea or guanidine hydrochloride, heat or other types of stress (45–47).

Aggregation and Fibrillation

Aggregation is used to describe either soluble or insoluble protein assemblies caused by either covalent or noncovalent interactions. The noncovalent interactions can occur between folded; associated, or unfolded proteins; aggregation. This self-association can occur because of changes in the environment such as pH, protein concentration, ionic strength, etc. (25). Aggregates on the other hand, are formed from unfolded or partly unfolded proteins (48). The aggregate formation may involve the formation of covalent bonds, for example, disulfide shuffling, or the formation of noncovalent bonds, for example, hydrophobic interactions (49), where the noncovalent aggregate can be disrupted by denaturing agents, for example, sodium dodecyl sulphate or guanidine hydrochloride (18).

These aggregates contain nonnative structures, for example, intermolecular β-sheet (50), and can cause irreversible changes to the unfolded species, such as precipitation, aggregation, or fibrillation (18,35,43), where precipitation is the macroscopic equivalent of aggregation (40,42). Aggregation is dependent not only on the protein concentration but also on the stress caused by shaking (49,51). The structure of the aggregated proteins can be more or less well defined, and an example of well-defined structures is the formation of insulin fibrils (52,53).

Adsorption

Apart from the unfolding of the protein, physical stability or degradation also includes undesirable adsorption to different surfaces and interfaces, which can induce unwanted

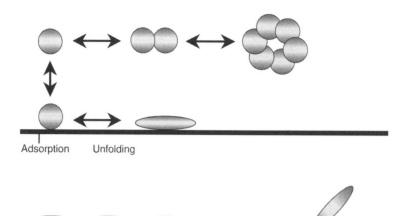

Figure 5 Changes of the conformation of proteins upon adsorption to surfaces. An example of the structural changes, where insulin is believed to adapt to the surface by changing the overall structure exposing the more hydrophobic residues buried in the interior of the protein.

structural changes in the solution (40). Upon adsorption at the surface, the protein structure undergoes a change from its globular configuration in solution to an extended chain structure, that is, surface denaturation (34,35,45). Proteins are amphiphilic molecules that adsorb at interfaces. They are also flexible molecules that adapt to their surroundings, accommodating changes in the environment that they are exposed to at the interface. Proteins readily adsorb at the interface in a manner dependent on bulk concentration, the diffusion coefficient through the solvent, affinity toward the interface, time, and available surface area (54,55). Upon adsorption, proteins may unfold, and this causes a rearrangement in the secondary and tertiary structure (31,56,57). Some proteins exhibit larger resilience against the structural rearrangement at the interface than others; these are often referred to as "hard" while those more structurally labile proteins are referred to as "soft" (58). The soft and less rigid proteins, for example, bovine serum albumin (BSA), unfold almost completely upon adsorption to surfaces (56,58).

An example of the structural changes is shown in Figure 5, where insulin is believed to adapt to the surface by changing the overall structure exposing the more hydrophobic residues buried in the interior of the protein (18,56,57,59,60).

Various surfaces occur during the production, purification, and preparation of proteins as well as in the formulation process, for example, exposure to glass surfaces in vials and air-liquid interfaces in the formulation. All these types of surfaces have various adsorption properties. A major distinction is made between hydrophilic and hydrophobic surfaces as well as air-liquid, liquid-liquid, and solid-liquid surfaces. Naturally, the type of interface also influences the observed structural changes (56,60,61).

Chemical Stability

The major pathways of chemical degradation are, among others, hydrolysis and oxidation as shown in Table 2. An unfolded polypeptide chain in a protein is more prone to chemical degradation than the native and folded protein (46). These chemical degradation reactions may be modifications involving changes in the covalent bonds, for example, deamidation, oxidation, or disulfide bond shuffling (47), and the reactions are usually irreversible (28). The breaking of peptide bonds is referred to as proteolysis and can often

Table 4 Sequences of Amino Acids, Which are Susceptible to Chemical Degradation and Formulation Strategies to Prevent Degradation (29,30,40,62)

Amino acid sequence	Mechanism of degradation	Formulation strategy
cys-cys	s-s reduction	Addition of surfactant, polyalcohols and other excipients
lys, -thr	Copper-induced cleavage	Chelating agents
glu, asp	Deamidation	pH 3–5
asp-pro, asp-tyr	Hydrolysis	pH > 7
asn, gln	Hydrolysis	
trp, met, cys, tyr, his	Oxidation	pH < 7
met	Oxidation	Protect from oxygen
trp	Photodegradation	Protect from light
cys, ser, thr, phe, and lys	Elimination	Acidic pH

lead to extensive configurational changes (23,28). In Table 4, the amino acids and amino acid sequences that are especially prone to chemical alterations or to cause physical alterations are listed. In addition, the formulation strategy to prevent degradation is included.

Hydrolysis most frequently occurs in the side chains of Asn, Gln, and the peptide bond at the C-terminal side of Asp and Pro. Hydrolysis involves the reaction of water and can lead to *deamidation*. The pH has a huge influence on the deamidation rates, since the rate is much slower at acidic pH than at neutral or alkaline pH (30). Deamidation does not always have an effect on the biological activity of the protein but it may affect, for instance, the clearance rate and thereby also the efficacy of the protein (30,62). *Oxidation* is one of the most common degradation pathways of proteins. The amino acids most likely to be influenced are those with sulphur (Cys and Met) and those with aromatic rings (His, Tyr, and Trp). The underlying mechanism involves oxygen and reactive oxygen species, which react with the protein or peptide. The reaction occurs with or without catalysts such as metal ions and it is pH dependent (30). The reaction is also catalyzed by light and is then referred to as *photodegradation or photooxidation*. The amino acids that primarily undergo photooxidation are Trp, Tyr, Phe, and Cys (63).

Other chemical degradation pathways include *β-elimination*, which can lead to racemization and disulphide exchange reactions. The amino acids that may undergo β-elimination include Cys, Ser, Thr, Phe, and Lys (40) and occur especially at alkaline pH (64). The *reduction and oxidation* of the disulphide bonds are often accompanied by a considerable change in the protein conformation (23,33). An example is the secondary structure of insulin that is disrupted or completely lost when the disulphide bonds are broken (23). The disulphide bond disruption or interchange can also result in an altered three-dimensional structure and therefore a possible loss of activity (40) or aggregation (29). For further details, the reader is directed to the following reviews and book chapters (30,40,62,65).

DELIVERY APPROACHES AND ADVANCES

For a successful formulation and delivery of peptides and proteins, it is crucial that the formulation scientist has a thorough knowledge of several factors: the physical and chemical stability of the drug compound, the content of well-defined and selective excipients in the formulation, an optimized storage stability, and naturally, the route of

Table 5 Examples of Formulation Types and Used Excipients

Formulation	Protein	Name and indication	Excipients
Liquid formulations			
Unbuffered solution for injection	Insulin glargine	Lantus (Sanofi-Aventis). Indication: diabetes mellitus	Zinc chloride, m-cresol, glycerol, hydrochloric acid, sodium hydroxide, water for injections, pH 4.0
Suspension for injection	Mixture of fast acting insulin and long acting insulin	Mixtard (Novo Nordisk). Indication: diabetes mellitus	Protamine sulphate, zinc, glycerol, disodium phosphate dehydrate, phenol, and metacresol
Liquid solution for inhalation	Dornase alfa	Pulmozyme (Roche). Indication: cystic fibrosis	Sodium chloride, calcium chloride hydrate, water for injection, pH 7.0
Liquid concentrate for IV administration	Rituximab, glycosylated IgG1-κ immunoglobulin	Mabthera (Roche). Indication: B-cell NHL	Sodium chloride, sodium citrate dehydrate, polysorbate 80 water for injection, pH 6.5
Solid formulations			
Kit for implant	Recombinant human bone morphogenetic protein-2 (rhBMP-2 or dibotermin α)	InductOs (Wyeth) Indication: induction of new bone at the site of implantation	Water for injection, glutamic acid, glycine, sodium chloride, sodium hydroxide polysorbate 80, saccharose, absorbable collagen sponge
Lyophilized powder for injection	Interferon β-1b	Betaferon (Schering AG). Indication: multiple sclerosis	Human albumin, dextrose, sodium chloride solution for reconstitution
Lyophilized powder for injection	Recombinant human antihemophilic factor VIII (rFVIII-SF)	Kogenate (Bayer). Indication: hemophilia A	Sucrose, histidine, glycine, sodium chloride, calcium chloride, water for injections, Ph. Eur.

Abbreviations: IV, intravenous; NHL, non-Hodgkin's lymphoma.

administration being well-chosen, meaning that the absorption barriers can be overcome in a successful manner.

Since the administration routes are mainly parenteral, the formulation has to be injectable. An injectable formulation requires specific excipients, ways of preparation and formulation types; liquid, suspension, or solid formulations. In the development of protein drugs, various formulation principles are used. In Table 5, examples of some of the formulation principles are given.

Liquid Formulations

Liquid formulations for parenteral use require preparation methods and composition that make the formulation stable and sterile. Other requirements for parenteral formulations are given by the European Pharmacopoeia such as tonicity, efficacy of the antimicrobial preservatives, and no content of endotoxins as well as the formulation being essentially free of particles (66). When preparing liquid formulations, the researcher distinguishes between whether the formulation should be a suspension or a homogeneous solution. The choice might depend on the drug properties. However, stability issues and pharmacological effect profiles should be considered as well. Suspensions are a much greater challenge to formulate than simple solutions and often freeze-dried simple solutions are chosen as opposed to suspensions (7). Wang (1999) gives an excellent review on the various excipients used in liquid formulations and their effect on the chemical and physical stability (18).

Solution

In liquid formulation, optimizing the pH, in essence, optimizing the hydrolytic stability is a major issue. It is important to study the stability especially in the range from pH 3 to 10 early on in the formulation process. The solubility depends on the pH value, as does the physical and chemical stability. There is usually a close relationship between optimum solubility and stability. Minimum solubility is observed around the pI values of the proteins. Typically, one would determine the pH range for obtaining the proper solubility and concentration for dosage and then optimize the stability afterwards (18,67).

The way to maintain the pH of the liquid solutions is to add an appropriate buffer system. This may also affect the overall stability of the formulation; for example, the rate of deamidation appears faster in phosphate and bicarbonate buffers than in sulfate, nitrate, acetate, chloride, and pyruvate buffers (30). The ionic strength of the solution changes as the buffer concentration and other excipients, for example, salts to adjust the tonicity, are added, and this has an influence not just on the stability but also on the solubility (18).

One of the major chemical degradation pathways is oxidation, and therefore the oxidative stability in solution has to be optimized. This can be done by choosing proper preparation procedures, storage temperature, and vials, or by addition of antioxidant. Preparing under inert gas, for example, nitrogen, packing in vials, and using stoppers that do not leach can minimize oxidation (18,30). The antioxidants are typically of three different types: true antioxidants, reducing agents, and chelating agents. Typical excipients and their function in formulations are shown in Table 6.

Physical stability can be optimized by selective choices to avoid adsorption to surfaces. For example, by avoiding unneeded agitation, minimizing the surplus air in the vials (exposure to the air-liquid interface), and adding excipients that are more surface-active than the protein itself. Regarding the increase of the competitive adsorption, some of the more frequently used excipients here are surfactants, for example, polysorbates. Cyclodextrin, albumin, or other proteins can also be used to prevent adsorption of the drug. However, the addition can also have adverse effects on the formulation. In the pharmaceutical product Eprex (Janssen-Cilag) containing the protein erythropoietin (EPO), human serum albumin (HSA) was exchanged for polysorbate 80, glycin was added, and the rubber stopper exchanged. One or more of these changes caused an increase in the immunogenicity (68,69).

There are two main mechanisms of solvent-induced stabilization of proteins: (*i*) strengthening of the protein-stabilizing forces or (*ii*) destabilization of the denatured state (18). The most tenable and widely accepted mechanism of protein stabilization in aqueous solution is the preferential interaction of proteins. Preferential interaction indicates that a protein prefers to interact with either water or the excipient. The two conventionally applied terms are: preferential hydration, which means that a protein prefers to interact with water, or preferential exclusion, which means that for example the excipient is

Table 6 Typical Excipients and Their Function in Formulations (18,29,30,73)

Formulation effect	Excipient type	Example
Antiadsorption	Surfactants	Polysorbate 80, poloxamer 188, dextran
	Polymer	PEG
	Other proteins	BSA and HSA
Oxidation protection	Antioxidants	Ascorbic acid, glutathione, propyl gallate, vitamin E
	Chelating agents	EDTA, citric acid, thioglycolic acid, hexaphosphate
Cryo (and lyo-) protectant	Sugars	Sucrose, lactose, glucose, maltose, trehalose
	Polyols	Inositol, ethylene glycol, glycerol, sorbitol, xylitol, mannitol
	Amino acids	Sodium glutamate, proline, α-alanine, β-alanine, glycine
	Polymers	PEG, dextran
	Salts	Succinate, magnesium sulfate, etc.
	Others	Betanine, ethanol, DMSO
	Ligand	Zink, phenol, calcium
pH	Buffer salts	Phosphate, bicarbonate, sulfate, nitrate, acetate, chloride, pyruvate
Stabilizers	Amino acids	Glycine, arginine, alanine, proline, aspartic acid, lysine
	Sugars	Trehalose
	Polyols	Cyclodextrin, mannitol, sorbitol
	Salts	Sodium sulfate, potassium phosphate
	Chelating agents	EDTA
Tonicity	Salts	NaCl and many other salts
	Other	Glycerol

Abbreviations: BSA bovine serum albumin; HSA, human serum albumin; EDTA, ethylenediaminetetraacetic acid; DMSO, dimethylsulfoxide; PEG, polyethylene glycol.

preferential excluded from the protein domain. In the presence of a stabilizing excipient, the protein preferentially hydrates and the excipients is preferentially excluded, that is, more water molecules are found at the surface of the protein than in the bulk (18,70). Since a denatured protein has a larger surface than a native protein, preferential exclusion of the excipient from the surface of the denatured protein is more unfavorable than adsorption to the surface of the native protein. Therefore, stabilization mainly arises from the destabilization of the denatured state (18,36).

In addition to the above-mentioned excipients and functions, preservation of formulations in multiple dose containers is also required. Therefore, antimicrobial preservatives such as phenol, methyl-, and propylparabens are added. Apart from their formulation function the excipients also interact specifically with the protein and can thereby cause alterations in its function and stability (7). For example, phenol has an influence on the stability and conformation of the insulin hexamer. The addition of phenol shifts the structure from the less stable T3 to the more stable R6 (71).

Suspension

Suspensions are solutions containing soluble protein, amorphous particles, crystals, or combinations thereof. However, the rationale for preparing and choosing this formulation type can be simple solubility problems such as if the desired dosage cannot be obtained in solution, or if there is stability issues. For example, can the chemical stability be increased in suspensions, and also from a purely pharmacological point, can the suspension pose as an adjustment of the release profile (7,72). On of the disadvantages is, however, that the preparation is more complex and can vary considerably.

The choice of excipients and the requirements that apply to liquid formulations also apply to suspensions. In addition, the particle size of both the amorphous and crystalline particles has to be controlled in a reproducible manner, as well as the distribution of these in the formulation, for instance, during filling and administration. The excipients need to keep the size distribution of the particles in the suspension should not disrupt distributions between crystalline and amorphous particles nor induce particle growth as such. Therefore, controls of the particle sizes are needed, for example, by dynamic light scattering. The choice of formulation as suspension adds on to the stability issues since the distribution of the particles and soluble drug needs to be constant, the particles resuspendable, injectable, and easy to use. The particles can be prepared by precipitation, crystallization and the process is heavily dependent on the excipients and external parameters such as temperature and time (7). There are only few examples of purely crystalline formulations, for example, insulin in Ultratard (Novo Nordisk) and growth hormone (rhGH) have shown to be able to formulate as long-acting crystals (72). The growth hormone product is a formulation of polyelectrolyte (polyarginine)-coated crystals of rhGH formed by complexation and crystallization. The release from this formulation is comparable to seven daily injections (72).

Solid Formulations

In the solid state proteins are frequently more stable, so formulations of solid dosage forms are often used to increase the stability. However, the process of making solids is still quite challenging.

Two frequently used methods are lyophilization (freeze-drying) and spray drying; common for both processes are the formation of particles that require hydration or reconstitution before use and the removal of water (solvent) from the liquid formulation. Therefore, the effects from the removal of water and the use of excipients to substitute the hydrogen bonds are a major issue. Pharmaceutically, freeze-drying is the most commonly used process for ensuring long-term storage stability of proteins (30,73,74). Freeze-drying of proteins enhances the physical stability by inducing a rigid protein structure, due to the reduced molecular mobility in the solid state compared to protein solutions. The aim of an optimized freeze-dried process is to obtain the protein in a solidified, freeze-dried cake, which fixes the protein in a rigid structure with low moisture content and with the durability to be stored over the desired period of time.

The freeze-drying process is divided into three stages: Freezing, primary drying (where the solvent is removed by sublimation), and secondary drying (where the residual solvent is removed by desorption). When freezing, ice crystals are formed and physically separated from the proteins (74). Lowering the temperature below the freezing point makes the bulk freeze. However, some of the water remains unfrozen and is adsorbed onto the proteins. Removing water during the freezing process increases the concentration of proteins, and of excipients if added. Primary drying is the step where the bulk water is removed (74). During the primary drying step, the ice crystals are removed from the bulk material by sublimation. In the secondary drying step, the unfrozen adsorbed water is removed. The amount of residual water can be up to 20% and is adsorbed to the cake. The residual water is removed by raising the temperature (74). Hereby, the water is removed by diffusion, flowing from a region with high concentration to a region with lower concentration. The water content ought to be reduced to a level that is optimal for the stability of the protein. This is typically less than 1 to 2 w/w % (74,75). However, the level of water can also be too low causing the protein hydration layer to be disrupted. This may result in conformational changes and aggregation (44).

The freeze-drying of proteins yields a dried powder containing the protein in a glassy phase often including amorphous excipients and residual water. The amorphous state is important for maximizing the stability after freeze-drying because this state allows maximal hydrogen bonding (73). The transition between the rubbery (glass-like) and glassy (solid-like) state is called the glass transition temperature (T_g). This parameter can be used to characterize the freeze-dried product. Raising the temperature above the T_g increases the mobility. Therefore, T_g should be as high as possible so that durable storage stability, preferably at room temperature, can be obtained. Also, the storage temperature can be increased with higher T_g values (73).

It is often necessary to add stabilizing excipients to stabilize proteins during the stress induced by a freeze-drying process. The stabilizing excipients can have cryoprotectant and/or lyoprotectant effects on the protein (75,76). Cryoprotection is generally believed to be accomplished by a preferential interaction. In the presence of a stabilizer, the protein thereby interacts preferentially with water, and the excipient is preferentially excluded (73). Lyoprotection effects can operate by the water-replacement theory. Stabilizing excipients can replace water by forming hydrogen bonds with the polar groups on the protein surface ensuring the protein conformation (77,78). Commonly used excipients are sugars, which have effects both during the freezing and drying processes. Furthermore, the addition of amino acids can act as cryoprotectants and/or lyoprotectants, some examples are shown in Table 6.

The addition of excipients generally lowers the T_g of the freeze-dried product when compared to the protein without added excipients. The T_g of proteins is high, above 150°C (75) and typically the T_g of excipients ranges from 50°C to 20°C. Therefore, formulation of proteins often includes stabilizing excipients, which decrease the T_g. The T_g of the freeze-dried product depends on the individual T_g and mass fraction of each compound in the solution. (75). When reducing sugars are used as protectants, they may react with the amino acid groups in the protein. This reaction is known as the Maillard reaction (described in 1912 by Maillard). The Maillard reaction occurs at high temperatures forming a browning carbohydrate complex (79). Some practical advice on how and what to take into account when formulating freeze-dried products can be found in Carpenter et al. (1997) (78) and Schwegman et al. (2005) (80).

Spray drying, is the process in which a liquid is transformed into dry particles by atomization. The process consists of a droplet formation step followed by evaporation of the liquid, typically, spraying of a liquid into hot air. The major concern when using biomacromolecules is the temperature applied and whether the protein can withstand the stress effects (81,82). Maa and Prestrelski (2000) review the different possibilities for preparing particles for pharmaceutical applications (82).

Advances in Delivery of Biotechnology-Based Pharmaceuticals

The use of advanced drug delivery systems for the delivery of biomacromolecules is typically either as particles or as complex liquid formulations. However, relatively few products have reached and are still on the market (83). Part of the developments is centered on exploiting new routes of administration and improving the bioavailability across the biological barriers. The quest for novel approaches to avoid barriers of adsorption and to improve delivery of biomacromolecules is an ever-evolving area. New materials are sought, exploited in search for improvement of the bioavailability or the possibility to deliver the proteins to new targets both locally and systemically.

Pulmonary Delivery

In the development of formulations for pulmonary delivery, control of the particle size is essential, since only particles below 5 μm are able to pass on to the deeper airways (8,84). The pulmonary route of delivery was first employed in 1925 with aqueous nebulization of insulin; however, the marketed product remains scarce (3). Shoyele et al. (85) list potential biomacromolecules that could be delivered through the lungs, but few have reached the market yet. An example is the treatment of cystic fibrosis (local) using Pulmozyme (Roche). It is an inhalation fluid containing dornase alfa in sterile water, pH ~7.0 (other excipients are calcium chloride and sodium chloride) (86). It was marketed in 1996 (3). Another product, Exubera (Pfizer), was withdrawn from the market in October, 2007, not due to safety or efficacy reasons, but because only few patients were treated with it (87). Exubera is a homogeneous insulin powder formulation containing sodium citrate (dihydrate), mannitol, glycine, and sodium hydroxide as excipients. The particle size is distributed so that a fraction of the total particle mass is emitted as fine particles capable of reaching the deep lung. Up to 45% of the 1 mg blister contents, and up to 25% of the 3 mg blister contents, may be retained in the blister (88), this will invariably cause variability in the delivered doses. Other companies were at this point in time still developing inhalable insulin formulations. Examples are Novo Nordisk (AERx), Alkemes (AIR), and MandKind Corporation (Technosphere®insulin), and some argue that the devices are potentially better while others say that their formulation is more rational (3,89). So in that respect, the potential for a viable inhalable protein formulation for systemic administration is still there.

Nasal Delivery

An alternative to the pulmonary route of administration is the nasal route, which is less demanding when it comes to formulation. With regard to, for example, particle size and simpler device development (5,90), examples are Minirin® (Ferring), desmopression, and Suprecur® (Sanofi-Aventis), buserelin, which are proteins formulated as nasal drops or nasal spray, where bioavailabilities of approximately 3% to 10% can be obtained. The formulations are just protein dissolved in purified water containing preservatives: chlorbutanol and benzalkonium chloride (91,92). However, more advanced delivery systems are also used, for example, chitosan formulations where bioavailabilities of 14% to 15% compared to subcutaneous administration can be obtained (90). A recent review by Illum (2007) gives more details on nanoparticulate systems used for nasal delivery (93) or consult Costantino et al. (2007) on the physiochemical and therapeutic aspects (5).

Oral Delivery

Oral delivery of biomacromolecules, especially peptides and proteins, poses a considerable challenge but also has great potential (94). A recent review on the formulation possibilities can be found in Mahato et al. (2003) (6). Examples of products on the market with desmopresin in oral or sublingual formulations are Minirin® (Ferring) melt tablets and tablets, Nocutil (Gebro Pharma), both with bioavailabilities of approximately 0.25% and 0.1% (95,96). However, the low bioavailabilities do tend to reduce the potential of biomacromolecules being delivered by this route, but intense research is taking place to increase the bioavailability. Alternative formulations are encapsulation into particles, for example, containing chitosan or thiomers or increasing the interaction with the intestinal mucus (10,11,97,98). The sublingual route is also used in Grazax® (ALK-Abelló), a melt tablet containing allergens of grass pollen, however, a systemic effect here is not expected (99).

Cutaneous Delivery

Delivery across the dermis (transdermal) or into the dermis (dermal) poses a considerable challenge for biomacromolecules. Formulation concepts are based on chemical enhancers, iontophoresis, or iontophoresis in combination with electroporation (100,101) or the formation of radio frequency–formed microchannels (102). A review on this topic as well as need-free injections can be found in Schuertz et al. (2005) (103).

Particle Encapsulation

Microparticles By encapsulation of protein in polymeric microspheres or solid microparticles, a sustained release profile can be obtained as well as a once-daily or once-weekly administration. For example, Zoladex (AstraZeneca), where goserelin is embedded in an absorbable lactid/glycolid copolymer, which releases goserelin continually over 28 days (104). Other examples of products based on polymeric microspheres are Lupron depot (TAP Pharmaceutical Products Inc), Pamorelin® (Ipsen Scandinavia), Sandostatin LAR depot (Novartis), and Decapeptyl (Debiopharm) (104–108). Some are formulated as implants releasing the drug compound over 28 days to one month (Zoladex), while others are suspensions, where a sustained-release is obtained. Nutropin depot, a depot formulation of growth hormone (rhGH) for once-weekly administration, is a formulation of micronized particles of rhGH embedded in biocompatible, biodegradable polylactide-coglycolide (PLG) microspheres (109), which was marketed in 1999 (by Genentech) and withdrawn from the market in 2004.

Microspheres are prepared by encapsulating the protein in a polymeric matrix either by solvent evaporation, coaservation, lyophilization, or spray drying. During the process, exposure to agitation, interfaces, and other types of denaturing stress should be minimized. Polymers introduced to prepare microspheres for controlled delivery of peptide and proteins can be either synthetic or purified from natural resources. The choice of material will depend on the desired release profile as well as the administration route, since many of the polymers are biodegradable. Some examples of polymers used are alginate, poly(lactic-co-glycolic acid) (PLGA), chitin, chitosan, or sodium hyaluronate. (9,110–113). The release mechanism from polymeric microspheres is diffusion, polymer degradation, or a combination of the two (111,114). However, one of the main drawbacks typically associated with the formulation of proteins in microspheres is the initial burst and the incomplete release of all the encapsulated protein (115,116). The amount of protein released from microspheres reaches approximately 28.2% to 54.7% for different formulations within the first day but with no subsequent release the following days (116). Thus, an incomplete release is exhibited. The incomplete release is likely to arise from noncovalent aggregates formed either within the microspheres or from the lyophilization process (116,117).

Nanoparticles Nanoparticles can be formed from surfactants, polymers, or polyamino acids. The concept is mainly that viable particles are formed, they can maintain their shape and use during preparation, they are stable, and the particles formed are in the nanometer range. An example of nanoparticles is the Medusa® concept by Flamel Technologies.

Nanoparticles of 10 to 50 nm are formed by poly L-glutamate grafted with a hydrophobic α-tocopherol (Medusa II) or of synthetic copolymer of natural leucine and glutamate amino acids (Leu hydrophobic and Glu hydrophilic) (Medusa I) (118,119). The amphiphilic character of the polyamino acid polymers drives the self-assembling of the nanoparticles in water; the poly-Leu chains are packed inside the structure, whereas those of Glu amino acids are exposed to water. The nanoparticles, which are 20 to 50 nm in diameter, are composed of 95% water and 5% Leu-Glu polymer. They are robust over a wide range of pH levels and can be stored as either stable liquid or stable dry forms (118,119). The Medusa I is used together with insulin in Basulin, and this formulation is the first controlled-release insulin formulation that uses recombinant human insulin rather than an insulin analog as in, for example, Lantus (Lilly) or Levemir (Novo Nordisk) (119). Other examples include the case of bone engineering (InductOs from Wyeth), where several different types of nanoparticulate systems have been tested (120). Solid lipid nanoparticles (SLN) are used for both parenteral and nonparenteral delivery, where mucosal membranes, blood-brain, and topical barriers may be surpassed (31,121). The encapsulations efficiencies vary immensely with the method of preparation and the excipients and protein used, but incorporation efficiencies from 1% to almost 100% can be obtained (31). The release from SLN can be a burst or an incomplete release, depending on the way the protein is incorporated (31).

One of the few potential successful sustained-release lipid formulations of biomacromolecules is the Depofoam™ concept by SkyePharma. It is different from the conventional liposomes by the increased surface area available, which makes the aqueous volume larger (122). It has been shown to successfully encapsulate (60–85%) and sustain the release of insulin, luteinizing hormone-releasing factor and others (123).

Chemical enhancers Another approach is a combination of particulate formation and enhancement of the delivery by use of enhancers that increase the ability of the biomacromolecules to cross membranes. Some examples are Eligen® and the SMART concept. The Eligen® technology employs low molecular weight compounds, for example, N-[8-(2-hydroxybenzoyl)amino]caprylat (SNAC) that interact weakly or noncovalently with the protein increasing its lipophilicity. Consequently, this increases the ability of the proteins to cross membranes and into the blood stream (12,13). The SMART concept of pH sensitive and membrane-destabilizing polymers enhances the uptake of biomacromolecules into the cytoplasm. These polymers undergo conformational changes as the pH changes in the endosome. The polymers are of the following types; pyridyl disulfide acrylate (PDSA) or poly(ethylarylic acid) (PEAA)(14,15).

Modification of Peptides and Proteins

Another approach to optimize the release and biological activity of protein drugs is to modify the drug compound itself (18). Protein conjugation is an expanding field in the search for ways to improve the efficacy of protein drugs (124). Conjugation can be defined as the covalent binding of one or more molecules to a drug molecule (125,126). Different conjugation strategies can be applied in the field of proteins. These include glycosylation (127,128) and attachment of fatty acids, i.e. acylation (129,130). Additionally, a large area of protein conjugation involves the attachment of polymers, for example, polyethylene glycol (PEG) (125,126). This invariably also leaves many choices and experiments as to which modifications to use and also subsequent formulation studies just with a modified protein. On the market are amino acid–substituted analogues, PEGylated and acylated proteins, for example, Proleukin (Novartis), Humalog (Lilly), NovoRapid (Novo Nordisk), Lantus® (Sanofi-Aventis), and Apidra® (Sanofi-Aventis), PEGylated: Neulasta (Amgen),

Pegasys (Roche), Somavert (Pfizer) and PegIntron (SP Europe), and acylated: Levemir (Novo Nordisk), and in Phase 3 trials Liraglutide (Novo Nordisk)(131).

Modification of the amino acid sequence The stability, biological activity, and distribution of proteins can be changed by alteration in the amino acid sequence. The main purpose is to increase or alter the pharmacological effect, but exchange of the chemical liable amino acids can also be employed. By altering the sequence, exchanging, or adding amino acids the pharmacological profile can be changed. Insulin has the alteration of proline at B28 to Asp, insulin aspart, NovoRapid (Novo Nordisk) and it has increased the onset of action to approximately 10 to 20 minutes after injection. This is due to the reduced tendency for insulin aspart to form hexamer, which increases the absorption rate upon injection (132–134). Similar profiles are obtained with insulin lispro, Humalog (Lilly), where Lis and Pro are exchanged at B28 and B29 and with insulin glulisin, Apidra[®] (Sanofi-Aventis), where Asp at position B3 is replaced by Lys, and Lys at position B29 is replaced by Glu (135–137).

A prolonged action can also be obtained, for example, insulin glargin, Lantus[®] (Sanofi-Aventis). It differs from native human insulin by three amino acids; Gly in position A21, and 2 Arg at the C-termial in the B-chain at position B31 and B32 (138,139). These alterations shift the pI of the protein from 5.4 to 7.0, which make the protein more soluble at acidic pH and insoluble at neutral pH. This leads to the formation of micro precipitates upon injection. The insulin is subsequently released slowly from the precipitate and absorbed from the injection site (138,139). The substitution at position A21 also alters the association properties, which makes the hexamer more stable. The release profile of insulin glargin is more flat, avoiding the peak concentrations seen for other insulin types (140). A prolonged effect and faster acting is also obtained in Proleukin (Novartis), where aldesleukin is produced as: nonglycosylated, containing no N-terminal alanine, and a replacement of Cys125 by Ser125 (141).

Modification by PEGylation Protein PEGylation is defined as the covalent conjugation of PEG to proteins (142). Conjugation of PEG, PEGylation, is now widely used due to its advantageous effects on therapeutic efficacy, low toxicity, relatively simple chemistry, and commercial availability. The main objective of protein PEGylation is to maintain the inherent therapeutic activity after modification while also optimizing the pharmacokinetic profile of the drug (125,126). In first generation PEGylation, typically small (2–5 kDa) PEG was randomly attached to the protein chain resulting in different PEGylated species with various PEGylation sites. The random attachment could potentially diminish biological activity (125). Second generation PEGylation includes improved PEGylated proteins using site-specific PEGylation with a better potential for preserving biological activity. Larger and sometimes branched PEGs are applied (20–40 kDa), and usually the proteins are monoPEGylated. The first PEGylated protein product to reach the market was adenosine deamidase (Adagen[®] by Enzon Inc.) in 1990. Adagen[®] contains multiple PEGylated isomers (143). The marketed products differ with respect to PEGylation site, size of PEG attached, and the number of PEGs attached.

Modification by acylation Acylation is the conjugation of an acylchain to the proteins (129,130). The rationale for acylating peptides is alteration in the circulation time and increased stability against degradation. One of the protein products on market is an insulin product, Levemir (Novo Nordisk). Determir has an increased circulation time due to the attachment to serum albumin; approximately 98% is bound (129,144,145). In Determir, a C-14 acylchain is attached to insulin at B29. Another product in Phase 3 trials is

Liraglutide, where a C-16 acylchain is attached to glucagons-like peptide (GLP-1) at position 26. For Liraglutide, the attachment of the acylchain decreases the enzymatic degradation, and thereby elimination in the kidneys. This results in prolonged half-life, also because of binding to serum albumin (130).

Modification by glycosylation Glycosylation is one of the naturally occurring modifications to the proteins (127,128). It describes the pattern of sugar moieties attached to the protein. It varies with the cell type used during the production. In other words, it is only human cells that produce the identical human proteins with regard to glycosylation pattern. It can be used in formulation to increase stability (146), but it is mostly the cause of differences between the produced drug compound and the naturally occurring protein. In the formulation of EPO, the alteration in the glycosylation patterns is thought to cause increased immunogenicity (69).

CHARACTERIZATION OF BIOTECHNOLOGICAL PHARMACEUTICALS

From the formulation point of view, the determination of, for instance, purity and structural changes of proteins when they are exposed to denaturing conditions, effects from addition of the excipients, effects from preparation of the drug delivery system, and stability are some of the main concerns. Major considerations, when choosing the methods for studying the stability of proteins, are the complexity of the formulation and the excipients used. In Table 7, a list of methods is given as well as a brief overview of the advantages and disadvantages of the method in a formulations study. For further insight into methods to examine protein formulations and structural stability, the reader is suggested to consult the following (124,147–149).

Structure Determination

Structural data is of high importance for peptide and protein characterization; however, data need to be obtained on highly purified samples. First of all, the primary structure can be determined by amino acid analysis, peptide mapping or Edman degradation, where the protein is degraded from the N-terminal and the sequence of amino acids determined subsequently. A similar procedure can be performed from the C-terminal. Protein modifications and posttranslational modifications such as glycosylations are thus identified. Furthermore, the primary structure along with effects from chemical degradation can also be determined by mass spectrometry (MS) (149,150).

The 3D structure of proteins, the secondary and tertiary structure, can be determined by Fourier transform infrared spectroscopy (FTIR), circular dichroism (CD), and fluorescence. The maintenance of the globular structure is essential for the biological and pharmacological activity of proteins. The assessment of structure can be complex and often several complementing methods are applied, for example, X-ray crystallography, nuclear magnetic resonance (NMR) as well as FTIR, CD, and fluorescence spectroscopy. Many of these methods can also be used after preparation of the formulation to determine alterations caused by addition of excipients. FTIR is often applied when studying structural changes in proteins induced by various factors and when studying proteins in different environments and in different sample forms, for example, in solid or solution (151–153). It is a sensitive technique and is often used to monitor the α-helix-β-sheet refolding that follows aggregation (48). CD is also

Table 7 Useful Methods for Determination of Protein Structure and Stability as Well as Characterization of the Formulation

Technique	Information obtained	Remarks
Structure and stability of the protein		
Amino acid analysis	Amino acid composition	Easily automated
Edman degradation	(Partial) amino acid sequence	Easily automated
MS	Accurate mass, chemical degradation	Requires expert personnel
Peptide mapping + mass spectroscopy	Amino acid sequencing, chemical degradation	Can be automated, but optimization and interpretation takes time
RP chromatography	Chemical degradation (various types), impurities, content of active compound and additives	Very versatile, can be automated, but protein analysis is generally not easy to optimize
SEC	Molecular size, aggregation, hydrolysis	Limited resolution
IEX	Relative molecular charge, chemical degradation with changes in charge	Limited resolution
AC	Integrity of affinity site, presence of multiple conformers with different affinities	Impossible to determine which structural changes have occurred
FFF	Molecular size, aggregation, hydrolysis	Milder technique than SEC
CE or CZE	Depending on matrix and set-up, same as the chromatographic methods above	Requires very little sample, but less established than HPLC
X-ray crystallography	3D structure of protein (in crystal)	Slow procedure, requires expert personnel
NMR	3D structure of protein	Slow procedure, requires expert personnel
FTIR	Protein secondary structure, crystallinity of the dry formulation	Can measure any physical state (gas, solution, solid) but requires high concentrations. Small volume, complex mixtures possible (drug delivery systems).
(FT-)Raman spectroscopy	Protein secondary structure (solution + solid state), local structure around certain absorbing amino acids, crystallinity of the dry formulation	Same as FTIR, can even be used for in-process control
CD	Protein secondary and tertiary structure in solution	Accurate protein concentration required for secondary structure, can only measure solutions
Fluorescence spectroscopy	Local structure around fluorophores, presence of fluorescent impurities	Easy to do, but interpretation difficult Trp, tyr, and phe in the amino acid sequence required

Table 7 Useful Methods for Determination of Protein Structure and Stability as Well as Characterization of the Formulation (*Continued*)

Technique	Information obtained	Remarks
DSC (solution)	Protein thermal stability	Protein thermal stability can also be measured with spectroscopic techniques, but with lower precision
DSC (solid state)	Crystallinity, glass transition	A must-have for lyophilized products
AUC	Protein size, aggregates	Not very common technique
ITC	Binding kinetics, interactions with excipients	–
Characterization of the formulation		
Rheology	Viscosity of formulation	Can be evaluated in various ways, important for injections
NIR	Water content, crystallinity, formulation structure	Can be used during in-process control. Interpretation difficult
TGA	Water content, melting point of formulation	–
Karl-Fischer titration	Water content	–
Surface tension	Protein adsorption	Often high volumes are required
TIRF	Protein adsorption	Modified proteins are required, fluorescence-based technique
EM, e.g., SEM, EM TEM, and CryoTEM	Imaging, particle form and integrity	–
AFM	Structure of adsorbed layers	Requires expert personnel
SAXS	Structure, unfolding and kinetics	Requires access to scarce facilities
SANS	Structure, unfolding and kinetics	Requires access to scarce facilities
DLS or SLS	Presence of large aggregates/impurities, determination of hydrodynamic radius of protein and self-assembly	Can be performed using stand-alone dedicated instruments, or in a more basic way using fluorescence and UV spectrometers
(SDS-)PAGE (gel electrophoresis)	Molecular size, aggregation and type of aggregates (noncovalent, cystein-bonded)	Simple, potentially high resolution
IEF	pI of protein, chemical degradation with changes in charge, and heterogeneity (e.g., of certain carbohydrates)	Simple, potentially very high resolution
Binding assays, e.g., ELISA	Binding site integrity, concentration determination	Sometimes limited precision, but very high sensitivity

Abbreviations: RP, reverse phase; SEC, size-exclusion chromatography, MS, mass spectrometry; FTIR, Fourier transform infrared spectroscopic; CD, circular dichroism; IEX, Ion-exchange chromatography; AC, affinity chromatography; FFF, field flow fractionation; CE or CZE, capillary electrophoresis; NMR, nuclear magnetic resonance; DSC, differential scanning calorimetry; TGA, thermogravitometric analysis; SEM, scanning electron microscopy; AUC, Analytical Ultracentrifugation; ITC, Isotherm titration calorimetry; NIR, Near-infrared spectroscopy; TIRF, Total Internal Reflectance Fluorescence spectroscopy; EM, Electron microscopy; TEM, transmission electron microscopy; Cryo TEM, cryo-transmission electron microscopy; AFM, atomic force microscopy; SAXS, small angle X-ray scattering; SANS, small angle neutron scattering; DLS, dynamic light scattering; SLS, static light scattering; IEF, isoelectric focusing.

used to determine structural alterations but only on liquid formulations (149), as it is more sensitive to the physical appearance of the solution such as light scattering. Fluorescence measurements on proteins are based on the fact that it is possible to excite the intrinsic fluorescent amino acid residues in protein, that is, tryptophan, tyrosine, and phenylalanine. Intrinsic tryptophan fluorescence in proteins is highly dependent on the local environment and in that respect, very useful for monitoring changes in the local protein conformation, that is, local tertiary structural changes (154). A distinction between three classes of tryptophan residues with different emission maximum (λ_{max}) is often applied, that is, deeply buried, close to the surface, and one on the surface (155,156). The span in the fluorescence maximum is often described from that of the "buried" in azurin (~ 308 nm) to that of the fully exposed in glucagon (~ 355 nm) illustrating the versatility of tryptophan fluorescence (156,157). For further reading on the specific methods, we suggest the following books and references (124,149,151,158,159).

Stability Determination

In a formulation study, alterations caused by either the process or the excipients are of interest. These alterations can be either chemical or physical in nature. The physical stability of formulations is assessed by determining the physical structure of a protein in the formulation, that is, by determining the changes in secondary, tertiary, and quaternary structure. This is often done by FTIR and CD, but differential scanning calorimetry (DSC) can also determine changes in the stability of the protein. DSC is useful for obtaining information on the folding thermodynamics of globular proteins (148,160), for example, the transition from native to denatured conformation and the unfolding of the different domains comprising the globular protein (161,162). It is also a frequently used technique for screening of the effectiveness of excipients as regards the thermal stress that the protein solution is exposed to in the DSC experiment (163). However, for accurate determination of the effects of excipients, a combination of methods is useful. For example, when Tween was added to a protein, the T_m value fell, which usually indicates a destabilization, where other tests did not indicate this destabilization (163,164). The α-helical structure is generally disrupted by the thermal denaturation, which also reflects change in the overall protein structure (165). In addition, methods like SDS-PAGE, light scattering, and others can also be used to assess physical changes such as aggregation. Chemical stability is often determined by, for example, HPLC or MS (150).

Characterization of the Formulation

The stability and suitability of the formulations also needs to be determined, for example, whether the viscosity of the formulation is suitable for the administration route and is stable over time. The water content is a parameter that often has a direct influence on the stability of solid formulations and may influence the appearance of freeze-dried products immensely. Karl-Fisher titration, thermogravitometric analysis (TGA), or DSC is normally used to determine the water content. Various microscopic techniques, where both macroscopic and microscopic appearance of formulation can be determined, such as particle appearance by scanning electron microscopy (SEM) or transmission electron microscopy (TEM), are usually only needed for special formulation. There are several other methods, but which one to choose depends entirely on the formulation and the critical parameters (149,150).

NUCLEIC ACID–BASED DRUGS

As described in the introduction to this chapter, nucleic acid–based therapeutics are attracting increasing interest. Gene replacement therapies and gene vaccines are no longer the only targets, as antisense oligonucleotides, which suppress or block expression of certain proteins, are now considered efficient and promising future therapeutics for clinical development. Currently, a number of DNA vaccines and oligonucleotides are in clinical trials for treatment of infectious diseases including AIDS/HIV infections, different stages and types of cancer, cardiovascular and neurological diseases, as well as genetic deficiency disorders, and autoimmune and metabolic diseases (1,166). To date, however, few products have been approved, one being Vitravene® (Ciba Vision/Isis Pharmaceuticals), an injectable that was approved by Food and Drug Administration (FDA) in 1998 for the treatment of cytomegalovirus retinitis in patients with AIDS (1,2). However, the drug has currently the marketing status of discontinued (167). Another product is Macugen® (Osi Eyetech), which is an aptamer RNA oligonucleotide, which binds to extracellular vascular endothelial growth factor (VEGF)(2,168). Other products are Gendicine® (Shenzhen SiBono GenTech) and H101/Oncorine® (Shanghai Sunway Biotech), which are both approved by the Chinese State FDA with the indication of cancer treatment supplementing chemotherapy. The latter two products are adenovirus vector–based p53 gene therapeutics (2,169).

Because of the high-sequence specificity of nucleic acid–based therapeutics, and thereby high potencies and low levels of off-target effects, the use of gene medicine seems promising. However, as for peptide and protein therapeutics, one of the major challenges is to efficiently deliver the nucleic acid–based drug to the target organ as well as to the intracellular target.

By nature, the nucleic acid therapeutics have a high negative charge density and are enzymatically labile hydrophilic biomacromolecules; thus, efficient delivery of these therapeutics faces similar challenges as the peptide and protein therapeutics. Irrespective of whether the nucleus (in the case of DNA delivery) or the cytoplasm (e.g., for siRNA delivery) of the cell is the intracellular target site, protection and targeting approaches are required to efficiently deliver the drug.

Although the siRNA duplexes used in gene silencing therapy are more resilient toward degradation by nucleases than single-stranded DNA, unmodified sequences of nucleic acids are inherently unstable in biological systems and need protection against degradation by either chemical modification or by use of a protecting delivery system. Chemical modifications to increase half-lives as well as binding affinities include sugar and backbone modifications, resulting in morpholino and peptide nucleic acid (PNA) analogs, sugar modifications by 2′-position modifications of the sugar moieties, resulting in formation of locked nucleic acids (LNA), heterocyclic modification as well as conjugations of fatty acids and cholesterol (170). Example of promising therapeutics is the HIF-1 α-antagonist developed from the LNA-platform and currently in clinical trials for treatment of solid tumors and lymphoma.

Parenteral administration is the primary route of testing delivery for nucleic acid therapeutics irrespective of whether systemic or local effects are desired. However, to some extent, pulmonary and oral routes are also investigated as potential routes for local targeting to treat cystic fibrosis or colonic tissue (171–173). For nonparenteral delivery, the use of pharmaceutical excipients in the formulation is critical. In addition, the production costs of nucleic acid therapeutic–containing drug delivery systems should be minimized. Even for intravenously or subcutaneously injected nucleic acid–based therapeutics, the use of protective carriers is most likely necessary, and advantageous as compared to injection of the naked RNA or DNA. Carriers can be divided into viral or nonviral carriers, with the viral vectors based on adeno- or retrovirus. As a result of the overall negative charge of the nucleotides, the nonviral carriers are most often based on positive carriers that complex with, encapsulate, or are even covalently conjugated to the siRNA. One of the most-studied carrier systems is liposomes, containing cationic lipids in which the biomacromolecule is encapsulated and which facilitate interaction with the cellular plasma membrane components. The liposomes may be modified by PEG. Thereby, a prolonged systemic circulation and passive targeting to inflammatory and cancer tissue are obtained due to the enhanced retention and permeability effect. In addition, active targeting moieties as for example folate or the vasculature targeting arginine-glycine-aspartate (RGD) peptide may be incorporated into the liposomal structure to achieve better delivery efficiencies (174). One of the main concerns with positively charged lipids and positively charged polymers such as polyethyleneimine (PEI) is their toxicity. However, the cationic charge provides the advantage of high loading efficiency but the disadvantage of tissue toxicity, thus surface modifications are necessary. Other approaches to deliver nucleic acids to the appropriate cellular interior are the use of cationic peptides conjugated or complexed with the nucleic acid (16,175), fusogenic lipids or protein sequences (176–178), and localizing sequences, such as the nuclear localizing signal (NLS) sequences that mediate nuclear entrance from the cytoplasm (179).

Since the chemistry used in nucleic acid drug research has reached the current level, the major limiting step is delivery of the therapeutic, and several technological challenges need to be overcome in terms of stability, efficient and controlled delivery as well as addressing safety. So the limited number of currently registered products is by no means indicative of failure of these potentially revolutionary types of drugs.

REGULATORY ASPECTS

Within the European Union, three possibilities of applying for a marketing authorization exist, the central procedure, the mutual recognition procedure, and the national procedure. The central procedure is compulsory for biotechnology-based pharmaceuticals, and the marketing authorization is granted by the European Medicines Evaluation Agency (EMEA) covering the EU member states. In the United States, regulatory control and review of biotechnology-based pharmaceuticals is administrated by the Center for Biologics Evaluation and Research (CBER) of the U.S. FDA. In contrast, a New Drug Application (NDA) is to be submitted for products to be approved by the Center for Drugs Evaluation and Research (CDER).

The purpose of the documentation for obtaining a marketing authorization is for the applicant to document a consistent quality, safety, and efficacy of the product, and to enable the regulatory agencies to evaluate that the risk-benefit ratio of the product is acceptable from a public health point of view. However, it is important to realize that the guidelines are guidelines and not legally binding documents. This means that the applicant must provide satisfactory documentation for the specific product, and the authorities may require additional documentation if considered necessary, even if this is not mentioned directly in a guideline.

Further information on European guidelines can be obtained on the EMEA homepage http://www.eudra.org/emea.html. The U.S. guideline can be found on the FDA homepage http://www.fda.gov/default.htm.

A special regulatory issue regarding biotechnology-based pharmaceuticals relates to the generic products or "follow-on protein products," as patent protections for a number of first-generation biotechnology-based protein products are about to expire. Because of the differences in complexity between small-molecule and follow-on protein products, the regulatory evaluation of biosimilarity for generic biotechnology-based proteins is a major challenge (180).

REFERENCES

1. Tauzin B. 418 Biotechnology Medicines in Testing Promise to Bolster the Arsenal Against Diseases. Medicines in Development, Biotechnology, 2006.
2. Walsh G. Biopharmaceutical benchmarks 2006. Nat Biotech 2006; 24(7):769–776.
3. Patton JS, Byron PR. Inhaling medicines: delivering drugs to the body through the lungs. Nat Rev Drug Disco 2007; 6:67–74.
4. Morishita M, Peppas NA. Is the oral route possible for peptide and protein drug delivery? Drug Discov Today 2006; 11(19–20):905–910.
5. Costantino HR, Illum L, Brandt G, et al. Intranasal delivery: physiochemical and therapeutic aspects. Int J Pharm 2007; 337:1–24.
6. Mahato RI, Narang AS, Thoma L, et al. Emerging trends in oral delivery of peptide and protein drugs. Crit Rev Ther Drug Carrier Syst 2003; 20(2–3):153–214.
7. Frokjaer S, Hovgaard L. Pharmaceutical Formulation Development of Pepides and Proteins. London: Taylor & Francis, 2000.
8. Shekunov BY, Cattopadhyay P, Tong HHY, et al. Particle size analysis in pharmaceutics: principles, methods and applications. Pharm Res 2007; 24(2):203–227.
9. Sarmento B, Ferreira DC, Jorgensen L, et al. Probing insulin's secondary structure after entrapment into alginate/chitosan nanoparticles. Eur J Pharm Biopharm 2007; 65:10–17.
10. Prego C, Fabre M, Torres D, et al. Efficacy and mechanism of action of chitosan nanocapsules for oral peptide delivery. Pharm Res 2006; 23(3):549–556.
11. Albrecht K, Bernkop-Schnürch A. Thiomers: forms, functions and applications to nano-medicine. Nanomedicine 2007; 2(1):41–50.
12. Malkov D, Angelo R, Wang H, et al. Oral delivery of insulin with the eligen(R) technology: mechanistic studies. Curr Drug Deliv 2005; 2:191–197.
13. Qi R, Pingel M. Gastrointestinal absorption enhancement of insulin by administration of enteric microspheres and SNAC to rats. J Microencapsul 2004; 21(1):37–45.
14. El-Sayed MEH, Hoffmann AS, Stayton PS. Rational design of composition and activity correlations for pH-responsive and glutathione-reactive polymer therapeutics. J Control Release 2005; 104:417–427.
15. Stayton PS, El-Sayed MEH, Murthy N, et al. Smart delivery systems for biomolecular therapeutics. Orthod Craniofacial Res 2005; 8:219–225.
16. Deshayes S, Morris M, Heitz F, et al. Delivery of proteins and nucleic acids using a non-covalent peptide-based strategy. Adv Drug Deliv Rev 2008; 60(4–5):537–547.
17. Deanda F, Smith KM, Liu J, et al. GSSI, a general model for solute-solvent interactions. 1. Description of the model. Mol Pharm 2004; 1(1):23–39.
18. Wang W. Instability, stabilization, and formulation of liquid protein pharmaceuticals. Int J Pharm 1999; 185(2):129–188.
19. Pauling L, Corey RB, Branson HR. The structure of proteins: two hydrogen-bonded helical configurations of the polypeptide chain. Proc Natl Acad Sci U S A 1951; 37:205–211.
20. Schultz GE, Schirmer RH. Principles of Protein Structure. New York: Springer-Verlag, 1979.
21. Pauling L, Corey RB. The structure of synthetic polypeptides. Proc Natl Acad Sci U S A 1951; 37:241–250.
22. Stickle DF, Presta LG, Dill KA, et al. Hydrogen bonding in globular proteins. J Mol Biol 1992; 226:1143–1159.
23. Linderstrøm-Lang KU, Schellman JA. Protein structure and enzyme activity. In: Boyer PD, Lardy H, Myrbäck K, eds. The Enzymes. New York: Academic Press Inc., 1959:443–510.
24. Chothia C. Principles that determine the structure of proteins. Ann Rev Biochem 1984; 53:537–572.

25. Brange J. Physical stability of proteins. In: Frokjaer S, Hovgaard L, eds. Pharmaceutical Formulation Development of Peptides and Proteins. London: Taylor & Francis, 2000:89–112.
26. Andrade JD. Principles of protein adsorption. In: Andrade JD, ed. Surface and Interfacial Aspects of Biomedical Polymers. New York: Plenum Press, 1985:1–80.
27. Brange J, Andersen L, Laursen ED, et al. Toward understanding insulin fibrillation. J Pharm Sci 1997; 86(5):517–525.
28. Brange J, Langkjaer L. Insulin structure and stability. In: Wang YJ, Pearlman R, eds. Stability and Characterisation of Protein and Peptide Drugs—Case Histories. New York: Plenum Press, 1993:315–350.
29. Parkins DA, Lashmar UT. The formulation of biopharmaceutical products. Pharm Sci Technol Today 2000; 3(4):129–137.
30. Cleland JL, Powell MF, Shire SJ. The development of stable protein formulations: a close look at protein aggregation, deamidation, and oxidation. Crit Rev Ther Drug Carrier Syst 1993; 10(4):307–377.
31. Almeida AJ, Souto E. Solid lipid nanoparticles as a drug delivery system for peptides and proteins. Adv Drug Deliv Rev 2007; 59(6):478–490.
32. Reubsaet JL, Beijnen JH, Bult A, et al. Analytical techniques used to study the degradation of proteins and peptides: physical instability. J Pharm Biomed Anal 1998; 17(6–7):979–984.
33. Kauzmann W. Some factors in the interpretation of protein denaturation. Adv Protein Chem 1959; 14:1–63.
34. Dickinson E. Proteins in solution and at interfaces. In: Goddard ED, Ananthapadmanabhan KP, eds. Interactions of Surfactants with Polymers and Proteins. Boca Ranton: CRC Press, 1993:295–317.
35. Dickinson E, Matsumura Y. Proteins at liquid interfaces: role of the molten globule state. Colloids Surf B Biointerf 1994; 3(1–2):1–17.
36. Shortle D. The denatured state (the other half of the folding equation) and its role in protein stability. FASEB J 1996; 10:27–34.
37. Jaenicke R. Protein stability and molecular adaptation to extreme conditions. Eur J Biochem 1991; 202(3):715–728.
38. Tanford C. Protein denaturation. Adv Protein Chem 1968; 23:121–282.
39. Bam NB, Cleland JL, Randolph TW. Molten globule intermediate of recombinant human growth hormone: stabilization with surfactants. Biotechnol Prog 1996; 12(6):801–809.
40. Manning M, Patel K, Borchardt RT. Stability of protein pharmaceuticals. Pharm Res 1989; 6(11):903–918.
41. Dobson CM. Unfolded proteins, compact states and molten globules. Curr Opin Struct Biol 1992; 2:6–12.
42. Lefebvre J, Relkin P. Denaturation of globular proteins in relation to their functional properties. In: Magdassi S, ed. Surface Activity of Proteins—Chemical and Physiochemical Modifications. New York: Marcel Dekker Inc., 1996:181–236.
43. Haynes CA, Norde W. Structures and stabilities of adsorbed proteins. J Colloid Interface Sci 1995; 169(2):313–328.
44. Wang W. Protein aggregation and its inhibition in biopharmaceutics. Int J Pharm 2005; 289:1–30.
45. Sadana A. Interfacial protein adsorption and inactivation. Bioseparation 1993; 3(5):297–320.
46. Fagain CO. Understanding and increasing protein stability. Biochim Biophys Acta 1995; 1252(1):1–14.
47. Chi EY, Krishnan S, Randolph TW, et al. Physical stability of proteins in aqueous solution: mechanism and driving forces in nonnative protein aggregation. Pharm Res 2003; 20(9):1325–1336.
48. Fink AL. Protein aggregation: folding aggregates, inclusion bodies and amyloid. Fold Des 1998; 3(1):R9–R23.
49. Katakam M, Bell LN, Banga AK. Effect of surfactants on the physical stability of recombinant human growth hormone. J Pharm Sci 1995; 84(6):713–716.
50. Dong A, Prestrelski SJ, Allison SD, et al. Infrared spectroscopic studies of lyophilization- and temperature-induced protein aggregation. J Pharm Sci 1995; 84(4):415–424.

51. Treuheit MJ, Kosky AA, Brems DN. Inverse relationship of protein concentration and aggregation. Pharm Res 2002; 19(4):511–516.
52. Vestergaard B, Groenning M, Roessle M, et al. A helical structural nucleus is the primary elongating unit of insulin amyloid fibrils. PloS Biol 2007; 5(5):1089–1097.
53. Nielsen L, Khurana R, Coats A, et al. Effect of environmental factors on the kinetics of insulin fibril formation: elucidation of the molecular mechanism. Biochemistry 2001; 40(20):6036–6046.
54. Andrade JD, Hlady V, Wei AP, et al. Proteins at interfaces: principles, multivariate aspects, protein resistant surfaces, and direct imaging and manipulation of adsorbed proteins. Clin Mater 1992; 11(1–4):67–84.
55. Cheesman DF, Davies JT. Physiochemical and biological aspects of proteins at interfaces. Adv Protein Chem 1954; 9:439–501.
56. Green RJ, Hopkinson I, Jones RAL. Unfolding and intermolecular association in globular proteins adsorbed at interfaces. Langmuir 1999; 15:5102–5110.
57. MacRitchie F. Proteins at interfaces. Adv Protein Chem 1978; 32:283–326.
58. Norde W. The behaviour of proteins at interfaces, with special attention to the role of the structure stability of the protein molecule. Clin Mater 1992; 11(1–4):85–91.
59. Pugnaloni LA, Dickinson E, Ettelaie R, et al. Competitive adsorption of proteins and low-molecular-weight surfactants: computer simulation and microscopic imaging. Adv Colloid Interface Sci 2004; 107(1):27–49.
60. Mollmann SH, Bukrinsky JT, Frokjaer S, et al. Adsorption of human insulin and Asp^{B28} insulin on a PTFE-like surface. J Colloid Interface Sci 2005; 286:28–35.
61. Norde W, Giacomelli CE. BSA structural changes during homomolecular exchange between the adsorbed and the dissolved states. J Biotechnol 2000; 79(3):259–268.
62. Goolcharran C, Khossravi M, Borchardt RT. Chemical pathways of peptide and protein degradation. In: Frokjaer S, Hovgaard L, eds. Pharmaceutical Formulation Development of Peptides and Proteins. London: Taylor & Francis, 2000:70–88.
63. Kerwin BA, Remmele RL. Protect from light: photodegradation and protein biologics. J Pharm Sci 2007; 96(6):1468–1479.
64. Violand BN, Siegel NR. Protein and peptide chemical and physical stability. In: Reid RE, ed. Peptide and Protein Drug Analysis. New York: Marcel Dekker, 2000:257–284.
65. Krishnamurthy R, Manning MC. The stability factor: importance in formulation development. Curr Pharm Biotech 2002; 3:361–371.
66. Council of Europe. European Pharmacopoeia. 5th ed. Strasbourg: Council of Europe, 2005.
67. Akers MJ, DeFelippis MR. Peptides and proteins as parenteral solutions. In: Frokjaer S, Hovgaard L, eds. Pharmaceutical Formulation Development of Peptides and Proteins. London: Taylor & Francis, 2000:145–177.
68. Hermeling S, Jiskoot W, Crommelin DJA, et al. Reaction to the paper: interaction of polysorbate with erythropoietin: a case study in protein-surfactant interactions. Pharm Res 2006; 23(3):641–642.
69. Schellekens H, Casadevall N. Immunogenisity of recombinant human proteins: causes and consequences. J Neurol 2004; 251(suppl 2):II/4–II/9.
70. Timasheff SN. Protein hydration, thermodynamic binding, and preferential hydration. Biochemistry 2002; 41(46):13473–13482.
71. Huus K, Havelund S, Olsen HB, et al. Ligand binding and thermostability of different allosteric states of the insulin zinc-hexamer. Biochemistry 2006; 45(12):4014–4024.
72. Govardhan C, Khalaf N, Jung CW, et al. Novel long-acting crystal formulation of human growth hormone. Pharm Res 2005; 22(9):1461–1470.
73. Arakawa T, Prestrelski SJ, Kenney WC, et al. Factors affecting short-term and long-term stabilities of proteins. Adv Drug Deliv Rev 2001; 46(1–3):307–326.
74. Tang X, Pikal MJ. Design of freeze-drying processes for pharmaceuticals: practical advice. Pharm Res 2004; 21(2):191–200.
75. Wang W. Lyophylization and development of solid protein pharmaceuticals. Int J Pharm 2000; 203:1–60.

76. Kett V, McMahon D, Ward K. Freeze-drying of protein pharmaceuticals—the application of thermal analysis. Cryo Letters 2004; 25(6):389–404.

77. Chang L, Shepard D, Sun J, et al. Mechanism of protein stabilization by sugars during freeze-drying and storage: native structure preservation, specific interaction, and/or immobilization in a glassy matrix? J Pharm Sci 2005; 94(7):1427–1444.

78. Carpenter JF, Pikal MJ, Chang BS, et al. Rational design of stable lyophilized protein formulations: some practical advice. Pharm Res 1997; 14(8):969–975.

79. Chobert J-M, Gaudin J-C, Dalgalarrondo M, et al. Impact of Maillard type glycation on properties of beta-lactoglobulin. Biotechnol Adv 2006; 24:629–632.

80. Schwegman JJ, Hardwick LM, Akers MJ. Practical formulation and process development of freeze-dried products. Pharm Dev Technol 2005; 10:151–173.

81. Shoyele SA, Cawthorne S. Particle engineering techniques for inhaled biopharmaceuticals. Adv Drug Deliv Rev 2006; 58:1009–1029.

82. Maa Y-F, Prestrelski SJ. Biopharmaceutical powders: particle formation and formulation considerations. Curr Pharm Biotechnol 2000; 1:283–302.

83. Degim IT, Celebi N. Controlled delivery of peptides and proteins. Curr Pharm Design 2007; 13:99–117.

84. Weers JG, Tarara TE, Clark AR. Design of fine particles for pulmonary drug delivery. Expert Opin Drug Deliv 2007; 4(3):297–313.

85. Shoyele SA, Slowey A. Prospects of formulating proteins/peptides as aerosols for pulmonal drug delivery. Int J Pharm 2006; 314:1–8.

86. Summary of Product Characteristics for Pulmozyme. Available at: http://www.produktresume. dk/docushare/dsweb/Get/Document-14730/Pulmozyme%2Cþinhalationsv%C3%83%C2% A6skeþtilþnebulisator%2Cþopl%C3%83%C2%B8sningþ1þmg-ml.doc. Accessed December 2007.

87. Scientific Discussion. Available at: http://www.exubera.com/content/con_index.jsp?setShowOn=../ content/con_index.jsp&setShowHighlightOn=../content/con_index.jsp. Accessed December 2007.

88. Scientific Discussion. Available at: http://www.emea.europa.eu/humandocs/PDFs/EPAR/ exubera/058806en6.pdf. Accessed December 2007.

89. Novo Nordisk A/S pipeline rFXIII Congenital deficiency. Available at: http://www. novonordisk.com/investors/rd_pipeline/rd_pipeline.asp?showid=5. Accessed December 2007.

90. Cheng YH, Dyer M, Jabbal-Gill I, et al. Intranasal delivery of recombinant human growth hormone (somatropin) in sheep using chitosan-based powder formulations. Eur J Pharm Sci 2005; 26:9–15.

91. Summary of Product Characteristics for Suprecur. Available at: http://www.produktresume. dk/docushare/dsweb/Get/Document-15675/Suprecur%2C+n%C3%A6sespray%2C+opl% C3%B8sning+0%2C15+mg-dosis.doc. Accessed December 2007.

92. Summary of Product Characteristics for Minirin. Available at: http://www.produktresume.dk/ docushare/dsweb/Get/Document-12804/Minirin%2C+n%C3%A6sespray%2C+opl%C3% B8sning+2%2C5+mikrog-dosis+og+10+mikrog-dosis.doc. Accessed December 2007.

93. Illum L. Nanoparticulate systems for nasal delivery of drugs: a real improvement over simple systems? J Pharm Sci 2007; 96(3):473–483.

94. Goldberg M, Gomez-Orellana I. Challenges for the oral delivery of macromolecules. Nat Rev Drug Disco 2003; 2:289–295.

95. Summary of Product Characteristics for Minirin. Available at: http://www.produktresume.dk/ docushare/dsweb/Get/Document-22023/Minirin%2C+smeltetabletter+60+mikrog% 2C+120+mikrog+og+240+mikrog.doc. Accessed December 2007.

96. Summary of Product Characteristics for Nocutil. Available at: http://www.produktresume.dk/ docushare/dsweb/Get/Document-22173/Nocutil%2C+tabletter+0%2C1+mg+og+0% 2C2+mg.doc. Accessed December 2007.

97. Sarmento B, Ribeiro AJ, Veiga F, et al. Oral bioavailability of insulin contained in polysaccharide nanoparticles. Biomacromolecules 2007; 8:3054–3060.

98. Delie F, Blanco-Prieto MJ. Polymeric particulates to improve oral bioavailability of peptide drugs. Molecules 2005; 10:65–80.

99. Summary of Product Characteristics for Grazax. Available at: http://www.produktresume.dk/docushare/dsweb/Get/Document-23337/Grazax%2C+smeltetabletter+75.000+SQ-T.doc. Accessed December 2007.

100. Badkar AV, Banga AK. Electrically enhanced transdermal delivery of a macromolecule. J Pharm Pharmacol 2002; 54:907–912.

101. Badkar AV, Smith AM, Eppstein JA, et al. Transdermal delivery of interfaron alpha-2B using microporation and iontophoresis in hairless rats. Pharm Res 2001; 24(7):1389–1395.

102. Levin G, Gershonowitz A, Sacks H, et al. Transdermal delivery of human growth hormone through RF-microchannels. Pharm Res 2005; 22(4):550–555.

103. Schuetz YB, Naik A, Guy RH, et al. Emerging strategies for the transdermal delivery of peptide and protein drugs. Expert Opin Drug Deliv 2005; 2(3):533–548.

104. Summary of Product Characteristics for Zoladex. Available at: http://www.produktresume.dk/docushare/dsweb/Get/Document-18419/Zoladex%2C+implantat+3%2C6+mg+og+10%2C8+mg.doc. Accessed December 2007.

105. Summary of Product Characteristics for Lupron Depot. Available at: http://www.accessdata.fda.gov/scripts/cder/drugsatfda/index.cfm?fuseaction=Search.Overview&DrugName=LUPRON%20DEPOT. Accessed December 2007.

106. Summary of Product Characteristics for Decapeptyl Depot. Available at: http://www.produktresume.dk/docushare/dsweb/Get/Document-11709/Decapeptyl+Depot%2C+pulver+og+solvens+til+injektionsv%C3%A6ske%2C+suspension%2C+3+%2C75+mg.doc. Accessed December 2007.

107. Summary of Product Characteristics for Pamorelin. Available at: http://www.produktresume.dk/docushare/dsweb/Get/Document-20482/Pamorelin%2C+pulver+og+solvens+til+injektionsv%C3%A6ske%2C+depotsuspension.doc. Accessed December 2007.

108. Summary of Product Characteristics for Sandostatin LAR. Available at: http://www.produktresume.dk/docushare/dsweb/Get/Document-18484/Sandostatin+LAR%2C+pulver+og+solvens+til+injektionsv%C3%A6ske%2C+suspension.+10+mg%2C+20+mg+og+30+mg.doc. Accessed December 2007.

109. Summary of Product Characteristics for Nutropin Depot. Available at: http://www.accessdata.fda.gov/scripts/cder/drugsatfda/index.cfm?fuseaction=Search.DrugDetails. Accessed December 2007.

110. Kang F, Jiang G, Hinderliter A, et al. Lysozyme stability in primary emulsion for PLGA microsphere preparation: effect of recovery methods and stabilizing excipients. Pharm Res 2002; 19(5):629–633.

111. Tracy MA. Development and scale-up of a microsphere protein delivery system. Biotechnol Prog 2005; 14:108–115.

112. Hahn SK, Kim SJ, Kim MJ, et al. Characterization and in vivo study of sustained-release formulation of human growth hormone using sodium hyaluronate. Pharm Res 2004; 21(8):1374–1381.

113. Kim SJ, Hahn SK, Kim MJ, et al. Development of a novel sustained release formulation of recombinant human growth hormone using sodium hyaluronate microparticles. J Control Release 2005; 104:323–335.

114. Tracy MA. Development and scale-up of a microshere protein delivery system. Biotechnol Prog 1998; 14:108–115.

115. Kwon YM, Baudys M, Knutson K, et al. In situ study of insulin aggregation induced by water-organic solvent interface. Pharm Res 2001; 18(12):1754–1759.

116. Kim HK, Park TG. Microencapsulation of human growth hormone within biodegradable polyester microspheres: protein aggregation stability and incomplete release mechanism. Biotechnol Bioeng 1999; 65(6):659–667.

117. Cleland JL, Mac A, Boyd B, et al. The stability of recombinant human growth hormone in poly(lactic-co-glycolic acid) (PLGA) microspheres. Pharm Res 1997; 14:4–5.

118. Chan Y-P, Meyrueix R, Kravtzoff R, et al. Review on Medusa (R); a polymer-based sustained release technology for protein and peptide drugs. Expert Opin Drug Deliv 2007; 4(4):441–451.

119. Flamel Technologies: technologies and products. Available at: http://www.flamel-technologies.fr/techAndProd/index.shtml. Accessed December 2007.

120. Kim K, Fisher JP. Nanoparticle technology in bone tissue engineering. J Drug Target 2007; 15(4):241–252.

121. Mehnert W, Mäder K. Solid lipid nanoparticles production, characterization and applications. Adv Drug Deliv Rev 2001; 47(2–3):165–196.

122. Ye Q, Asherman J, Stevenson M, et al. DepoFoam(TM) technology: a vehicle for controlled delivery of protein and peptide drugs. J Control Release 2000; 64(1–3):155–166.

123. Howell SB. Clinical application of a novel sustained-release injectable drug delivery system: Depofoam™ technology. Cancer J 2001; 7(3):219–227.

124. Pelton JT, McLean LR. Spectroscopic methods for analysis of protein secondary structure. Anal Biochem 2000; 277(2):167–176.

125. Veronese FM, Pasut G. PEGylation, successful approach to drug delivery. Drug Discov Today 2005; 10(21):1451–1458.

126. Veronese FM, Morpurgo M. Bioconjugation in pharmaceutical chemistry. Farmaco 1999; 54:497–516.

127. Solá RJ, Griebenow K. Chemical glycosylation: new insights on the interralation between protein structural mobility, thermodynamic stability, and catalysis. FEBS Let 2006; 580: 1685–1690.

128. Solá RJ. Rodríguez-Martínez JA, Griebenow K. Modulation of protein biophysical properties by chemical glycosylation: biochemical insights and biomedical implicationsw. Cell Mol Life Sci 2007; 64:2133–2152.

129. Soran H, Younis N. Insulin detemir: a new basal insulin analogue. Diabetes Obes Metab 2006; 8:26–30.

130. Knudsen LB, Nielsen PF, Huufeldt PO, et al. Potent derivatives of glucagon-like peptide-1 with pharmacokinetic properties suitable for once daily administration. J Med Chem 2000; 43:1664–1669.

131. Novo Nordisk A/S pipeline Vagifem®. Available at: http://www.novonordisk.com/investors/ rd_pipeline/rd_pipeline.asp?showid=4. Accessed December 2007.

132. Jars MU, Hvass A, Waaben D. Insulin aspart (Asp^{b28} Human insulin) derivatives formed in pharmaceutical solutions. Pharm Res 2002; 19(5):621–628.

133. Setter SM, Corbett CF, Campbell RK, et al. Insulin aspart: a new rapid-acting insulin analog. Ann Pharmacother 2000; 34:1423–1431.

134. Scientific Discussion. Available at: http://www.emea.europa.eu/humandocs/PDFs/EPAR/ Novorapid/272799en6.pdf. Accessed December 2007.

135. Heise T, Nosek L, Spitzer H, et al. Insulin glulisine: a faster onset of action compared with insulin lispro. Diabetes Obes Metab 2007; 9:746–753.

136. Scientific Discussion. Available at: http://www.emea.europa.eu/humandocs/PDFs/EPAR/ Humalog/060195en6.pdf. Accessed December 2007.

137. Scientific Discussion. Available at: http://www.emea.europa.eu/humandocs/PDFs/EPAR/ apidra/121804en6.pdf. Accessed December 2007.

138. Wang F, Carabino JM, Vergara CM. Insulin glargine: a systematic review of a long-acting insulin analogue. Clin Ther 2003; 25(6):1541–1577.

139. Scientific Discussion. Available at: http://www.emea.europa.eu/humandocs/PDFs/EPAR/ Lantus/061500en6.pdf. Accessed December 2007.

140. Campbell RK, White JR, Levien T, et al. Insulin glargine. Clin Ther 2001; 23(12):1938–1957.

141. Summary of Product Characteristics for PROLEUKIN® (aldesleukin). Available at: http:// www.pharma.us.novartis.com/product/pi/pdf/proleukin.pdf. Accessed December 2007.

142. Katre NV. The conjugation of proteins with polyethylene glycol and other polymers—altering properties of proteins to enhance their therapeutic potential. Adv Drug Deliv Rev 1993; 10: 91–114.

143. Summary of Product Characteristics for Adagen®. Available at: http://www.accessdata.fda. gov/scripts/cder/drugsatfda/index.cfm?fuseaction=Search.DrugDetails. Accessed December 2007.

144. Hussar DA. New drug: varenicline, tatrate, insulin glulisine, and insulin detemir. J Am Pharm Assoc 2006; 46(4):524–527.

145. Jones MC, Patel M. Insulin detemir: a long-acting insulin product. Am J Health Syst Pharm 2006; 63:2466–2472.

146. Solá RJ, Al-Azzam W, Griebenow K. Engineering of protein thermodynamic, kinetic, and colloidal stability: chemical glycosylation with monofunctional activated glycans. Biotechnol Bioeng 2006; 94(6):1072–1079.

147. Herron JN, Jiskoot W, Crommelin DJA. Physical Methods to Characterize Pharmaceutical Proteins. New York: Plenum Press, 1995.

148. Freire E. Differential scanning calorimetry. In: Shirley BA, ed. Protein Stability and Folding— Theory and Practice. Totowa, NJ: Humana Press, 1995:191–218.

149. Jiskoot W, Crommelin DJA. Methods for Structural Analysis of Protein Pharmaceuticals. Arlington, VA: American Association of Pharmaceutical Scientists, 2005.

150. Baudys M, Kim SW. Peptide and protein characterization. In: Frokjaer S, Hovgaard L, eds. Pharmaceutical Formulation Development of Peptides and Proteins. London: Taylor & Francis, 2000:41–69.

151. Jackson M, Mantsch HH. The use and misuse of FTIR spectroscopy in the determination of protein structure. Crit Rev Biochem Mol Biol 1995; 30(2):95–120.

152. Cooper EA, Knutson K. Fourier transform infrared spectroscopy investigations of protein structure. In: Herron JN, Jiskoot W, Crommelin DJA, eds. Physical Methods to Characterize Pharmaceutical Proteins. New York: Plenum Press, 1995:101–143.

153. Haris PI, Severcan F. FTIR spectroscopic characterization of protein structure in aqueous and non-aqueous media. J Mol Catal 1999; 7(1–4):207–221.

154. Burnett GR, Rigby NM, Clare Mills EN, et al. Characterization of the emulsification properties of 2S albumins from sunflower seed. J Colloid Interface Sci 2002; 247(1):177–185.

155. Burstein EA, Vedenkina NS, Ivkova MN. Fluorescence and the location of tryptophan residues in protein molecules. Photochem Photobiol 1973; 18(4):263–279.

156. Vivian JT, Callis PR. Mechanisms of tryptophan fluorescence shifts in proteins. Biophys J 2001; 80(5):2093–2109.

157. Eftink MR. Fluorescence techniques for studying protein-structure. Methods Biochem Anal 1991; 35:127–205.

158. Anderson GJ. Circular dichoism and Fourier transform infra-red analysis of polypeptide conformation. In: Reid RE, ed. Peptide and Protein Drug Analysis. New York: Marcel Dekker, 2000:753–774.

159. Lakowicz JR. Principles of Fluorescence Spectroscopy. 2nd ed. New York: Kluwer Academic/ Plenum Publishers, 1999.

160. Freire E. Statistical thermodynamic analysis of the heat capacity function associated with protein folding-unfolding transitions. Comments Mol Cell Biophys 1989; 6(2):123–140.

161. Robertson AD, Murphy KP. Protein structure and the energetics of protein stability. Chem Rev 1997; 97:1251–1267.

162. Ma C-Y, Harwalkar VR. Thermal analysis of food proteins. Adv Food Nutr Res 1991; 35:317–366.

163. Bam NB, Cleland JL, Yang J, et al. Tween protects recombinant human growth hormone against agitation-induced damage via hydrophobic interactions. J Pharm Sci 1998; 87(12): 1554–1559.

164. Kasimova MR, Milstein SJ, Freire E. The conformational equilibrium of human growth hormone. J Mol Biol 1998; 277(2):409–418.

165. Moriyama Y, Kawasaka Y, Takeda K. Protective effect of small amounts of sodium dodecyl sulfate on the helical structure of bovine serum albumin in thermal denaturation. J Colloid Interface Sci 2003; 257(1):41–46.

166. Potera C. Antisense—down, but not out. Nat Biotech 2007; 25(5):497–499.

167. Summary of Product Characteristics for Vitravene®. Available at: http://www.accessdata.fda.gov/ scripts/cder/drugsatfda/index.cfm?fuseaction=Search.DrugDetails. Accessed December 2007.

168. Summary of Product Characteristics for Macugen®. Available at: http://www.accessdata.fda. gov/scripts/cder/drugsatfda/index.cfm?fuseaction=Search.DrugDetails. Accessed December 2007.

169. Pearson S, Jia H, Kandachi K. China approves first gene therapy. Nat Biotech 2004; 22:3–4.
170. Swayze EE, Bhat B. The medicinal chemistry of oligonucleotides. In: Crooke ST, ed. Antisense Drug Technology. Principles, Strategies and Applications. Boca Raton: CRC Press, 2006:143–182.
171. Birchall J. Pulmonary delivery of nucleic acids. Expert Opin Drug Deliv 2007; 4(6):575–578.
172. Hardee GE, Tillman LG, Geary RS. Routes and formulations for delivery of antisense oligonucleotides. In: Crooke ST, ed. Antisense Drug Technology. Principles, Strategies and Applications. Boca Raton: CRC Press, 2006:217–236.
173. Behlke MA. Progress towards in vivo use of siRNAs. Mol Ther 2006; 13(4):644–670.
174. MacLachlan I. Liposomal formulations for nucleic acid delivery. In: Crooke ST, ed. Antisense Drug Technology. Principles, Strategies and Applications. Boca Raton: CRC Press, 2006: 237–270.
175. Foged C, Nielsen HM. Cell penetrating peptides for drug delivery across membrane barriers. Expert Opin Drug Deliv 2008; 5(1):105–117.
176. Kaneda Y. Virosomes: evolution of the liposome as a targeted drug delivery system. Adv Drug Deliv Rev 2000; 43(2–3):197–205.
177. Oliveira S, van Rooy I, Kranenburg O, et al. Fusogenic peptides enhance endosomal escape improving siRNA-induced silencing of oncogenes. Int J Pharm 2007; 331(2):211–214.
178. Wasungu L, Hoekstra D. Cationic lipids, lipoplexes and intracellular delivery of genes. J Control Release 2006; 116(2):255–264.
179. Escriou V, Carriere M, Scherman D, et al. NLS bioconjugates for targeting therapeutic genes to the nucleus. Adv Drug Deliv Rev 2003; 55(2):295–306.
180. Woodcock J, Griffin J, Behrman R, et al. The FDA's assessment of follow-on protein products: a historical perspective. Nat Rev Drug Disco 2007; 6(6):437–442.

8

Veterinary Pharmaceutical Dosage Forms

Michael J. Rathbone
Griffith University, Gold Coast Campus, Queensland, Australia

Todd P. Foster
Pfizer Animal Health, Kalamazoo, Michigan, U.S.A.

INTRODUCTION

Animals provide us with companionship (e.g., dogs and cats), recreation (e.g., horses), food (e.g., cattle and pigs), and manual labor (whether an elephant carrying logs in Thailand or a hunting dog retrieving a downed pheasant in South Dakota). Just like humans these animals receive medicines to keep them healthy, and the reasons for producing single-dose veterinary dosage forms is the same as those in humans; to permit delivery of an active in a form that is effective, safe, and able to be handled and administered by the end user. However, when one extends that comparison to long-acting dosage forms, the reasons for developing such a system differs between humans and animals. In the case of humans, the reasons for developing a drug into a long-acting delivery system include the reduction of dose frequency to improve patient compliance, or to improve the efficiency of therapy and thereby improve the health of the patient. In contrast in the veterinary field, the major reasons for developing a drug into a long-acting drug delivery system is to minimize animal handling to reduce the stress to animals from repeated administration and to reduce the cost of treatment in terms of money and time spent by the end user on drug administration. These reasons do not impact on the science used to develop such dosage forms, but they do impact heavily on the outcomes such as the size, shape, volume administered, etc. of the dosage form.

The primary purpose of this chapter is to provide a basic background in the design and evaluation of veterinary dosage forms. It will describe both basic and advanced dosage forms from the perspective of their application. The basic dosage forms are described according to their pharmaceutical characteristics, whereas the descriptions of advanced drug delivery systems are organized according to routes of administration. Throughout this chapter we will provide comparisons between the formulations used for humans and animals. In addition we will highlight factors that influence the development of veterinary dosage forms and describe some of the relevant issues pertaining to the development of veterinary dosage forms.

Human Vs. Veterinary Formulation Science

In the simplest approach the development of pharmaceuticals for humans and animals are the same. The process involves (*i*) selection of the active pharmaceutical ingredient (API) with good physicochemical properties for development and determine that it is efficacious and safe, (*ii*) design dosage form and packaging, (*iii*) produce clinical supplies for efficacy and safety testing, (*iv*) collect registration stability data on the API and drug product, (*v*) scale-up and transfer API and drug product methods in to commercial facilities, (*vi*) ensure methods to verify that quality are validated and in place, and (*vii*) file for approval with regulatory agencies. Some other less obvious similarities include very similar regulatory requirements (e.g., International Conference on Harmonization for humans and the Veterinary International Conference on Harmonization for animals); United States is the major profit market for both disciplines and the importance of intellectual property.

Probably the most important difference is the added focus in veterinary medicine with food-producing animals of ensuring no unsafe drug or metabolite residues exist in the food being consumed. This involves extensive ADME and safety characterization. Other more subtle differences include animal health clinical programs often less complicated, smaller, and quicker to conduct; drug product price sensitivity for livestock (i.e., animals not treated if product is too costly and not an economical advantage); and often no need for animal modeling because of the ability to use the target species in a humane and cost-effective testing manner.

Essentially the same approaches and disciplines are applied to the development of veterinary dosage forms as those that are applied to human dosage form development. Physical pharmacy alongside biopharmaceutical and pharmacokinetic principles are all used in the same manner, and detailed descriptions of the theory and principles of these topics can be found elsewhere in this book. However, in the animal, both within and between species, there are vast differences in weight, size, physiology, anatomy, and the way individual animals pharmacokinetically handle drugs. Thus, although the same scientific principles are used to develop both human and veterinary dosage forms, the outcomes are very different. In modern day pharmaceutics, in the human field, nanotechnology and microtechnology are the approaches commonly taken to improve drug delivery to improve absorption or to give sustained depot delivery, respectively. In the veterinary field, such systems are infrequently used, and "macro" delivery systems often rule the day. Chewable dog treats with medications are macro tablets. Feed additives placed in food or water dose thousands of cattle a day or even millions of chickens. These situations often are not considered by the graduate students or formulation scientist, but it offers a different set of opportunities to their human counterparts, allowing for innovative solutions to difficult formulation issues.

Another aspect that we will discuss in this chapter is the means by which the dose is administered (the administration method). In the human field the very young and the very old need assistance in delivering the dosage form, but this represents a small percentage of the patient population. Nevertheless, as those experienced in the field will tell administration to these patients can be fraught with difficulty. Imagine, therefore, the challenge presented where the entire population needs assistance in the administration process. This problem falls on the formulator and is overcome by designing purpose-built applicators and by developing the delivery system with this problem in mind.

The Patient

Animals can be conveniently divided into two broad categories: food-producing animals and companion animals. Food-producing animals include cattle, sheep, swine, and poultry, together with fish and any other animal from which meat or other products such as eggs or milk are obtained. Companion animals are those that are considered pets and include dogs, cats, and horses. Birds, lizards, rabbits, etc. can be considered companion animals; however, they are sometimes classified as "exotic" animals. Because the latter species represent only a small proportion of the companion animal market, dosage forms that have been developed for the more common species (e.g., dogs and cats), or indeed, for humans, are often adapted for use in the exotic species since the markets are not usually large enough to warrant development of such specialized products.

A Perspective of the Market

Animal Health Pharmaceuticals and Biologicals Sales

The market for animal health products is often divided into two main areas: pharmaceuticals and biologicals. In simple terms, pharmaceuticals are medicines to treat and cure animals, while biologicals are vaccines to prevent diseases. However, things can get muddled. Protein drugs like bovine growth hormone are not vaccines but often can be called a biological and may be classified as pharmaceuticals. Sometimes a third class is nutritionals, which cover products like selenium supplements for livestock or vitamins for companion animals. Medicinal and nutritional feed additives can be another designation. In addition there is the pet food and pesticide/herbicide industries and their respective products. Therefore, it is important when examining sales figures for companies that an understanding of what is being reported is clear. For example, in 2001, the reported animal health market was $17 billion (this figure includes pharmaceuticals, biologicals, feed additives, and nutritionals) (1). In 2006, the market was reported to be $16.1 billion for those areas not including nutritionals (2). While areas like companion animal pharmaceuticals have grown, and in the last couple of years there has been market growth, during the last 10 years the total market has been fairly flat.

The top 15 animal health companies represent over 80% of the total $16.1 billion market. The top five companies with their 2006 sales were Pfizer ($2.3 billion), Merial ($2.2 billion), Intervet ($1.4 billion), Bayer ($1.1 billion), and Novartis ($0.95 billion). The Bayer and Novartis figures include some environmental health sales (2).

Additional ways to examine sales are via species (e.g., swine, cattle, poultry, dogs, cats), region (e.g., United States, Europe, Asia), or therapeutic areas (e.g., anti-infectives, parasiticides, anti-inflammatories).

Challenges in the Market

Many changes and challenges are occurring in the veterinary market. Some of these issues include (*i*) consolidation of companies, which reduces the amount of R&D dollars spent on discovering new molecules, resulting in fewer new chemical entities (NCEs) being discovered and approved, (*ii*) a relatively flat market for years coupled with less real dollars spent on R&D today, (*iii*) a reduction in spending on livestock R&D as the companion animal area has become a focus as it is thought to be more lucrative, (*iv*) a curtailing of R&D on antibiotics because of antibiotic resistance that some attribute to the overuse in veterinary medicine, (*v*) the appearance of less product line extensions via drug delivery as a consequence of less overall R&D dollars, and (*vi*) a higher risk in developing certain new medicines because of a consolidation of farms resulting for certain species (e.g., swine, chickens) in the profitable U.S. market being controlled by only a few companies. (This means that if you cannot get those companies to buy your new product, you will not be able to recoup your investment.)

Scientific Challenges

Each product that is developed must exhibit acceptable safety, efficacy, and stability profiles, each feature being built into the product through dosage form design based on sound scientific principles. However, the manner in which these are addressed and the additional challenge of residual drug remaining at the administration site must be taken into account when developing a dosage form for an animal. Safety aspects apply to both the user and the animal. Efficacy trials may involve many more participants compared with human trials, and must often encompass different breeds, seasons, and geographical locations to evaluate the effect of these on product efficacy. As mentioned before, the final design of the product must take into account the means by which the product will be administered to the animal by the end user. The maximum size of any veterinary delivery system, for example, may not be determined by the anatomical constraints of the animal, but rather by the physical dimension of the administration device. Thus the final dosage form can often be much smaller than the formulation scientist first envisages, resulting in lower dose-loading capacity and fewer capabilities of the delivery system than first imagined.

Chemical stability can be a major issue. Neither farm sheds nor farm vehicles (typical storage places for purchased veterinary pharmaceuticals) have cold storage facilities or even air conditioning, therefore assuming that a product can be stored below 20°C or in the fridge for the duration of its lifetime prior to administration is an unreasonable assumption. Dosage forms must therefore be stable to elevated heat conditions and hot/cold heat fluctuations. Where appropriate packaging must offer more than just physical protection, it is the formulation scientist's responsibility to determine and demonstrate if moisture protection needs to be addressed through relevant packaging, but this can add cost to the final product.

Physical stability is also an issue. Farmers do not have the time to premix individual doses of suspensions, nor constantly "shake the bottle" between administrations to some several hundred individual cows of their herd. Thus, for example, in the case of suspensions, the final product physical characteristics are often a balance between retardation of sedimentation and ease of flow to draw up into the syringe. Thus a critical evaluation of existing suspension products by a formulation scientist new to the field may draw false conclusions as to the need for an improved product based on ease of administration since there is more than pharmaceutical elegance involved in developing the perfect veterinary formulation. Indeed, a farmer is less interested in what the product looks like compared with its efficacy profile, ease of use, ease of administration, ease of removal, tissue residue profile, and time it takes to herd, administer, and release his animals back into the paddock. Veterinary formulation scientists may therefore trade off pharmaceutical elegance to improve other features, provided the efficacy and safety profile is acceptable and not altered during storage.

A final issue relating to veterinary dosage forms designed for long action is assurance of safety and efficacy after administration at the terminal end of its shelf life. Data is often generated to demonstrate that a drug product is stable under normal storage conditions for two years; however, a long-acting veterinary dosage form may be designed to deliver drug for up to six months. If such a product is purchased close to its accepted shelf life period, what assurances are there that this product will remain safe and effective when it is administered to the animal and becomes subjected to the biological environment of high moisture and elevated temperatures (40°C). This is an interesting problem, and maybe such delivery systems should be subjected to the normal shelf life storage conditions for two years, followed by a further period (dictated by the proposed duration of the product) of 40°C/75% RH. Such a procedure could assure both users and regulatory authorities alike that the product is safe and effective under label stated storage conditions, for the approved duration as stated on the label as well as after administration regardless of when the product is purchased within the label-approved shelf life period of the product. Acceptance limits may need to be proposed wider, but can be justified based on the demonstration of comparative efficacy and safety to freshly manufactured product.

Literature

Prior to the last decade there have been few major review articles or other important literature published on the development of veterinary dosage forms. Of worthy note was the book *Development and Formulation of Dosage Forms*, edited by G.E. Hardee and J.D. Baggot, which has recently been republished with additional chapters as a second edition (3), several articles (4–11), and a special issue of the *Journal of Controlled Release* (12).

However, in the last decade a wealth of information has been published, which has resulted in the provision of a valuable resource to the veterinary formulation scientist. An overview of these publications is provided in Table 1. Other journal reviews (20–26) or book chapters (27–30) have added to this wealth of knowledge.

Key Advantages

The formulation of veterinary dosage forms is a challenging process, but it can oftentimes be aided by opportunities. Some of these are discussed below.

The Animal

One of the greatest advantages that a veterinary formulation scientist has compared with his human counterpart is the availability of the target species from day one of the research and development process. Products can, therefore, be tailored directly to the intended species. Appropriately designed animal studies can be used to rapidly develop meaningful in vitro–in vivo relationships, screen lead formulations, and generally provide an insight into the behavior of the dosage form within a biological environment it will ultimately be exposed to during use. The use of animals early in product development phases assures the development of appropriate and meaningful in vitro test procedures.

Manufacturing Process

Because, in general, large numbers of animals (and often large body weight animals) are used in research trials, large-scale manufacturing equipment tends to be used early in the R&D process to manufacture the large amount of product that is required. This offers the advantage that scale-up issues are minimized.

Human Drugs for Animals

Animals are often used to test human drugs during early development. In that respect data are gained without any cost to the eventual animal health drug. Several analogs might be considered for humans and a veterinary use takes the "backup" drug. Or, after a number of years on the market for humans, some drugs end up being used for animal applications.

Metabolism and Distribution

While understanding the ADME characteristics of a drug for humans is very important, it is extremely important for drugs used in food-producing animals. Metabolism and

Table 1 List of Major Review Articles or Other Important Articles on Formulation of Veterinary Drug Delivery Systems

Book/special journal issues title	Book/ journal	Publisher/ journal	Editor(s)	Date of publication	Topics covered	Reference
Development and formulation of dosage forms	Book	Marcel Dekker, New York	G. E. Hardee and J. D. Baggott	1998 (2nd ed)	Veterinary Drug Availability, Basis for Selection of the Dosage Form, Formulation of Veterinary Dosage Forms, Protein/Peptide Veterinary Formulations, Formulation of Vaccines, Administration Devices and Techniques, Specification Development and Stability Assessment, Bioavailability Bioequivalence Assessments, Development and Formulation of Dosage Forms, Design of Preclinical Studies	3
Controlled release veterinary drug delivery: biological and pharmaceutical considerations	Book	Elsevier Science BV	M. J. Rathbone and R. Gurny	2000	Mechanisms of Drug Release, Intravaginal Veterinary Drug Delivery Systems, Controlled Release Drug Delivery Systems for Estrous Control of Domesticated Livestock, In Vitro Drug Release Testing, Stability Testing, Biopharmaceutical and Pharmacokinetic Principles, Intraruminal Controlled Release Products, Postruminal Drug Delivery Systems and Rumen-Stable Products, Ocular Veterinary Drug Delivery Systems, Controlled Release Products for the Control of Ectoparasites of Livestock, Controlled Drug Delivery and the Companion Animal, Controlled Release Vaccines, USA Regulatory Aspects Pertaining to Controlled Release Veterinary Drug Delivery Systems	13
Veterinary drug delivery, part I	Journal	Advanced Drug Delivery Reviews	Michael J. Rathbone	1997	Intraruminal Devices, Rumen-Stable Delivery Systems, Ocular Drug Delivery Systems, Intravaginal Veterinary Drug Delivery Systems	14

Veterinary drug delivery, part II	Journal	Advanced Drug Delivery Reviews	Michael J. Rathbone and S. Cady	1999	Long-Acting Control of Ectoparasites (Collar Technologies for Companion Animals), Growth Promoting Implants in Farmed Livestock, Pulsatile Release from Subcutaneous Implants, Somatotropin Delivery to Farmed Animals, Vaccine Delivery to Animals	15
Veterinary drug delivery, part III	Journal	Advanced Drug Delivery Reviews	Michael J. Rathbone and L. Witchey-Lakshmanan	2000	DNA Vaccines in Veterinary Medicine, DNA Vaccines for the Treatment of Diseases of Farmed Animals, Application of DNA Vaccine Technology to Aquaculture, Transcutaneous Immunization of Domestic Animals, Applications of Genetic Engineering in Veterinary Medicine, Bone Morphogenetic Proteins	16
Veterinary drug delivery, part IV	Journal	Advanced Drug Delivery Reviews	Michael J. Rathbone and L. Witchey-Lakshmanan	2001	Transdermal Patches for Veterinary Applications, Potential for Skin Penetration Enhancement, Aquaculture, Bovine Mastitis and Intramammary Drug Delivery, Veterinary Dental Drug Delivery, Drug Delivery System Design for the Control of the Estrous Cycle in Cattle	17
Veterinary drug delivery, part V	Journal	Advanced Drug Delivery Reviews	Michael J. Rathbone	2002	Zoological Pharmacology, Drug Administration to Poultry, Applying the Biopharmaceutics Classification System to Veterinary Pharmaceutical Products (in 2 Parts), Vaccine Development, Immunological Aspects of Controlled Antigen Delivery, Pharmaceutical Challenges in Veterinary Product Development	18
Veterinary drug delivery	Journal	Journal of Controlled Release	Michael J. Rathbone and Terry L. Bowersock	2002	In Situ Forming Injectables, Bacterial Ghosts, Dermal Peptide Antigens, Various Research Papers	19

distribution throughout the animal needs to be clearly delineated since drug and metabolite levels are used to set withdrawal periods for animals. Withdrawal period is the time for which edible items such as milk, eggs, and meat are not allowed to be marketed after an animal receives a treatment. Because this is so important, early in development of veterinary pharmaceutical there are scientists trying to understand the ADME parameters that then aid the formulation scientist in designing the formulations.

Environmental Assessment

Because animals eliminate administered drugs and their metabolites directly into the environment via feces and urine, the decomposition of these products in water, via sunlight, and in various types of soil must be evaluated. In some cases even their effect on certain insects must be studied. Because of this regulatory requirement, an increased focus on the understanding of drug degradation pathways is conducted, which may not be undertaken for drugs used to treat humans.

Key Challenges

Challenges in designing and developing dosage forms for animals are similar to those for humans. However, there are also specific issues that necessitate additional exploration and understanding. Issues can range from ensuring product stability to using inexpensive excipients and manufacturing methods to produce cost-effective products. They can encompass product-specific issues relating to a given delivery device to broad issues such as antimicrobial resistance. Some of the challenges a veterinary formulation scientist may encounter are discussed further below.

Interspecies and Intraspecies Differences

One of the most obvious differences and challenges is caused by the wide variety in both anatomy and physiology within and between species. Excellent reviews on differences between various animals and humans have been published (31,32). Others have studied specific differences in gastrointestinal physiology compared with those of humans (33,34), the effect of age and body size in dogs on drug absorption (35–39), or the value of dogs in modeling human drug absorption (40). These interspecies and intraspecies differences present formulation issues to those developing a product that must span different breeds or even species.

The end user can often successfully deal with solutions or suspensions that contain the same amount per volume and which can be administered at different volumes for different-sized animals. However, these liquid products are sometimes not so easy to transfer across species, as palatability becomes an issue. For example, cats are known to lack a gene allowing them to taste sugar/sweets, so a sweet formulation for dogs will not gain the same acceptance in cats. Solid dosage forms can be challenging as a wide range of dosing amounts are often needed between species, and administering a handful of tablets to a large dog may not be a viable option. One feasible alternative is to consider developing single- or double-scoring tablets. For farmed animals, a solution is to develop a flexible product that can be produced in different sizes during the manufacturing process. The TimeCapsule (Fig. 1) achieves this through its simple formulation approach and flexible manufacturing process.

Formulation

A good understanding of physicochemical properties of the active is required. An awareness of the drug and product stability profile (sensitivity to moisture, oxygen, light),

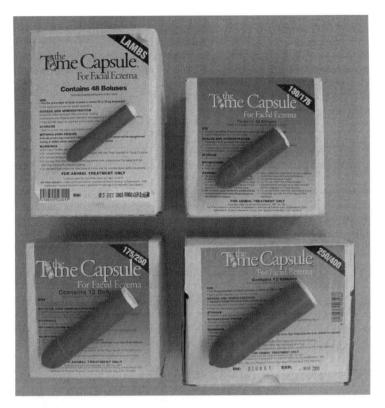

Figure 1 Various sized TimeCapsule intraruminal bolus administered to a range of sheep and cattle of different age and weight.

active forms like polymorphs and crystal form, hygroscopicity, powder characteristics (like density, flow, compression indices) are all important to study. Fundamental pharmacokinetic understanding is also similar with the added requirement in veterinary medicine to consider drug and metabolite residue levels. Ensuring formulations are effective and safe for animals is the same goal as new formulations developed for humans; however, a number of unique scientific and logistical/marketing formulation challenges exist with veterinary medicines.

Logistical/marketing Logistically, the time allotted for formulation scientists to design and develop formulations is considerably less than in the human health care arena. Reasons include the ability to get into the test subject very quickly (less time to recruit study subjects), less complex clinical study designs, which saves time, the need to understand ADME so that residue limits and withdrawal times can be set, and the pressure of less ultimate profit from the new product, resulting in the need to complete things quicker and less expensively to make the new medicine a profitable endeavor. Moving a compound from discovery through to filing takes approximately 7 years in the veterinary arena, while in human health care it takes around 10 years.

Other logistical/marketing-type problems center around cost of goods and the price an owner/producer will pay. All companies developing new animal medicines will from the beginning be examining the cost of goods (contributed by API, formulation excipients, manufacturing processes, packaging) and comparing that price with what the customer will pay. Developing a dosage form that is profitable remains one of the biggest challenges to the veterinary formulation scientist today.

Formulation design and development The challenges for developing a specific dosage form type vary, and, again, are quite similar to those dosage forms developed for humans. Some unique challenges with particular dosage forms are mentioned further in this chapter when discussing specific dosage forms. However, three examples are given in this section to highlight the potential formulation challenges associated with palatability, in-use stability (often called "broached" stability), and large package sizes.

While sweet, sour, bitter, salty, and umami (if one believes in the L-glutamine theory) are the tastes associated with human taste receptors, similar knowledge is not readily available for animals. The area of taste acceptance understanding for animals is ripe for research, with only a few published articles (41). Mainly through trial and error with flavorings (e.g., fish, meat), chewable delivery systems have become popular for dogs and cats. One frequently debated problem is whether laboratory animals can accurately represent the ultimate patient. It is thought that the owner-animal relationship (i.e., the bond) can affect the results and that is hard to simulate with laboratory animals. Additionally, one-time use medication is different from daily administration of drugs, where the animal may eventually tire of that "bad"-tasting solution or tablet. Sometimes it may have nothing to do with the active's taste or the formulation; a side effect like nausea due to the active could result in the animals not liking the dosage form. The important point to remember is that while designing a palatable formulation, the challenges could be quite difficult, lengthy, and resource consuming.

In-use or broached stability is the period of time a product can be used after the initial packaging is opened. It is particularly important in the veterinary field for liquid products. In the treatment of animal health, particularly in the farmed animal arena, numerous animals are often treated all at the same time; thus, the designing of multiple dose vials is more common than for human health care. This then leads to the question of how long after initial use can the contents of that bottle or vial be used. It is therefore important to understand chemical, physical, and microbiological stability of that broached container. Typically this involves withdrawing a representative amount from the container (e.g., 50% or 75%), then placing the reminder on stability. For microbiological testing, the USP Preservative Effectiveness Testing is often used. The aim is to develop a product that achieves the maximum time that a regulatory authority will allow to enable the most flexible for marketing of the product. While 28 days for sterile products is the maximum allowed in Europe, other sterile products may be 30 days or longer in various countries, and with oral solutions, periods of 6 months could be obtained if the data supports it.

Large package sizes are also more common in animal products compared with human medicines. Like the in-use stability issue, this is due to the large number of animals treated at one time. This could mean containers of 100 mL up to 25 L. Upon first glance, this may not appear to be problematic, but, larger packages take up more space and you may not have enough room in your good manufacturing practice (GMP)-controlled registration stability chambers to accommodate your test batches. Or, when making the registration stability batches you have to now manufacture much larger batch sizes to get suitable samples for stability testing, meaning, more API is required. These larger packages may not fit into secondary packages (i.e., cartons), which give protection during shipping. However, you still need to ensure package integrity during shipping. In fact, your drug may be classified in certain countries as being hazardous and your packaging must be safety tested (e.g., drop tested, leak tested). These are unique challenges that a formulation scientist needs to be aware of and address during the R&D process of a veterinary pharmaceutical.

Analytical

Similarity is seen between human and animal health products in analytical testing conducted to assure the quality attributes of the final product. The validation of these assays is identical in that linearity, precision, accuracy, robustness, and reproducibility are all required. Two examples of analytical areas that may differ include stability and in vitro drug testing.

Stability testing The unique stability testing requirements for animal health products include stability protocols that account for package size, extremes in exposed temperatures, in-use or broach packages, blending with other components (e.g., feeds), and compatibility with unique dosing devices.

As mentioned above, veterinary dosage forms can be very large and packaging of multiple doses achieved through the use of large packages. This presents substantial demands upon stability test chambers due to the sheer volume of product that must be stored. Appropriate sampling-size protocols can aid in the solution of this issue.

While regulatory requirements throughout the world for stability testing are very similar between veterinary and human products, sometimes the practical use of the product will dictate product development to withstand lower or higher temperatures. This impacts heavily on the products' stability requirements, which must be addressed and overcome by the formulator during the development stages of the product. How often in drug development for humans do you need to consider the cold winters of Wyoming and that the physical stability of that oil suspension may be different or the drug distribution of the steroid implant from the ear may be slower due to reduced ear temperature?

Broached packages have been discussed previously, but another "in-use" period that demands consideration is when products such as feed additives are mixed with the feeds. Good knowledge of how long your new drug can withstand high mineral, high water content (corn can have $\geq 15\%$ water content) is essential. Equally difficult may be the actual potency assay development as you try to extract the active and degradants from these complex feeds.

Some unique delivery devices are used in animal health as discussed later in this chapter. Knowing the compatibility of the formulation with these devices and whether any deleterious components are extracted from the devices is required. One example would be the rubber or silicone seals in oral drenching guns. Numerous manufactures of these guns exist, and each gun should be examined to be sure that as product contacts the seals those components are not removed that will either affect dosing accuracy and ease or be toxic to the animals receiving the product.

In vitro drug release testing The physical size of some veterinary dosage forms particularly encountered for livestock; the very large quantities of incorporated drug (usually in gram rather than milligram quantities); the very long delivery periods (weeks and months for veterinary products compared with hours or days for human products); the diverse physicochemical properties of the incorporated drug; and the unique shapes and geometries and unique release mechanisms can present difficulties in the development and validation of in vitro drug release tests for veterinary dosage forms. The aim is always to use compendial methods (like the USP-specified apparatus and conditions); however, some scientifically justified deviations from these specifications may be justified on a case-by-case basis to successfully develop a regulatory meaningful assessment method. Large vessels are being introduced, but some tolerance to nonaqueous-based media must be forthcoming. Acknowledgment of the final test capabilities is required by developers. If no in vitro–in vivo correlation can be shown when using a modified test or test conditions, then the test must remain a simple monitor of manufacturing consistency, and not be argued to show biological relevance and used as a surrogate for formulation, site, or manufacturing changes.

Residues

Three areas will be covered with respect to this topic in this chapter: residues within food-producing animals, residues within the environment, and antimicrobial resistance.

Two major disciplines work together to establish allowable residues in animal food products. The first discipline involves those who assess safety of drugs and metabolites who determine whether the compounds have effects on humans and at what dose. This is achieved through testing on mice, rats, dogs, monkeys, or other lab animals that can serve as models for humans. The effects on genes, the potential for causing cancer, and the ability of the drug to be teratogenic are all explored. The potential to cause harm to various organs such as the liver, kidneys, lungs, and heart is also conducted. Studies are conducted with various doses and ideally a "no effect level" (NOEL) with respect to safety is determined. The second discipline involves the pharmacokineticist to study the distribution and elimination of the administered compounds and its metabolites. This typically involves a full tissue residue analysis to be performed, first with radiolabeled drug to determine the sites of deposition, then with nonradiolabeled drug to prove it in the final formulation. By understanding where the drug and metabolites will distribute (i.e., where they might accumulate) and the rate of elimination (i.e., how long they will be around and at what concentrations), the second set of key information is determined. This information is then married with the safety findings and additional safety margins applied to determine the drug's allowable daily intakes (ADIs). From all these data a "tissue withdrawal" time is determined to inform the farmer of when the animal is fit for slaughter. Obviously, the shorter the withdrawal time is for the product, the more desirable the overall product profile. This applies to all food, including meats, milk, and eggs. Approved withdrawal times for all marketed products are located in the Compendium of Veterinary Products (42). For those wanting more detailed information, several good review articles are available (43–46).

The residue potential for the environment is also studied. Both the active drug and metabolites could be studied. A focus is on livestock and other animals (e.g., chickens, turkeys, fish) that eliminate waste on to the ground or into the water. The rate of degradation of the drug is examined in water at different pHs and when exposed to light. The adsorption of these drugs on to certain soils is also studied. The goal is to determine the degradation rate to nontoxic compounds. Also examined are the effects on certain aquatic life to gauge toxicity. Dependent on the drug, even soil bacteria can be evaluated during this phase. An excellent review article is available along with VICH (International Cooperation on Harmonisation of Technical Requirements for Registration of Veterinary Medicinal Products) report (47–49).

Antimicrobial resistance has been a hotly debated issue during the last 15 years. One issue that brought it to the forefront was the use of fluroquinolones in poultry in the mid-1990s. The use of the product in such a large number of animals was purported to increase antimicrobial resistance. While data was presented on both sides of the argument, ultimately the fluoroquinolone poultry product was withdrawn from the market, a decision that was upheld in a U.S. court. To get an antimicrobial approved for food-producing animals in the United States, the sponsor must use FDA-CVM Guidance 152 (50) and follow the guidance to show the benefit of the product and to rank its potential for causing antimicrobial resistance. Again, this process represents an additional hurdle that is placed on the development of animal health products that is not encountered with human drug product development.

Regulatory Considerations

Both human and animal health products need to be safe, efficacious, and of defined quality. For major markets in the world, both animal and human products need to be manufactured in GMP facilities. For human products, regulatory requirements are set for the areas of toxicity, safety, dosing intervals, therapeutic effect, stability, manufacturing, etc. Veterinary products not only include all of the above but are also required to address tissue residue, handler safety, and environmental assessment, particularly if the product is for food-producing animals. If producing a new antimicrobial agent for food-producing animals, the issue of antimicrobial resistance also needs to be addressed. Details about these special requirements were covered in section "Residue" of this chapter.

Unique Products

There are some very unique formulations or delivery systems that are used to treat animals, each of which present unique development challenges. For example, the large feed-additive market dictates that drugs must be stable in a wide variety of feeds even if those feeds have grains containing 10% moisture or more. Or, sometimes those same feeds are fortified with minerals that have the capability of catalyzing drug oxidation degradation pathways. Feed additives are often diluted to parts per million levels, and you need to ensure adequate homogeneity when the local feed-mill blends the product with coarse feeds. Appropriate analytical methods need to be developed to extract the active from those feeds.

  The pour-on or spot-on tick/flea products can also present unique challenges to the formulator. With these products there is a need to deliver accurate amounts of active topically and, depending on the mechanism of action, one may wish for the active to stay on the skin or in the hair follicles and be effective for one month or longer. The challenge is that these products must also be inherently safe for children when they pet their dog, or, for example, to the other cattle that may lick the hides of their field mates.

DOSAGE FORM DESIGN

In this section, our objective is to briefly describe the dosage forms used in animals. This topic has been expertly covered in the book by Hardee and Baggot (3), and the reader is referred to this book for a comprehensive insight.

Solids

The primary solid dosage forms for veterinary medicine include tablets, capsules, and feed additives.

Tablets

Because animals cannot self-administer, tablets as a single-unit dosage form are used less often in veterinary medicine compared with human medicine. However, they are still a prevalent dosage form. Tablets are used in a wide variety of indications, with several species, are available in a large size range, and are manufactured by several different processes. The primary species treated with tablets are dogs and cats; however, for some indications, cattle and sheep may receive a large tablet (often referred to as a bolus).

  The major indications for tablets in dogs and cats would be those diseases that mirror those seen in humans. These would include the therapeutic areas of anticonvulsants, anti-inflammatories, antimicrobials, antitussives (there is a treatment for coughing dogs), antispasmodics (there is a treatment for cats with upset stomachs/diarrhea), behavior modification (e.g., separation anxiety in dogs), cardiovascular, diuretics, thyroid hormone replacement, laxatives, muscle relaxants, nutraceuticals (e.g., antioxidants, glucosamine/chondroitin), sedatives, vitamin and mineral supplements (e.g., multivitamins, calcium), and parasiticides.

In general, the manufacturing process used for the majority of these tablets are the same as those used for humans and are discussed elsewhere (chap. 13, vol. 1). Direct compression and granulation (wet, dry) are both used. Chewable tablets can also be made by these methods or sometimes are molded via excursion and cut into appropriate sizes. The terms "chewable tablets" and "treats" are sometimes confusing. One way to classify is to state that chewable tablets that are made by direct or granulation processes are then called tablets. This would be similar to the mannitol-based chewable tablets prevalent for humans. The term treat is used for the more soft tablets that are produced via extrusion or cast molding.

Tablets can be coated to differentiate the product by color, to help mitigate offensive-tasting compounds, or to prevent dusting in the bottle (which minimizes handler safety issues). Again, the same coating techniques used for human products are utilized.

The relative size of the tablets for companion animals are somewhat similar to those used for humans. Tablets are manufactured large enough for pet owners to handle but small enough to "push" down the throat or hide in foods. Sizes from 80-mg weight up to 1- to 2-g weight are appropriate for use in animals. The tablet sizes for cattle, sheep, and horses are larger to incorporate the larger amount of active and facilitate administration. These tablets are typically called boluses and are often oblong for easier administration. Approximate weights are several grams to 8 g. To minimize the number of product presentations (i.e., tablet strengths), scoring of tablets can be used. Product presentations also include the bottle counts or blister cards and both can be used for animal health products. Child-resistant packaging is frequently considered for products used for cats and dogs.

Tablets are mainly formulated as immediate release types with once- to twice-daily dosing for the course of therapy depending on the disease being treated. Because of the faster gastrointestinal tract motility in dogs and cats, it is fairly difficult to achieve once-daily dosing unless the pharmacokinetic properties of the drug (i.e., a drug with a longer half-life) allow it. Thus, an important area of current research is that of achieving once-daily dosing through retention of the dosage form in the stomach. The use of fast-dissolving tablets (in the mouth) to minimize degradation in the gastrointestinal tract and facilitate ease of use is also of interest. Schering-Plough markets a rapidly disintegrating tablet (Zubrin®) for osteoarthritic dogs and, according to the label, the tablet is placed in the mouth and which is kept shut for approximately four seconds to aid tablet dispersion.

The following examples of anti-inflammatory agents illustrate some tablet products that are used in animal health: Amtech® Phenylbutazone Tablets; Aspirin Bolus; Canine Aspirin Chewable Tablets for Large Dogs; EtoGesic® (etodolac); Deramaxx® Chewable Tablets (deracoxib); Rimadyl® Caplets and Chewable Tablets (carprofen); Medrol® (prednisone); and Zubrin (tepoxalin).

Capsules

Like tablets, capsules are mainly used for dogs and cats, but there are some vitamin and mineral supplement capsules formulated for cattle. There are three main treatment areas using capsules as the dosage form: nutraceuticals, vitamins and minerals, and antimicrobials.

While the typical gelatin capsules used for humans can be used for veterinary medicine if the doses are small (e.g., sizes no. 000, no. 00), there are very large veterinary capsules that range in sizes from no. 13 (2–3 g) to no. 7 (14–24 g). Interestingly, Capsuline manufactures DOGCaps™ and CATCaps™, which are capsules containing beef, chicken, or bacon flavoring in the shells to entice dogs and cats to consume the products. These may be good capsules to hide small tablets that a finicky pet will not consume.

There are fewer capsule animal health products on the market when compared with the human health care market. This is somewhat surprising since capsules are often thought to take less time to develop (blending and flow are the important steps compared with tablets where blending, flow, compression, and sometimes coating are needed). Since time to develop the formulation is often the rate-limiting step for product approval, one may have thought that more capsules would have been developed for the veterinary market. One possible reason for there not being more animal health capsule formulations is that the eating action of cats and dogs would result in capsules being split and spill their contents. If the drug contained in the capsule is associated with a bad taste, then the cat or dog will be more careful to accept that product on a subsequent occasion.

Formulation development of capsule products involves the key areas of (*i*) blending active with bulking excipients, (*ii*) forming a free-flowing granulation, which results in good content uniformity, and (*iii*) ensuring drug stability in the capsule.

While the majority of the capsule products are hard shell gelatin products, two soft elastic capsules are marketed that contain fish oils/omega-3 and vitamin K_1. Some products on the market include vitamin K_1 Oral Capsules, 3V CAPS® series of products by DVM, which contain fish and cod liver oils, BioStart™ Capsules for Adult Cattle (contains vitamins; minerals; rumen and intestinal bacteria, yeast, enzymes), Vita Charge® Gel Cap (a 21-g capsule for cattle containing a mixture of *Aspergillus oryzae*, vitamins, and minerals), Aller G-3™ Capsules (omega-3), Cosequin® (glucosamine, chondroitin capsules that can be opened and flavored granules sprinkled on food), and Antirobe® Capsules (clindamycin hydrochloride).

Feed Additives

Feed additives are useful dosage forms for treating large numbers of animals simultaneously. Cattle, poultry, and swine are the main species to receive feed additives. The dosage forms include solid powders, which are mixed with feeds and liquids that are mixed in the feeds. Products that can be placed into the drinking systems could also be classified as feed additives. They would usually be a solution but could be a soluble powder that is reconstituted before being added to the drinking system.

People typically associate feed additives with solid powders (containing the actives) that are placed into the feed. It is important to understand the designation of type A, B, or C feed additives. Medicated type A feeds are the products containing one or more animal drugs that are sold to feed mills or producers and are intended to be mixed into feeds. Medicated type B feeds are feeds that contain type A or another type B plus a substantial quantity of nutrients (not less than 25% of the total weight) and are intended to be mixed with feeds and additional nutrients to make the feed that the animals consume. The important point is that medicated type B feeds are not to be fed directly to the animals. Type C is the final diluted feed that is fed to animals. This medicated type C feed can be offered directly to the animal or top dressed on to the animal's normal daily rations.

Challenges with developing feed additives reside in blend homogeneity and stability. The type A medicated feeds may contain concentrations of 1% or less (sometimes down to 0.05%). With concentrations of 0.05% achieving homogeneous products is important. These type A medicated feeds are usually formulated with a "carrier" such as rice hulls or calcium carbonate. Ideally the active will be milled or micronized to a similar particle size as the carrier to help insure blend uniformity. These carriers then help facilitate the blending of the type A with type B and C feeds by providing a greater surface area. Because type B and C feeds will consist of ground grains, the particle sizes will be large but obtaining content uniformity is necessary to ensure proper dosing. Often dilution down to several parts per million is required. In addition, a robust formulation is required as the blending equipment and capabilities of feed mills will vary.

A second major challenge is to ensure adequate stability. While maintaining stability in the type A medicated feed (sometimes called Premix) may not be difficult, when blending in to type B and C, stability must be ensured. Because these feeds may include numerous metals (like copper that catalyzes oxidation) and contain grains with high moisture content, accelerated potency loss is possible. Additionally, type B medicated feeds may be stored for several months while they are being used on a daily basis to mix the final feeds. Storage can be in hot, moist grain bins or sometimes in the open where the sun and rain can further cause problems.

Finally, there are other challenges like minimizing dust. Most often mineral oil is added to feed additives to prevent the type A feed from being lost in to the air, which cannot only reduce potency but also potentially be a safety issue for the feed operators. A solid feed additive is definitely a challenging dosage form to develop.

For feed additives that are soluble powders, the key challenge is designing a powder that will readily go into solution and be stable when blended with the feed. Whether a soluble powder or a ready-to-use solution that is mixed with feeds, obtaining a homogenous blend is again important. For those solutions that are added to water systems, ensuring that no complexation occurs with minerals in the water or adsorption to pipes is important. These can happen because the drug may be in concentrations of parts per million or less. A dose-metering device is hooked into the water system to continuously add the drug solution at a prescribed rate.

The major uses for feed additives are as vitamin/mineral supplements, electrolyte replacements, and antimicrobials/progestins (for increased rate of weight gain and improved feed efficiency in livestock). The vitamin/mineral supplements are numerous and include cobalt, cooper, iodine, manganese, multiple vitamins/minerals, vitamin A, vitamin K, vitamin E, selenium, and zinc. Electrolyte replacements include Calf Quencher and Bluelite®Swine Formula, while products for weight gain include MGA®200 Premix and MGA500 Liquid Premix.

Liquids

The previously discussed dosage forms had a solid physical appearance. This section will explore those that are classified as liquids. The three main liquid dosage forms are those administered via the mouth, injected, or placed on the skin.

Oral Liquids

Oral liquids would typically be aqueous, nonaqueous, or blends to create a solution. In some cases they may be a suspension if it is difficult to find a vehicle that completely solubilizes the active or yields chemical stability. The liquid may be used directly "as is" from the container or, if sold in a concentrated form, is diluted before administration. Oral liquids may be given directly to the animal or, if administering to many animals, placed in drinking water or even dispersed among feed.

Oral liquids are probably one of the easier dosage forms to develop. The main challenges are finding a vehicle that results in adequate chemical stability while achieving a solution. Many prefer to develop a solution instead of a suspension because of the added requirement with the latter of insuring physical stability, namely the ease of resuspendability. The first vehicle choice will be water. A good understanding of the pH and temperature effects on solubility are needed to ensure no precipitation of the marketed product when exposed to abrupt changes in temperature or pH. Having a twofold or above cushion with solubility will help avoid crystallization during product storage. Use of a buffering agent may be appropriate for an oral liquid if the solubility-pH curve is very sharp and slight changes in pH have a dramatic effect on solubility.

If water does not solubilize the drug, a cosolvent system is next explored. Vehicles to consider include ethanol, propylene glycol, polyethylene glycol (low molecular weight), glycerin, and triacetin as examples. These can be used alone or in combination to give a truly nonaqueous system. In some cases cosolvents with oleaginous vehicles may be utilized to solubilize the drug.

If a solution is not achieved, a suspension may be developed. The main challenge is to achieve a product that uniformly and easily resuspends. This needs to happen at room temperature and for livestock products even at very low temperatures. Whether developing a suspension for oral or parenteral use, the issue of resupendability is equally important. The key is achieving appropriate particle-to-particle interaction to yield a flocculated system. With the appropriate surface charges of the particles, interaction will occur resulting in flocs that settle in the vehicle but do not compact in the bottom of the bottle. This might result in sedimentation volumes of 30% to 70%, which then, with little energy (e.g., shaking), will resuspend. Besides achieving floc formation, using a vehicle of appropriate viscosity to allow uniform dosing is also important. For aqueous systems, this could mean using a cellulose (such as carboxymethylcellulose) to enhance viscosity so that after shaking the product stays uniform for sufficient time to allow dosing.

An oral liquid product for animals is quite often a multiple-use product. If the container is going to be opened and closed several times with storage time between uses, then a preservative should be used. These should be soluble in the vehicle and result in the formulation meeting the Preservative Efficacy Test as outlined in the pharmacopoeias (USP, EP, BP, JP). Examples of preservatives for oral liquids include benzoic acid, sodium or potassium benzoate, and sorbic acid. The vehicles ethanol, glycerin, and propylene glycol can also be good preservatives themselves. If treating companion animals, a flavoring agent may also be required.

As mentioned above, liquid dosage forms are one of the easier products to develop especially solutions. It is also fairly easy to manufacture requiring a tank, mixer, and bottle-filling line. The main challenge with a suspension is ensuring homogeneity throughout the filling process. This can be done by mixing the product throughout filling; however, careful study of suspension uniformity when product levels drop below the mixing blades is required.

The uses of oral liquids is quite varied and in some cases rather unique in veterinary medicine. For example, propylene glycol is marketed to treat ketosis in dairy cows where it is mixed with the solid feeds or given as a drench. A formulation consisting of vegetable oil, polyethylene glycol, and other ingredients is sold as Bloat Drench™ to be given as a drench (a large oral dose of liquid medicine) in cattle to treat bloating. Oral liquid products are available as antacids, anticoccidials, anti-inflammatories, antimicrobials, and antitussives. They are used in dental care, as diuretics, for electrolyte replacement, growth promotants in cattle, as laxatives, and as vitamin/mineral supplements. All species are treated with oral liquid products.

Parenteral Liquids

The uses of parenteral products for animals and the development process of these are nearly identical to those products used for humans. The sterile dosage form types include solutions, suspensions, emulsions, and lyophilized powders. Any dosage form must be chemically, physically, and microbiologically stable, sterile, easy to inject, cause minimal pain and irritation upon injection, and packaged in appropriate vial sizes. Multiple-use vials are more common in animal health to treat herds/flocks).

One somewhat different, but critical, parameter in animal health sterile products compared with human health care products is the irritation and residue at the injection site. For companion animals, the pain upon injection should be minimal, and any lasting reactions that cause either pain or visual lumps to a pet will not be tolerated by many owners. For food-producing animals such as cattle, pigs, and poultry, the added challenge is that of ensuring the residue levels at the injection site have been depleted adequately by the time the animal is harvested. The formulation scientist thus may need to carefully observe the viscosity and polarity of the vehicle as they can affect residue times. Volumes injected and the route can also have an impact. Oftentimes subcutaneous administration is used instead of intramuscular administration to minimize residues in the tissue and potential damage to meat (i.e., muscle).

Parenteral liquids are used as analgesics, general and local anesthetics, antihistamines, anti-inflammatories (steroidal and nonsteriodal), antimicrobial agents, antiprotozoal, antitussives, andrenergics, anticholinergics, antiparasiticides, blood substitutes, diuretics, euthanasia agents, electrolyte replacements, hematinics, hormone replacements (e.g., insulin, gonadotropins), milk production enhancer, immunostimulants, muscle relaxants, respiratory stimulants, sedatives, and vitamins/mineral supplements. All species are treated with injectable liquids, including off-label exotic animal uses.

Representative dosage forms that are sterile solutions include the many vitamin/ mineral supplements such as multiple vitamins (Vta-15™ injection for horses, Mineral Max™ for cattle), antibiotics like oxytetratcyclines (Oxybiotic™-200) or florfenicol (Nuflor® Injectable Solution), anti-inflammatories (Ketoprofen Sterile Solution), and unique products like an artificial blood substitute for dogs, called Oxyglobin® Solution. Sterile suspensions include antibiotics like Excenel® RTU or Sterile Suspension (ceftiofur hydrochloride). Freeze-dried products for reconstitution prior to administration include Solu-Delta-Cortef® (prednisolone sodium succinate) in a unique Act-O-Vial system (Fig. 2), where the sterile water is pushed through an orifice into the sterile powder chamber. Other freeze-dried products are Naxcel® (ceftiofur sodium) and many of the vaccines (which are not discussed in this chapter). Some powders may be dry filled and then reconstituted to form a sterile liquid for injection [Polyflex® (ampicillin)]. There are even available a few sterile emulsions like BO-SE® containing selenium and vitamin E as the oleaginous component with water and vitamin E plus vitamin AD that has vitamins E, A, and D_3 in an aqueous emulsion.

Dermal/Transdermal Liquids

Probably the first thought for liquids for dermal and transdermal application is in animals used to treat ticks, fleas, and mites in dogs, cats, and cattle. But, there are other

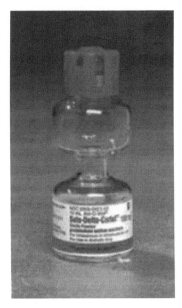

Figure 2 Act-O-Vial system that allows sterile water to be pushed through an orifice into a chamber containing sterile powder.

applications such as antifungals, anti-inflammatories, antimicrobials, antiseptics, antipruritics, teat dips/udder washes, otic/ocular preparations, and miscellaneous items like egg dips and wart removers. The last two refer to Gentadip, a gentamicin sulfate solution for dipping turkey eggs before hatching to reduce or eliminate organisms such as *salmonella* or *mycoplasma*, and Wartsoff® to remove warts from cow teats.

Dermal/transdermal liquids are normally solution dosage forms. The viscosities can vary and may often increase to the point of being called gels, ointments, or creams. With the less viscous liquids for dermal/transdermal use, designing the delivery device may be one of the greater challenges during development. The spot-ons (e.g., tubes), sprays (e.g., pump/pressurized containers), or even impregnated collars to deliver antiparasiticides to cats and dogs would be good examples of challenging-to-develop dosage forms. Designing the delivery system to provide adequate coverage of the fur/skin, for example, with a spray can be difficult. Then, obtaining long enough activity can be critical because frequent administration is not wanted. The fipronil active in Frontline® is a good example. It is thought that the ability of fipronil to diffuse slowly out of the hair follicles and sebaceous oils gives flea and tick prevention for at least one month. A good understanding of how the active and formulation contributes to the duration of efficacy is important for topical products. Other issues to consider with these special packaged products include egress/ingress of solvents (including water) from plastic tubes and diffusion of active from collars during storage.

The liquid products used to treat parasites topically are typically called pour-ons. Example products include ivermectin (Ivomec® Pour-on for Cattle; Top Line™) that can treat gastrointestinal roundworms, lungworms, cattle grubs, mites, lice, and horn flies. These are administered with special squeeze bottles that have dose-metering cups or application guns and are applied in a narrow line from the withers to the tail head in cattle.

Antifungal liquid dermal products include Clotrimazole Solution USP and Micazole Lotion or Spray 1%, which are used in cats and dogs. Topical antibiotics include Gentamicin Spray. The antiseptics are isopropyl alcohol based and contain hydrogen peroxide, chlorhexidine, iodine, or benzalkonium chloride. Teat dips and udder washes to prevent bacterial contamination during milking generally contain iodine or chlorhexidine.

Intramammary Drug Delivery

The intramammary route for drug delivery is primarily used for the treatment of mastitis in cows and can be classified according to two main areas: for the treatment of animals lactating and dry (nonlactating). A once-only administration is beneficial to both these areas since it reduces handling of the animal. Each approach offers specific challenges to the delivery of an active agent. For example, the requirements for drug delivery to lactating cattle requires that the active ingredient be removed from the mammary gland or milk as soon as possible after the treatment period has elapsed so that there is no issue with regard to the presence of drug in the milk. In contrast, intramammary delivery in dry cows would allow for the formulation to be developed so that the drug persists for a longer period after the treatment period has elapsed. Dry cow applications, therefore, lend themselves more readily to controlled drug delivery applications since the prolonged exposure of the infected site to drug improves the efficacy of treatment, and the concerns for drug residues in milk are not an issue.

Various formulation types have been explored for the intramammary route and include water- and ointment-based systems, oil-based systems, encapsulated systems, polymeric aqueous systems, and vaccines and recombinant therapies.

Long-Acting Formulations

The reasons for developing a long-acting product for animals differ from those typically associated with their human counterparts. In the case of animals, the reasons to develop long-acting preparations include reduction of stress to the animal, reduced herding, and reduced labor costs. In the human field, drugs incorporated into long-acting formulations need to possess certain physicochemical properties such as high potency and low dose. These characteristics do not necessarily need to be inherent with a drug that is intended to be incorporated into a long-acting formulations developed for an animal. Because of the size of the final dosage form, less potent actives with higher dose sizes can be incorporated into a long-acting formulation designed for use in an animal. Finally, durations of delivery contrast markedly between human products and animal products. In general, human long-acting preparations are designed for 12 to 24 hours, perhaps days, whereas veterinary preparations are designed to last for weeks or months. A useful review article on long-acting parenterals for veterinary medicine has been published by Medlicott et al. (51).

Parenteral Long-Acting Dosage Forms
Solutions and suspensions
Solutions Several solution dosage forms exist for administration to an animal. For example, Ivomec injection (Merial, Harlow, Essex, U.K.) is a solution of 1% w/w ivermectin in propylene glycol and glycerol formal, which is given subcutaneously at approximately 200 µg/kg in cattle and 300 µg/kg in pigs. This injection is given once a month for the treatment of endoparasites. The main reason the injection is so long lasting

is that the half-life of ivermectin in cattle is long and the potency of the compound is high, allowing even trace levels of the drug in the blood to be effective. The half-life of the drug combined with its formulation into a nonaqueous vehicle (which allows for the creation of a depot at the site of injection) prolongs the action of the drug for over a month. Similar results are also seen with the doramectin and moxidectin products, since they are of the same drug classification and exhibit similar half-life profiles.

In the area of antibiotics, florfenicol and oxytetracycline have been developed as long-acting injectables. Nuflor® injection (florfenicol) was developed by Schering-Plough to replace a chloramphenicol product, which needed to be administered at frequent intervals to combat bovine respiratory disease, or shipping fever. The dose of florfenicol is approximately 20 mg/kg; however, its solubility is low in most solvents. Therefore to improve the drug's solubility, the formulators devised a complex nonaqueous cosolvent system, which allowed for sufficient drug to be administered once every two days. The solvents added to the formulation include propylene glycol, polyethylene glycol, and *n*-methyl pyrrolidone, which allows for dosing at 48-hour intervals.

Suspensions Oxytetracycline has been formulated to combat shipping fever (i.e., bovine respiratory disease). The development of the Liquamycin® LA by Pfizer has been well documented in the literature (52). In this case, tetracyclines were well known to also be insoluble, as well as irritating, upon injection. To alleviate this problem, formulators identified 2-pyrrolidone as a solubilizer and developed methods of chelating the oxytetracycline with magnesium ion to reduce the irritation upon injection. The theory was to prepare a solution of drug that was close to saturation so that upon injection the drug would slowly deposit a fine precipitate creating, in effect, a drug suspension depot at the injection site. This depot formulation would reduce the irritation and necrosis, which had been previously observed. The resulting formulation succeeded in reducing the irritation and provided release of drug over two to three days.

A unique approach to minimizing tissue residues and thus withdrawal periods is used with Pfizer's ceftiofur product Excenel Sterile Suspension for bovine respiratory disease. This one-time administered oil-based suspension is injected into the middle section of the ear. During slaughter the ears of cattle are not put into the food chain. The product is also used for swine, but for that species is given intramuscularly.

Implants Implants are cylindrical rod-shaped delivery systems that contain drugs incorporated into lactose, cholesterol, polyethylene, or silicone rubber delivery matrices. They are typically 2 to 4 mm in diameter and up to approximately 20 mm in length. Drugs can be incorporated into the implant by homogenously distributing them throughout the entire cylinder, or as a coat that covers the surface of the cylinder. Lactose-based implants are shorter acting ($\sim$40 days) compared with cholesterol-based implants ($\sim$80 days). Silicone rubber matrices provide the longest duration of release for estrogens ($\sim$200–400 days). The actual duration is very dependent on the physicochemical drug characteristics, especially solubility. The amount of drug released from these delivery systems is greatest initially and slowly decreases with time, and release kinetics are typically described by either first-order kinetics or a square-root-of-time mechanism.

Simple compressed pellets (i.e., small tablets) is the technology used to manufacture products for weight gain in range cattle. Depending on the drug and size of the animal, anywhere from 4 to 8 of these pellets are introduced with a single-trochar administration into the ear. Estradiol benzoate (EB), progesterone, and trenbolone acetate are the drugs used in this technology. A range of doses and actives are marketed under the tradename Synovex® by Fort Dodge Animal Health.

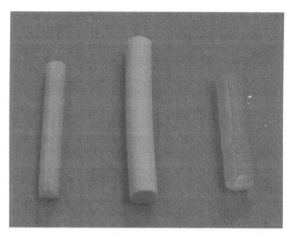

Figure 3 Subcutaneous implants (*left* to *right*: Crestar implant, Compudose 400 implant, and Syncro-Mate-B implant).

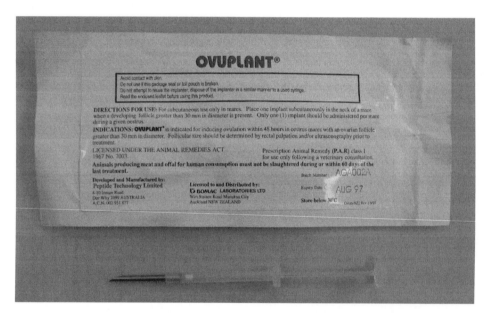

Figure 4 Ovuplant, a small white implant (2×3 mm^2) packaged in its applicator.

Compudose is a silicone implant composed of a drug-free silicone cylinder coated with a layer of silicone containing 20% dispersion estradiol (Fig. 3). It has a surface area of 4.84 cm^2 and has been shown to release drug by a square-root-of-time mechanism. Different release durations are achieved by manufacturing the product with coatings of different thickness. It has been coated with oxytetracycle to minimize reactions at the injection site and enhance implant retention. The Crestar implant (Fig. 3) is an ear implant that also uses silicone as the polymeric matrix, but in this case it contains 3 mg norgestomet homogeneously distributed throughout the entire cylinder.

Ovuplant (Fig. 4) is a cylindrical subcutaneous implant containing the synthetic GnRH analog Deslorelin [6-D-tryptophan-9-(*N*-ethyl-L-prolinamide)-10-desglycinamide]. The implant is 2.3 mm in diameter and 3.6 mm in length and contains 2.1 mg of Deslorelin acetate in an inert matrix. The implant is biocompatible and becomes absorbed overtime and therefore does not need removal after administration.

Syncro-Mate-B comprises a norgestomet/Hydron implant (Fig. 3). It measures 3×18 mm^2, contains 6-mg norgestomet, and weighs approximately 0.125 g. During manufacture the implants are encased within a protective plastic sheath and packaged in individually sealed foil packaging. A specially designed applicator is then used to administer them under the skin of the outer surface of the ear of cattle.

Although implants are a useful dosage form for administering drugs to farmed animals, they are not so well accepted in the small animal field as they can be felt through the skin, a feature that pet owners do not like.

In situ forming gels An in situ forming gel system based on sucrose acetate isobutyrate (SAIB) has been investigated for veterinary applications. SAIB is a fully esterified sucrose molecule. It is a low molecular weight material that has many properties associated with polymeric materials; however, it is a nonpolymer, and dilution with only small amounts of solvents such as alcohol results in an easily injectable solution. Formulations are manufactured by a simple process of weighing and mixing SAIB, diluting solvent, and adding drug and mixing. The resultant formulation is a hydrophobic, low-viscosity liquid that rapidly increases in viscosity after intramuscular injection as the solvent diffuses away leaving behind a SAIB-drug matrix, which releases drug by diffusion through the highly viscous SAIB, accompanied by degradation of SAIB to sucrose and the aliphatic acids from which the sucrose ester was prepared.

Microspheres Intramuscular injections comprising a microsphere formulation manufactured from poly(DL-lactide) have been described for veterinary applications. Microspheres have been formulated to deliver progesterone (1.25 g) and estradiol (100 mg) continuously for a duration of 12 to 14 days. Other microsphere products have been developed, which contain various active ingredients including ivermectin, estradiol, moxidectin, and vitamin B_{12}.

The production of the microspheres is affected by multiple factors such as the type of polymer and solvent being used and the drug being encapsulated. High yields, lower residual solvent content, and better control of microsphere size distributions are all extremely important in large-scale commercial production of such. Also, extremely important in the production of microspheres is sterility and pyrogenicity and the need to use sterile water for injection in the manufacturing process. Lastly, any products using steroids, especially estrogens, also add significant regulatory and environmental concerns as does the large amount of nearly pure wastewater generated. Several microsphere products have been commercialized for use in animal health (Fig. 5). These include Proheart[R]6, a 180-day moxidectin in microspheres for heartworm in dogs (Fort Dodge Animal Health, Wyeth, Madison, New Jersey, U.S.); SMART Shot[R], a 150-day vitamin B_{12} PLGA microsphere product for cattle (Stockguard, New Zealand); and Celerin[R], a 150 day EB PLGA microsphere product for cattle (PR Pharmaceuticals, Colorado, U.S.).

Intraruminal Bolus Formulations

Intraruminal drug delivery systems are products administered to, and retained in, the rumen of ruminant animals (e.g., cattle, sheep) and formulated to deliver drugs over extended periods (months). Many controlled-release intraruminal drug delivery systems have been developed over the last few decades, and for extensive reviews on intraruminal drug delivery the reader is referred to Refs. 11, 13, and 14.

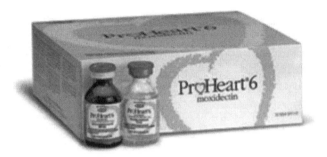

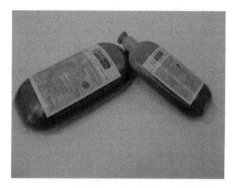

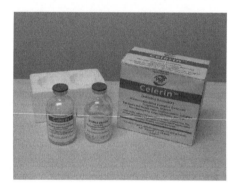

Figure 5 Proheart®6, SMART Shot®, and Celerin® microsphere products used in veterinary animal health.

Cardinal has outlined several key design features that are required of a controlled-release intraruminal drug delivery system (13). These include the inherent need to (*i*) design the delivery system around a balling gun (an administration device for discharging a rumen bolus down the throat of an animal) to allow for oral administration, (*ii*) design the delivery system with a shape compatible with passage down the esophagus, (*iii*) design the device with some mechanism that allows for long-term retention in the rumen of the animal (i.e., prevents regurgitation), and (*iv*) incorporate some form of controlled-release technology that allows for the long-term delivery of the drug (up to 180 days).

Intraruminal boluses are cylindrical or elongated capsule-shaped devices that are typically 7- to 16-cm long and 1 to 3 cm in diameter, dependant on the species for which they are intended. They must be designed to provide some mechanism for long-term

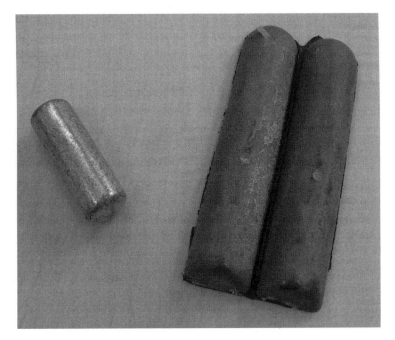

Figure 6 Rumbul Bullet (*left*) and Rumetrace Magnesium Capsule (*right*) heavy density products.

retention in the rumen of the animal. Two methods are commonly employed to retain devices in the rumen. The first involves the incorporation of components that provide an overall device density of greater than 2 g/cm^3. This condition ensures that the device will remain at the bottom of the reticulo-rumen cavity and will not be regurgitated. The TimeCapsule bolus (Fig. 1), which contains high amounts of the active ingredient zinc oxide, is an example of this approach. Zinc oxide is a dense powder, and this property affords sufficient density to the product to retain in it the rumen. Other examples of heavy density products include the Rumbul Bullet and Rumetrace Magnesium Capsule (Fig. 6), which erode to completion following administration. In the case where the product does not erode, incorporation of a density element such as iron or sintered iron block in the product allows for prolonged retention in the rumen. The Ivomec SR bolus is an example of this approach (Fig. 7).

Alternatively, device retention can be achieved by using a design that leads to a significant expansion of the device in at least one dimension following its introduction into the reticulo-rumen cavity. The Captec device (Auckland, New Zealand) is an example of a technology that uses this method for retention (Fig. 8). The Captec device incorporates polymeric "wings" that are constrained by a water-soluble tape during administration. Upon passage into the rumen, the tape dissolves allowing the wings to expand, thereby preventing regurgitation. This "winged-cylinder" design has also been utilized for the Rumensin ABC and the Monensin RDD (Fig. 8) devices. As an alternate to the opening wings, a device in the form of a large trilaminate sheet, approximately 21 × 10 cm^2 (Paratect Flex), serves as another example of the change in shape approach. The sheet is rolled into a cylinder and constrained with a water-soluble adhesive tape, which following administration dissolves to allow the device to unroll. The unrolled device has dimensions that are greater than those of the esophageal channel, thereby preventing device regurgitation. Interestingly the tape was composed of multiple layers, special water-soluble adhesives, and was also perforated to enhance the rate of water penetration once the device reaches the rumen. It was found that it was critical that the tape released

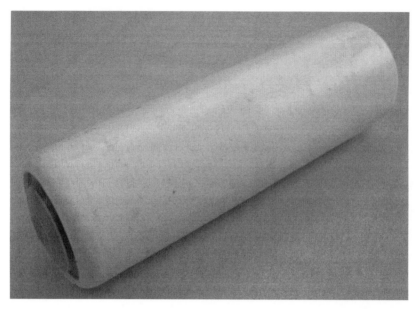

Figure 7 Ivomec SR bolus.

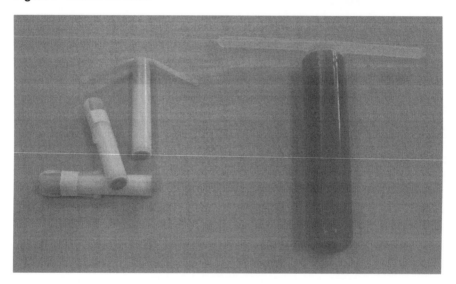

Figure 8 Captec device (*left*) and Monensin RDD (*right*) products that utilize a change in geometry (plastic wings) to impel retention to the rumen delivery system.

and permitted the device to unroll within the first hour or two following administration to ensure that the device was not regurgitated. For these reasons, the design of the tape was as difficult as the design of the controlled-release matrix. This serves as an example of the range of issues, sometimes unusual, the veterinary formulation scientist will encounter, and must solve, when developing a product for animal health.

Intravaginal

The processes of designing, developing, optimizing, and assessing a long-acting intravaginal veterinary drug delivery system has been discussed by Rathbone et al.

Table 2 Factors Affecting Design of an Intravaginal Veterinary Drug Delivery System

Factor affecting design	Factor influences	Factor influenced by
Applicator design	Dimensions and geometry of delivery system Ease of use Animal comfort End-user acceptance	Size and shape of vaginal cavity Dimensions and geometry of delivery system
Retention rate	Overall efficacy of delivery system	Retention mechanism Dimensions and geometry of delivery system
Retention mechanism	Ease of use Retention rate	Dimensions and geometry of delivery system
Dimensions	Release rate Ease of use Animal comfort End-user acceptance	Size and shape of vaginal cavity Applicator design Desired release rate
Geometry	Release rate Ease of use Animal comfort End-user acceptance	Size and shape of vaginal cavity Applicator design Desired release rate
Irritation (mucopurulent discharge production)	End-user acceptance Release rate	Dimensions and geometry of delivery system Polymer used to manufacture delivery system Drug incorporated into delivery system Presence or absence of additives
Removal	Ease of use End-user acceptance Animal comfort	Retention mechanism Dimensions and geometry of delivery system
Damage to vaginal mucosa and cervix	Applicator design Removal mechanism Retention mechanism	Dimensions and geometry of delivery system
Environmental considerations	End-user acceptance Environment Regulatory acceptance Optimal drug load	Polymer Method of disposal Drug load Residue
Release characteristics	Efficacy of delivery system	Polymer used to manufacture delivery system Drug incorporated into delivery system Presence or absence of additives Manufacturing process

(13,20,21). Several factors affect the design and development of an intravaginal veterinary drug delivery system. These are listed in Table 2 (13).

The drugs used in intravaginal veterinary delivery systems are synthetic and natural hormones used to control the estrous cycle (progesterone, methyl acetoxy progesterone, fluorogestone acetate, and EB). Other drugs (melatonin, prostaglandin $F_{2\alpha}$, and a variety of other synthetic progestagens) have been shown to be systemically absorbed from the

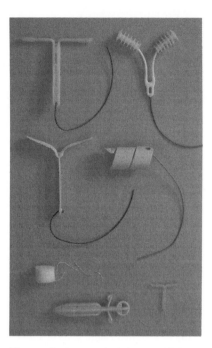

Figure 9 Intravaginal inserts (CIDR 1380 Insert, CueMate, PCL Intravaginal Insert, PRID, sponge, CIDR Pig Insert, and CIDR-G).

vagina of farmed animals. Polymers utilized in intravaginal veterinary delivery systems have included polyurethane, silicone, and polycaprolactone.

An intravaginal delivery system is usually designed and optimized for a given species; therefore its design features that provide retention, safety, etc. may not be as effective in a second species. This may be for several reasons including differences in vaginal size and structure as well as different dosage requirements.

Several drug delivery systems of intravaginal veterinary delivery systems are commercially available (Fig. 9), and include

- The PRID (progesterone-releasing intravaginal device), which consists of a stainless steel spiral covered with a silicone elastomer, with micronized progesterone (1.55 or 2.25 g) uniformly dispersed throughout.
- The CIDR 1380 Cattle Insert, which is a T-shaped delivery system comprising a nylon spine that gives form to the device, over which a layer of silicone is cured, and 1.38 g (10%w/w) of USP grade micronized progesterone is dispersed homogeneously throughout it.
- Several sponge delivery systems made from polyurethane and impregnated with a potent progestagen. They are cylindrical in shape with a string (tail) fitted to aid removal at the end of treatment period.
- The CIDR-G (Controlled Internal Drug Release–Goat), which is a T-shaped intravaginal device with a body, wings, and tail for use in sheep and goats, comprises a preformed nylon spine that has a filament of flexible nylon molded to it (tail). The body and wings of the preformed spine are coated with silicone, which is impregnated with 0.3 g (9% w/w) of USP grade micronized progesterone.

- The CueMate, which is a wishboned-shaped delivery system comprising a polyester spine that gives form to the device onto which progesterone impregnated silicone pods can be attached. These pods are manufactured by injection molding at high temperatures.
- The Pig CIDR, which contains 2 g of progesterone that is homogeneously dispersed throughout a silicone matrix cured at low temperatures (below 120°C) over a polyester spine.
- The PCL Intravaginal Insert, which is a T-shaped delivery system comprising a single-mold polycaprolactone polymeric insert impregnated with progesterone that is manufactured by injection molding at very low molding temperatures (around 80°C).

Collars and Spot-Ons

Collar technologies for animals such as dogs and cats have been formulated for the prolonged topical control of ectoparasites. The collar is worn by the animal and the active ingredient is slowly delivered from the device, permeates the fur of the animal, and kills the ectoparasites. Collars offer the advantages of ease of use and an extended duration of action, which can be up to six months after only one application.

These collar technologies can be divided into (*i*) matrix devices, (*ii*) reservoir devices, and (*iii*) mechanical devices. Matrix devices in which the active agent is blended directly into the polymer itself represent the most commonly used technology. The vinyl collar is an example of a matrix collar. Others include elastomeric and wax-based devices. In some cases the devices contain additives, which increase the overall percentage of active agent delivered. A reservoir technology comprises dispersed or dissolved active in a vehicle that is encapsulated in a solid or mesh-like casing. Mechanical systems including ultrasonic devices, which emit sound waves, designed to disrupt the flea life cycle; topical pumps, which deliver small quantities of a dissolved active agent; and chambered devices designed to physically entrap the flea inside the collar have also been formulated.

More recently spot-on products have been developed, which have a long action due to the inherent properties of the active ingredient. Commercially available topical liquids include Ex-spot® (permethrin), Advantage® (imidacloprid), and Frontline (fipronil). These products are very easy to use and, because of the potency of the active ingredient, require only a few drops per treatment to be administered on the back of the animal. These products are mainly used for dogs and cats and have a duration as long as one month.

Excellent overviews on the collar and spot-on technologies have been published by Witchey-Laskmanan (15).

APPLICATORS

As mentioned previously, normally animals cannot self-medicate (exceptions are feed additives, insect dusters) and innovative solutions must be devised by the veterinary formulation scientists to assure that their final products can be administered safely, quickly, and easily by the end user. Thus the means of administration must be carefully considered and be part of the product development process (53).

Applicators vary considerably between route of administration and volume/capacity for delivery and are available for intravaginal (Fig. 10), intraruminal (Fig. 11), and for subcutaneous implants (Fig. 12).

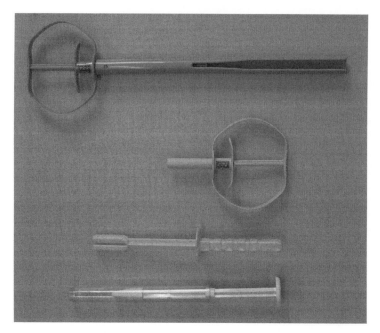

Figure 10 Intravaginal applicators available in either a single-handed (*upper two applicators*) or a double-handed (*lower two applicators*) design.

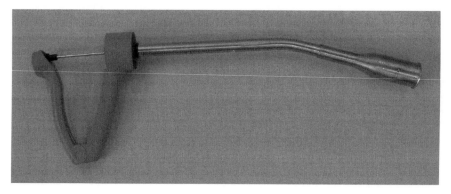

Figure 11 Intraruminal balling gun.

Intravaginal

Intravaginal inserts are administered with applicators that are available in either a single-handed (Fig. 10) or a double-handed design. Each commercially available intravaginal insert has a specifically designed applicator associated with it, which is used to administer that particular intravaginal insert. Obviously single-handed applicators are more convenient and quicker to use compared with two-handed applicators. Each is designed to allow a folded intravaginal insert to be located into the applicator and has some mechanism to push out the loaded insert after the applicator has been lubricated and inserted into the vagina of the animal.

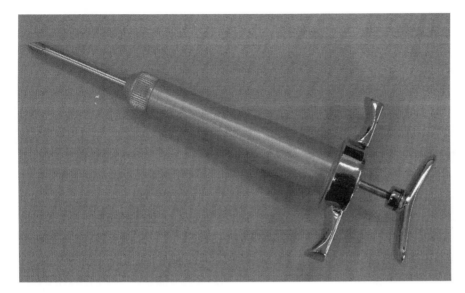

Figure 12 Subcutaneous implanter device.

Intraruminal

Rumen devices are administered with a balling gun or equivalent. A balling gun has a cup or suction-type mechanism to hold the bolus in place, a long rodlike tool designed to move the device through the oral cavity, and a means to expel the bolus from the cup upon placement at the upper end of the esophagus (Fig. 11). Several commercial designs of balling guns are available. Associated with this is the need to provide a bolus shape compatible with passage down the esophagus.

Injections and Implants

Injections
Liquid injection formulations can readily be administered to animals through conventional syringes and needles. Small animals use the same gauge as humans do (e.g., 27 to 32 gauge). In contrast, large animals require larger needle gauges to ensure they penetrate the hair and skin and do not break during use (e.g., 14 to 21 gauge). Fortunately large animals are less needle shy than humans. Larger bore needles do offer the formulator some additional formulation benefits as more viscous preparations can, theoretically, be administered through a larger bore needle. Volumes administered are much greater than those administered in humans (up to 10 mL subcutaneously in cattle), which again, affords the formulator some scope in the dosage form design. A major challenge when formulating a product for injection is the mass of active that needs to be incorporated into the dosage form. An in-depth knowledge of solubility science is required for this area of veterinary formulation science.

The physical characteristics of the dosage form require tailoring around the injectability profile of the product. Ease of administration is a key marketing and use characteristic and should be borne in mind during the development of such a dosage form. To understand syringing acceptability for products in development, Foster has categorized liquid formulations into five model formulations representing a wide range of viscosity and Newtonian and non-Newtonian systems. These model formulations were then tested

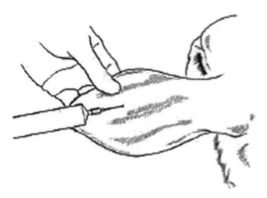

Figure 13 Administration to the middle third of the ear of a cow.

by veterinarians using 14 to 21 gauge needles and 3 to 35 cc syringes. The veterinarians determined whether the product could be withdrawn from a vial and injected through the syringe/needle combination. New products in development then need only to be classified as being similar to one of the five model formulations, and immediate understanding of how acceptable veterinarians will find the syringing of the product will be known (54).

As mentioned previously in this chapter, the availability of the animal in veterinary dosage form development is an opportunity that the formulation scientist can capitalize upon. They can be used to advantage in the development of injectable formulations since injectability depends not only on the internal diameter of the needle, the viscosity of the preparation, and the syringe characteristics, but also on the environment of the injection site, something that is difficult to model on the bench.

Administration sites are a great consideration when developing an injectable formulation for large animals. Intramuscular injections are less popular than the subcutaneous route as meat damage can occur, which can devalue the animal at slaughter.

Often the ear has been chosen as the site for administration since it represents an inedible portion of the carcass (except for swine in certain regions of the world) and is discarded on slaughter, accessible to the administrator, well perfused with blood, and administration is relatively pain free and, therefore, provides minimal distress to the animal. Pfizer's one-time administered cephalosporin for cattle (Excenel®) is administered into the middle third of the ear (Fig. 13). This minimizes tissue residue and was considered unique and granted a U.S. patent (55).

Implants

Implants are a favored subcutaneous delivery system for veterinary formulation scientists as it affords long release of drug, and in contrast to its human counterparts, animals better tolerate the rather invasive administration procedures that are associated with implants. An example of a commercially available subcutaneous implanter is shown in Figure 12.

Intramammary

For intramammary application, the storage container comes with its applicator nozzle attached. The external design and diameter of the nozzle is such that it permits ease of insertion into the teat. Its length can vary depending on where in the teat the preparation is destined to be delivered, but generally nozzle lengths provide access through the teat

Table 3 Medicines Used for Humans Now Being Used to Treat Animal Maladies

Product (drug)	Year (company)	Indication (species)
Hypercard (diltiazem)	2000 (Arnolds)	Hypertrophic cardiomyopathy (cat)
Vetmedin (pimobendan)	2000 (B.I.)	Congestive heart failure (dog)
Gastrogard (omeprazole)	1999 (Merial)	Gastric ulcers (horse)
Vasotop (ramipril)	1999 (Intervet)	Hypertrophic cardiomyopathy (cat)
Anipryl (selegiline)	1998 (Pfizer)	Cognitive dysfunction syndrome and hyperadrenocorticism (dog)
EtoGesic (etodolac)	1998 (Fort Dodge)	Pain and inflammation (dog)
Selgian (selegiline)	1997 (Ceva)	Hyperadrenocorticism (dog)
Clomicalm (clomipramine)	1997 (Novaritis)	Separation anxiety (dog)

canal into the gland itself. The teat opening constrains the maximum external dimensions of the nozzle. This in turn dictates the maximum internal diameter of the nozzle through which the preparation is delivered. In practice, this results in a relatively small internal dimension; thus intramammary products must still be designed carefully to ensure the correct flow characteristics to ensure optimal ease of administration and physical stability.

HUMAN AND ANIMAL HEALTH CROSSOVER

Crossing over use of human health care medicines to animals does happen especially when treating companion animals. Table 3 shows examples of products originally formulated for use in humans that have crossed over and are also now being used in animals.

Injectable products are generally good dosage forms for (almost) direct transition to use in animals. If dosing volumes are acceptable for the animals being treated, the direct use in animals can be pursued. Immediate-release tablets appear attractive candidates, but might prove difficult, particularly if there are palatability issues with the product. This can be overcome by instructions for pushed administration down the animal's throat or to hiding it in food or treats. Even so, it should be realized that the shorter gastrointestinal tract transit time for dogs and cats could result in inadequate absorption. Also, in both cases (injectables or oral immediate-release tablets) there may be different extents of drug metabolism or different drug absorption mechanisms in animals compared with that in humans; so these aspects need to be considered and examined. A good understanding of pharmacokinetic parameters in the different species is important when attempting to cross over human medicine to animals. Other dosage forms like topical delivery systems can be even more problematic since the transdermal absorption process will change depending on the skin thickness and components, amount of hair, and the solvent and penetration enhancers used. Similarly, ocular formulations, oral films, and oral controlled-release tablets need to be studied carefully if a switch from use in humans to animals is desired.

CONCLUDING REMARKS

Veterinary medicine offers many challenges to the scientist developing new dosage forms and medicines. These challenges arise from the diverse nature of the field, which covers a multitude of animal species that differ in size, habits, social behavior, etc.; farm management practices in which farmers may not have any direct contact with their flock or herd for many weeks or even months; and anatomical and physiological constraints that are peculiar to an individual animal species. These factors present the formulation scientist with a unique opportunity to develop innovative solutions to challenging and demanding delivery problems.

In the food animal pharmaceutical business, there are many issues that make the development of a veterinary dosage form particularly challenging. For example, the profit margins associated with the raising and selling of farmed animals are rather slim. As a result, it is not atypical for only a few cents per dose to make a large difference to the farmer's overall profit. Therefore, the formulation scientist must produce a product under considerable cost constraints. In addition, the product manufacturers must also accept that their profit margins will be slim. However, this situation can be used to justify the development of a controlled-release formulation for a drug that is administered on multiple occasions. This is because every visit of the veterinarian is associated with the cost of their time and expertise. This, together with the cost of rounding up individual animals for treatment, results in a cheap delivery formulation becoming an expensive treatment. Thus the more frequently a product needs to be administered (e.g., once a day vs. once a season), the overall cost of the treatment effectively increases. Innovative adjustments in a once-a-day administration to make it a one-time-only administration can vastly improve the costs of the overall treatment. Moreover, the development of a more complex controlled-release delivery system that delivers the active agent over an entire season has the potential to open huge areas of the market, allowing the handling of the animals only once, when they are turned to pasture.

The companion animal market is somewhat different in that the potential cost and profit margins associated with a product developed for a companion animal can be much higher compared with one developed for the food animal market. First, the companion animal owner does not own, and therefore does not have to treat, several hundred animals in their herd or flock. Rather, the outlay is directed toward a single animal. Second, the price of the delivery system is not determined by the profitability of the animal, but by the arbitrary value of the animal to the owner. Theoretically, therefore, the companion animal market will support the development of more complex and expensive dosage forms. Whether developing new products for livestock or companion animals, the challenges are always exciting and the scientific problem solving conducted to bring new medicines to the market can be fulfilling to the pharmaceutical scientists working in the veterinary medicine arena.

REFERENCES

1. Animal Pharm 2001 Report. Animal Pharm, 69-77 Paul Street, London.
2. Vetnosis Limited 2006 Report. Vetnosis Limited (Former Animal Health business of Wood Mackenzie), 74-77 Queen Street, Edinburgh.
3. Hardee GE, Baggott JD, eds. Development and Formulation of Dosage Forms. 2nd ed. New York: Marcel Dekker, 1998.
4. Chien YW. Controlled administration of estrus-synchronizing agents in livestock. In: Chien YW, ed. Novel Drug Delivery Systems; Fundamentals Developmental Concepts Biomedical Assessments. New York: Marcel Dekker, 1982:413–463.
5. Pope DG, Baggot JD. Special considerations in veterinary formulation design. Int J Pharm 1983; 14:123–132.
6. Chien YW. Implantable therapeutic systems. In: Robinson JR, Lee VHL, eds. Controlled drug delivery. New York: Marcel Dekker, 1987:481–522.
7. Baggott JD. Veterinary drug formulations for animal health care: an overview. J Control Release 1988; 8:5–13.

8. Carter DH, Luttinger M, Gardner DC. Controlled release parenteral systems for veterinary applications. J Control Release 1988; 8:15–22.
9. Koestler RC, Janes G, Miller JA. Pesticide delivery. In: Kydonieus A, ed. Treatise on Controlled Drug Delivery. New York: Marcel Dekker, 1992:491–543.
10. Arnold RG. Controlled release new animal drugs. J Control Release 1988; 8:85–90.
11. Cardinal JR, Witchey-Lakshmanan LC. Drug delivery in veterinary medicine. In: Kydonieus A, ed. Treatise on Controlled Drug Delivery. New York: Marcel Dekker, 1992:465–489.
12. Baggot JD. Special issue on veterinary drug delivery. J Control Release 1988; 8:3–91.
13. Rathbone MJ, Gurny R, eds. Controlled Release Veterinary Drug Delivery: Biological and Pharmaceutical Considerations. The Netherlands: Elsevier Science BV, 2000.
14. Rathbone MJ (Theme Editor). Veterinary drug delivery. Part I. Special theme issue. Adv Drug Deliv Rev 1997; 28(3):91pp.
15. Rathbone MJ, Cady SM (Theme Editors). Veterinary drug delivery. Part II. Special theme issue. Adv Drug Deliv Rev 1998; 38(2):83pp.
16. Rathbone MJ, Witchey-Lakshmaman L (Theme Editors). Veterinary drug delivery. Part III. Special theme Issue. Adv Drug Deliv Rev 2000; 43(1):92pp.
17. Rathbone MJ, Witchey-Lakshmaman L (Theme Editors). Veterinary drug delivery. Part IV. Special theme issue. Adv Drug Deliv Rev 2001; 50(3):147pp.
18. Rathbone MJ (Theme Editor). Veterinary drug delivery. Part V. Special theme issue. Adv Drug Deliv Rev 2002; 54(6):97pp.
19. Rathbone MJ, Bowersock T, (Guest Editors). Veterinary drug delivery (special issue). J Control Release 2002; 85(1–3):284pp.
20. Rathbone MJ, Macmillan KL, Inskeep K, et al. Fertility regulation in cattle. J Control Rel 1997; 54:117–148.
21. Rathbone MJ, Macmillan KL, Jöchle W, et al. Controlled release products for the control of the estrous cycle in cattle sheep goats deer pigs and horses. Crit Rev Ther Drug Carrier Syst 1998; 15:285–380.
22. Rathbone MJ, Martinez MN. Linking human and veterinary health: trends directions and initiatives. AAPS PharmSci 2002; 4 (article 32). Available at: http://www.aapsj.org/view.asp?art=ps040432
23. Rathbone MJ, Martinez MN. Modified release drug delivery in veterinary medicine. Drug Discov Today 2002; 7:823–829.
24. Rotehn-Weinhold A, Dahn M, Gurny R. Formulation and technology aspects of controlled drug delivery in animals. Pharm Sci Technol Today 2000; 3:222–231.
25. Matschke C, Isele U, van Hoogevest P, et al. Sustained release injectables formed in situ and their potential use for veterinary products. J Control Release 2002; 85:1–15.
26. Jalava K, Hensel A, Szostak M, et al. Bacterial ghosts as vaccine candidates for veterinary applications. J Control Release 2002; 85:17–25.
27. Cady SM, Steber WD. Controlled delivery of somatotropins. In: Sanders LM, Hendren P, eds. Protein Delivery: Physical Systems. New York: Plenum Press, 1997:289–317.
28. Ferguson TH. Peptide and protein delivery for animal health applications. In: Park K, ed. Controlled Drug Delivery. Washington, DC, U.S.A.: American Chemical Society, 1997:289–308.
29. Robinson JR, Rathbone MJ. Mucosal drug delivery—rectal uterine and vaginal. In: Mathiowitz E, ed. Encyclopedia of Controlled Drug Delivery. New York: John Wiley and Sons, 1999.
30. Rathbone MJ, Witchey-Lakshmanan L, Ciftci KK. Veterinary applications of controlled release drug delivery. In: Mathiowitz E, ed. Encyclopedia of Controlled Drug Delivery. New York: John Wiley and Sons, 1999:1007–1037.
31. Sutton S. Companion animal physiology and dosage from performance. Adv Drug Deliv Rev 2004; 56:1383–1398.
32. Kararli TT. Comparison of the gastrointestinal anatomy physiology and biochemistry of humans and commonly used laboratory animals. Biopharm Drug Dispos 1995; 16:351–380.
33. Dressman JB. Comparison of canine and human gastrointestinal physiology. Pharm Res 1986; 3:123–131.
34. Dressman JB, Yamada K. Animal model for oral drug absorption. In: Welling, PG, Tse FLS, Dighe S, eds. Pharmaceutical Bioequivalence. New York: Marcel Dekker, 1991:235–266.

35. Hernot DC, Dumon HJ, Biourge VC, et al. Evaluation of association between body size and large intestinal transit time in healthy dogs. Am J Vet Res 2006; 67:342–347.
36. Weber MP, Stambouli F, Martin LJ, et al. Influence of age and body size on gastrointestinal transit time of radiopaque markers in healthy dogs. Am J Vet Res 2002; 63:677–682.
37. Weber MP, Martin LJ, Biourge VC, et al. Influence of age and body size on orocecal transit time as assessed by use of the sulfasalazine method in healthy dogs. Am J Vet Res 2003; 64:1105–1109.
38. Hernot DC, Biourge VC, Martin LJ, et al. Relationship between total transit time and faecal quality in adult dogs differing in body size. J Anim Physiol Anim Nutr (Berl) 2005; 89:189–193.
39. Weber MP, Martin LJ, Dumon HJ, et al. Influence of age and body size on intestinal permeability and absorption in healthy dogs. Am J Vet Res 2002; 63:1323–1328.
40. Chiou WL, Jeong HY, Chung SM, et al. Evaluation of using dog as an animal model to study the fraction of oral dose absorbed of 43 drugs in humans. Pharm Res 2000; 17:135–140.
41. Thrombre AG. Oral delivery of medications to companion animals: palatability considerations. Adv Drug Deliv Rev 2004; 56:1399–1413.
42. Compendium of Veterinary Products. 10th ed. Port Huron, Michigan: AJ Bayley (publisher), North American Compendiums, 2007: 501–554.
43. FDA-Center for Veterinary Medicine Guidance Documents. General principles for evaluating the safety of compounds used in food-producing animals Document No. 3. Version July 2006.
44. VICH Guidance Documents. Studies to evaluate the safety of residues of veterinary drugs in human food: general approach to testing. Document GL 33. Version October 2002.
45. Concordet D, Toutain PL. The withdrawal time estimation of veterinary drugs revisited. J Vet Pharmacol Ther 1997; 20:380–386.
46. Reeves PT. Residues of veterinary drugs at injection sites. J Vet Pharmacol Ther 2007; 30:1–17.
47. Robinson JA. Assessing environmental impacts of veterinary products: lessons from VICH. Drug Inf J 2007; 41:169–185.
48. VICH 2000 Environmental Impact Assessment (EIAs) for Veterinary Medicinal Products (VMPs)—Phase I. Topic GL6 (Ecotoxicity Phase I). CVMP/VICH/592/98-Final. Available at: http://wwwemeaeuropaeu/pdfs/vet/vich/059298enpdf.
49. VICH 2004 Environmental Impact Assessment for Veterinary Medicinal Products—Phase II. GL 38 (Ecotoxicity Phase II). CVMP/VICH/790/03-Final. Available at: http://www. emeaeuropaeu/pdfs/vet/vich/079003enpdf.
50. FDA Center for Veterinary Medicine Guidance Documents. Guidance for Industry: Evaluating the Safety of Antimicrobial New Animal Drugs with Regard to Their Microbiological Effects on Bacteria of Human Health Concern. Document No. 152. Version October 2003.
51. Medlicott NJ, Waldron NA, Foster TP. Sustained release veterinary parenteral products. Adv Drug Deliv Rev 2004; 56:1345–1365.
52. Aguiar AJ, Armstrong WA, Desai SJ. Development of oxytetracycline long-acting injectable. J Control Release 1987; 6:375–385.
53. Cook, DW. Administration devices and techniques. In: Hardee GE, Baggott JD, eds. Development and Formulation of Dosage Forms. 2nd ed. New York: Marcel Dekker, 1998:305–356.
54. Leatherman MW, Stultz TD, Foster TP. Using flow rates to predict syringeability acceptance of veterinary parenteral formulations. Poster presentation at AAPS Annual Meeting, San Diego, CA, 1994.
55. Brown SA. Administration of an injectable antibiotic in the ear of an animal. U.S. patent 6 074 657. 2000.

9

Target-Oriented Drug Delivery Systems

Vijay Kumar
*Division of Pharmaceutics, College of Pharmacy, The University of Iowa,
Iowa City, Iowa, U.S.A.*

INTRODUCTION

Although the idea of drug targeting to a specific site in the body was first introduced almost a century ago by Paul Ehrlich (1), the field has emerged as an important area of research only in the past 40 years or so. The advent of recombinant deoxyribonucleic acid (DNA) technology and progress in biochemical pharmacology and molecular biology have not only provided a clearer elucidation of pathogenesis of many diseases and identification of various types of surface cell receptors but also enabled the production of several new classes of highly potent protein and peptide drugs (e.g., homo- and heterologous peptidergic mediators and sequence-specific oligonucleotides) (2). For these new drugs, and for some conventional drugs (e.g., antineoplastic agents) that have narrow therapeutic windows and require localization to a particular site in the body, it is essential that they be delivered to their target sites intact, in adequate concentrations, and in an efficient, safe, convenient, and cost-effective manner. Most drug therapies currently available provide little, if any, target specificity. The selective delivery of drugs to their pharmacological receptors should not only increase the therapeutic effectiveness but also limit side effects and increase safety.

In this chapter, various target-specific drug delivery systems and biological events/ processes that influence drug targeting are discussed.

RATIONALE FOR TARGETED DRUG DELIVERY

Most drugs, after administration in a conventional immediate- or controlled-release dosage form, freely distribute throughout the body, typically leading to uptake by cells, tissues, or organs other than where their pharmacological receptors are located. Figure 1 illustrates the distribution, metabolism, and elimination pathways of drugs following administration by different routes. The lack of target specificity for the most part can be attributed to the many barriers that the body presents to a drug. For example, a drug taken orally (most drugs are administered by this route, if possible) must withstand large

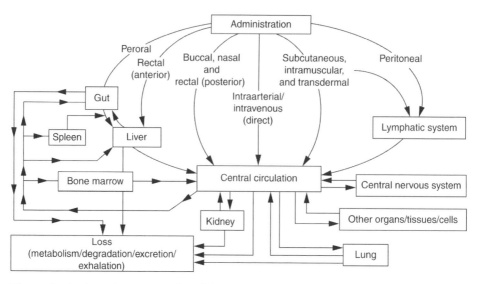

Figure 1 A schematic representation of drug disposition in the body.

fluctuations in pH as it travels along the gastrointestinal (GI) tract as well as resist the attack by the enzymes that digest food and metabolism by microflora that reside there. To be systemically active, the drug must then be absorbed from the GI tract into the blood before it passes its region of absorption in the tract. Once in the blood, it needs to survive inactivation by metabolism and extraction (first-pass effects). To produce its therapeutic effect(s), the drug must then be able to selectively access and interact with its pharmacological receptor(s). The concentration of drug at the active site must also be adequate. Administration of drugs by parenteral routes avoids GI-associated problems, but deactivation and metabolism of the drug and dose-related toxicity are frequently observed. Furthermore, of all the paths the drug may take following administration, which one will produce the drug at its desired destination in adequate concentrations cannot be predicted. In addition, there are many diseases, such as rheumatoid arthritis, diseases of the central nervous system, some cancers, and intractable bacterial, fungal, and parasitic infections that are poorly accessible. To treat these diseases, high doses and frequent administration of drugs are often required, which lead to toxic manifestations, inappropriate pharmacodisposition, untoward metabolism, and other deleterious effects.

Table 1 lists the reasons for targeting drugs to their sites of action (3). Thus, a target-oriented drug delivery system offers potential to supply a drug selectively to its site(s) of action(s) in a manner that provides maximum therapeutic activity by preventing degradation or inactivation during transit to the target sites, protecting the body from adverse reactions because of inappropriate disposition, and delivering drugs in adequate concentrations and in predetermined, controlled-release kinetics. For drugs that have a low therapeutic index, targeted drug delivery may provide an effective treatment at a relatively low drug concentration. Other requirements for target-oriented drug delivery include that (*i*) the delivery system should be nontoxic, nonimmunogenic, and physically and chemically stable in vivo and in vitro; (*ii*) the drug carrier must be biodegradable (degradation products must also be safe) or readily eliminated without problems; and (*iii*) the preparation of the delivery system must be reasonably simple, reproducible, and cost effective.

Table 1 Reasons for Site-Specific Delivery of Drugs

Pharmaceutical
    Drug instability as delivered from conventional formulation
    Solubility
Biopharmaceutical
    Low absorption
    High membrane binding
    Biological instability
Pharmacokinetic and pharmacodynamic
    Short half-life
    Large volume of distribution
    Low specificity
Clinical
    Low therapeutic index
    Anatomical or cellular barriers
Commercial
    Drug presentation

Source: From Ref. 3.

BIOLOGICAL PROCESS AND EVENTS INVOLVED IN DRUG TARGETING

Drug targeting has been classified into three types: (*i*) first-order targeting—this describes delivery to a discrete organ or tissue, (*ii*) second-order targeting—this represents targeting a specific cell type(s) within a tissue or organ (e.g., tumor cells versus normal cells and hepatocytic cells versus Kupffer cells), and (*iii*) third-order targeting—this implies delivery to a specific intracellular organelle in the target cells (e.g., lysosomes) (4). Basically, there are three approaches for drug targeting. The first approach involves the use of biologically active agents that are both potent and selective to a particular site in the body (magic bullet approach of Ehrlich). The second approach involves the preparation of pharmacologically inert forms of active drugs, which, upon reaching the active sites, become activated by a chemical or enzymatic reaction (prodrug approach). The third approach utilizes a biologically inert macromolecular carrier system that directs a drug to a specific site in the body where it is accumulated and effects its response (magic gun or missile approach). Regardless of the approach, the therapeutic efficacy of targeted drug delivery systems depends on the timely availability of the drug in active form at the target site(s) and its intrinsic pharmacological activity. It is important that the intrinsic pharmacokinetic properties of the targeted delivery system be the same as that of the free drug. Figure 2 shows a schematic representation of possible anatomical and physiological pathways that a drug may follow to reach its target site(s) (5). As is depicted by this figure, a drug can selectively access, and interact with, its pharmacological receptors, either passively or by active processes. Passive processes rely on the normal distribution pattern of a drug-drug carrier system, whereas the active pathways use cell receptor–recognizing ligand(s) or antibodies ("homing" or "vector" devices) to access specific cells, tissues, or organs in the body. Various biological processes and events that govern drug targeting are briefly discussed in the following sections.

Cellular Uptake and Processing

Following administration, low molar mass drugs can enter into or pass through various cells by simple diffusion processes. Targeted drug delivery systems often contain

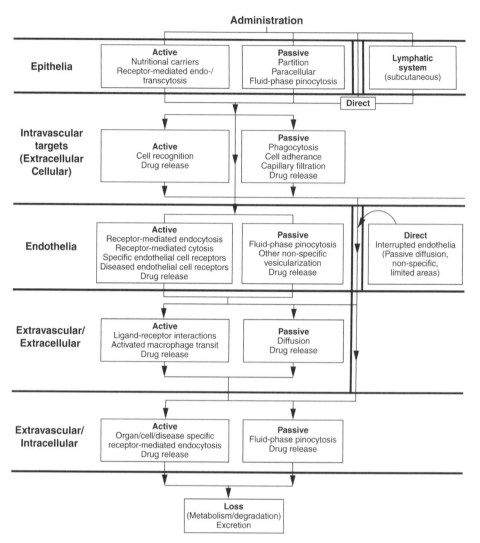

Figure 2 Anatomical and physiological pathways for site-specific delivery. *Source*: From Ref. 5.

macromolecular assemblies and hence cannot enter into cells by such simple processes. Instead, they are taken up by a process called endocytosis, which involves internalization of the plasma membrane, concomitant with engulfment of the extracellular material. It is divided into two types: phagocytosis and pinocytosis. The former refers to the capture of particulate matter, whereas the latter represents engulfment of fluids. Various (endocytic) mechanisms by which macromolecules can enter into the cell have recently been reviewed by Bareford and Swaan (6).

Figure 3 illustrates the phagocytic and pinocytic processes. Phagocytosis is carried out by specialized, immunologically incompetent cells of the mononuclear phagocyte system (MPS) called phagocytes. The latter are present in the liver (Kupffer cells), lungs (alveolar interstitial), spleen, lymph nodes, thymus, gut, bone marrow, brain, connective tissue, and serous cavities. Phagocytosis is mediated by the adsorption of specific blood components [e.g., immunoglobulin G (IgG), complement C3b, and fibronectin] called opsonins and relevant receptors located on macrophages. Certain serum proteins, such as

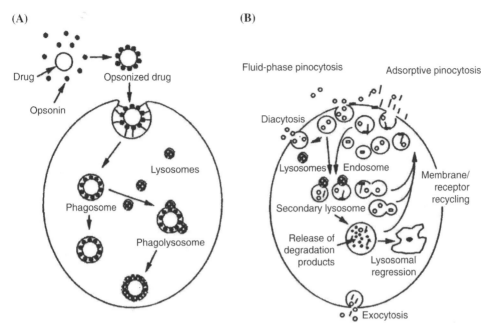

Figure 3 (**A**) Phagocytic and (**B**) pinocytic uptake of drugs.

immunoglobulin A (IgA) and secretory IgA (sIgA), called dysopsonins impart a high degree of hydrophilicity, leading to significantly decreased uptake by cells (7,8). Thus, the extent to which a drug is opsonized, and by what plasma protein, determine the uptake mechanism. This in turn depends on the size and surface characteristics of the particles (9). In general, smaller-size particles are better taken up by cells. Interactions between the colloidal/particulate carriers and blood components mostly involve long-range electro-static, van der Waals, and short-range hydrophobic types (10,11). Changes in the glycoprotein levels have also been suggested to cause variations in the opsonization of administered particles and, consequently, their ultimate distribution in the body (12). Particles with higher hydrophilic surface characteristics, for example, through coatings/ coupling with polymers, such as polyethylene glycols (PEGs), poloxamers, or poloxamines, also undergo opsonization to a lesser extent and, consequently, exhibit decreased phagocytic uptake (13–16). This offers opportunity to target drugs to cells other than those of the reticuloendothelial system (RES), because the longer the drug stays in the central circulation, the greater the chances of uptake by other cells. Nonspecific phagocytic uptake of particles, triggered by particle size and hydrophilic coatings (17) and mediated by membrane components (18), has also been reported.

Following ingestion, the phagocytic vacuole (or phagosome) fuses with one or more lysosomes to form phagolysosomes (or secondary lysosomes) (Fig. 3A). It is here that the digestion of particles by lysosomal hydrolases (e.g., proteinases, glycosidases, phospholipases, phosphatases, and sulfatases) occurs, making the drug available to exert its therapeutic effect. The internal pH of lysosomes ranges between 4.5 and 5.5.

Compared with phagocytosis, pinocytosis is a universal phenomenon in all cells, including phagocytes. Unlike phagocytosis, which is mediated by the serum opsonin, pinocytosis does not require any external stimulus. Pinocytosis is divided into two types: fluid-phase pinocytosis and adsorptive pinocytosis (Fig. 3B). Fluid-phase pinocytosis is a nonspecific, continuous process. It serves as a means to transport macromolecular constructs lacking targeting ligands through epithelia, some endothelia, and into various blood cells. Molecules taken up by this route avoid direct binding with the membrane constitutes. Adsorptive pinocytosis, in contrast, refers to internalization of macromolecules that bind to the cell surface membrane. If the macromolecule adheres to a general cell surface site, then uptake is referred to as simply nonspecific pinocytosis. However, if it binds to a specific cell receptor site, then the process is called receptor-mediated pinocytosis. Before membrane internalization, the pinocytic substrate often patches into domains or areas of the membrane called coated pits. Coated pits have a cytoplasmic coat consisting of clathrin and other proteins such as caveolin-1. Once internalized, the pinocytic vesicles can interact among themselves or with vesicles of other intracellular origins, such as endosomes and lysosomes. Endosomes are rich in pinocytic receptors. The pH within endosomes ranges between 5.0 and 5.5. The mild internal acidic pH condition induces dissociation of the receptor–drug carrier complex, freeing the receptor for recycling. Endosomes also help in routing engulfed substrates to their appropriate intracellular destinations. Substrates (macromolecules) internalized by the clathrin receptor–mediated mechanism (known to occur with targeting ligands such as transferrin, mannose-6-phosphate, and riboflavin) are believed to remain intact in the endosome and are usually transferred to the lysosome, where their digestion by acid hydrolases occurs. Ligands such as folic acid and low-density lipoproteins (LDL) support caveolin-assisted endocytosis. Substrates internalized by this pathway are transferred to nonlysosomal compartments, such as endoplasmic reticulum. In some cells, for example, endothelial cells, the endosomes, instead of transferring their contents to the lysosome, release them outside the cell. This process is termed diacytosis or retroendocytosis and can achieve a vectorial translocation of substances (19). In cells, such as secretory polymeric IgG in the neonatal gut, polymeric IgA in hepatocytes, and LDL in endothelia, the secondary lysosome transports its contents to the other side of the membrane by a process called transcytosis. The secondary lysosome can also regress to form residual bodies that continue to retain nondegraded macromolecules.

Nonspecific pinocytic uptake appears to be dependent on the size (molar mass and configuration), charge, and hydrophobicity of the pinocytic substrates. Polycation macromolecules have increased pinocytic uptake in rat yolk sacs and rat peritoneal macrophages cultured in vitro, compared with neutral and anionic macromolecules (20–22). Recently, positively charged hydroxypropyl methacrylamide conjugates have also been reported to accumulate in greater amounts in cells than their negatively charged counterparts (23). The rate of pinocytic uptake in different cells has also been reported to increase with an increase in hydrophobicity of the substrates. The molecular size of the pinocytic substrate is also detrimental to the movement of macromolecules from one compartment to another.

The receptor-mediated form of endocytic uptake, compared with nonspecific pinocytosis, provides a more rapid means of cellular uptake (24,25). It has been identified for a wide variety of physiological ligands, such as metabolites, hormones, immunoglobulins, and pathogens (e.g., virus and bacterial and plant toxins). Several endosomotropic receptors identified in cells are listed in Table 2 (5).

A number of cell-adhesive ligands, such as proteins and peptides containing tripeptide Arg-Gly-Asp (RGD) sequence and intercellular adhesive molecules (e.g., ICAM-1) antibody, have also been investigated for targeting drugs to cancer and other diseases (e.g., autoimmune) (26). RGD specifically binds to the integrin receptors ($\alpha_v\beta_5$ or $\alpha_v\beta_e$) present on cells.

Table 2 Distribution of Some Endosomotropic Receptors

Cell	Receptor for
Hepatocytes	Galactose-terminated (neo)glycoproteins, LDL, polymeric IgA, high-density lipoprotein, epidermal growth factor, transferrin
Macrophages (Kupffer cells)	Galactose (particles), mannose-fucose, acetylated LDL, AMPC, complement factors
Leukocytes	Chemotactic peptide, complement C3b, IgA
Basophils, mast cells	IgE
Fibroblasts	Transferrin, epidermal growth factor, LDL, mannose-6-phosphate, transcobalamine II, AMPC, mannose
Mammary acinar	Growth factor
Enterocytes	Maternal IgG, dimeric IgA, transcobalamine-B_{12}/intrinsic factor
Renal tubular cells	Low molar mass proteins (cationic)
Endothelia	
Blood/brain	Transferrin, insulin
Diaphragm, lung, heart	Albumin
Liver	Monomeric negatively charged proteins, Man/GlcNAc-terminated (neo)glycoproteins, Fc receptor

Abbreviations: LDL, low-density lipoproteins; IgA, immunoglobulin A; AMPC, α_2-macroglobulin-protease complex.
Source: From Refs. 5 and 409.

Compared with phagocytosis, fluid-phase pinocytic capture of molecules is relatively slower, being directly proportional to the concentration of macromolecules in the extracellular fluid. It is also dependent on the size of macromolecules; in general, lower molar mass fractions are captured faster than the higher molar mass fractions. The magnitude of the rate of capture by adsorptive pinocytosis is higher than that by fluid-phase pinocytosis and relates to the nature of substrate-membrane interactions.

Transport Across the Epithelial Barrier

The oral, buccal, nasal, vaginal, and rectal cavities are all internally lined with one or more layers of epithelial cells. Depending on the position and function in the body, epithelial cells can be of varied forms, ranging from simple columnar, to cuboidal, to squamous types. Irrespective of their morphological differences, these cells are extremely cohesive. The lateral membrane of these cells exhibits several specialized features that form intercellular junctions (tight junction, zonula adherens, and gap junction), which serve not only as sites for adhesion but also as seals to prevent flow of materials through the intercellular spaces (paracellular pathway) and to provide a mechanism for intercellular communication. Below the epithelial cells is a layer of connective tissue called the lamina propria, which is bound to epithelium by the basal lamina. The latter also connects epithelium to other neighboring structures. The luminal side of the epithelium is covered with a more or less coherent, sticky layer of mucus. This is the layer that first interacts with foreign materials (e.g., food, drugs, bacterial organisms, and chemicals).

Various transport processes used by low molar mass drugs to cross the epithelial barrier lining oral, buccal, nasal, vaginal, and rectal cavities include passive diffusion, carrier-mediated transfer systems, and selective and nonselective endocytosis. Additionally, polar materials can also diffuse through the tight junctions of epithelial cells (the paracellular route). Evidence also exists that suggests that macromolecules (particulate and soluble), including peptides and proteins, can reach the systemic circulation, albeit in small amounts, following administration by these routes. This offers potential in certain therapies, such as immune reactions and hormone replacement treatments. Both passive- and active-transport pathways may occur simultaneously. Passive transport is usually higher in damaged mucosa, whereas active transport depends on the structural integrity of epithelial cells.

Harris (27) reported that nasal administration of biopharmaceuticals (polypeptides) resulted in bioavailabilities of the order 1% to 20% of administered dose, depending on the molar mass and physiochemical properties of the drug. It is widely accepted that macromolecules with a molar mass of less than 10,000 can be absorbed from the nasal epithelium into the systemic circulation in sufficient amounts without the need for added materials, except for bioadhesives (28). Larger molecules, such as proteins [e.g., interferon, granulocyte colony-stimulating factor (G-CSF), and human growth hormone], however, require both a penetration enhancer (e.g., bile salts and surfactants) and a bioadhesive. Since the entire dose passes through one tissue, these flux enhancers may cause deleterious effects to the nasal mucosa and muciliary function. Cyclodextrins (29) and phospholipids (30) have been reported to significantly increase the absorption of macromolecules without causing any damage to the nasal mucosal membrane. The phospholipid approach is particularly attractive in that phospholipids are biocompatible and bioresorbable and thus pose no threat of toxicity. Lectin isolated from *Bandeiraea simplicifolia* has been shown to be almost exclusively specific to the M cells of nasal-associated lymphoid tissue and hence offers potential for targeting the upper respiratory tract (31,32).

The transport of macromolecules across intestinal epithelium may occur by cellular vesicular processes involving either fluid-phase pinocytosis or specialized (receptor-mediated) endocytic processes (33). Matsuno et al. (34) reported that spheres of 20 nm in diameter, when given orally to suckling mice, pass through the epithelial layer and become localized in the omentum, the Kupffer cells of the lumen, the mesenteric lymph nodes, and even the thymic cortex. Studies with poly(alkylcyanoacrylate) nanocapsules smaller than 300 nm in size suggest that particles can also pass intact through the intestinal barrier by the paracellular route (35). Harush-Fenkel et al. (36) reported a reduced permeation of positively and negatively charged poly(ethylene glycol)-D,L-polylactide (PEG-PLA) nanoparticles (size 89.6 ± 4 nm and 96.4 ± 3 nm, respectively) through the apical plasma membrane of the polarized epithelial cells of the GI tact. This was attributed, in part, to the mucosal barrier and low endocytosis rates at the apical side of the membrane. Both cationic and anionic nanoparticles were reported to enter the cells mainly by the clathrin-mediated endocytic pathway; the positively charged particles showed increased uptake than the negatively charged counterparts. A significant amount of nanoparticles transcytosed and accumulated in the basolateral membrane. Some anionic but not cationic nanoparticles routed through the lysosomal degradative pathway. These results suggested that positively charged particles show potential not only for delivering drugs to epithelia but also for transcytosing drugs in the blood circulation.

The M cells found in Peyer's patches have also been suggested to transport particles. These are specialized absorptive cells known to absorb and transport indigenous bacteria (i.e., *Vibrio cholerae*); macromolecules, such as ferritin and horseradish peroxidase; viruses; and carbon particles, from the lumen of the intestine to submucosal lymphoid tissue (33,37,38). It has been reported that hydrophobic, negatively charged or neutral particles of size smaller than 5 μm are better taken up by M cells; particles smaller than 1 μm in size accumulate in the basal medium, while larger particles remain entrapped in the Peyer's patches (39). Transport of absorbed materials to the systemic circulation through lymph fluid and by lymphocytes has also been suggested to be possible. An increase in the lymph flow or a decrease in the blood supply could make lymphatic uptake of particles important (37). Since Peyer's patches are more prevalent and larger in young individuals and drastically decrease with increasing age, the transport by this route is of significance in younger individuals (40). Lectins [e.g., Ulex europaeus agglutinin 1 (UEA-1)] show high specificity for sugar residues of glycoconjugates present on cell surfaces and are thus useful for drug and antigen targeting nasal, intestinal, cecal, and other epithelia M cells (41).

Various physicochemical, physiological, and biochemical factors that can influence the absorption of drugs, including peptides and proteins, from the GI tract have been reviewed (39,42–44). A variety of penetration enhancers have been found useful in improving intestinal absorption of peptides and other macromolecular drugs. These include chelators (e.g., ethylene diamine tetraacetic acid and citric acid); natural, semisynthetic, and synthetic surfactants (e.g., bile salts, derivatives of fusidic acid, sodium lauryl sulfate, polyoxyethylene-9-laurylether, and polyoxyethylene-20-cetylether); fatty acids and their derivatives (e.g., sodium caprate, sodium laurate, and oleic acid); and a variety of mixed micelle solutions (45,46). It must be noted that the sensitivity of penetration enhancers varies depending on the regions; a general rank order suggested for different regions is rectum > colon > small intestine > stomach. Although considerable progress has been made, the bioavailabilities of macromolecules (peptides/proteins) delivered via these routes are often suboptimal because of their poor absorptions and stabilities (45,47).

Absorption of drugs from the buccal cavity occurs via transcellular and paracellular pathways; the latter being the predominant route of absorption. Drugs administered in the oral cavity avoid the hepatic first-pass effect and reach the systemic circulation through the reticulated vein and jugular vein (48). A number of hydrophilic macromolecules, such as peptides, oligopeptides, and polysaccharides, have been investigated. However, there is little evidence to suggest that soluble or particulate macromolecules can be transported across the buccal mucosa (49). Recently, it has been suggested that lectins or lectin-like molecules, which can bind to cell surface glycoconjugates, or systems containing ligands specific to endogenous lectins located on epithelial surface, could be used to target and improve delivery by this route (41,48).

The absorption of drugs from the rectal cavity has been studied in some detail (50). Muranishi et al. (51) have shown that a significant increase in the absorption and lymphatic uptake of soluble and colloidal macromolecules can be achieved by pretreating the rectal mucosal membrane with lipid–nonionic surfactant mixed micelles. They found no evidence of serious damage of the mucosal membrane. Davis (47) suggested that the vaginal cavity could be an effective delivery site for certain pharmaceuticals, such as calcitonin, used for the treatment of postmenopausal osteoporosis. Working with a human ex vivo uterine perfusion model, Bulletti et al. (52) demonstrated that drugs, when delivered vaginally, first undergo uterine pass effect, suggesting that the vaginal route can be used to target drugs to the uterus.

Extravasation

Many diseases result from the dysfunction of cells located outside the cardiovascular system. Thus, for a drug to exert its therapeutic effects, it must exit from the central circulation and interact with its extravascular-extracellular or extravascular-intracellular target(s). This process of transvascular exchange is called extravasation, and it is governed by the permeability of blood capillary walls. The main biological features that control permeability of capillaries include the structure of the capillary wall under normal and pathophysiological conditions and the rate of blood and lymph supply. Physicochemical factors (of drugs/macromolecules) that are of profound importance in extravasation are molecular size, shape, charge, and hydrophilic-lipophilic balance (HLB) characteristics.

The structure of the blood capillary wall varies in different organs and tissues (53,54). It consists of a single layer of endothelial cells joined together by intercellular junctions. Each endothelial cell, which, on an average, is 20 to 40 µm long, 10 to 15 µm wide, and 0.1 to 0.5 µm thick, contains 10,000 to 15,000 uniform, spherical vesicles called plasmalemmal vesicles. These vesicles range in size between 60 and 80 nm in diameter. About 30% of these vesicles are located within cytoplasm, while the remaining 70% open on the luminal side of the endothelial cell surface. Plasmalemmal vesicles are believed to be involved in the pinocytic transport of substances across the endothelium (53). Because they contain low density of anionic sites, plasmalemmal vesicles have also been suggested as the sites where extravasation of anionic proteins occurs (53). Fusion of plasmalemmal vesicles leads to the formation of transendothelial channels. The endothelial cells are covered, on the luminal side, with a thick layer (10–20 nm) of a glycosaminoglycan (GAG) coating. This layer continues into the plasmalemmal vesicles and into transendothelial channels, and is believed to be involved in cell adhesion, the stabilization of receptors, cellular protection, and the regulation of extravasation. It also provides microdomains of differing charge or charge density on the endothelial cell surface. On the external side, the endothelium is supported by a 5 to 8 nm thick membrane called the basal lamina. Below the basal lamina, a connective tissue lining called the adventia lies.

Depending on the morphology and continuity of the endothelial layer and the basement membrane, blood capillaries are divided into three types: continuous, fenestrated, and sinusoidal (54). A schematic illustrating the differences in their structures is shown in Figure 4 (55). Continuous capillaries are common and widely distributed in the body. They exhibit tight interendothelial junctions and an uninterrupted basement membrane. Fenestrated capillaries show interendothelial gaps of 20 to 80 nm at irregular intervals. Sinusoidal capillaries show interendothelial gaps of up to 150 nm. Depending on the tissue or organ, the basal membrane in sinusoidal capillaries is either absent (e.g., in liver) or present as a discontinuous membrane (e.g., in spleen and bone marrow).

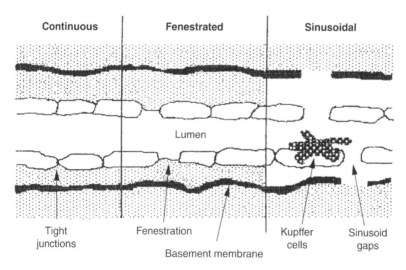

Figure 4 The endothelial barrier. *Source*: From Ref. 55.

Numerous variations in the microvasculature bed (i.e., arterioles, capillaries, and venules) exist, which can affect permeability. For example, venular portions of the capillaries have thin endothelial cells (170 nm), with frequent interendothelial discontinuities. The gap in about 30% venular junctions is about 6 nm. Arterioles, in contrast, have endothelial cells that are linked by the tight junctions and communicating junctions, whereas the capillary endothelium contains only occluding junctions. Communicating gaps are small and rare in muscular venules and are absent in capillaries and pericytic venules. Endothelial cells in capillaries have more vesicles than those in arterioles ($1000/\mu m^3$ vs. $190/\mu m^3$). The intercellular sealing is strong in arterioles, well developed in capillaries, and particularly loose in venules. Furthermore, capillaries and venules have more transendothelial channels.

The transport of macromolecules across endothelium has been extensively reviewed (53,56,57). Macromolecules can traverse the normal endothelium by passive processes, such as nonspecific fluid-phase transcapillary pinocytosis and passage through interendothelial junctions, gaps, or fenestrae, or by receptor-mediated transport systems. Passive extravasation is affected by regional differences in capillary structure, the disease state of the tissue or organ, the number and size of the microvascular surface area, and the physicochemical characteristics of the macromolecules. In general, the transfer of macromolecules across endothelium decreases progressively with an increase in molecular size. Low molar mass solutes and a large number of macromolecules, up to 30 nm in diameter, can cross the endothelium under certain normal and pathophysiological conditions (37). For proteins, the threshold restricting free passage through the glomerular endothelium is at a molar mass between 60,000 and 70,000. Molecules with a molar mass of greater than 70,000 are predominantly retained in the blood until they are degraded and excreted. Certain hydrophilic polymers, such as poly(vinylpyrrolidone) (PVP), dextran, PEG, and N-(2-hydroxypropyl)methacrylamide (HPMA), exhibit much greater hydrodynamic radii compared with proteins of the same molar mass, and consequently, the threshold molar mass restricting glomerular filtration is lower than that for proteins (25,000 for PVP, 50,000 for dextran, and 45,000 for HPMA) (58).

Because of the presence of anionic sites on the endothelium and on the glycocalyx layer, anionic macromolecules show a significantly slower rate of extravasation compared with neutral and cationic macromolecules (59–61). Regional differences in the capillary structure and the number and size of the microvascular surface area determine the flux of macromolecules in the interstitium (37). For example, organs such as the lung with very large surface areas have a proportionately large total permeability and, consequently, a high extravasation. Renal endothelium has a thick basement membrane and contains anionic groups (on the epithelial surface) and heparin sulfate proteoglycan (on the basement membrane). Thus, extravasation through this membrane largely depends on the charge, shape, size, and lipophilic-hydrophilic balance characteristics of the macromolecules. Intestinal endothelium, although fenestrated, is highly restrictive to passage of macromolecules. The absolute rate of extravasation varies considerably from one region to another within the alimentary canal. There is a large difference in permeation of solute macromolecules with a radius of less than 6 nm and no decrease in the permeation for molecules with a radius between 6 and 13.5 nm (62). The lung endothelium, which is nonfenestrated and has vesicles with a size of 50 to 100 nm, is more selective to the passage of macromolecules; the lymph/plasma ratio was decreased from 0.7 to 0.25 when the molecular radius of the macromolecule increased from 3.7 to 11.0 nm (63). Skeletal muscle, adipose tissue, liver, and myocardial endothelia all show extravasation as a function of macromolecular size. The endothelium of the brain is the tightest of all endothelia in the body. It is formed by continuous, nonfenestrated endothelial cells, which show virtually no pinocytic activity. There are, however, certain regions of the brain (e.g., choroid plexus) that have fenestrated endothelium. Macromolecules, such as horseradish peroxidase, reach the cerebrospinal fluid by this route. Also, certain pathophysiological conditions, such as osmotic shocks, thermal injury, arterial hypertension, air or fat embolism, hypovolemia, and traumatic injury, cause transcapillary leakage and onset of pinocytic activity. This may have some implications in extravasation of macromolecules across the blood-brain barrier.

The blood capillaries in solid tumors are dense, disorganized, and tortuous. However, because of increased levels of vascular endothelial growth factor, bradykinin, nitric oxide, and peroxy nitrite, all of which are known to promote angiogenesis and degradation of basement membrane and extracellular matrix, the vasculature in solid tumors is high and leaky. In general, macromolecules with a molar mass of up to 300,000 are capable of extravasation from blood vessels within experimental solid tumor, whereas molecules with a molar mass ranging between 70,000 and 150,000 extravasate mainly from the vascular plexus around solid tumors. The pH within the tumor mass is slightly lower than that of the normal tissue (pH 6.5 vs. 7.4), because of the production of lactic acid and hydrolysis of ATP caused by the hypoxic conditions (64).

The changes in the permeability of capillaries as a result of inflammation are believed to be due to the effect of histamine, bradykinin, and a variety of other mediators (56). Damaged capillaries, in general, show increased openings (ranging in size between 80 and 140 nm) in the endothelium and, hence, increased transport activity. Inflamed tissues also show changes in the glycocalyx layer (lining the luminal side of the endothelium), which causes increased vesicular trafficking and, consequently, increased extravasation of blood-borne materials. Other factors that can affect extravasation include metabolic changes, which are mediated through a reduced oxygen concentration and an increased carbon dioxide concentration.

Soluble macromolecules permeate the endothelial barrier more readily than particulate macromolecules. The rate of movement of fluid across the endothelium appears to be directly related to the difference between the hydrostatic and osmotic forces.

Receptor-mediated transport systems include both the fluid-phase and constitutive and nonconstitutive endocytosis or transcytosis. Ghitescu et al. (65), using 5-nm gold-albumin particles, showed that particles are first adsorbed onto specific binding sites of the endothelia (examined in lung, heart, and diaphragm) and then transported in transcytotic vesicles across the endothelium by receptor-mediated transcytosis and, to a lesser extent, by fluid-phase processes. In case of LDLs, it was reported that particles pass through sinusoids, enter the space of Disse, and then are processed into the liver hepatocytes after interaction with the apolipoprotein ligands located on the surface of the hepatocytes (66). These results suggested that particles can be directed to other cells in the liver by altering the surface with ligands specific for the plasma membrane of those cells. Table 2 lists various receptors and the cells that have them.

Lymphatic Uptake

Following extravasation, drug molecules can either reabsorb into the bloodstream directly by the enlarged postcapillary interendothelial cell pores found in most tissues (67) or enter into the lymphatic system and then return with the lymph (a constituent of the interstitial fluid) to the blood circulation (Fig. 5). Also, drugs administered by subcutaneous, intramuscular, transdermal, and peritoneal routes can reach the systemic circulation by the lymphatic system (Fig. 1).

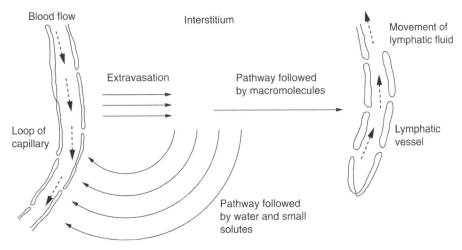

Figure 5 Schematic representation of extravasation and lymphatic drainage. *Source*: From Ref. 58.

Similar to blood capillaries, the lymphatic capillaries consist of a single layer of endothelial cells joined together by intercellular junctions. The diameter of small pores is 12 nm, whereas large pores range between 50 and 70 nm. The rate of formation of lymph depends on the hydrostatic pressure of blood and the permeability of the capillary wall. As blood enters the arterial end of the capillary, the hydrostatic pressure increases and, consequently, extravasation of water, electrolytes, and other blood-borne substances (e.g., proteins) occurs. By the time blood reaches the venular end of the capillary, the hydrostatic pressure drops, and some water and other low molar mass (<10,000) substances are reabsorbed. However, there is a net excess of extravasation over reabsorption, which results in accumulation of excess lymph in the tissues. This accumulation of excess fluid causes an increase in the interstitial pressure, which forces the lymph to enter the lymphatic system (68). Following absorption in the peripheral capillary bed, the lymph is transported (by large lymph capillaries) to the regional lymph node where lymphocytes are added. The lymph is then taken to the next node up the chain and, finally, into the great vein.

Factors known to influence the clearance of drugs from interstitial sites, following extravasation or parenteral interstitial or transepithelial administration, include size and surface characteristics of particles, formulation medium, the composition and pH of the interstitial fluid, and disease within the interstitium (69–73). Soluble macromolecules smaller than 30 nm can enter the lymphatic system, whereas particulate materials larger than 50 nm are retained in the interstitial sites and serve as a sustained-release depot. The use of lipids or oils in a formulation and the presence of a negative surface charge facilitate the absorption of particles into the lymphatic system. Moghimi (74) reported that the inclusion of methoxypoly(ethylene glycol) into the liposomal bilayer can control the rate of drainage as well as lymphatic distribution following subcutaneous administration.

Solid tumors, in general, lack lymphatic drainage (75). Therefore, macromolecular drugs that enter tumor interstitium, by extravasation, remain there. This mechanism is commonly referred to as the tumor-enhanced permeability and retention (EPR) effect (76,77). Tumor-associated proteolytic enzymes may then release the trapped drug in the tumor interstitium. The released drug is then able to penetrate readily through cell membranes and reach its intracellular targets. Active angiogenesis, high vascular density,

extensive production of vascular mediators (bradykinin, nitric oxide, vascular permeability factor, vascular endothelial growth factor, prostaglandins, collagenase, and
peroxinitrite) that facilitate extravasation, and defective vascular architecture have all
been identified as important factors affecting the EPR effect. Possible exploitation of this
phenomenon in selective tumor therapy has been discussed in detail by Seymour (58) and
Maeda (76). Studies reported by Maeda and coworkers (77–80) show that, in general, EPR
effect can lead to 10 to 15 times higher drug concentrations in tumor tissue than in plasma
and about 10 times higher tumor concentration than in normal tissue after 24 hours of
intravenous administration. It is suggested that drug molecules/delivery systems that
remain in circulation for prolonged periods (at least six hours), by avoiding renal
elimination or adsorption onto the vessel, can achieve this effect. Recently, Vlerken et al.
(81) reported 10 to 100 times higher accumulation of drug concentration in the vicinity of
tumor mass following intravenous administration.

The direct delivery of drugs into lymphatics has also been proposed as a potential
approach to kill malignant lymphoid cells located in lymph nodes.

PHARMACOKINETIC AND PHARMACODYNAMIC CONSIDERATIONS

When a drug is administered, it is readily distributed to various compartments by blood.
The relative amounts of drug available at the target (response compartment) and nontarget
(toxicity compartment) sites determine the therapeutic effect and toxicities relative to that
effect. In conventional therapy, the natural distribution characteristics of the drug
determine the ratio of therapeutic response to the toxic effects.

Targeted drug delivery systems are designed to maximize therapeutic response by
delivering a drug selectively to its pharmacological site(s). Several factors determine the
availability of a drug at the target site (82,83). These include the rates of (*i*) input of
targeted drug into the body plasma, (*ii*) distribution of targeted drug to the active site,
(*iii*) release of active drug from the targeted drug at the site of action, (*iv*) removal
(elimination) of the targeted drug and free drug from the target site, (*v*) diffusion or
transport of the targeted drug and free drug from the active site to nontarget sites, and
(*vi*) blood and lymph flow to and from the target site. The release of free drug from the
targeted drug delivery system may occur either passively or by an active mechanism
mediated by an internal or external stimulus (e.g., pH, temperature, and enzymes). In
enzyme-mediated mechanisms, the rate of release of free drug depends on the activity and
concentration of the enzyme involved, whereas in processes that are selective but
nonspecific to the local chemical characteristics of the active site, the rate of release of
drug varies with the concentration of the targeted drug available at the site. Thus,
depending on the rate of distribution of targeted drug delivery to active site(s) and the rate
of elimination of targeted drug from the active site (with respect to the rate of delivery to
this site), a drug may or may not be available at the target site in sufficient amounts to
produce the desired pharmacological effect (82). The rate of distribution of targeted drug
delivery system to the target site depends on the rate of blood flow, whereas the
permeability of endothelium, the rates of blood and lymph flow to and from the target site,
and the rate of release of free drug determine the removal of targeted delivery and free
drug from the active site. The product of blood flow and concentration of the species in
the blood provides the upper limit of distribution of targeted drug or free drug to a specific
tissue or organ in the body. The inability of macromolecules or charged species to cross
membrane barriers can limit their access to and removal from the target sites. The binding

of the targeted drug delivery system or drug within the target site reduces the concentration available for removal. Thus, for drugs that are active only in the free form, the binding reduces the effective amount required to produce the desired therapeutic effect.

On the basis of the assumption that the transport of targeted drug delivery from the target site to the rest of the body occurs by diffusion, convection or transport processes, Levy (84) predicted that drug elimination from the target site will be much more rapid than drug elimination from the body as a whole, the duration of the bolus dose administration will be much shorter than that of the conventionally administered dose, and the rate of elimination of targeted drug from the site of action will not be affected by changes in biotransformation and excretion kinetics or other processes, such as the liver perfusion rate, that determine the systemic clearance of a drug. Further, if there is a large difference between the rates of drug elimination from the active site and that from the body, if the ratio of the effective dose at the active site to that in body plasma is small, and if elimination at the target site does not represent biotransformation, then the drug in the body will gradually accumulate if the targeted drug delivery system is continuously administered. As a result, the pharmacological effect will gradually increase. However, because the drug amount in the body plasma will continue to increase, the drug-targeting selectivity may be lost. Thus, to maintain the selectivity of drug targeting, the drug delivery system must be designed such that it provides a very low continuous input relative to the rate of elimination of drug from the body (84).

In conventional delivery, the pharmacological response of a drug is assumed to be linearly related to the drug concentration in the plasma. This relationship between concentration and effect is much more complex in targeted drug delivery. It can vary in different organs or tissues, depending on access, retention (maintenance of adequate levels of targeted delivery and free drug at the active site), and timing of release of drug within the site. The various approaches used to quantitate targeted drug delivery systems have been reviewed by Gupta and Hung (85). These authors suggested that the overall drug-targeting efficiency (T_e*), which represents selectivity of a delivery system for the target tissue (T), compared with n nontarget tissues (i), can be reliably calculated according to the following expression:

$$T_e^* = \frac{(AQU_0^\infty)_T \times (\text{weight or volume})_T}{\sum_{i=1}^{n} (AQU_0^\infty)_i \times (\text{weight or volume})_i}$$

where $(AQU_0^\infty)_T$ is the area under the amount of drug (Q) in a tissue versus time curve. Q can be obtained, at any time t, by the relationship $Q = C \cdot V$ (or $C \cdot W$), where C is the concentration of drug at time t, and V and W are the volume and weight, respectively, of the tissue.

A comprehensive discussion of pharmacokinetic/pharmacodynamic modeling in drug targeting has been recently reviewed in a book chapter by Proost (86).

TARGETED DRUG DELIVERY SYSTEMS

As noted in section "Biological Process and Events Involved in Drug Targeting," three strategies have been used to achieve drug targeting. These include use of site-specific, pharmacologically active molecules (magic bullet approach); preparation of pharmacologically inert agents that are activated only at the active site (prodrugs); and use of biologically inert carrier systems that selectively direct drugs to a specific site in the body (magic gun/missile or drug carrier approach). In this section, prodrugs and drug carrier delivery systems are discussed in detail.

Prodrugs

A prodrug is a pharmacologically inert form of an active drug that must undergo transformation to the parent compound in vivo by either a chemical or an enzymatic reaction to exert its therapeutic effects. The theory and practice of prodrugs have been reviewed by Notari (87). Stella and Himmelstein (88,89) have critically reviewed the use of prodrugs in site-specific delivery, and the recent development in targeted prodrug design to optimize drug delivery has been described by Han and Amidon (90). For a prodrug to be useful in site-specific delivery, it must exhibit adequate access to its pharmacological receptor(s). Also, the enzyme or chemical agent responsible for reactivating the prodrug should show major activity only at the target site. Furthermore, the enzyme should be in adequate supply to produce the required level of drug to manifest its pharmacological effect. Finally, the active drug produced in situ must remain at the target site and not leak out into the systemic circulation, which could lead to adverse effects. Thus, prodrugs are designed to alter the absorption, distribution, and metabolism of the parent compound and, thereby, to increase its beneficial effects and decrease its toxicity.

Table 3 lists some commonly used types of prodrugs and their methods of regeneration (91). Many of these prodrugs are simple esters and can be reactivated in vivo by an esterase enzyme. Prodrugs containing an amide bond can be regenerated by peptidases, but their use in vivo has had varying degrees of success. The chemically reconvertible prodrugs frequently lack selectivity of activation at the target sites and thus

Table 3 Prodrug Modifications and Method of Regeneration

Tissue	Characteristics	Characteristics
R–OH (alcohols and phenols)	Alkyl esters and half esters	Enzymes
	Phosphate and sulfate esters	Enzymes
	Sulfoacetyl, dialkyl aminoacyl	Enzymes
	Acyloxyalkyl ethers and thioethers	Enzymes
	Carbamates	Enzymes
R–COOH	Alkyl and glyceryl esters	Enzymes
	Acyloxyalkyl and lactonyl esters	Enzymes
	Alkoxycarbonyloxyalkyl esters	Enzymes
	(2-oxo-1,3-dioxolenyl)alkyl esters	Enzymes
	Amides and amino acid derivatives	Enzymes
R–NH$_2$, R$_2$NH, and R$_3$N	Enamines, Schiff bases, Mannic bases, and oxalzolidines	Chemical
	Amides and peptides	Enzymes
	Hydroxymethyl derivatives	Chemical
	Hydroxymethyl esters	Enzymes
	Soft quaternary ammonium salts	Enzymes
	Carbamates	Enzymes
R–CHO and >C=O	Enol esters	Enzymes
	Thiazolidines and oxazolidines	Chemical
R–C(O)–NH$_2$ and imides	Hydroxymethyl derivatives	Chemical
	Hydroxymethyl esters such as acetate and phosphates	Enzymes
	Mannich bases	Chemical

Source: From Ref. 91.

offer little opportunity for drug targeting. A detailed discussion of prodrugs listed in Table 3 can be found in book chapters by Stella (92) and Roche (93).

Numerous reports of prodrugs in the literature show improved drug effects. Prodrugs that have shown some measure of success for site-specific delivery include L-3,4-dihydroxyphenylalanine (L-dopa) to the brain (94), dipivaloyl derivative of epinephrine to the eye (95), γ-glutamyl-L-dopa to the kidney (96), β-D-glucoside dexamethasone and prednisolone derivatives to the colon (97), thiamine-tetrahydrofuryldisulfide to red blood cells (98), and various amino acid derivatives of antitumor agents, such as daunorubicin (DNR) (99,100), acivicin (101), doxorubicin (101), and phenylenediamine (101), to tumor cells.

The selective delivery of drugs to the brain has been, and continues to be, one of the greatest challenges. Only highly lipid-soluble drugs can cross the blood-brain barrier. Prodrugs with high lipid solubility can be used, but they may show increased partitioning to other tissues and thereby cause adverse reactions. For example, L-dopa, the precursor of dopamine, when administered orally, readily partitions throughout the body, including the brain. Its conversion to dopamine in the corpus striatum produces the therapeutic response, whereas its conversion in the peripheral tissues results in many undesirable side effects. Although many of these side effects can be overcome by additional administration of an inhibitor of aromatic amino acid decarboxylase, such as carbidopa (this does not penetrate into the brain and thereby permits the conversion of L-dopa to dopamine in the brain, but prevents its transformation in the peripheral tissues), the direct delivery of dopamine to the brain constitutes an attractive alternative. One approach that has been used is a prodrug carrier system developed by Bodor and Simpkins (102). This approach is based on the observation that certain dihydropyridines readily enter the brain, where they are oxidized to the corresponding quaternary salts. The latter, owing to difficulty in crossing the blood-brain barrier, remain in the brain. The formation of quaternary salts in the peripheral tissues, on the other hand, rapidly accelerates their removal by renal or biliary mechanisms. This results in a significant buildup of the quaternary salt concentration in the brain and a significant reduction in systemic toxicity. Chemical or enzymatic hydrolysis of the quaternary salt (in the brain) then slowly releases the drug in the cerebrospinal fluid, allowing the therapeutic concentration to be maintained over some period. Examples of drugs that have been investigated using this approach include pralidoxime iodide (2-pyridine aldoxime methyl iodide) (103), phenylethylamine (104), dopamine (105), 3'-azido-2',3'dideoxyuridine (AZddU) (106), and 3'-azido-3'-deoxythymidine (AZT; zidovudine) (106–108).

Recently, new prodrug strategies aimed at targeting a specific enzyme or a specific membrane transporter or both, facilitated by simultaneous use of gene delivery engineered to express the requisite enzyme or transporter, have been developed and proposed to be especially useful in cancer chemotherapy (90).

The use of polymeric prodrugs has also been the subject of intense research recently. Various synthetic strategies to prepare prodrugs and their use in passive and active targeting have been reviewed by Khandare and Minko (109). An excellent review covering prodrugs of anthracyclines in cancer chemotherapy has been reported by Kratz et al. (110). Selected polymer-drug conjugate systems are also discussed in this chapter later.

Drug Carrier Delivery Systems

Drug carrier delivery systems employ biologically inert macromolecules to direct a drug to its target site in the body. These are divided into two types: particulate and soluble macromolecular. Depending on the carrier system, the drug can be either molecularly entrapped within the carrier matrix or covalently linked to the carrier molecules. The major advantage of drug carrier delivery systems is that the distribution of drugs in the body depends on the physicochemical properties of the carrier, not those of drugs. Thus, targeting can be manipulated by choosing an appropriate carrier or by altering the physicochemical properties of the carrier. As outlined by Tomlinson and reproduced in Table 4 (37), there are, however, several other factors that must be considered in the pharmaceutical development and clinical use of both soluble macromolecular and particulate biotechnical and synthetic site-specific systems.

Table 4 Considerations in the Pharmaceutical Development and Clinical Use of Both Soluble Macromolecular and Particulate Biotechnical and Site-Specific Drug Delivery Systems

---

Specification/activity

I. Pharmaceutical development
    A. Production
       Purity
       Evaluation of novel production safety hazard (e.g., sparkling with particulate)

    B. Characterization
       Indentity
       Conformation
       Size
       Size distribution
       Charge, aggregation
       Density
       Surface configuration, homogeneity of attachment moieties
       a. Polymers
       b. Ligands
       c. Spacers

    C. In vitro functionality
       Drug-loading efficiency
       Drug release
       Retention of recognition

    D. Stability
       Characteristics of the breakdown products
       a. In storage formulation
       b. In biological fluids

    Parameter to be assessed on storage
       a. Chemical stability
       b. Character
       c. In vitro functionality
       d. Sterility and functionality
       e. Colloidal character (e.g., aggregation, size, charge)
       f. Surface properties (including conformation and epitopic character)

II. Safety pharmacology (nonhuman)
    A. General considerations
       General safety
       Sterility and pyrogenicity
       a. Major organ function tests
       b. Acute and subacute toxicity studies

Table 4 Considerations in the Pharmaceutical Development and Clinical Use of Both Soluble Macromolecular and Particulate Biotechnical and Site-Specific Drug Delivery Systems (*Continued*)

B. Potential novel toxicities
   MPS uptake
   Uptake in specialized immune
   Depression/exhaustion of MPS

   a. Bone marrow
   b. Bacterial and viral infections
   c. Immunological depression
   d. Hemorrhagic and endotoxin shock
   e. Altered drug response

Low-level activation of MPS

   a. Interleukin-I
   b. Amyloidosis
   c. Hyperplastic liver foci
   d. Altered stem cell kinetics
   e. Altered drug metabolism
   f. Altered response to drug

C. Biotechnics: for biotechnics (and specifically monoclonal antibodies), factors affecting safety include
   Hybridoma background

   a. Murine-murine
   b. Human-human
   c. Interspecies 9chimerics

Contaminants

   a. General safety
   b. Pyrogens
   c. Sterile
   d. Free of hazardous viruses
   e. Free of detectable deoxyribonucleic acid

Interaction with the host

   a. Immunogenicity
   b. Cross-reactivity
   c. Hypersensitivity
   d. Anti-idiotypic response to normal cell
   e. Immune complex disease
   f. Potential MPS toxicity

D. Specific specificity
   Issues include altered drug disposition/metabolism and the need for a tier assessment of safety to include knowledge on

   a. Pathology of lymphoid tissues
   b. Antibody and cell-mediated immunity
   c. Host cell resistance
   d. Phagocytic cell function
   e. Immune/immunotoxicity reaction
   f. Testing
   g. Antigen specificity
   h. Complement binding

Table 4 Considerations in the Pharmaceutical Development and Clinical Use of Both Soluble
Macromolecular and Particulate Biotechnical and Site-Specific Drug Delivery Systems (*Continued*)

III. Metabolism
   A. Issues here include species-specific metabolism (related to novel pattern of drug release at
      receptor sites and possible use of novel paracrine- and endocrine-like peptidergic mediators.
      These could manifest themselves in novel:
      Dose response
      Absorption sites/rates
      Bioavailabilities (at receptors)
      Organ, tissue, cell disposition
      Disease-dependent release
      Excretion routes/rates

IV. Efficacy
   A. Major considerations in the clinical development of a site-specific system, relating to effect,
      utility, and efficacy could include:
      Novel pharmacokinetic and disposition
      Novel modalities of cell/tissue/receptor exposure
      Utilization of novel cellular transport processes
      Species-specific drugs and delivery modalities
      Novel drug interactions
      Novel drug metabolism
      Local versus general distribution
      Biphasic drug action
      Chronopharmacoloy
      New routes of administration: transmucosal; specific regional uptake in gastrointestinal tract
      New pattern of drug release: bolus/first order; pulsatile; feedback control; disease-related
         release of drug (Analytical techniques will need to encompass the identification of very
         low levels of site-specific systems and their degradation and metabolic products.)

V. Extended nonclinical development:
   A. These parallel activities will include:
      Reproductive toxicology
      Chronic toxicology
      Selection of market formulation
      Definition of marketed specifications
      Development of implementation of market-related scale up
      Confirmation of specification following scale up

Abbreviation: MPS, mononuclear phagocyte system.
Source: From Ref. 37.

Targeting with drug carrier systems can be divided into three types: passive, active,
and physical (58,111). Passive targeting relies on the natural distribution pattern of
the drug–drug carrier system. For example, particles with a diameter of 5 μm or less are
readily removed from the blood by macrophages of the RES when administered
systemically. This natural defense mechanism of the RES thus provides an opportunity to
target drugs to macrophages if they are encapsulated in or conjugated with an appropriate
carrier system. Mechanical filtration of particulate carriers larger than 5 to 7 μm by
capillary blockage has also been exploited to target drugs to the lungs by the venous
supply and to other organs through the appropriate arterial supply. Thus, by controlling
the rate of drug release, one can achieve the desired therapeutic action in the targeted

organ. Passive targeting also includes delivery of drug carrier systems directly to a discrete region in the body (e.g., different regions of the GI tract, eye, nose, knee joints, lungs, vagina, rectum, and respiratory tract).

Active targeting employs a deliberately modified drug carrier/drug molecule capable of recognizing and interacting with a specific cell, tissue, or organ in the body. Modifications of the carrier system may include a change in the molecular size, alteration of the surface properties, incorporation of antigen-specific antibodies, or attachment of cell receptor–specific ligands (e.g., glucose, transferrin, and folic acid) (111–115).

Physical targeting refers to delivery systems that release a drug only when exposed to a specific microenvironment, such as a change in pH or temperature, or the use of an external magnetic field (111).

A brief discussion of particulate and soluble macromolecular delivery systems is presented in the following sections.

Particulate Drug Delivery Systems

Particles ranging in sizes from 10 nm to 300 μm have been proposed for drug targeting. They can be introduced directly into the central circulation by intra-arterial or intravenous injection or delivered to a given body compartment, for example, by injection into a joint or by administration using an aerosol to the lungs and nose. Subcutaneous and intraperitoneal administration routes have also been used to deliver drugs to the lymphatic system (Fig. 1) and regional lymph nodes. Some suggested uses of particulate drug delivery systems in drug targeting are presented in Table 5 (37).

Particulate drug delivery systems can be monolithic (i.e., containing a homogeneous mixture of drug and the core material), capsular (in which the drug is surrounded by the carrier material), or emulsion (in which the drug is dispersed in a suspension of the carrier material) types. Passive targeting of particulate drug delivery systems depends on the size, shape, charge, and surface hydrophobicity of the particles. A relationship between particle size and biological targeting, after intravascular injection, is schematically depicted in (Fig. 6) (111). In general, particles larger than 7 μm are mechanically filtered by the smallest capillaries of the lungs, and particles smaller than 7 μm in diameter (between 2 and 7 μm) may pass the smallest lung capillary beds and be entrapped in the capillary network of the liver and spleen. Chiles et al. (116) reported that particles of 15 μm were homogeneously distributed throughout the lung, whereas particles of 137 μm exhibited a more peripheral distribution. Larger particles can also be injected intra-arterially. In this case, particles lodge in the first capillary bed they encounter (first-order targeting). For example, administration into the mesenteric, portal, or renal artery leads to entrapment of particles in gut, liver, or kidneys, respectively. For organs bearing solid tumors, this approach may lead to localization of the drug in the tumor cells. Particles between 0.05 and 2 μm in size are rapidly cleared from the bloodstream by macrophages of the RES (primarily by the Kupffer cells of the liver) after intravenous, intra-arterial, or intraperitoneal administration. This natural targeting to the liver offers opportunities for the treatment of tropical diseases (e.g., leishmaniasis) and fungal infections (e.g., candidiasis). Because of the dominant role of Kupffer cells, other cells of the RES play a small role in removing particles from the blood. Since the fenestrae of the liver endothelium have a diameter of 0.1 μm, particles smaller than 0.1 μm (<100 nm) can pass through the sieve plates of the sinusoid and become localized in the spleen and bone marrow.

Negatively charged particles are more rapidly cleared from the blood than neutral and positive ones (117). The clearance rate of particles by the RES is inversely related to

Table 5 Some Uses for Particulate Drug Delivery Systems

Target site /purpose (particle size)	Disease/therapy
Direct administration to discrete compartments (0.005–100 μm)	
Eye	Infection
Lung	Allergy
Joints	Arthritis
Gastrointestinal tract	Crohn's disease, immunization
Intralesional	Tumor
Cerebral ventricles	Infection
Interstitial administration (0.005–100 μm)	
Subcutaneous	Lymph node targeting (e.g., some cancers)
Intramuscular	Depot for anesthetics, proteins
Intravascular targets	
Diseased macrophages (0.1–1.0 μm)	Parasitic, fungal, viral, enzyme storage disease; autoimmune disease; gene therapy
Other blood cells (0.1–1.0 μm)	Cancerous, platelets, gene therapy (bone marrow erythroblasts), immune cells (vaccination/adjuvant), antivirals
Circulating depot (0.1–1.0 μm)	Anti-infective, antileukemics, antithrombotics, antivirals, release of polypeptides and protein drugs
Capillary filtration (>1.0 μm)	Cancer, emphyma, thrombi: drug acting on local endothelia
Extravascular targets	
Macrophages activation (0.1–1.0 μm)	Abnormal cells (e.g., cancerous and virally infected)
Discontinuous endothelia (<0.15 μm)	
Basement membrane	Spleen
Parenchymal cells	Liver
Diseased endothelia	Rheumatoid arthritis, malignant hypertension, myocardial infarct, transluminal angioplasty
Ex vivo (>0.5–50 μm)	
Cells	Cell targeting (e.g., for gene therapy)

Source: From Ref. 37.

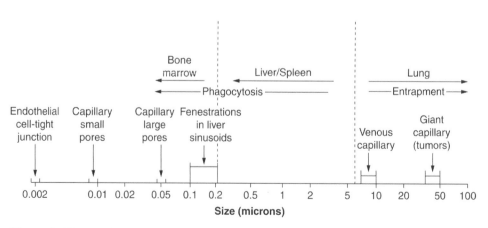

Figure 6 The vascular bed and passive targeting. *Source*: From Ref. 111.

the load of the particles; that is, the rate of clearance of a larger dose of microparticulate is slower than that for a smaller dose (118).

The targeting of drugs to sites in the body other than the RES (e.g., parenchymal cells or tumor cells of the liver or monocytes in the blood) has been extensively studied. In vitro studies show that this can be achieved by linking particles to monoclonal antibodies (118–121) or to cell-specific ligands [e.g., desialylated fetuin (122), glycoproteins (123), native immunoglobulins (124), folic acid (115), and heat-aggregated immunoglobulins (125)] or by alterations of the particles' surface characteristics [e.g., by using bioadhesives (126), water-soluble polymers, such as PEG, or nonionic surfactants (13)] so that they are not recognized by the RES as being foreign (active targeting) (111). Changes in the surface properties can prevent particles from adhering to the macrophages and, consequently, their endocytic uptake. This allows the particles to distribute to other parts of the body where they do not normally localize (Table 6) (13,127,128).

Other approaches used to avoid RES uptake of particles include incorporation of ferromagnetic materials, such as carboxyl iron powder and Fe_3O_4 (129); formulation of particles in oils (130); and the use of an appropriate carrier capable of degrading and releasing the drug into the surrounding tissues with slight changes in temperature (131) or in pH (131) conditions. The approach involving magnetic materials has been successfully used in humans in the therapy of carcinoma of the prostate and bladder (132). It allows maneuvering of the delivery system with external magnetic fields. The particle-in-oil approach has been used by Sezaki et al. (130) in the treatment of VXZ carcinoma in rabbits and cystic hygroma in pediatric patients. They reported a significant increase in the survival rate of the rabbits and the management of 22 cases of pediatric cystic hygroma when treated with a bleomycin-gelatin microsphere-oil emulsion. Free bleomycin had no effect on these tumors.

The various particulate drug carrier systems that have been investigated can be grouped into the following classes.

Polymeric microparticles and nanoparticles Colloidal particles ranging in size from 1 to 1000 nm (1 μm) are called nanoparticles, and those larger than 1 μm but small enough to remain suspended in water are classified as microparticles. They can be composed of either a homogeneous polymer-drug matrix or a central drug core surrounded by a polymer shell, commonly referred to as microspheres/nanospheres and microcapsules/nanocapsules, respectively. Polymers can be either natural (e.g., albumin, gelatin, alginate, collagen, and chitosan) or synthetic [e.g., poly(lactic acids), poly(caprolactone), poly(methyl methacrylates), and poly(alkylcyanoacrylates)] in origin. The most commonly practiced methods to prepare microparticles and nanoparticles include direct

Table 6 Uptake of Polystyrene Microsphere (60-nm diameter) in Rat Organs Following IV Injection

System	Liver	Spleen	Blood[a]	Femurs
Uncoated control	47.4^b + 2.6 (7)	1.05 + 0.65 (4)	3.7 + 0.28 (7)	0.059 + 0.002 (3)
Coated with poloxamer 338	3.5 + 1.1 (2)	0.39 + 0.015 (2)	39.2 + 5.4 (2)	0.142 + 0.057 (2)
Coated/uncoated ratio	0.073	0.36	10.6	2.4

[a]Blood volume taken as 6.5 mL/100 g body weight.
[b]Percentage uptake at one hour.
Source: From Ref. 13.

polymerization of monomers and dispersion of preformed polymers. The former includes direct emulsion, micelle, and interfacial polymerization approaches. The emulsion polymerization method involves heating a mixture of monomer and active agent(s) in an aqueous or a nonaqueous phase that contains an initiator, a surfactant (employed usually in excess of its critical micelle concentration), and a stabilizer. Vigorous agitation is employed during the emulsion formation to produce particles smaller than 100 μm. The smaller particle size assures good tissue tolerance, uptake, and transfer, and causes no foreign body reaction. Examples of carrier systems prepared by the emulsion polymerization approach include poly(alkyl methacrylate) nanoparticles, which exhibit excellent adjuvant properties for vaccines (133), and poly(alkylcyanoacrylate) nanoparticles (134), which are biodegradable. The main advantage of emulsion polymerization is that higher molar mass polymers are usually formed at a faster rate and a lower temperature. A major disadvantage, however, is that the product cannot be readily freed from the residual monomers. Micellar polymerization differs from emulsion polymerization only in that the monomers and active agent(s) are contained within the micelles formed by a suitable concentration of a surfactant before the polymerization is commenced. This allows very little, if any, increase in particle size as polymerization proceeds. In interfacial polymerization, monomers react at the interface of two immiscible liquid phases to produce a film that encapsulates the dispersed phase. The process involves an initial emulsification step in which an aqueous phase, containing a reactive monomer and a core material, is dispersed in a nonaqueous continuous phase. This is then followed by the addition of a second monomer to the continuous phase. Monomers in the two phases then diffuse and polymerize at the interface to form a thin film. The degree of polymerization depends on the concentration of monomers, the temperature of the system, and the composition of the liquid phases.

Non-polymerization approaches commonly practiced to prepare microparticles and nanoparticles are polymer precipitation, solvent evaporation, and salting out methods. The precipitation method is used to encapsulate hydrophilic drugs and frequently yields particles with a narrow polydispersity index. The solvent evaporation approach is applicable to both hydrophobic and hydrophilic drugs. Typically, the polymer, optionally with a surface-modifying agent, is dissolved in an appropriate nonaqueous solvent (usually, methylene chloride, chloroform, or ethyl acetate). The drug is then dissolved or suspended in the solution and an oil-in-water (o/w) emulsion is prepared by mixing it with a large volume of water containing an emulsifier [e.g., poly(vinyl alcohol) or a surfactant] under vigorous stirring (to produce smaller-size oil droplets). The solvent is then removed to produce the particles. To produce nanosize particles, a high-shear mixer, ultrasonicator, or microfluidizer can be used. Addition of a water-miscible organic solvent (e.g., acetone) has also been used to produce smaller-size particles. It has been suggested that the rapid diffusion of a water-miscible organic solvent into the aqueous and organic phases generates interfacial turbulence, which spontaneously results in a large interfacial area, leading to the formation of smaller-size droplets. Removal of the organic solvent produces the particles. One of the disadvantages of the o/w method is poor entrapment efficiency of the moderately and highly soluble drugs. To overcome this problem, an oil-in-oil (o/o) emulsion or a double emulsification (w/o/w) method can be used. The o/o type emulsion is prepared by using a volatile organic solvent and mineral oil. The w/o/w emulsion approach is especially useful for encapsulating large doses of hydrophilic drugs, peptides, proteins, and vaccines. The salting out/solvent displacement method eliminates the use of chlorinated organic solvents and large amounts of surfactants. The coacervation (phase separation) approach involves heating or chemical denaturation and desolvation of natural proteins or carbohydrates. As much as 85% of water-soluble drugs can be entrapped within a protein matrix by freeze drying the emulsion prepared in this manner. For water-insoluble drugs, a microsuspension emulsion procedure has been suggested as a method of choice to achieve high drug payloads. Various processing parameters that can affect the preparation of micro- or nanoparticles include the concentration and nature of the surfactant, the number of homogenization cycles, the addition of excipient to the inner water phase, the drug concentration, and the oil-water phase ratio.

Micro- or nanoparticles, for use in drug targeting, must be produced as sterile, freeze-dried, free-flowing powders. They can be administered either systemically or by an intramuscular route. Drugs can either be encapsulated or molecularly entrapped within the polymer matrix or conjugated on the particle surfaces. As is obvious from Table 5, the major use of micro- and nanoparticles, including magnetic particles, has been in tumor therapy (135–143). Particle-in-oil emulsions have been used as lysosomotropic systems. After subcutaneous administration, the oily product is readily taken up by the lymphatic system (130). Numerous examples of biodegradable polymeric micro- and nanoparticles, with potential applications in medical imaging, gene therapy, and drug targeting specific cells or tissues, have been reported (136–139,144–146). Nanoparticles can carry high doses of drug or agent (up to 45% of particle weight), with an entrapment efficiency of over 95%. Studies also show that solid lipid particles can be used to target antineoplastic and gene-therapeutic agents to the brain (143,147) and to increase the permeation of glucocorticoids through the human epidermis (148). Peracchia et al. (149) reported that PEG conjugated poly(cyanoacrylate) nanoparticles, following intravenous administration, accumulated in larger amounts in the spleen than in the liver, offering an interesting perspective for targeting drugs to tissues other than the liver. The release of drugs from particulate carriers can occur by surface erosion, disintegration, hydration, or breakdown (by a chemical or an enzymatic reaction) of the particles. These and other factors that can affect the release of drugs are presented in Table 7.

Liposomes Liposomes are versatile, efficient, and, probably, the most extensively studied class of carrier systems. Several liposomal formulations are currently either in preclinical/clinical trials or commercially available (e.g., Doxil®/Caelyx®, Myocet®, AmBisome®, and DaunoXome®). A comprehensive review of the preparation, analysis, drug entrapment, and interactions with the biological milieu, including drug targeting, can be found in a compendium entitled *Liposome Technology*, edited by Gregoriadis (150,151). There are several books (152–155), book chapters (156–160), and review articles (161–168) that cover various aspects of liposome technology.

The important attributes of liposomes as a drug carrier are that (*i*) they are biologically inert and completely biodegradable; (*ii*) they pose no concerns of toxicity, antigenicity, or pyrogenicity, because phospholipids are natural components of all cell membranes; (*iii*) they can be prepared in various sizes, compositions, surface charges, and so forth, depending on the requirements of a given application; (*iv*) they can be used to entrap or encapsulate a wide variety of hydrophilic and lipophilic drugs, including enzymes, hormones, vitamins, antibiotics, and cytostatic agents; (*v*) drugs entrapped in liposomes are physically separated from the environment and are thus less susceptible to degradation or deactivation by the action of external media (e.g., enzymes or inhibitors); and (*vi*) liposome-entrapped drugs offer new possibilities for drug targeting, since entrapped drugs follow the fate of liposomes and are released only at the site of liposome destruction.

The drug-loading capacities of liposomes depend on the properties of the drug, phospholipids, and other additives used. Typically, hydrophobic drugs are solubilized

Table 7 Factors Affecting the Release of Drugs from Particulate Carriers

Drugs
  Position in the particle
  Molecular mass
  Physiochemical properties
  Concentrations
  Drug carrier interaction
  Diffusion, desorption from surface, low exchange

Particles
  Type and amount of matrix material
  Size and density of the particle
  Capsular or monolithic
  Extent and nature of any cross-linking, denaturation of polymer
  Presence of adjuvants
  Surface erosion, particle diffusion and leaching
  Total disintegration of particles

Environmental
  Hydrogen ion concentration
  Polarity
  Ionic strength
  Presence of enzymes
  Temperature
  Microwave
  Magnetism
  Light

Source: From Ref. 3.

with lipid(s) in an organic solvent that is then dried and subsequently hydrated to yield liposomal drug formulations. The loading of hydrophilic drugs is limited by their aqueous solubility. By submitting the liposome-drug solution to several freeze-thaw cycles, the entrapment efficiency of water-soluble drugs can be increased. However, this is possible only at high lipid concentrations (169). The loading of cationic (or anionic) drugs can be significantly improved by using liposomes containing negatively (or positively) charged lipids. Gabizon (170) reported that the entrapment efficiency can be increased from 10% for neutral liposomes to 60% for charged liposomes. Other approaches to increase entrapment efficiency involve the use of transmembrane pH gradients and dehydration and rehydration of vesicles (DRV). In general, liposomes with low internal pH tend to accommodate a higher loading of cationic drugs, whereas a high intraliposomal pH enables increased entrapment of negatively charged (anionic drugs) and amphiphilic drugs (171). The dehydration-rehydration method allows entrapment of drugs in a concentration range of 50% to 85% (172,173). This method is easy to scale up, and the liposome vesicles containing drug, including protein, can be freeze dried and reconstituted with saline solution without affecting the entrapped drug. Proteins, sugar residues, and antibodies can also be incorporated into liposomes. Other approaches used include physical adsorption, incorporation during liposomal preparation, and covalent attachment (direct or through a spacer) to the active drug or an inert additive (e.g., polymer) incorporated into the liposomal membrane (167,174,175).

After intravenous administration, liposomes are rapidly removed from blood, primarily by cells of the RES, and, foremost, by the liver (Kupffer cells). The half-lives of liposomes in the bloodstream may range from a few minutes to many hours (up to 72 hours) (176), depending on the nature and compositions of the lipids, surface properties, and size of the liposomal vesicles. In general, smaller unilamellar vesicles (SUVs) show much longer half-lives in the blood than multilamellar vesicles (MLVs) and large unilamellar vesicles (LUVs). Negatively charged liposomes are cleared more rapidly from the circulation than corresponding neutral or positively charged liposomes. Also, the uptake by the spleen is greater for negatively charged liposomes than for positive or neutral liposomes. The SUVs can penetrate 0.1-μm fenestrations located in the endothelium of discontinuous (sinusoidal) capillaries lining the liver, spleen, and bone marrow (177) and reach the underlying parenchymal cells. The endothelium of the hepatic sinusoid contains openings larger than 0.1 μm in diameter, and this may allow penetration of MLVs and LUVs. An increase in the liposome dose causes a relative decrease in liver uptake and, consequently, an increase in blood levels and, to some extent, in spleen and bone marrow uptake (177). Prolongation of the blood clearance times of the liposomes by blocking the RES uptake has been used to increase the likelihood of liposomes to interact with vascular endothelial cells and circulating blood cells.

Irrespective of size, liposomes, when injected intraperitoneally, partially accumulate in the liver and spleen. It has been suggested that transport of liposomes from the peritoneal cavity to the systemic circulation and eventually to tissues occurs by lymphatic pathways. Local injection of larger liposomes leads to quantitative accumulation at the site of injection. The slow disintegration of the carrier releases the drug, which then diffuses into the blood circulation. Smaller liposomes, on the other hand, enter the lymph nodes and blood circulation and eventually accumulate in the liver and spleen.

Since the RES is the natural target, liposomes have been extensively investigated as carriers for the treatment of liver and RES organ diseases (passive targeting). Belchetz et al. (178) reported that liposome-entrapped glucocerebroside, when administered intravenously in patients suffering with Gaucher's disease, reduced the liver size significantly. The effect is attributed to the penetration ability of the liposomal drug into the cells. The native enzyme had no effects because of its inability to penetrate the cells. A similar finding was reported in patients suffering with glycogenesis type II disease following administration of amyloglycosidase entrapped in liposomes (179). Encapsulation of antimonial drugs within liposomes has increased the efficacy by 800- to 1000-fold compared with the free drug against experimental visceral and cutaneous leishmaniasis in rats (180–182). Bakker-Woudenberg et al. (183) found an about-90-fold increase in the therapeutic efficacy following administration of liposome-encapsulated ampicillin compared with free ampicillin against Listeria monocytogenes infection.

The rapid clearance of liposomes by cells of the RES system can be avoided by creating a highly hydrated layer on the surface of the liposomes by coating/grafting with water-soluble polymers [e.g., PEG, surfactants (e.g., poloxamers)] or by including phosphatidylinositol or gangliosides to create a highly hydrated shell. Moghimi (74) reported that the inclusion of methoxypoly(ethylene glycol) into the liposomal bilayer can control the rate of drainage as well as lymphatic distribution following subcutaneous administration. Liposomal vesicles containing 6.7 mol% PEG (molar mass 2000) were noted to drain faster from the site of application than 15mol% PEG (molar mass 350). The latter, however, showed greater retention in the regional lymph nodes. Conjugation of nonspecific IgG to the distal end of PEG, however, dramatically increased the lymph node retention of the faster-draining PEG-containing vesicle.

Liposomes have also been used for delivering immunomodulating agents to macrophages, the immunologically competent extravascular cells that contribute to host defense mechanisms. Activated macrophages are capable of selectively killing tumor cells, thereby leaving normal cells unharmed. Fidler et al. (184) have shown that lymphokines (e.g., interferon), muramyl dipeptide, and a lipophilic derivative of muramyl tripeptide, encapsulated within liposomes, are highly effective in activating antitumor functions in rodent and human macrophages in vitro and in mouse and rat in vivo. Dose-response measurements show that these preparations induce maximum levels of macrophage activation at a significantly lower dose than needed for equivalent activation by the nonencapsulated preparation (185–187). Roerdnik et al. (157) reported a 50% to 60% increase in the tumoricidal activity of muramyl dipeptide when encapsulated within liposomes compared with free drug against B-16 melanoma cells in vitro. The free drug gave a maximum activity of 30% cytotoxicity versus a 250- to 1000-fold increase in potentiation of muramyl-induced cytotoxicity because of encapsulation within liposomes. Saiki et al. (188,189) and Sone et al. (190) have found that encapsulation of more than one agent within the same liposome produces synergistic activation of macrophages in vitro and in vivo. The activation of macrophages, in general, requires phagocytosis of the liposome, followed by a lag period of four to eight hours before tumoricidal activity is expressed (186). Since no participation of macrophage surface receptors is required, the tumoricidal activity of macrophages results from the interaction of immunomodulating agents with intracellular targets (191).

Liposomes have been extensively studied as carriers for a variety of antineoplastic drugs. Mayhew and Rustum (192) demonstrated that liposomes containing doxorubicin [adriamycin (ADR)] are 100 times more effective compared with free drug against the liver metastasis of the M5076 tumor. Liposomal encapsulation of amphotericin B, a potent, but extremely toxic, antifungal drug, also resulted in much reduced toxicity, while it maintained potency (193). Rosenberg et al. (194) and Burkhanov et al. (195) have reported that liposomes prepared by using autologous phospholipids obtained from tumor cells are taken up by the tumor cells two to six times better than a control egg lecithin liposome.

Liposomes containing specific targeting molecules, such as tumor-specific antibodies or cell receptor–specific ligands (e.g., glycolipids, lipoproteins, lectin, folic acid, and amino sugars), have been prepared to provide liposomes with increased direct transport properties (115,167,176,196,197). These cell-specific targeting molecules can be either adsorbed on or covalently attached, directly or by a spacer, to the outer surface of the liposomal membrane. The use of spacers enables binding of considerable quantities of targeting molecules without affecting its specific binding properties or the integrity of the liposomes.

Temperature- and pH-sensitive liposomes have been investigated for targeting drugs to primary tumors and metastases or sites of infection and inflammation (198). The basis for the temperature-sensitive drug delivery is that at elevated temperatures, above the gel to liquid crystalline phase transition temperature (T_c), the permeability of liposomes markedly increases, causing the release of the entrapped drug. The release rate depends on the temperature and the action of the serum components, principally the lipoproteins. Weinstein et al. (199) investigated the effect of heating on incorporation of [3H]methotrexate, administered in the free form and encapsulated in 7:3 (w/w) dipalmitoyl and distearoyl phosphatidylcholine liposomal vesicles, in L1210 tumors implanted in the hind feet of mice. They found about a 14% increase in [3H]methotrexate incorporation from the liposomal form, compared with the free drug, after heating. This approach has been extended to a bladder transitional cell carcinoma, implanted in the hind legs of C3H/Bi mice (200), and for delivery of cisplatin (cis-diamminedichloroplatinum) selectively to tumors (201).

The pH-sensitive liposomes consist of mixtures of several saturated egg phosphatidylcholines and several N-acylamino acids. The release of drug is suggested to be a function of acid-base equilibrium effected by the interaction between ionizable amino acids and N-acylamino acid headgroups of the liposomes. There appears to be a close relation between T_c and pH effect (198). Recently, long-circulating pH-sensitive liposomal formulations have been prepared using PEG and a terminally alkylated poly(N-isopropylacrylamide)-methacrylic copolymer. Incorporation of PEG renders hydrophilicity, causing liposomes to avoid RES uptake and, consequently, stay in circulation for a longer period (202). The fusogenic peptide–based pH-sensitive liposomes containing folate and transferrin ligands have been described for intracellular targeting (113).

Liposomes also offer potential for use as carriers to transfer genetic materials to cells. Nicolau et al. (203) reported that a recombinant plasmid containing the rat preproinsulin I gene, encapsulated in large liposomes, when injected intravenously, resulted in the transient expression of this gene in the liver and spleen of the recipient animals. A significant fraction of the expressed hormone was in physiologically active form. Recently, liposomes have also been used to block the initial binding of human immunodeficiency virus (HIV) to host cells (157). This binding takes place between a glycoprotein (gp 120) on the virus coat and the CD4 receptor on the surface of T-helper lymphocytes and other cells. Antiviral drugs, such as zalcitabine (2′,3′-dideoxycytidine)-5′-triphosphate (204) and AZT (205), have also been incorporated into liposomes and studied for their antiviral activities.

The incorporation of magnetic particles in liposomes, combined with an externally applied magnetic field, has recently demonstrated in vivo the ability to selectively target a specific organ, that is, one kidney over the other (206). The use of liposomes for targeting and to increase the bioavailability of antibiotics has been recently reviewed (207). Ocular drug targeting by liposomes is another important area of research (208). Several oral liposomal formulations for drug delivery and immunization have also been described (209–213).

Niosomes Niosomes are globular submicroscopic vesicles composed of nonionic surfactants. They can be formed by techniques analogous to those used to prepare liposomes (214). To predict whether the surfactant being used will produce micelles or bilayer niosome vesicles, an arbitrary critical packing parameter (CPP) can be used, that is, $v/a \cdot l$, where v and l are specific volume and length of the hydrophilic portion of the surfactant and a is the area of the hydrophobic segment of the surfactant (215). A CPP value of 0.5 or less favors the formation of micelles, whereas a value between 0.5 and 1.0 favors the formation of vesicles. The various types of nonionic surfactants used to prepare niosomes include polyglycerol alkylethers (216), glucosyl dialkyl ethers (217), crown ethers (218), and polyoxyethylene alkylethers (218). Similar to liposomes, niosome vesicles can be unilamellar, oligolamellar, or multilamellar. A variety of lipid additives, such as cholesterol, can be incorporated in the niosome bilayer. Incorporation of cholesterol in the niosome bilayer enhances the stability of niosomes against the destabilizing effects of plasma and serum proteins and decreases the permeability of the vesicle to the entrapped solute (219). Niosomes are osmotically active and require no special conditions for handling and storage.

Niosomes have been investigated as drug carriers in experimental cancer chemotherapy and in murine visceral leishmaniasis (219). When compared with free drug, niosomal forms of methotrexate, after intravenous administration by the tail vein in mice, exhibited prolonged lifetimes in the plasma and produced increased methotrexate levels in the liver and the brain. In addition, encapsulation within niosomes caused a reduction in the metabolism and urinary and fecal excretion of methotrexate (220,221). Polysorbate 80, a nonionic surfactant that does not form niosomes, when coadministered with free methotrexate, provided reduced efficacy compared with methotrexate encapsulated in niosomes (221). This suggests that it is essential for surfactants to have a vesicular structure to effect enhanced targeting of drugs. Niosomal delivery has also been reported for 5-fluorouracil (222).

The delivery of doxorubicin to the S180 sarcoma (tumor) in mice by using niosomes as a carrier has been studied by Rogerson (223). Much higher tumor drug levels were reported with niosomes containing 50% cholesterol than with free drug or drug encapsulated in cholesterol-free niosomes. The initial serum drug concentrations were higher following administration of free drug, but between two and six hours after administration, the concentrations dropped and were lower than those observed by using niosomal drugs, suggesting a rapid metabolism or distribution of free drug from the vascular system.

Niosomes containing stibogluconate have been found to be as effective as the corresponding liposomal drugs in the visceral leishmaniasis model. Free drug showed reduced efficacy (224).

Lipoproteins A lipoprotein is an endogenous macromolecule consisting of an inner apolar core of cholesteryl esters and triglycerides surrounded by a monolayer of phospholipid embedded with cholesterol and apoproteins. The functions of lipoproteins are to transport lipids and to mediate lipid metabolism. There are four main types of lipoproteins (classified on the basis of their flotation rates in salt solutions): chylomicrons, very-low-density lipoprotein (VLDL), LDL, and high-density lipoprotein (HDL). These differ in size, molar mass, and density, and have different lipid, protein, and apoprotein compositions. The apoproteins are important determinants in the metabolism of lipoproteins—they serve as ligands for lipoprotein receptors and as mediators in lipoprotein interconversion by enzymes.

Lipoproteins have been suggested as potential drug carriers (225) because (i) they are natural macromolecules and thus pose no threats of any anti-immunogenic response; (ii) unlike other particulate carriers, lipoproteins are not rapidly cleared from the circulation by the reticuloendothelial system; (iii) the cellular uptake of lipoproteins is by high-affinity receptors; (iv) the inner core of a lipoprotein, which comprises triglycerides and cholesterol, provides an ideal domain for transporting highly lipophilic drugs, whereas amphiphilic drugs can be incorporated in the outer phospholipid coat of the core; (v) drugs incorporated in the core are protected from the environment during transport, and the environment is protected from the drug; and (vi) drugs located in the core do not affect the specificity of the ligand(s) present on the surface of the particle for binding to various cells.

Several methods are known to entrap or incorporate drugs into lipoproteins. The three most commonly practiced procedures include (225) (i) direct addition of an aqueous solution of a drug to the lipoprotein; (ii) transfer of a drug from a solid surface (e.g., the wall of a glass tube, glass beads, or small siliceous earth crystals) to the lipoprotein; and (iii) delipidation of lipoprotein with sodium desoxycholate or an organic solvent, followed by reconstitution with drug-phospholipid microemulsion or drug alone.

The use of LDL and other lipoproteins in drug targeting has been reviewed (225,226). Damle et al. (227) have shown that radiopharmaceuticals, such as iopanoic acid, a cholecystographic agent, could be incorporated in chylomicron remnants by esterification with cholesterol and used for liver imaging. About 87% of the chylomicron remnant–loaded iopanoic acid accumulated in the liver within 0.5 hours after administration, compared with 31% accumulated by using a saline solution containing the same amount of the drug. The LDLs have been used as a carrier to selectively deliver chemotherapeutic agents to neoplastic cells. The rationale is that tumor cells, compared with normal cells, express higher amounts of LDL receptors and can thus be selectively targeted with LDL. Thus, Samadi-Baboli et al. (228) have shown that LDL loaded with 9-methoxyellipticin incorporated in an emulsion containing dimyristoylphosphatidylcholine and cholesteryl oleate exhibited much higher activity than free drug against L1210 and P388 murine leukemia cells in vitro. The eradication of the L1210 cells by the drug-LDL complex occurred exclusively by an LDL receptor mechanism. The LDL-drug complex showed higher cytotoxicity against cells preincubated with lipoprotein-deficient serum than those incubated in fetal serum, confirming that higher LDL expression on the cells leads to a higher uptake of LDL. Another study (229) indicated that acrylophenon antineoplastic molecules, when incorporated within LDL, can be delivered selectively to cancer cells without being entrapped in other blood proteins and cleared by the reticuloendothelial cells.

Kempen et al. (230) synthesized a water-soluble cholesteryl-containing trigalactoside, tris-gal-chol, which when incorporated in lipoproteins allowed the utilization of active receptors for galactose-terminated macromolecules as a trigger for the uptake of lipoproteins.

LDL and HDL have also been chemically modified to provide new recognition markers so that they can be selectively targeted to various types of cells in the liver (225,226). Lactosylated LDL and HDL, which contain D-galactose residues as a ligand, can be prepared by incubating the corresponding protein with lactose (D-galactosyl-D-glucose) and sodium cyanoborohydride. Incubation of LDL with acetic anhydride produces the acetylated LDL. When injected intravenously in rats, both lactosylated LDL and HDL and acetylated LDL are rapidly cleared from the circulation by the liver (Table 8). Lactosylated LDL is specifically taken up by the Kupffer cells, whereas lactosylated HDL is mainly cleared by the parenchymal cells. Acetylated LDL shows a higher accumulation in endothelial and parenchymal cells than in Kupffer cells. Thus, lactosylated HDL can be used to deliver antiviral drugs to parenchymal cells, whereas lactosylated LDL may serve as a carrier for immunomodulators, antivirals, and antiparasitic drugs to Kupffer and parenchymal cells. Acetylated LDL, on the other hand, is suitable for targeting anti-infective drugs to parenchymal and endothelial liver cells. Both Kupffer and endothelial cells have been implicated in HIV infections (231).

Activated carbon (charcoal) Activated carbon is commonly used as an adsorbent. It has a microporous structure and possesses a large surface area for adsorption. Drugs or chemicals adsorbed on activated carbon particles exist in dynamic equilibrium with nonadsorbed drugs. The aqueous suspensions of activated carbon, available commercially

Table 8 Distribution of Acetylated LDL, Lactosylated LDL, and Lactosylated HDL over Liver Cell Types

	Percentage of total liver uptake ($n = 3$)		
	Acetylated LDL	Lactosylated LDL	Lactosylated HDL
Parenchymal cells	38.8 ± 5.8	31.8 ± 4.9	98.1 ± 0.6
Kupffer cells	7.4 ± 1.7	57.1 ± 1.9	1.0 ± 0.5
Endothelial cells	53.8 ± 5.7	11.1 ± 3.2	0.9 ± 0.2

Abbreviations: LDL, low-density lipoproteins; HDL, high-density lipoproteins.
Source: From Ref. 225.

under the trade name Actidose® with Sorbitol and Actidose®-Aqua (Paddock Laboratories, Inc., Minneapolis, MN), have been accepted for oral use in humans to remove toxic substances. Studies in mice have shown that activated carbon, following oral administration, can be taken up M cells that line the lumen of the intestine and subsequently transported through the Peyer's patches to the submucosal lymphoid tissue (232).

Activated carbon, when injected into tissues, is taken into the lymphatic capillaries and becomes localized in the regional lymph nodes. However, when administered into a cancerous pleural or abdominal cavity, it was adsorbed onto cancer and serosal surfaces. Takahashi (233) reported that mitomycin (MMC) binds reversibly to activated carbon with desorption rates of 90 > 4.8% and 107.2 > 7.3% in saline and Ringer's solutions, respectively. Activated carbon adsorbs 20 to 500 times more MMC than what is considered to be effective for cancer cells. The acute toxicity, evaluated in vivo in non-tumor-bearing and tumor-bearing humans and animals, showed an increase in the median lethal dose (LD50) value with an increase in the activated carbon amount. When administered peritoneally in non-tumor-bearing rats, activated carbon–MMC particles (equivalent to 5.0 mg of MMC) were observed in the lymphatic system and deposited in the omentum and peritoneum cavities. In tumor-bearing rats, particles were observed in lymph nodes of the omentum, para-aorta, perirenal, and thoracic 10 minutes after administration. There were no particles in the lymph nodes displaced by tumor tissues at a terminal stage, suggesting that the administered activated charcoal–MMC particles are delivered to distant lymph nodes with metastasis through the lymph vessels. In rabbits, MMC was delivered only to the lymphatic system (233). Patients with advanced gastric cancer, when injected locally with activated carbon–MMC combined with intraperitoneal hyperthermic hypoosmolar infusion, showed significantly reduced lymph node and peritoneal recurrences compared with those who were treated surgically, improving the one- and two-year survival rates to 91.2% and 72.1% versus 78.9% and 45.5% for the control patients, respectively (234).

Studies in dogs indicated that MMC–activated carbon, when injected into the gastric wall, is taken up primarily by the lymphatic system and transported rapidly to the regional lymph nodes, with drug activity being retained (233). A similar observation was made by Ito et al. (235) following an administration of activated charcoal–MMC suspension into the subserosal space. In both the studies, compared with a MMC solution, a significant inhibition of lymph node metastasis was noted with MMC–activated charcoal. In humans, both early stomach cancers and advanced cancers of Borrmann I type either decreased by more than 50% in size or completely disappeared following the local injection of MMC–activated charcoal. No significant effect was noted in advanced cancers with Borrmann II, III, and IV types. High drug activity was demonstrated in regional lymph nodes for a prolonged period. The drug in the peripheral blood was scarce. Patients tolerated about a five times larger dose of the anticancer agent when presented in the activated charcoal–adsorbed form than in free form (233). It appears that activated carbon might be a potential carrier for lymphatic delivery, or to peritoneal or pleural cavities, the most common sites in cancer metastasis. Minimal side effects are expected, since constant low concentrations of drug are maintained in the general circulation. Recently, the use of MMC adsorbed on activated carbon particles against advanced, unresectable esophageal cancer has been reported (236). The median survival time following four weekly intratumoral injections was 16 weeks.

Liu et al. (142) investigated the effect of different particle sizes of activated carbon (0.14–0.24, 0.4–0.6, and 0.7–1.5 μm) on lymphatic distribution following intrapleural administration in healthy immune competent rats, immune competent rats following pneumonectomy, and nude rats with metastatic lung cancer. The activated carbon particles were suspended in aqueous solutions containing 50, 20, and 9 mg of charcoal, poly(vinyl pyrrolidone), and sodium chloride, respectively, and administered into the pleural space of rats. The particles were cleared by the regional thoracic lymphatic system through the parietal pleura three hours after injection and reached the regional lymph nodes in all three animal models. However, particles ranging in size from 0.7 to 1.5 μm provided better lymph distribution than two smaller–size ranges particles, suggesting that large-size particles are effective for intralymphatic targeting following intraperitoneal administration.

Colloidal activated carbon bound to methotrexate, following intratumoral administration of a weekly dose of 30 mg/kg, has also been found to be effective against human colon carcinoma (LoVo) implanted into the backs of BALB/c nude mice (237).

Cellular carriers Erythrocytes, leukocytes, platelets, islets, hepatocytes, and fibroblasts have all been suggested as potential carriers for drugs and biological substances. They can be used to provide slow release of entrapped drugs in the circulatory system, to deliver therapeutic agents to a specific site in the body, as cellular transplants to provide missing enzymes and hormones (in enzyme-hormone replacement therapy), or as endogenous cells to synthesize and secrete molecules that affect the metabolism and function of other cells. Because these carriers are actual endogenous cells, they produce little or no antigenic response, and when old or damaged, they, like normal cells, are removed from the circulation by macrophages. Another important feature of these carriers is that, once loaded with drug, they can be stored at 4°C for several hours to several days, depending on the storage medium and the entrapment method used. Various targeting strategies involving cells as a carrier have been recently reviewed by Roth et al. (238).

Since erythrocytes, platelets, and leukocytes have received the greatest attention, the discussion that follows will be limited to these carriers. Fibroblasts (239) and hepatocytes (240) have been specifically used as viable sources to deliver missing enzymes in the management of enzyme deficiency diseases, whereas islets are useful as a cellular transplant to produce insulin (241,242). Recently, various specific cell types (e.g., dendritic cells and endothelial progenitor cells) transduced with gene therapy vectors ex vivo have also been investigated for treating human diseases (238,243). The use of cell carriers, such as mesenchymal progenitor cells, monocytes, myeloma cells, and T cells, to deliver oncolytic viruses (e.g., measles virus, vesicular virus, and coxackievirus A21) to sites of myeloma tumor growth has been reviewed by Munguia et al. (244).

Erythrocytes Erythrocytes are biconcave, disk-shaped blood cells (with pits or depressions in the center on both sides), the primary function of which is to transport hemoglobin, the oxygen-carrying protein. The biconcave shape of the erythrocyte provides a large surface volume ratio and thereby facilitates exchange of oxygen. The average diameter of erythrocytes is 7.5 μm, and thickness at the rim is 2.6 μm and in the center is about 0.8 μm. The normal concentration of erythrocytes in blood is approximately 3.9 to 5.5 million cells per microliter in women and 4.1 to 6 million cells per microliter in men. The total life span of erythrocytes in blood is 120 days. Erythrocytes show a net negative surface charge (owing to the presence of carboxylic groups of sialic acids), which prevents erythrocytes from agglutinating in the presence of IgG. The plasmalemmal membrane that surrounds the cell contains equal weights of lipids (major components: phospholipids, cholesterol, and glycolipids) and proteins (glycophorin, ankyrin, and protein 4.1), in addition to some carbohydrates. The latter is responsible for some of their surface antigenic properties.

Erythrocytes have been suggested as potential carriers for a number of biologically active substances, including drugs, proteins, peptides, nucleic acids, and enzymes (245–253). They can be used as storage depots for sustained drug release or potentially be modified to permit targeting specific cell types in the blood (e.g., direct targeting cells in leukemia) (254). Although constrained to move within blood vessels, erythrocytes can exit from blood vessels into tissues (255), potentiating their use as carriers in treating inflammations. Destruction of microbubbles with ultrasound can rupture the microvessels and, consequently, deliver the drug-loaded cells to the tissue (256). Erythrocytes loaded with ferromagnetic particles have also been prepared and successfully used in targeting ibuprofen and diclofenac to inflamed tissue (252,257). Since erythrocytes are removed from the circulation by the RES, especially by cells located in the spleen and the liver, they offer potential in the treatment of lysosomal storage diseases, hepatic tumors, and parasitic diseases of the RES (248). Erythrocytes have also been investigated for treating metabolic and immunological disorders (258,259), including AIDS (260). Studies show that subjecting the erythrocytes to thermal shock, oxidative compounds, neuraminidase, or proteolytic enzymes prior to use can improve targeting RES (253), while coating with IgG and IgM antibodies causes their uptake by spleen and liver, respectively (253). Stabilization of drug-loaded cells by cross-linking the membrane with glutaraldehyde (261), bis(sulfosuccinimidyl) suberate (262), and 3,3′-dithiobis(sulfosuccinimidyl propionate) (262) has also been suggested to increase RES uptake.

The release of drugs can occur from the intact cell or following its hemolysis. The size and polarity of the drug molecules are the determining factors controlling the release from the intact cells (263). For drug-targeting purposes, drugs that show no release from the intact cell have been suggested as the best candidates (248).

Several methods have been used to incorporate exogenous substances within erythrocytes (246,248,250,251). These include hypotonic hemolysis, dielectric breakdown, endocytosis, osmotic pulse, and entrapment without hemolysis. Of these, hypotonic hemolysis is most commonly used. It involves placing the cells in a hypotonic solution containing the drug or chemical substance to be incorporated. As a result, the cell swells. When the internal (osmotic) pressure exceeds a critical value (150 mOsm), the cell ruptures and releases its content in the external medium. Just before the cell lysis, the cell membrane transiently develops pores ranging in diameter from 200 to 500 Å. Substances present in the external medium enter into the cell through these pores at this time too. Restoration of the tonicity of the surrounding medium to isotonic conditions reseals the pores/ruptured cell membrane, causing entrapment of substances present in the external medium. This is the fastest and simplest method of drug incorporation and works efficiently for encapsulation of low molar mass (<130,000) substances. The major disadvantages of the method, however, are that (*i*) it requires a relatively large amount of the starting material (owing to the large extracellular volume compared with the small intracellular volume); (*ii*) a substantial percentage of the cellular content of erythrocyte enzymes and hemoglobin is lost during lysis; and (*iii*) a small change in ionic strength of the external medium may cause a significant alteration in the structure of the cell membrane (owing to the loss of membrane polypeptides) and, consequently, a decrease in the life span of the erythrocytes.

Several modifications in the foregoing method (hypotonic hemolysis) have been made to circumvent the disadvantages noted above (246,248). For example, the loss of enzymes and hemoglobin during lysis can be reduced by preswelling the erythrocytes in 0.6% NaCl solution before subjecting them to a very hypotonic lysis containing the substance to be loaded. The morphological and structural integrity of the resealed erythrocytes can also be preserved by hemolyzing and resealing erythrocyte cells in a dialysis tube. The dialysis approach allows a slow and gradual decrease in the ionic strengths and, consequently, preserves the elasticity of the erythrocyte membrane. Other advantages of the dialysis method are that (*i*) entrapped materials do not leak out to an appreciable extent, (*ii*) the use of a high hematocrit during dialysis allows more efficient encapsulation, and (*iii*) erythrocytes with appreciably higher drug percentages can be prepared. Several factors can influence the optimal encapsulation of the drug and the integrity of the erythrocytes and need to be properly optimized, including the composition of the buffer solution, centrifugation speed, osmolarity of the hypotonic buffers, the hematocrit, the temperature during hemolysis and resealing, the time of resealing, and the nature of the lysis procedure.

The dielectric breakdown method involves application of a high-intensity electric pulse (a few kV) for a short duration (20–160 μsec) to a suspension of erythrocytes in isotonic or slightly hypotonic solution. Hemolysis is typically achieved at 0°C to 4°C for half an hour to one hour. It occurs as a result of dielectric breakdown of the cell membrane, which in turn causes a reversible change in the permeability of the membrane. An increase in the temperature to 37°C initiates the resealing process, and the original membrane resistance and impermeability of the erythrocytes are restored within minutes at this temperature. A major advantage of this method is that the size of the pore during lysis and hence the permeability of the membrane can be controlled by appropriate manipulations of the electric pulse intensity, pulse duration, or ionic strength of the pulsation medium.

The loading of drugs in erythrocytes by endocytosis typically involves incubating the intact or resealed erythrocytes with the substance to be entrapped for 30 minutes at 37°C in the presence of varying amounts of membrane-active agents, such as primaquine or chlorpromazine, in a buffer solution. Drugs can also be loaded by incubating the erythrocytes with amphotericin B in an isotonic solution and then with the drug to be loaded for 30 minutes, each at 37°C (264). In the osmotic pulse method, dimethyl sulfoxide (DMSO) is used to create a transient osmotic gradient across the cell membrane. In a typical experiment, erythrocytes are incubated in an isotonic solution of DMSO and then diluted with an isotonic solution containing the substance to be loaded. The second step establishes an immediate DMSO concentration gradient across the cell membrane, making it possible for the DMSO to diffuse out of the cell and for water and the dissolved chemical substance to enter into the cell. Post dilution with a DMSO-free isotonic solution causes all the DMSO to diffuse out and the cells to resume their original shape. Other methods used to load drugs within erythrocytes include chemical-induced isotonic lysis of cells (265) and the use of anesthetic agents, such as halothane (266). The latter method avoids the use of both isotonic and hypotonic solutions.

Platelets Platelets are nonnucleated, discoid or elliptical cells that originate from the fragmentation of giant polyploid megakaryocytes located in the bone marrow. The average diameter of the platelet is 1.5 μm. Each platelet is surrounded by a trilaminar membrane, and its cytoplasm contains a dense body (δ-granule), a surface-connected canalicular system, microchondrion, α-granules, a lysosome, peroxisomes, glycogen, and a dense tubular system. The normal platelet count ranges from 1.5 to 4.0×10^{10}/dL of blood. Once they enter the blood, platelets have a total life span of about 10 days. Although the primary role of platelets is in controlling hemorrhage, they are also involved in immune reactions, inflammation, maintenance of vascular wall integrity, and the evolution of vascular diseases (e.g., vasculitis and atherosclerosis) (267,268).

Platelets have been used as a carrier for several biological substances and drugs useful in the management of various hematological diseases (267). Platelets can accumulate drugs by selective active transport. Certain drugs, such as angiotensin, hydrocortisone, imipramines, vinca alkaloids (vinblastine and vincristine), and many others, are known to bind platelets. The first clinical trial of platelet-loaded vinca alkaloids in the treatment of idiopathic thrombocytopenic purpura, an autoimmune disorder characterized by decreased platelet counts, was reported by Ahn et al. (269). The platelets were loaded with vinblastine and vincristine separately by incubation at 37°C in the dark for an hour. Following removal of the unbound drug, the platelets were resuspended in the donor's plasma and then infused to the patients over a period of 30 minutes. They found that patients treated with platelet-loaded alkaloids, compared with free drugs, required fewer treatments to provide a long-lasting remission from the disorder, without any form of maintenance therapy. Despite its success, the technique has several limitations, such as the tedious preparation and high cost for platelet-drug production, and is thus restricted to those patients refractory of readily available therapies. The use of vinca-loaded platelets has also been reported in the management of autoimmune hemolytic anemia (270), an autoimmune disease of red cells in which they become sensitized with autoantibodies of IgG and are cleared by macrophages, and of various malignant disorders of the MPS (e.g., malignant histiocytosis, Rosai Dorfman syndrome, hairy cell leukemia, monocytic leukemia, familial erythrophagocytic lymphohistiocytosis, and other platelet-phagocytosing tumors) (271,272).

Leukocytes   Leukocytes are white blood cells involved in the cellular and humoral defense of an organism against foreign materials. They are grouped into two classes: polymorphonuclear leukocytes, which comprise neutrophils, eosinophils, and basophils; and mononuclear leukocytes that include lymphocytes and monocytes. Of these, neutrophils and lymphocytes have been suggested as potential cellular carriers.

Neutrophils constitute about 60% to 80% of the total blood leukocyte level. They are spherical, with a diameter ranging between 12 and 15 μm. Their total life span is about six to seven hours. They are known to carry a wide range of digestive enzymes and carrier proteins. Unlike erythrocytes, which are constrained to move within blood vessels, neutrophils can leave the capillaries and accumulate in large numbers at localized areas of disease. This property, their ready availability (the average production per day in adults is 1×10^{11}), and their highly pure form make them very attractive as a natural drug carrier. Segal et al. (273) reported that neutrophils containing ^{111}In-oxinate complex as a radiolabel marker, when administered intravenously in patients with abscesses and inflammation, preferentially accumulated at the diseased sites. Gainey and McDougall (274) successfully used this approach for the detection of acute inflammation in children and adolescents. Neutrophils could also be used as carriers for drugs that are effective in the treatment of pyrogenic infections, including diseases such as ulcerative colitis, acute arthritis, and other infections.

Sioux and Teissie (275) loaded propidium iodide in 70% leukocytes in whole blood using the dielectric breakdown method. The entrapped drug showed a half-life of longer than four hours at 4°C and 37°C. When compared with the nonpulsed cells, leukocytes loaded with the drug showed 10 times more accumulation in the inflammation area than in control areas.

Lymphocytes are of two sizes: smaller lymphocytes, with a diameter of 6 to 8 μm; and larger lymphocytes, with a diameter up to 18 μm. They are found not only in blood but also in lymph and in every tissue of the body. Larger lymphocytes are believed to be cells that differentiate into T- and B-lymphocytes when activated by specific antigens. The life span of lymphocytes may vary from a few days to many years. Lymphocytes have been suggested as potential carriers for transporting macromolecules, particularly DNA, to other cells. Low molar mass exogenous substances can be introduced into lymphocytes by electrical breakdown methods.

Soluble Macromolecular Drug Delivery Systems

Soluble macromolecules of both natural and synthetic origins have been used as drug carriers. When compared with the particulate carriers, soluble macromolecules (*i*) encounter fewer barriers to their movement around the body and can enter into many organs by transport across capillary endothelium or in the liver by passage through the fenestration connecting the sinusoidal lumen to the space of Disse; (*ii*) penetrate the cells by pinocytosis, which is a phenomenon universal to all cells and which, unlike phagocytosis, does not require an external stimulus; and (*iii*) can be found in the blood many hours after their introduction (particulate carriers, in contrast, are rapidly cleared from the blood by the RES). The fate of soluble macromolecules in animals and humans, with special reference to the transfer of polymers from one body compartment to another, has been reviewed by Drobnik and Rypacek (67).

Macromolecular drugs, in general, can be divided into four types: (*i*) polymeric drugs—these represent macromolecules that themselves display pharmacological activity and polymers that contain therapeutically active groups as an integral part of the main chain, (*ii*) macromolecule-drug analogs—these are derivatives of drugs that require no separation from the macromolecule to fulfill their therapeutic actions, (*iii*) macromolecular prodrugs (or macromolecule-drug conjugates)—these represent drugs that must be detached from the macromolecule at the target site(s) to exert their therapeutic effects, and (*iv*) noncovalently linked macromolecule-drug complexes. In this section, only macromolecule-drug conjugates are discussed.

A general configuration of an ideal macromolecule-drug conjugate is shown in Figure 7 (276). The drug can be attached to the macromolecule (or polymer chain) either directly or by a spacer and may present as a pendant or terminal (not shown in Fig. 7) group. The macromolecule-drug conjugate may also contain a homing or vector device (e.g., antibodies or receptor-specific ligands) to achieve selective access to, and interaction with, the target cell and a moiety for controlling physical and chemical properties of the conjugate. The use of a spacer arm to attach a drug to a macromolecule enhances both configuration and drug-receptor interaction efficiencies.

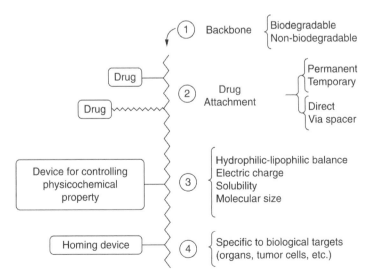

Figure 7 A schematic representation of an ideal macromolecule-drug conjugate. *Source*: From Ref. 276.

Depending on the chemical functional groups present on the drug and on the macromolecule, a variety of methods can be used to prepare covalently linked macromolecule-drug conjugates. The most commonly used coupling reactions are shown in Figure 8. Proteinaceous compounds can be conjugated by using the free thiol groups of cysteine, whereas the coupling between carboxylic acid–containing macromolecules and amine drugs, or vice versa, is achieved by the carbodiimide method. Polysaccharides can be attached to amine drugs by a dialdehyde intermediate, prepared by using periodates. The covalently linked antibody-toxin conjugates are typically prepared by using the N-succinimidyl-3-(2-pyridyldithio)propionate (SDPD) reagent. It is important that the coupling reaction being used does not adversely affect the therapeutic

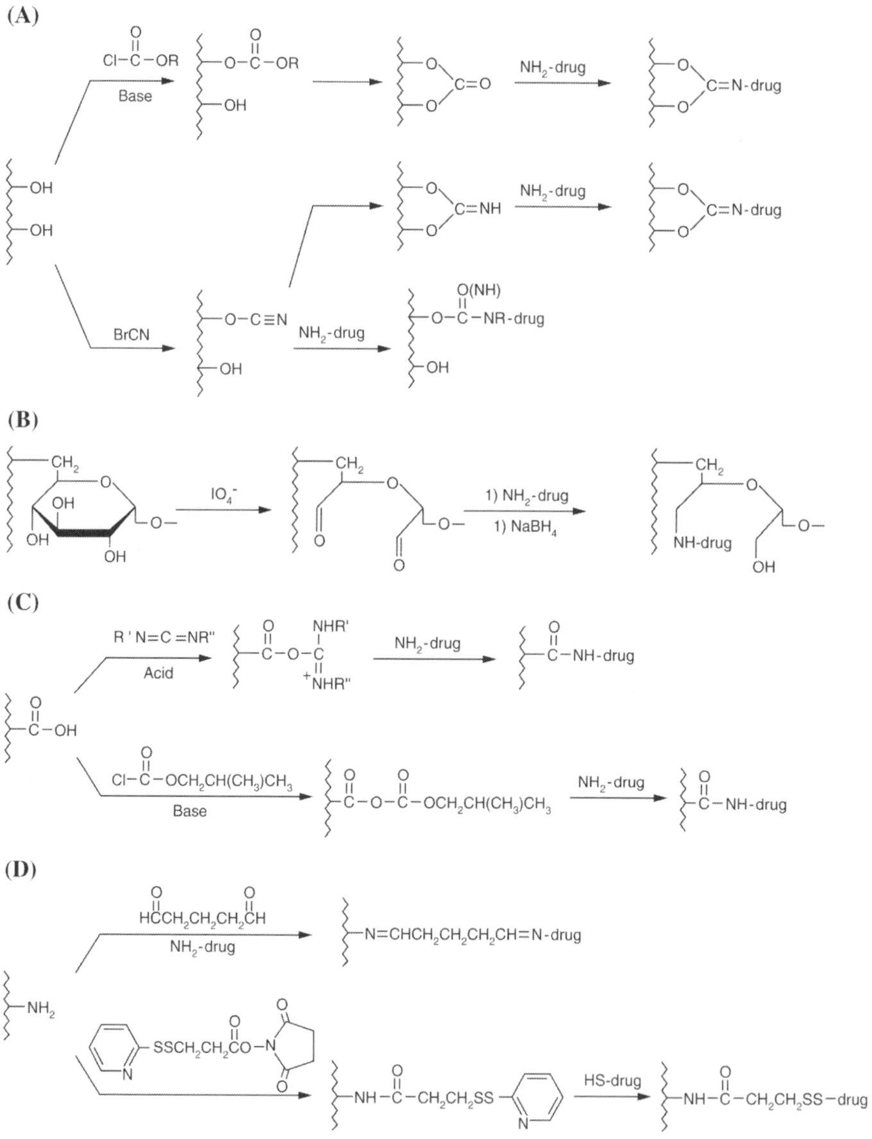

Figure 8 Commonly used coupling methods for the preparation of macromolecule-drug conjugates. Functional groups of the drug and macromolecule are interchangeable with each other.

activity of the drug. The preparation of ester-linked conjugates is typically achieved by activating the carboxylic acid group with a water-soluble or water-insoluble carbodiimide [e.g., 1-ethyl-3-(dimethylaminopropyl) carbodiimide and N,N'-dicyclohexylcarbodiimide, respectively], optionally in the presence of a base catalyst [e.g., 4-(dimethylamino) pyridine], followed by a reaction with an alcohol group–containing agent. The use of a mixture of carbodiimide and N-hydroxysuccinimide has also been extensively used (277).

The fate of macromolecular drug conjugates in vivo depends on their distribution and elimination properties. In general, the plasma half-life of a macromolecule-drug conjugate depends on its molar mass, ionic nature, configuration, and interaction tendencies in the physiological milieu. It has been reported that macromolecules with molar mass less than 40,000 are cleared rapidly, while those with molar mass higher than 40,000 remain in the circulation for prolonged periods. Although the RES is the natural target, other organs in the body can be targeted as well. Because many tumors possess vasculature that is hyperpermeable to macromolecules, soluble macromolecules also serve as potential drug carriers in the treatment of cancers. Present evidence suggests that the greatest levels of tumor accumulation are achieved by using macromolecules that carry a negative charge. Several excellent reviews that describe the distribution of soluble macromolecules in biological systems have been published (37,56,58,67,278).

The choice of a macromolecular carrier depends on the intended clinical objectives and the nature of the therapeutic agents being used. In general, the properties of an ideal soluble carrier system include the following (276,279): (*i*) the carrier and its degradation products must be biodegradable (or, at least, should not show accumulation in the body), the carrier must be nontoxic and nonantigenic and must not alter the antigenicity of the therapeutic agents being transported; (*ii*) the carrier must have an adequate drug-loading capacity; that is, the carrier must have functional groups for chemical fixation of the therapeutic agent; (*iii*) the carrier must remain soluble in water when loaded with drug; (*iv*) the molar mass of the carrier should be large enough to permit glomerular filtration but small enough to reach all cell types; (*v*) the carrier-drug conjugate must retain the specificity of the original carrier and must maintain the original activity of the therapeutic agent until it reaches the targeted site(s); (*vi*) the carrier-drug conjugate must be stable in body fluids but should slowly degrade in extracellular compartments or in lysosomes; and (*vii*) for lysosomotropic drug delivery, the macromolecule should not interfere with pinosome formation at the cell surface and subsequent intracellular fusion events. Furthermore, the macromolecule-drug linkage must be sensitive to acid hydrolysis or degradation by specific lysosomal enzymes.

Various natural and synthetic soluble macromolecules that have been investigated together with their uses are listed in Table 9. Natural polymers are monodisperse (i.e., same chain lengths), have rigid structures, and are biodegradable. The rigid structures may facilitate interactions between the determinant groups on the natural polymer and the binding region of immunoglobulin. Synthetic polymers, by contrast, are less immunogenic and can be better tailor-made to predetermined specifications (i.e., molecular size, charge, hydrophobicity, and their capacity for drug loading can be optimized). They are also easier and cheaper to produce in large quantity and high purity, and the chemistry to load drugs is much less laborious. In addition, they are more robust and are thus more stable during manipulation and storage. Another interesting field that is developing is the design of polymers that mimic biopolymers (280). These synthetic polymers have properties similar to those of proteins and RNA and present new opportunities to design new novel structures with desirable functions, including drug therapy. A detailed discussion of some natural and synthetic soluble carrier systems follows.

Table 9 Suggested Soluble Macromolecular Drug Delivery Systems

Carrier	Targets/disease/therapy
Proteins	
Antibodies, antibody fragments (e.g., collagen specific drug-toxin conjugates)	Injured sites of blood vessels' walls, tumor cells
Albumin-drug conjugates	Cancer cells (lysosomotropic)
Glycoproteins	Hepatocyte-specific agents (infectious disease, especially viruses)
Lipoproteins	Liver/cancers of ovaries and gonads
Lectins	General carrier/recognition ligands
Hormones (toxin-drug-hormone conjugate)	Tumors
Dextrans (e.g., enzyme-drug-dextran conjugates)	Tumors
Deoxyribonucleic acid (drug-conjugate; lysosomotropic carrier)	Cancer cells
Synthetic polymers	
Poly(L-lysine)and polyglutamic acid	Carrier for targeting cancer
Poly(L-aspartic acid)	Hydrolyzable targeting carrier for cancer
Polypeptide-mustard conjugates	Lung targeting, tumor targeting
N-(2-hydroxypropyl)methacrylamide copolymers	Lysosomotropic carrier for cytotoxics
Pyran copolymers	Lysosomotropic carrier for cytotoxics

Source: From Ref. 37.

Antibodies Antibodies are circulating plasma proteins of the globulin group. They are produced by plasma cells that arise as a result of differentiation and proliferation of B-lymphocytes. Antibodies interact specifically with antigenic determinants (molecular domains of the antigens) that elicit their formation. In humans, there are five main types of antibodies, commonly designated as IgG, IgA, 1gM, IgE, and IgD. Of these, IgG is the most abundant. It constitutes 75% of the serum immunoglobulins and is the only immunoglobulin that crosses the placental barrier and is incorporated in the circulatory systems of the fetus, thereby protecting a newborn from infection. The basic structure of the immunoglobulin molecule consists of two identical heavy (long) chains, each with a molar mass of 50,000, and two light (short) chains with a molecular mass of 23,000 (Fig. 9). These chains are held together by noncovalent forces as well as by disulfide linkages. Each chain also contains interchain disulfide linkages. In addition, each chain contains a region of a constant amino acid sequence and a region of variable amino acid sequence. Antibodies belonging to the same class share the constant region in their heavy chains and may have κ- or λ-type light chains. The ends of the constant region (carboxyl ends) of the heavy chains form the Fc region, which is responsible for binding to Fc receptors present on many cells. The specificity of a particular antibody is determined by amino acid sequences of the variable region that are similar in the light and heavy chains. The ends of the variable region, referred to as amino (NH_2) terminals, serve as the binding sites for antigens.

The use of antibodies for active targeting of drugs to specific cell types in vivo has long been recognized (281–285). They have been extensively explored as carriers in cancer diagnosis and in targeting drugs, toxins, and other therapeutic agents to tumor cells. Monoclonal antibodies of defined class and antigen specificity can be obtained in a highly purified form and in virtually unlimited amounts by immunizing mice with human tumor cells, followed by hybridizing their spleen cells with myeloma cells and, subsequently, screening the hybridoma cells for the formation of antibodies that bind only

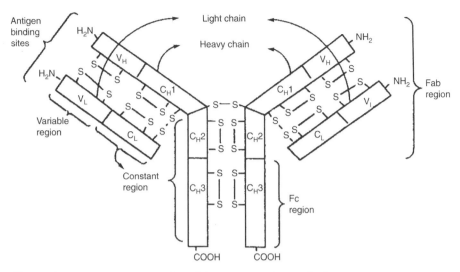

Figure 9 Schematic representation of the structure of an antibody.

to immunizing tumor cells. The clinical usefulness of a given antibody in drug targeting, however, depends on its degree of cross-reaction with normal tissues and its affinity to target antigens. The presence of free antigens in the general circulation is also an important determinant in drug targeting, because an antibody specific to these antigens would combine with it prematurely, thereby lowering site specificity. To improve specificity of action and to aid penetration into the target site (e.g., tumor cells), antibodies have been broken enzymatically to Fab′ fragments (Fig. 9) and used in drug targeting. The various cytotoxic drugs that have been investigated by using antibodies as a carrier include alkylating agents [e.g., chlorambucil (286) and trenimon (287)]; antimetabolites (e.g., methotrexate) (288,289); antitumor drugs (e.g., daunomycin and doxorubicin) (290,291); and toxic proteins [e.g., A-chains of diphtheria toxin (292) and ricin (293)]. Depending on the nature of the drug, the antibody-drug conjugates can be prepared by a carbodiimide, mixed anhydride, periodate, or glutaraldehyde-mediated coupling reaction (Fig. 8) (291,294–296). Diphtheria toxin has been linked to antibodies by using either a homobifunctional (e.g., glutaraldehyde) or heterobifunctional (e.g., toluene diisocyanate) agent, or through disulfide groups by using the SPDP reagent. Antibodies, in general, are fairly robust molecules and are little affected by chemical manipulations during conjugate synthesis. However, a method that works well with one monoclonal antibody may not necessarily produce the same (intended) conjugated product with another monoclonal antibody. Further, the number and distribution of ε-lysine residues vary from one antibody to another, leading to different degrees of substitution of cytotoxic drugs. Rowland et al. (297) found that four monoclonals recognizing different human tumor–associated antigens, when conjugated using an active azide derivative of a vinca alkaloid, produced vindesine–monoclonal antibody conjugates with a drug/antibody conjugation ratio varying from 3:1 to 10:1, depending on the antibody used. The percentage activity of the vindsine-monoclonal conjugate coupled at 6:1 was 98%, whereas the conjugate with a drug/antibody ratio of 4:1 showed only 2% activity. Recently, the preparation of a highly cytotoxic C-10 methyldisulfanyl-propanoyl taxoid conjugated with monoclonal antibodies (298) and doxorubicin conjugated to murine and humanized anti-B-cell antibody LL1 (DOX-LL1) (299) against epidermal growth factor receptor (EGFR)-expressing A431 tumor xenografts and Raji lymphoma cells, respectively, in SCID mice has been reported; the former showed a complete inhibition of EGFR-expressing tumor, while the latter resulted in survival of all animals for 180 days.

Samokhin et al. (300) demonstrated that biotinylated red blood cells complexed with biotin antihuman collagen antibodies (by an avidin cross-linking molecule) bind efficiently and specifically to collagen-coated surfaces and can thus be used to deliver drugs to injured sites of blood vessel walls. Biotinylated antibodies specific to tumor-associated ganglio-N-triosylceramide (GalNAcβ1→4GalNAcβ1→4GlcIβ1→ceramide) have been prepared and found very effective in killing tumor cells that express ganglio-N-triosylceramide (301).

Antibodies have also been adsorbed or covalently linked to a variety of other carrier systems, such as liposomes (167,302), erythrocytes (303,304), and microparticles and nanoparticles, to selectively target them to a specific site in the body. In recent years, bispecific antibodies, which are designed to bind to two epitopes of either the same or different antigen (e.g., a cytotoxic drug and a cell receptor such as CD3), have also been used to target cytotoxic drugs, such as radionuclides, drugs, and toxins, to tumors. Interested readers are referred to several excellent reviews published recently (305,306).

Deoxyribonucleic acid DNA has been suggested as a potential carrier for drugs that show a strong affinity for DNA and that can be released from DNA by a simple equilibrium process or after digestion of DNA by extra- or intracellular enzymes. This approach has been extensively investigated in chemotherapy for a number of malignant disorders, because (*i*) DNA complexed with drugs acts as a lysosomotropic drug system; (*ii*) DNA itself is a potent inducer of pinocytosis and is easily degraded by lysosomal hydrolases; and (*iii*) compared with normal cells, tumor cells exhibit higher endocytic activity. To avoid clearance by the RES, DNA-drug complexes are usually administered intraperitoneally (307).

The DNA forms stable complexes with doxorubicin (ADR) and DNR. Doxorubicin and DNR, although structurally similar, show distinctly different properties: ADR is more toxic and active than DNR in the treatment of various human solid tumors; the apparent binding affinity of ADR to DNA is about 1.8 times higher than that of DNR to DNA. Trouet et al. (308) found the ADR-DNA complex to be more active than ADR, DNR, or DNR-DNA in subcutaneously inoculated leukemic mice, whereas the DNR-DNA complex showed the highest activity against intravenously inoculated leukemic cells. Similar results have been reported in other tumor models. A pharmacokinetics study in patients revealed an enhanced uptake into leukemic cells and a reduction in distribution volume, cardiotoxicity, and rates of plasma clearance following administration of DNA conjugates compared with the free drug (309).

DNA has also been tested as a carrier for ethidium bromide, a drug used in the treatment of protozoal diseases. When compared with free drug, the DNA-bound drug showed decreased toxicity and higher therapeutic efficacy in mice infected with *Trypanosoma cruzi* (310).

A major advantage of DNA as a carrier is that no chemical synthesis or manipulations are needed to obtain DNA-drug complex. The efficacy of the DNA-drug complex depends on stability in the bloodstream, endocytic behavior of normal and tumor cells, presence of extracellular deoxyribonuclease activity in the tumor tissues, and capillary barriers that separate normal and tumor cells from the bloodstream.

Low molar mass proteins Low molar mass proteins, such as lysozyme, have been recently suggested as a potential carrier for targeting drugs to the kidney (311). The rationale is that these endogenous proteins, when administered intravenously, rapidly, and extensively, accumulate in the proximal tubule cells of the kidney (312). Following glomerular filtration, the proteins are endocytosed into the cells and are taken to lysosomes, where their hydrolysis into amino acids occurs by the lysosomal enzymes, causing the release of free drug. The released drug can either act locally or be transferred into the tubular lumen of the kidney. This approach showed effective specific delivery of captopril to the kidney in a recent study (313).

Transferrins Transferrins are iron-binding proteins. They are responsible for transporting iron to sites in the body where it can be absorbed. They are taken up by cells by an endocytic process involving interaction between transferrin and the transferrin receptor via clatherate-coated pits (314). Because of high levels of transferrin receptors present on the surface of tumor cells, transferrin has been investigated as a carrier to target drugs to tumors. Studies show that conjugation of transferrin to antineoplastic agents may overcome cardiotoxicity and drug-resistant problems. CRM107, a mutant of diphtheria toxic, when conjugated to transferrin and administered intratumorally in patients with malignant brain tumors, has been found to be highly selective in killing tumor cells that express high levels of transferrin receptors. Patients, who received high doses of the conjugate, developed neurological deficit due to damage of the endothelial cells (315). Using rats and nude mice bearing subcutaneous U251 gliomas, it was found that systemic administration of chloroquine, an antimalarial drug, can prevent toxicity of transferrin-CRM107 without compromising the activity of the drug (316).

Glycoproteins Glycoproteins are endogenous substances consisting of a polypeptide backbone, with oligosaccharides as side chains. Each oligosaccharide chain contains monosaccharide residues and has sialic acid as the terminal group. The exact sequence of carbohydrate groups varies in different glycoproteins. The sialic acid groups from the terminal carbohydrate residues can be removed by treatment with the enzyme neuraminidase. When the sialic acid groups are removed, the resulting asialoglycoproteins are readily recognized and cleared by certain cells of the liver, depending on the sugar residues exposed. Hepatocytes recognize and internalize mainly galactose- and N-acetylgalactosamine-terminated glycoproteins, whereas Kupffer cells and endothelial cells recognize fucose-, mannose-, or N-acetylglucosamine-terminated glycoproteins. Kupffer cells also endocytose particulate material to which galactose groups are attached. Thus, asialoglycoproteins covalently linked to drug, protein, or diagnostic agent can be used as hepatocyte-specific carriers (317).

A variety of glycoconjugates (also known as neoglycoproteins), such as mannosylated albumin, lactosylated albumin, galactosylated poly(L-lysine), ficoll (a polycarbohydrate), and galactosylated poly(hydroxymethylacrylamide) (317–319) have been prepared. These, like glycoproteins, are readily recognized by various liver cell types. The rationale for using asialoglycoproteins as a carrier for antiviral drugs is that the sugar residues (e.g., mannose, fucose, and galactose) on the carrier are capable of recognizing lectin receptors on the T lymphocytes and thus enhance targeting of antiviral drugs.

Albumin Albumin is available in highly pure and uniform form and exhibits low toxicity and good biological stability. It has been used as a carrier for methotrexate and a variety of antiviral drugs [amantadine, floxuridine (5-fluorodeoxyuridine), and cytarabine (cytosinc arabinoside)] to treat macrophage tumors and infections caused by DNA viruses growing in macrophages. Heavily modified albumins are known to be readily endocytosed by cells of the macrophage system. After penetration into the cell, albumin is digested by lysosomal enzymes, causing the release of free drug. Albumin (bovine and murine)-methotrexate conjugates as well as galactosylated albumin-methotrexate systems exhibit improved liver targeting, or higher and more prolonged serum levels and decreased excretion rates, than the free drug. When administered intraperitoneally into L1210 tumor–bearing mice, the methotrexate-albumin conjugate produced increased localization of methotrexate in the ascitic fluid and elevated intracellular methotrexate levels (320,321). It was also more effective, compared with free drug, in reducing the number of metastases in female (C57BL/6 × DBA/2)F mice bearing subcutaneously implanted Lewis lung carcinoma (322). Whiteley et al. (323) examined the mechanism of the therapeutic activity of the conjugate by using the methotrexate transport–resistant strain of Reuber hepatoma H35 cells. They found no suppression of the tumor growth, suggesting that the observed increased therapeutic activity of the conjugate occurs either through the transport of free drug following its extracellular release from the albumin or the conjugate invokes a specific transport system to penetrate the cell. Fibrosis of the liver results from extracellular matrix deposition caused by activation of hepatic stellate cells (HSCs), making this cell type an important target. However, antifibratic drugs are not effectively taken up by HSCs. The recent finding that albumin modified with mannose-6-phosphate does selectively target these cells in animals may offer promise to much more efficiently treat fibrosis of the liver (324).

The conjugates of antiviral drugs have been investigated to treat ectromelia, a virus known to infect Kupffer cells of the liver (325). Albumins containing a variety of carbohydrate residues (e.g., lactosyl, galactosyl, and mannosyl) as terminal groups have also been chemically prepared and used as carriers to selectively deliver antitumor and antiviral drugs to the liver cells (317,319). The homing of negatively charged albumins to the lymphatic system has recently been proposed as a method of facilitating the distribution of anti-HIV-1 agents (326).

Hormones Hormones, such as human placental lactogen, human chorionic gonadotropin, epidermal growth factor, and melanotropin, have been suggested as carriers to deliver toxins (e.g., ricin and diphtheria toxin) and antineoplastic agents (e.g., daunomycin) to cancer cells (327–329). The rationale is that cancer cells frequently possess receptors for hormones. Thus, drugs covalently linked to hormones can be selectively targeted to these cells. Other reasons include that (*i*) hormones are easy to obtain in a chemically pure form, (*ii*) they are not bound by Fc receptors on macrophages, and (*iii*) they cause no allergic reactions since hormones from different species are structurally similar (327).

Dextran and other polysaccharides Dextrans are colloidal, hydrophilic, and water-soluble substances produced from sugar by microorganisms of the lactobacillaceae family or by cell-free systems containing dextran sucrase. Pharmaceutical and commercial dextrans of different molecular weights are produced by controlled hydrolysis and repeated fractionation of native dextran. Dextrans are inert in biological fluids and do not affect cell viability. Colloidal dextrans of 40,000, 70,000, and 110,000 molar masses can be used in the prevention of thromboembolic diseases in high-risk surgical patients (330). The immunogenicity of dextran increases with increasing molar mass and branching. Dextrans of molar mass equal to or smaller than 45,000 are completely excreted in the urine within 48 hours following intravenous administration, whereas those with a molar mass higher than 45,000 remain in the blood for a long period. However, they are eventually cleared by the RES cells. Dextrans are slowly hydrolyzed in vivo into soluble sugars (the major products being isomaltose and isomaltotriose) by dextranase, an enzyme found in the intestinal mucosa and in RES cells (331). Despite their removal, administration of large doses of dextran can cause a storage problem.

Dextrans have been used as carriers for a variety of drugs and enzymes, including antimicrobial agents (e.g., ampicillin, kanamycin, and tetracycline), cytostatic agents [e.g., MMC, methotrexate, bleomycin, DNR, daunomycin, and cytarabine (cytosine-1-(3-D-arabinoside))], cardiac drugs (e.g., alprenolol and procainamide), peptides and proteins (e.g., asparaginase, carboxypeptidase α- and β-amylase, and insulin), enzyme inhibitors (e.g., pancreatic trypsin inhibitor) (332), and antineoplastic agents (333). Drugs or enzymes can be coupled to dextrans either directly or through a spacer (e.g., γ-aminobutyric acid, ε-aminocaproic acid, and ω-caprylic acid), via activated intermediates produced from reactions with alkali metal periodates, cyanogen bromide, carbodiimide, or chloroformate (Fig. 8), depending on the nature of the drug and carrier molecules. The direct esterification reaction can be used to link organic acids to dextrans. Drugs coupled to dextran by hydrolyzable covalent linkages are more efficacious than free drugs or drug-dextran conjugates containing nonhydrolyzable covalent linkages. Studies have also revealed that direct substitution of drugs to antibody (four to six moles of a drug per mole of antibody) causes a significant loss of antibody activity, whereas antibody-dextran conjugates of drugs, with and without a spacer, show increased stability, longer duration of activity, reduced toxicity, and enhanced cell selection activity (drug targeting). The antitumor activity of dextran-MMC conjugates against B16 melanoma has been shown to be molar mass dependent (334). Modifications of dextran-drug conjugates by an appropriate choice of linkage have permitted the synthesis of a variety of cationic and anionic forms. In vivo studies in mice bearing subcutaneous sarcoma 180 showed that cationic forms clear much more quickly from the bloodstream than anionic forms, accumulating primarily in liver and spleen, with little uptake into tumor tissues. Anionic conjugates with molar mass ranging between 10,000 and 50,000, on the contrary, show greater tumor accumulation (following intravenous administration) and are thereby more effective in the treatment of a subcutaneous tumor. This probably occurs because of prolonged residence time of anionic conjugates in the bloodstream. γ-Cyclodextrin has also been reported to produce site-directed inclusion complexes with several cytotoxic drugs (335).

Other polysaccharides that have been suggested as potential carriers in drug targeting are chondroitin sulfate, heparin sulfate, dermatin sulfate, hyaluronic acid, and keratin sulfate. All are highly water soluble, linear polyanions composed of 1:1 mixture of uronic acid and hexosamine. These are commonly called GAGs and are generally biocompatible, nonimmunogenic, and biodegradable. They contain carboxylic and sulfate groups, in addition to primary and secondary hydroxyl groups, and thus provide additional sites for drug attachment. Since polyanions interact with cell membranes, it is proposed that the use of GAGs may facilitate transport to drugs into the interior of cells (336). O-palmitoylamylopectin, another polysaccharide, has been used to coat liposomes to alter their distribution in vivo.

Synthetic polymers Synthetic polymers are versatile and offer promise for both targeting and extracellular-intracellular drug delivery. Of the many soluble synthetic polymers known, the poly(amino acids) [e.g., poly(L-lysine), poly(L-aspartic acid), and poly (glutamic acid)], poly(hydroxypropylmethacrylamide) copolymers (polyHPMAs), and maleic anhydride copolymers have been investigated extensively, particularly in the treatment of cancers. A brief discussion of these materials is presented.

Poly(amino acids) Both anionic [e.g., poly(L-aspartic acid) and poly(glutamic acid)] and cationic [e.g., poly(L-lysine)] poly(amino acids) have been suggested as potential drug carriers. Poly(L-lysine) is a homopolymer consisting of repeating units of L-lysine. It exhibits some affinity for cancer cells and possesses antimicrobial and antiviral properties. It also shows some activity against murine tumors. The covalently linked methotrexate conjugate of poly(L-lysine), prepared by the carbodiimide method, penetrated Chinese hamster ovary cells faster and was more effective than free drug (337). A poly(D-lysine)-methotrexate conjugate, by contrast, had no effect, because it is resistant to degradation by intracellular enzymes. In vitro growth inhibition studies revealed that the poly(L-lysine)-methotrexate conjugate was more effective against five cell lines of human solid tumors than five cell lines of lymphocytes (338).

Poly(amino acids) can be covalently linked to DNR by a nucleophilic substitution reaction of the 14-bromo derivative of the drug (338). This method avoids alteration or modification of the amino sugar moiety of the drug. When compared with free drug, the poly(L-aspartic acid)-DNR conjugate prepared by this method was less toxic to HeLa cells in vitro but more effective against P388 leukemia, Gross leukemia, and MS-2 sarcoma in vivo. The corresponding conjugate of poly(L-lysine) showed markedly reduced activity overall. This was attributed to the more stable amide linkage in the poly(L-lysine) conjugate compared with that of the poly(L-aspartic acid) conjugate (339).

Hurwitz et al. (340) used a hydrazide derivative of poly(glutamic acid) as a carrier for daunomycin. This was less toxic than free drug against mouse lymphoma in vitro, but it was as effective, or more effective, against the same lymphoma in vivo.

Poly(L-lysine) has also been suggested as a carrier for pepstatin, a specific inhibitor of the lysosomal proteinase cathepsin D, responsible for causing muscle-wasting diseases, such as muscular dystrophy (341).

Poly(hydroxypropylmethacrylamide) copolymer   PolyHPMA is a nonbiodegradable, non-immunogenic, biocompatible polymer. It has been extensively investigated as a plasma expander and as a carrier for a variety of drugs, including anthracycline antibiotic antitumor agents (e.g., doxorubicin and DNR), alkylating agents (e.g., sarcolysin and melphalan), chlorin e[6] (phytochlorin), and mesalamine (5-aminosalicylic acid) (342), and several drug conjugates of polyHPMA conjugates [doxorubicin (343), camptothecin (344), paclitexol (345), and platinate (346)] have recently entered the phase I/II clinical trials. PolyHPMA is cleared from the circulation depending on the molar mass. The molar mass threshold permitting renal excretion was 45,000. In general, the lower the molar mass, the faster the clearance rate. Larger molar mass polymers are more susceptible to capture by RES cells and have little chance of passing the basement membrane and other natural barriers.

PolyHPMA has been linked to drugs by oligopeptidyl linkages (e.g., Gly-Phe-Leu-Gly) (278). These linkages undergo degradation by lysosomal enzymes, causing the release of free drug. The digestibility of oligopeptides by lysosomal enzymes depends on the length and detailed structure of the oligopeptide sequence and follows the order tetrapeptide > tripeptide > dipeptide. It is important that the oligopeptide linkage used to attach a drug to the polymer not be susceptible to degradation during transit in the bloodstream. The Gly-Phe-Leu-Gly tetrapeptide sequence fulfills this and the intra-lysosomal digestibility criteria.

Targeting a specific cell has been accomplished by attaching appropriate cell receptor–specific ligands to polyHPMA. Thus, polyHPMA derivatized with glycyl-glycyl-galactosamine (Gly-Gly-GalNH$_2$), when injected into the bloodstream of rats, was very efficiently removed by the liver parenchymal cells and taken into the lysosomes. Only 5% to 10% hydroxypropyl residues substitution was needed to achieve maximal targeting (279). It has been suggested that the presence of low levels of side chains decreases the pinocytic uptake, which in turn causes targeting residues to achieve maximum targeting. More complex targeting systems, such as the use of melanocyte-stimulating hormone (347) and antibodies (121), have also been investigated.

To obviate the accumulation of polyHPMA in the body (polyHPMA copolymers are not biodegradable), low molar mass fractions (small enough to pass through the glomerular filter) of polyHPMA have been cross-linked by diamine-containing oligopeptidyl sequences and used as drug carriers (121). Similar to non-cross-linked polyHPMA, these are also cleared from the circulation in a molar mass–dependent fashion. In vivo studies in rats revealed the appearance of lower molar mass polymer chains in the urine 8 to 24 hours after intravenous administration.

PolyHPMA copolymers containing galactosamine–chlorin e^6 (phytochlorin) and anti-Thy 1.2 antibody-chlorin e^6 have been developed as targetable polymeric photoactivable drugs (348). Compared with polyHPMA–chlorin e^6, the polyHPMA-galactosamine-chlorin e^6 conjugate was found to be more active against human hepatoma cell line (PLC/PRF/5; Alexander cells) in vitro. The polyHPMA-anti-Thy 1.2 antibody-chlorin e^6 conjugate was prepared in two ways—one was linked by N^ε-amino groups of lysine residues, and the other by oxidized carbohydrate. Compared with the nontargeted conjugate, both showed higher activity toward mouse splenocytes. The polyHPMA-anti-Thy 1.2 antibody-chlorin e^6 conjugate linked by oxidized carbohydrate was the most active in its photodynamic effect on the viability of splenocytes and the suppression of the primary antibody response of mouse splenocytes toward sheep red blood cells in vitro.

Maleic anhydride copolymers Examples of this class of drug carriers include styrene–maleic anhydride (SMA) and divinyl ether–maleic anhydride (DIVEMA) copolymers. Both SMA and DIVEMA have been suggested as potential carriers for neocarzinostatin (NCS), a naturally occurring antitumor antibiotic, and other antitumor agents (e.g., macromycins and actinoxanthin) (349). NCS is more potent than many conventional antitumor drugs (e.g., MMC and doxorubicin). It is composed of a protein (molar mass 12,000) and a low molar mass cytotoxic chromophore. Following release from the protein, the chromophore enters neighboring cells and interacts with the DNA and eventually kills the cells. Despite its higher antitumor activity, NCS cannot be used clinically because (*i*) it is nonspecific in its action, causing severe toxicity, including bone marrow suppression, and (*ii*) it is rapidly cleared ($t_{1/2} = 1.8$ minutes) by urinary excretion following intravenous administration.

Maeda and Matsumura (350) synthesized SMA conjugates of NCS (also known as zinostatin stimalamer) by reacting the two amino groups (one belonging to Ala-I and the other to Lys20 residues) on NCS, with the anhydride group of SMA at a pH of 8.5 for 10 to 12 hours. Compared with free NCS, the SMA-NCS conjugate was retained longer in the blood circulation ($t_{1/2} = 19$ minutes in mice) and, consequently, promoted accumulation of NCS in peripheral tumor tissues (by up to eightfold in a solid sarcoma 180) (Fig. 10). The SMA-NCS conjugate was also effective against lymphatic metastases (350). Various vasoactive agents can be used to modulate the rates of extravasation and, consequently, penetration of SMA-NCS in tumor tissue (351). A multi-institutional phase II clinical trial of SMA-NCS, formulated in an oily lipid contrast medium, lipiodol (an ethyl ester of iodinated poppy seed oil, 37% w/w in iodine content, used clinically as a lymphographic agent), completed in Japan in 1990, revealed that tumor/blood ratio was greater than 2500 following intra-arterial administration of this formulation. The results of the first pilot study (total number of patients 44) showed detectable tumor shrinkage in 95% of the cases (352). Of 21 patients, 9 showed a 40% to 99% reduction in tumor mass within one to five months, and extensive necrosis was seen in biopsy specimens. Mean

(A)   (B)

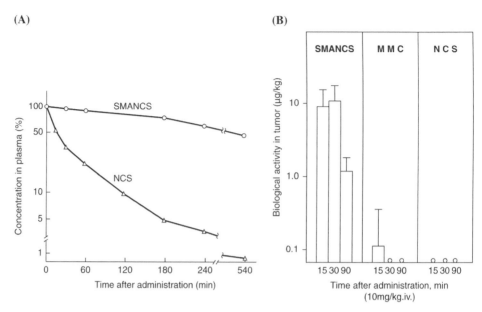

Figure 10 (**A**) Plasma concentration of SMA-NCS and NCS in human after an intravenous bolus injection. (**B**) Intratumor concentration of SMA-NCS, NCS, and MMC. SMA-NCS exhibits a much higher and more prolonged tumor concentration than MMC and NCS. All drugs were given as an intravenous bolus at 10 mg/kg to rabbits bearing VX-2 tumor in the liver (assayed by antibacterial activity). *Abbreviations*: SMA, styrene–maleic anhydride; NCS, neocarzinostatin; MMC, mitomycin. *Source*: From Ref. 80.

survival rate was greater than 18 months for the treated patients, compared with 3.7 months for the controls. In a parallel study, 24 patients with tumors other than hepatoma were included, and SMA-NCS was administered by various arterial routes (353). The results showed a regression of the tumors in six of nine patients with metastatic liver cancer, four of four with adenocarcinoma of the lung, and one of three patients with unresectable gallbladder tumors. Since 1995, SMA-NCS/lipiodol has been accepted in Japan for use to treat primary hepatoma. Selective tumor uptake and some pharmacological characteristics of SMA-NCS, along with some other macromolecular conjugates, have been reviewed by Griesh et al. (354).

SMA-NCS can also be used to activate macrophages, natural cells, and T cells and to induce interferon-γ production (80). A DIVEMA-NCS conjugate, on the contrary, exhibited cytotoxic activity (on a molar basis) in vitro against eight cell lines and bone marrow cells similar to that observed with free NCS (355). In vivo toxicity data indicated about a 1.7-fold higher LD50 value for the conjugate than for NCS. Studies also revealed a lower distribution of the conjugate than that for NCS in bone marrow and spleen cells and, to some extent, in other organs. The biological activity of DIVEMA-NCS in plasma was about 2.2 times higher than that of NCS. Because of reduced acute toxicity, DIVEMA-NCS showed a 10 times higher antitumor activity than NCS at a high dose. At lower doses, there was no difference in the antitumor activities of DIVEMA-NCS and free NCS. The relatively low antitumor activity of DIVEMA-NCS, compared with SMA-NCS, has been attributed to its rapid clearance from the circulation (355).

The DIVEMA copolymer has also been covalently linked to methotrexate (356). This polymer spontaneously released methotrexate from the polymer backbone by hydrolysis. The DIVEMA-methotrexate conjugate (molar mass 22,000) was more effective against L1210 leukemia and Lewis lung carcinoma at optimal equivalent doses than either DIVEMA or NCS alone or the combination of DIVEMA and NCS. As such, DIVEMA also shows various biological properties. It is a well-known interferon inducer and shows activity against several solid tumors and viruses. It also possesses antibacterial, antifungal, anticoagulant, and anti-inflammatory properties and is capable of stimulating macrophage activation. Biological studies have revealed that the toxicity of DIVEMA increases with an increase in its molar mass. Low molar mass pyrans stimulate phagocytosis, whereas high molar mass copolymers decrease the rate of uptake. The inhibition of polymer metabolism also increases with an increase in the molar mass (357).

TARGETING IN THE GASTROINTESTINAL TRACT AND TO OTHER MUCOSAL SURFACES

The alimentary canal has been and continues to be the preferred route for drug administration for systemic drug action. Thus, there is a growing interest in developing oral dosage forms that can either (*i*) exert a therapeutic effect at a specific site in the GI tract (see Ref. 42 for diseases of the GI tract) or (*ii*) allow systemic absorption of drugs or prodrugs utilizing a specific region of the alimentary canal, without being affected by the GI fluid, pH fluctuations, enzymes, and microflora, while traveling along the GI tract. The various anatomical, physiological, physicochemical, and biochemical features of various regions of the alimentary canal, including intestinal transporters that influence drug targeting and possible formulation approaches that can be used, have been reviewed by Ritschel (43) and Oh et al. (358) The theoretical rationale and potential for targeting various microflora that reside in the GI tract as possible therapeutic and prophylactic strategies has been recently described by Jia et al. (359).

Depending on the site in the GI tract where drug release is sought, a variety of approaches can be used. Bioadhesive polymers are used to prepare adhesive tablets and films for use in the buccal cavity and other regions of the alimentary canal (360). These polymers adhere to a biological tissue for an extended period, thereby providing increased local therapeutic effect or prolonged maintenance of therapeutic amounts of drug in the blood. Examples of bioadhesive polymers commonly used include hydroxypropylcellulose, poly(acrylic acid) (Carbopol®), and sodium carboxymethylcellulose. Enteric polymers (e.g., cellulose acetate phthalate, hydroxypropylcellulose acetate phthalate, polyvinyl acetate phthalate, methacrylate–methacrylic acid copolymers, and others), which remain insoluble in the stomach but dissolve at higher pH of the intestine, are used to deliver drugs to the small intestine. Enteric coating also prevents drugs from degradation by gastric fluid and enzymes and protects the gastric mucosa from the irritating properties of certain drugs. Using coating solutions containing a mixture of cellulose acetate phthalate, Eudragit® S100 (Röhm Pharma GmbH, Darmstadt, Germany), and Eudragit L30D and an acidic coating system containing succinic acid in a solution of ethylcellulose (Aquacoat) and hydroxypropylcellulose, Klokkers-Bethke and Fisher (361) developed a novel multiunit delivery system capable of targeting both the lower part of the bowel and the colon. Drug delivery to the stomach can be achieved using hydrodynamically balanced (floating) dosage forms (362). Because of lower bulk density, such dosage forms stay buoyant in the stomach, thereby resisting gastric emptying. Drug delivery systems that contain inflatable chambers (these become gas filled at body temperature) or solids (e.g., carbonates and bicarbonates) that form gases when in contact with gastric fluid also stay buoyant and are used to target drugs for release in the stomach

(363). A variety of techniques have been advocated for drug targeting the small intestine, including the use of polysaccharide swellable hydrogels (364).

Targeting drugs to the colon is of significance not only for local treatment of colonic diseases, such as ulcerative colitis, irritable bowel syndrome, and colon cancer, but also for drugs that are not well absorbed from other regions of the GI (365,366). Some examples of drugs that have shown enhanced efficacy upon delivery to colon are aminosalicylates, corticosteroids, and immunosuppressive agents. The successful delivery to the colon can be achieved by using prodrugs or by drug entrapment within or by coating with polymers that undergo enzymatic degradation in the colon. A number of pH-dependent polymers, such as enteric polymers (e.g., Eudragit S in Asacol®, from Proctor & Gamble Pharmaceuticals, Inc., Ohio, U.S., under license from Medeva Pharma Schweiz AG) have also been used to deliver drugs to the colon. However, because of a small difference in the pH of the small and large intestines and the fact that pH in the proximal and distal bowel, cecum, and colon can vary from 2.9 to 9.2, (frequently between 5.9 and 9.2), in patients with inflammatory bowel disease, ulcerative colitis, and Crohn's disease (367–371), such preparations may fail to produce the intended dose in the colon. The prodrug approach relies on the ready susceptibility of the prodrug carrier–drug linkages to enzymatic hydrolysis (e.g., hydrolysis of glycosides by glycosidases). Over 400 distinct microbial species, predominantly anaerobic, exist in the colon. They produce enzymes responsible for hydrolysis and redox reactions. Examples of hydrolytic enzymes are β-glucuronidases, β-xylosidase, and β-galactosidase and those of reductive enzymes include nitroreductase, azoreductase, and deaminase. Sinha and Kumaria (372) recently reviewed and listed several examples of prodrugs evaluated for colon-specific delivery. Macromolecule-based prodrugs are advantageous in that they remain intact and excreted with feces and hence pose no concerns of toxicity. Of particular importance are azo polymers [e.g., azo-linked poly(acrylic acid), poly(ester-ester), and copolymers of methylmethacrylate and 2-hydroxyethyl methacrylate] (373–380). They have been used as a coating material or as a macromolecular prodrug carrier. The azo linkage is resistant to proteolytic digestion in the stomach and small intestine but degrades in the colon by the indigenous microflora [concentration 10^{11}–10^{12} CFU/mL vs. mainly gram-positive $<10^3 - 10^4$ CFU/mL microflora present in the upper part of GIT (381)] to produce the corresponding amines, causing the release of free drug. Several hydrogel formulations using azo-cross-linked polymers have also been developed (382–385), but they may be limiting because of the low drug-loading capability. It has been reported that differences in the redox potential between the colon and the other regions of the upper GI tract (stomach, -65 mV; proximal small intestine, -67 ± 90 mV; distal small intestine, -196 ± 97 mV; and colon, -415 ± 72 mV), caused by microflora present in the respective segments, make these polymers susceptible to degradation in the colonic environment (372). Targeting in the colon is specifically important for polypeptide delivery, because there are no digestive enzymes in the colon, and the duration of residence is longer in the colon than in other regions of the GI tract [esophagus, 9–15 seconds; stomach, 0.4–4.5 hours; duodenum, jejunum, and ileum, 1–4 hours; cecum and colon, 4–16 hours; and rectum, 2–8 hours (43)]. Targeting in the colon is also feasible by pH and time-dependent pulsatile systems (386–388). The use of lectins (plant or microbial origin), neoglycoconjugates, and a number of natural polysaccharides (e.g., chitosan, pectin and its salts, chondroitin sulfate, cyclodextrin, dextrans, guar gum, inulin, amylose, and locust bean gum) as colon-specific drug carriers has been recently reviewed by Minko (389) and Sinha and Kumria (372). A number of colonic microflora are known to secrete polysaccharidases (e.g., β-D-glucosidase, amylase, pectinase, etc.), which can degrade polysaccharides and release the drug. Lectins, the naturally occurring proteins, are bioadhesives and show high specificity for sugar residues (e.g., D-Gal, GalNac, GlcNAc, α-D-Man, α-D-Glc, and Gal) attached to proteins and lipids of epithelial cells. They can trigger vesicular uptake by epithelial cells (41) and are hence ideally suited to target drugs to the intestine and buccal cavity. Lectins are also found on the epithelial cell surfaces and can hence be targeted as well by using synthetic polymers (e.g., HPMA) bearing sugars as ligands (390). Bridges et al. (391) reported that proximal regions of the gut showed greater accumulation of polymers bearing galactose, while fucose-containing polymers were more specific to distal regions of the gut. Uptake of polymeric particles in the inflamed colon has been found to be size dependent.

Rectal delivery, depending on the position of the dosage form in the rectum, can be used to target either the systemic circulation or the liver. For systemic targeting, the dosage form should be placed and located directly behind the internal rectal sphincter, whereas targeting the liver requires the dosage form to be placed in the ampulla recti (about 12–15 cm up the rectum) (50).

Targeting esophageal mucosa and other regions of the GI tract can also be achieved by using bioadhesive magnetic granules (392). The various parameters that influence targeting a specific site using bioadhesive magnetic granules include the composition of the formulation, the amount of the magnetic material in the granules, and the magnitude of the magnetic field. This approach can be used for local chemotherapy of esophageal cancer and for other diseases in the alimentary canal.

Although most drugs are absorbed from the intestine by the blood capillary network in the villi, they can also be taken up by the lymphatic system, predominantly by M cells that reside in the Peyer's patch regions of the intestine. Uptake of particles by M cells may involve specific fluid-phase pinocytosis or receptor-mediated phagocytosis. Various intestinal-uptake mechanisms of particles and their implications in drug and antigen delivery have been reviewed by O'Hagan (393) and Rieux (39). Peyer's patches have also been implicated in the regulation of the secretory immune response. Wachsmann et al. (394) reported that an antigenic material encapsulated within a liposome, when administered perorally, was taken up by these M cells and exhibited better saliva and serum IgA (primary and secondary) immune response than a simple solution of antigen (Fig. 11). In an attempt to demonstrate the use of microparticles as potential oral

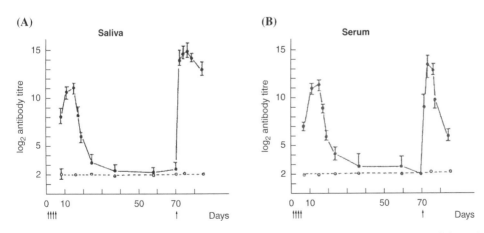

Figure 11 Saliva and serum IgA (primary and secondary) responses following orally administered soluble antigen *Streptococcus mutans* cell wall extract (*open circles*, soluble antigen; *solid circles*, liposome-encapsulated material) (phosphotidylcholine, phosphotidic acid, cholesterol). *Source*: From Ref. 394.

immunological adjuvants, O'Hagan et al. entrapped ovalbumin, a model, but poor, immunogen, into polyacrylamide (2.55-μm diameter) (395), poly(butyl-2-cyanoacrylate) (3 μm and 100 nm) (396), and poly(D,L-lactide-co-glycolide) (397–399) particles and found significantly elevated sIgA and systemic IgG antibody responses in rats compared with soluble antigen, following oral administration. These studies show that micro-particles can be used as potential oral adjuvants for the induction of long-term immune responses (393). Various issues pertaining to the uptake and targeting of particles by the oral route have been recently described by Florence (400).

MECHANICAL PUMPS

The mechanical pump approach employs miniature mechanical devices, such as implantable and portable infusion pumps and percutaneous infusion catheters, to deliver drugs into appropriate blood vessels or to a discrete site in the body. When compared with the conventional drug therapy, these devices offer several advantages: (*i*) the rate of the drug infusion can be better controlled; (*ii*) a relatively large volume of relatively dilute drug solutions can be administered; (*iii*) the drug dose can be readily changed, stopped, or alternated with other drugs, or a placebo when required; and (*iv*) the drug can be directed into a vascular site or body cavity using the drug-delivery cannula (e.g., hepatic arterial chemotherapy, intrathecal morphine infusion for pain control, intraventricular and intraarticular treatment of central nervous system tumors, intravenous infusions of heparin in thrombotic disorders, and intravenous infusions of insulin in type II diabetes). Several excellent review articles describing design and applications of infusion and implantable pumps in drug therapy, particularly insulin therapy, have been published (401–406). Drugs such as floxuridine (5-fluorodexyuridine) and zidovudine (azidothymine; AZT) have also been investigated for delivery using an implantable pump (407).

SUMMARY

The field of targeted drug delivery has grown rapidly in the last three to four decades. Several delivery systems based on passive, active, and physical targeting strategies have been explored. The two approaches that have received the most attention include prodrugs and polymer-carried drug delivery systems. Prodrugs are pharmacologically inert forms of the active drug that must be converted to their active form (i.e., parent drug) by either a chemical or an enzymatic reaction at the site of action. As our understanding of active sites becomes clearer, this approach should lead to the production of drugs that have a targeting moiety built into the structure. Currently, several examples of prodrugs exist that show promise for site-specific drug delivery.

Polymer macromolecule–carried drug delivery systems are of two types: particulate and soluble macromolecular. Particulate drug delivery systems, owing to their rapid clearance from the central circulation by the RES system, offer the greatest promise for use in combating diseases of the RES system. Several of these systems [e.g., phase I/II interferon α-2 and weekly liposome-encapsulated all-*trans*-retinoic acid in patients with advanced renal cell carcinoma (408)] are currently undergoing clinical trials. Various strategies to avoid uptake of particles by the RES have also been developed. This may provide opportunities to deliver drugs to cellular targets within the vasculature and to sites other than the RES.

Soluble macromolecular (natural and synthetic) systems are frequently used as lysosomotropic agents. Because of their ability to extravasate, they have been extensively explored for treating cancer and other remotely located diseases. The recent advent of the hybridoma technology and the progress made in identifying target-specific antibodies and ligands that enable ready target selectivity have provided additional impetus to design and develop site-specific delivery systems. An antibody-directed delivery system (Rituxan®, Genetech, Tech., California, U.S.) has been approved by FDA for the treatment of follicular or low-refractory, CD20-positive, non-Hodgkin's lymphoma. Several of these systems have been proved very effective in animals, and it remains to be seen how these results will be translated in clinical trials; (e.g., SAMCNS in Japan and polyHMPA copolymer–anthracycline conjugates in the United Kingdom have been completed or are in progress).

As our understanding of the drug action and pathogenesis of various diseases becomes clearer, more rational approaches to the design of therapeutic systems with functions that selectively target the disease, or deliver the drug to its intended site of action, with no or with reduced side effects, will emerge. The advent of the control of gene expression has already provided several new classes of biopharmaceuticals, including peptidergic mediators and sequence-specific oligonucleotides, and efforts are continuing to deliver them to their sites of action exclusively.

REFERENCES

1. Ehrlich P. Collected Studies on Immunity. London and New York: John Wiley & Sons, 1906.
2. Tomlinson E. Impact of the new biologics on the medical and pharmaceutical sciences. J Pharm Pharmacol 1992; 44(suppl 1):147–159.
3. Tomlinson E. Microsphere delivery systems for drug targeting and controlled release. Int J Pharm Tech Prod Mfr 1983; 4:49–57.
4. Widder KJ, Senyei AE, Ranney DF. Magnetically responsive microspheres and other carriers for the biophysical targeting of antitumor agents. Adv Pharmacol Chemother 1979; 16: 213–271.
5. Tomlinson E. (Patho)physiology and the temporal and spatial aspects of drug delivery. In: Tomlinson E, Davis SS, eds. Site-Specific Drug Delivery. Cell Biology, Medical, and Pharmaceutical Aspects. Chichester, U.K.: John Wiley & Sons, 1986: 1.
6. Bareford LM, Swaan PW. Endocytic mechanisms for targeted drug delivery. Adv Drug Deliv Rev 2007; 59:748–758.
7. Patel HM. Serum opsonins and liposomes: their interaction and opsonophagocytosis. Crit Rev Ther Drug Carrier Syst 1992; 9:39–90.
8. Absolom DR. Opsonins and dysopsonins: an overview. Methods Enzymol 1986; 132:281–318.
9. Ahsan F, Rivas IP, Khan MA, et al. Targeting to macrophages: role of physicochemical properties of particulate carriers-liposomes and microspheres on the phagocytosis by macrophages. J Control Release 2002; 79:29–40.
10. Jeon SI, Lee JH, Andrade JD. Protein–surface interactions in the presence of polyethylene oxide. II. Effect of protein size. J Colloid Interface Sci 1991; 142:159–166.
11. Jeon SI, Lee JH, Andrade JD, et al. Protein–surface interactions in the presence of polyethylene oxide. I. Simplified theory. J Colloid Interface Sci 1991; 142:149–158.
12. Vanoss CJ, Gillman CF, Bronson PM, et al. Opsonic properties of human-serum alpha-1 acid glycoprotein. Immunol Commun 1974; 3:329–335.
13. Davis SS, Douglas SJ, Illum L, et al. Targeting of colloidal carriers and the role of surface properties. In: Gregoriadis G, Senior J, Poste G, eds. Targeting of Drugs with Synthetic Systems. New York: Plenum Press, 1986:123.
14. Illum L, Davis SS, Jones PDE. Surface coated microspheres to minimize capture by the reticuloendothelial system. Polym Preprints 1986; 27:25–26.
15. Illum L, Davis SS. Targeting of colloidal particles to the bone-marrow. Life Sci 1987; 40:1553–1560.

16. Saito K, Ando J, Yoshida M, et al. Tissue distribution of sialoglycopeptide bearing liposomes in rats. Chem Pharm Bull 1988; 36:4187–4191.

17. Moghimi SM, Porter CJ, Muir IS, et al. Non-phagocytic uptake of intravenously injected microspheres in rat spleen—influence of particle size and hydrophilic coating. Biochem Biophys Res Commun 1991; 177:861–866.

18. Hsu MJ, Juliano RL. Interaction of liposomes with the reticuloendothelial system. 2. non-specific and receptor-mediated uptake of liposomes by mouse peritoneal macrophages. Biochim Biophys Acta 1982; 720:411–419.

19. Hopkins CR. Site-specific drug delivery-cellular opportunities and challenges. In: Tomlinson E, Davis SS, eds. Site-Specific Drug Delivery, Cell Biology, Medical and Pharmaceutical Aspects. Chichester, U.K.: John Wiley & Sons, 1886:27.

20. Duncan R, Cable HC, Rypacek F, et al. Targeting of soluble crosslinked N-(2-hydroxypropyl) methacrylamide copolymers in vivo—a potential drug delivery system. Biochem Soc Trans 1984; 12:1064–1065.

21. Duncan R, Cable HC, Rejmanove P, et al. Tyrosinamide residues enhance pinocytic capture of N-(2-hydroxypropyl)methacrylamide copolymers. Biochim Biophys Acta 1984; 799:1–8.

22. Kooistra T, Duursma A, Bouma JMW, et al. Effect of size and charge on endocytosis of lysozyme derivatives by sinusoidal rat liver cells in vivo. Biochim Biophys Acta 1980; 631:439–450.

23. Mitra A, Nan A, Ghandehari H, et al. Technetium-99m-labeled N-(2-hydroxypropyl) methacrylamide copolymers: synthesis, characterization, and in vivo biodistribution. Pharm Res 2004; 21:1153–1159.

24. Vyas SP, Sihorkar V. Endogenous carriers and ligands in non-immunogenic site-specific drug delivery. Adv Drug Deliv Rev 2000; 43:101–164.

25. Vyas SP, Singh A, Shirokar V. Ligand-receptor-mediated drug delivery: an emerging paradigm in cellular drug targeting. Crit Rev Ther Drug Carrier Syst 2001; 18:1–76.

26. Dunehoo AL, Anderson M, Majumdar S, et al. Cell adhesion molecules for targeted drug delivery. J Pharm Sci 2006; 95:1856–1872.

27. Harris AS. Biopharmaceutical aspects of the intranasal administration of peptides. In: Davis SS, Ilium L, Tomlinson E, eds. Delivery Systems for Peptides. New York: Plenum Press, 1986:191.

28. Ilium L, Farraj NF, Critichley H, et al. Nasal administration of gentamicin using novel microsphere delivery system. Int J Pharm 1988; 46:261–265.

29. Hermans WAJJ, Deurloo MJM, Romeyn SG, et al. Nasal absorption enhancement of 17β-estradiol by dimethyl-β-cyclodextrin in rabbits and rats. Pharm Res 1990; 7:500–503.

30. Fisher AN, Farraj NF, O'Hagan DT, et al. Effect of L-cu-lysophosphatidylcholine on the nasal absorption of human growth hormone in three animal species. Int J Pharm 1991; 74:147–156.

31. Giannasca PJ, Boden JA, Monath TP. Targeted delivery of antigen to hamster nasal lymphoid tissue with M-cell-directed lectins. Infect Immun 1997; 65:4288–4298.

32. Kumar P, Timoney JF, Sheoran AS. M cells and associated lymphoid tissue of the equine nasopharyngeal tonsil [comment]. Equine Vet J 2001; 33:224–230.

33. Pusztai A. Transport of proteins through the membranes of the adult gastrointestinal tract—a potential for drug delivery. Adv Drug Deliv Rev 1989; 3:215–228.

34. Matsuno K, Schaffner T, Gerbel HA, et al. Uptake by enterocytes and subsequent translocation to internal organs, EG, the thymus, of percoll microspheres administered per OS to suckling mice. J Reticuloendothelial Soc 1983; 33:263–273.

35. Damge C, Aprahamian M, Balboin G, et al. Polyalkylcyanoacrylate nanocapsules increase the intestinal absorption of a lipophilic drug. Int J Pharm 1987; 36:121–125.

36. Harush-Frenkel O, Rozentur E, Benita S, et al. Surface charge of nanoparticles determines their endocytic and transcytotic pathway in polarized MDCK cells. Biomacromolecules 2008; 9:435–443.

37. Tomlinson E. Theory and practice of site-specific drug delivery. Adv Drug Deliv Rev 1987; 1:87–198.

38. Ermak TH, Giannasca PJ. Microparticles targeting to M-cells. Adv Drug Deliv Rev 1998; 34:261–283.

39. des Rieux A, Fievez V, Garinot M, et al. Nanoparticles as potential oral delivery systems of proteins and vaccines: a mechanistic approach. J Control Release 2006; 116:1–27.

40. Ritschel WA. Microemulsions for improved peptide absorption from the gastrointestinal tract. Methods Find Exp Clin Pharmacol 1991; 13:205–220.

41. Bies C, Lehr CM, Woodley JF. Lectin-mediated drug targeting: history and applications. Adv Drug Deliv Rev 2004; 56:425–435.

42. Dressman JB, Bas P, Ritschel WA, et al. Gastrointestinal parameters that influence oral medications. J Pharm Sci 1993; 82:857–872.

43. Ritschel WA. Targeting in the gastrointestinal tract: new approaches. Methods Find Exp Clin Pharmacol 1991; 13:313–356.

44. O'Hagan DT. Microparticles and polymers for the mucosal delivery of vaccines. Adv Drug Deliv Rev 1998; 34:305–320.

45. Lee VHL, Yamamoto A. Penetration and enzymatic barriers to peptide and protein absorption. Adv Drug Deliv Rev 1990; 4:171–207.

46. Muranishi S. Absorption enhancers. Crit Rev Ther Drug Carrier Syst 1990; 7:1–33.

47. Davis SS. Delivery systems for biopharmaceuticals. J Pharm Pharmacol 1992; 44(suppl 1): 186–190.

48. Smart JD. Lectin-mediated drug delivery in the oral cavity. Adv Drug Deliv Rev 2004; 56:481–489.

49. Merkle HP, Anders R, Sandow J, et al. Drug delivery of peptides: the buccal route. In: Davis SS, Ilium L, Tomlinson E, eds. Delivery Systems for Peptide Drugs. New York: Plenum Press, 1986:159.

50. Ritschel WA, Ritschel GB, Ritschel BEC, et al. Rectal delivery system for insulin. Methods Find Exp Clin Pharmacol 1988; 10:645–656.

51. Muranishi SS, Takada K, Yoshikawa H, et al. Enhanced absorption and lymphatic transport of macromolecules via the rectal route. In: Davis SS, Ilium L, Tomlinson E, eds. Delivery Systems for Peptide Drugs. New York: Plenum Press, 1986:177.

52. Bulletti C, deZiegler D, Flamigni C, et al. Targeted drug delivery in gynecology: the first uterine pass effect. Hum Reprod 1997; 12:1073–1079.

53. Petrak K, Goddard P. Transport of macromolecules across the capillary walls. Adv Drug Deliv Rev 1989; 3:191–214.

54. Williams PL, Warwick R, eds. Gray's Anatomy. Oxford, U.K.: Churchill Livingston, 1980.

55. Davis SS, Ilium L. Colloidal delivery systems opportunity and challenges. In: Davis SS, Tomlinson E, eds. Site-Specific Drug Delivery: Cell Biology, Medical and Pharmaceutical Aspects. Chichester, U.K.: John Wiley & Sons, 1986:93.

56. Joyner WJ, Kern DF. Microvascular permeability to macromolecules and its dynamic modulations. Adv Drug Deliv Rev 1990; 4:319–342.

57. Takakura Y, Mahato RI, Hashida M. Extravasation of macromolecules. Adv Drug Deliv Rev 1998; 34:93–108.

58. Seymour LW. Passive tumor targeting of soluble macromolecules and drug conjugates. Crit Rev Ther Drug Carrier Syst 1992; 9:135–187.

59. Kern DF, Bell DR, Blumenstock FA. The effect of charge on albumin permeability and uptake in the lung. Microvasc Res 1983; 25:241.

60. Lanken PN, Hansen-Flaschen JH, Sampson PM, et al. Passage of uncharged dextrans from blood to lung lymph in awake sheep. J Appl Physiol 1985; 59:580–591.

61. Pietra GG, Fishman AP, Lanken PN, et al. Permeability of pulmonary endothelium to neutral and charged macromolecules. Ann N Y Acad Sci 1982; 401:241–247.

62. Arturson G, Granath K. Dextrans as test molecules in studies of functional ultrastructure of biological membranes—molecular weight distribution analysis by gel chromatography. Clin Chim Acta 1972; 37:309–322.

63. Taylor AE, Granger DN. Exchange of macromolecules across the microcirculation. In: Handbook of Physiology. Vol 6. Ohio, U.S.A.: Oxford Press, 1984:467–520.

64. Wike-Hooley JL, Haveman J, Reinhold HS. The relevance of tumour pH to the treatment of malignant disease. Radiother Oncol 1984; 2:343–366.

65. Ghitescu L, Fixman A, Simionescu M, et al. Specific binding sites for albumin restricted to plasmalemmal vesicles of continuous capillary endothelium: receptor-mediated transcytosis. J Cell Biol 1986; 102:1304–1311.

66. Vasile E, Simionescu M, Simionescu N. Visualization of the binding, endocytosis, and transcytosis of low-density lipoprotein in the arterial endothelium in situ. J Cell Biol 1983; 96:1677–1689.

67. Drobnik J, Rypacek F. Soluble synthetic polymers in biological systems. Adv Polym Sci 1984; 57:1–50.

68. Hall JG. The lymphatic system in drug targeting: an overview. In: Gregoriadis G, Poste G, eds. Targeting of Drugs—Anatomical and Physiological Considerations. New York: Plenum Press, 1985:15.

69. Moghimi SM, Bonnemain B. Subcutaneous and intravenous delivery of diagnostic agents to the lymphatic system: applications in lymphoscintigraphy and indirect lymphography. Adv Drug Deliv Rev 1999; 37:295–312.

70. Moghimi SM, Hawley AE, Christy NM, et al. Surface engineered nanospheres with enhanced drainage into lymphatics and uptake by macrophages of the regional lymph nodes. FEBS Lett 1994; 244:25–30.

71. Moghimi SM, Rajabi-Siahboomi AR. Advanced colloid-based systems for efficient delivery of drugs and diagnostic agents to the lymphatic tissues. Prog Biophys Mol Biol 1996; 65:221–249.

72. Oussoren C, Zuidema J, Crommelin DJA, et al. Lymphatic uptake and biodistribution of liposomes after subcutaneous injection. II. Influence of liposomal size, lipid composition and lipid dose. Biochim Biophys Acta 1997; 1328:261–272.

73. Phillips WT, Klipper R, Goins B. Novel method of greatly enhanced delivery of liposomes to lymph nodes. J Pharmacol Exp Ther 2000; 295:309–312.

74. Moghimi SM. The effect of methoxy-PEG chain length and molecular architecture on lymph node targeting of immuno-PEG liposome. Biomaterials 2006; 37:136–144.

75. Noguchi Y, Wu J, Duncan R, et al. Early phase of tumor accumulation of macromolecules: a great difference in clearance rate between tumor and normal tissues. Jpn J Cancer Res 1998; 89:307–314.

76. Maeda H. The enhanced permeability and retention (EPR) effect in tumor vasculature: the key role of tumor-selective macromolecular drug targeting. Adv Enzyme Regul 2001; 41:189–207.

77. Maeda H, Matsumura Y. Tumoritropic and lymphotropic principles of macromolecular drugs. Crit Rev Ther Drug Carrier Syst 1989; 6:193–210.

78. Maeda H, Matsumura Y, Oda T, et al. Cancer selective macromolecular therapeutics: tailoring of antitumor protein drugs. In: Feeney RE, Whitaker JR, eds. Protein Tailoring for Food and Medical Uses. New York: Marcel Dekker, 1986:353–382.

79. Matsumura Y, Maeda H. A new concept for macromolecular therapeutics in cancer chemotherapy: mechanism of tumoritropic accumulation of proteins and the antitumor agent SMANCSs. Cancer Res 1986; 46:6387–6392.

80. Maeda H. SMANCS and polymer–conjugated macromolecular drugs: advantages in cancer chemotherapy. Adv Drug Deliv Rev 1991; 6:181–202.

81. van Vlerken LE, Duan Z, Seiden MV, et al. Modulation of Intracellular ceramide using polymeric nanoparticles to overcome multidrug resistance in cancer. Cancer Res 2007; 67: 4843–4850.

82. Boddy A, Aarons L. Pharmacokinetic and pharmacodynamic aspects of site-specific drug delivery. Adv Drug Deliv Rev 1989; 3:155–163.

83. Boddy A, Aarons L, Petrak K. Efficiency of drug targeting—steady state considerations using a 3-compartment model. Pharm Res 1989; 6:367–372.

84. Levy G. Targeted drug delivery—some pharmacokinetic considerations. Pharm Res 1987; 4:3–4.

85. Gupta PK, Hung CT. Quantitative evaluation of targeted drug delivery systems. Int J Pharm 1989; 56:217–226.

86. Proost JH. Pharmacokinetic/pharmacodynamic modeling in drug targeting. In: Molema G, Meijer DKF, eds. Drug-Targeting Organ-Specific Strategies. Weinheim, Germany: Wiley-VCH Verlag GmbH, 2001:333–370.

87. Notari RE. Prodrugs kinetics: theory and practice. In: Bundgaard H, Hansen AB, Koford H, eds. Optimization of Drug Delivery. Copenhagen, Denmark: Munksgaard, 1982:117.

88. Stella VJ, Himmelstein KJ. Prodrugs and site-specific drug delivery. J Med Chem 1980; 23:1275–1282.

89. Stella VJ, Himmelstein KJ. Critique of prodrugs and site-specific drug delivery. In: Bundgaard H, Hansen AB, Kofod H, eds. Optimization of Drug Delivery. Copenhagen, Denmark: Munksgaard, 1982:134.

90. Han HK, Amidon GL. Targeted prodrug design to optimize drug delivery. AAPS PharmSci 2000; 2:1–11.

91. Gardner CR, Alexander J. Prodrug approaches to drug targeting: past accomplishments and future potential. In: Buri P, Gumma A, eds. Drug Targeting. Amsterdam, The Netherlands: Elsevier Science Publishers, 1985:145.

92. Stella VJ. Prodrugs: an overview and definition. In: Higuchi T, Stella V, eds. Prodrugs in Novel Drug Delivery Systems. Washington, DC: American Chemical Society, 1975:1.

93. Roche EB, ed. Design of Biopharmaceutical Properties Through Prodrugs and Analogs. Washington, DC: American Pharmaceutical Association, 1977.

94. Cotzias GC, VanWoert MH, Schiffer LM. Aromatic amino acids and modifications of parkinsonism. N Engl J Med 1967; 276:374–379.

95. Hussain A, Truelove JE. Prodrug approaches to enhancement of physicochemical properties of drugs IV: novel epinephrine prodrug. J Pharm Sci 1976; 65:1510–1512.

96. Wilk S, Mizoguchi H, Orlowski M. Gamma-glutamyl dopa: a kidney-specific dopamine precursor. J Pharmacol Exp Ther 1978; 206:227–232.

97. Friend DR, Chang GW. Drug glycosides: potential prodrugs for colon-specific drug delivery. J Med Chem 1985; 28:51–57.

98. Stella VJ, Mikkelson TJ, Pipkin JD. Prodrugs: the control of drug delivery via bioreversible chemical modification. In: Juliano RL, ed. Drug Delivery Systems: Characteristics and Biomedical Applications. New York: Oxford University Press, 1980:112.

99. Baurain R, Masquelier M, Deprezedcampeneere D, et al. Amino acid and dipeptide derivatives of daunorubicin. 2. cellular pharmacology and anti-tumor activity on L1210 leukemic-cells in vitro and in vivo. J Med Chem 1980; 23:1171–1174.

100. Masquelier M, Baurain R, Trouet A. Amino acid and dipeptide derivatives of daunorubicin. 1. Synthesis, physicochemical properties, and lysosomal digestion. J Med Chem 1980; 23: 1166–1170.

101. Chakravarty RK, Carl PL, Weber MJ, et al. Plasmin activated prodrugs for cancer chemotherapy. 1. Synthesis and biological activity of peptidylacivicin and peptidylphenylenediamine mustard. J Med Chem 1983; 26:638–644.

102. Bodor N, Simpkins JW. Redox delivery system for brain-specific, sustained-release of dopamine. Science 1983; 221:65–67.

103. Shek E, Higuchi T, Bodor N. Improved delivery through biological membranes. 3. delivery of N-methylpyridinium-2-carbaldoime chloride through the blood-brain barrier in its dihydropyridine prodrug form. J Med Chem 1976; 19:113–117.

104. Bodor N. Targeting of drugs to the brain. Methods Enzymol 1985; 112:381–396.

105. Bodor N, Farag HH. Improved delivery through biological membranes. 13. Brain specific delivery of dopamine with a dihydropyridinne-reversible-pyridinium salt type redox delivery system. J Med Chem 1983; 26:528–534.

106. Chu CK, Bhadti VS, Doshi KJ, et al. Brain targeting of anti-HIV nucleosides—synthesis and in vitro and in vivo studies of dihydropyridine derivatives of 3′-azido-2′,3′-dideoxyuridine and 3′azido-3′-deoxythymidine. J Med Chem 1990; 33:2188–2192.

107. Palomin E. Delivery of drugs through dihydropyridine carriers. Drugs Future 1990; 15:361–368.

108. Brewster ME, Anderson W, Bodor N. Brain, blood, and cerebrospinal-fluid distribution of a zidovudine chemical delivery system in rabbits. J Pharm Sci 1991; 80:843–846.

109. Khandare J, Minko T. Polymer-drug conjugates: progress in polymeric prodrugs. Prog Polym Sci 2006; 31:359–397.

110. Kratz F, Warnecke A, Schmid B, et al. Prodrugs of anthracyclines in cancer chemotherapy. Curr Med Chem 2006; 13:477–523.
111. Illum L, Davis SS. Passive and active targeting using colloidal carrier systems. In: Buri P, Gumma A, eds. Drug Targeting. Amsterdam, The Netherlands: Elsevier Science Publishers, 1985:65.
112. Dufes C, Schatzlein AG, Tetley L, et al. Niosomes and polymeric chitosan based vesicles bearing transferrin and glucose ligands for drug targeting. Pharm Res 2000; 17:1250–1258.
113. Kakudo T, Chaki S, Futaki S, et al. Transferrin-modified liposomes equipped with a pH-sensitive fusogenic peptide: an artificial viral-like delivery system. Biochemistry 2004; 43: 5618–5628.
114. Li H, Sun H, Zhong MQ. The role of the transferrin–transferrin-receptor system in drug delivery and targeting. Trends Pharmacol Sci 2002; 23:206–209.
115. Lu Y, Low PS. Folate-mediated delivery of macromolecular anticancer therapeutic agents. Adv Drug Deliv Rev 2002; 54:675–693.
116. Chiles C, Hedlund LW, Kubek RJ, et al. Distribution of 15-MU and 137-MU diameter microspheres in the dog lung in the axial plane. Invest Radiol 1986; 21:618–621.
117. Kim CK, Lee MK, Han JH, et al. Pharmacokinetics and tissue distribution of methotrexate after intravenous injection of differently charged liposome-entrapped methotrexate to rats. Int J Pharm 1994; 108:21–29.
118. Ahmad I, Allen TM. Antibody-mediated specific binding and cytotoxicity of liposome-entrapped doxorubicin to lung cancer cells in vitro. Cancer Res 1992; 52:4817–4820.
119. Hurwitz E, Adler A, Shouval D, et al. Immunotargeting of daunomycin to localized and metastatic human colon adenocarcinoma in athymic mice. Cancer Immunol Immunother 1992; 35:186–192.
120. Affleck K, Embleton MJ. Monoclonal antibody targeting of methotrexate(MTX) against MTX-resistance tumor cell lines. Br J Cancer 1992; 65:838–844.
121. Seymour LW, Al-Shamkhani A, Flanagan PA, et al. Synthetic polymers conjugated to monoclonal antibodies—vehicle for tumor targeted drug delivery. Sel Cancer Ther 1991; 7:59–73.
122. Gregoriadis G, Neerunjun ED. Homing of liposomes to target cells. Biochem Biophys Res Commun 1975; 65:537–544.
123. Juliano RI, Stamp D. Lectin-mediated attachment of glycoprotein-bearing liposomes to cells. Nature 1976; 261:235–238.
124. Gregoriadis G, Meehan A, Mah MM. Interaction of antibody-bearing small unilamellar liposomes with target free antigen in vitro and in vivo—some influencing factors. Biochem J 1981; 200:203–210.
125. Weissman G, Bloomgarden D, Kaplan R, et al. A general method for introduction of enzymes by means of immunoglobulin-coated liposomes, into lysozomes of deficient cells. Proc Natl Acad Sci U S A 1975; 72:88–92.
126. Kaplan MR, Calef B, Bercovivi T, et al. The selective detection of cell-surface determination by means of antibodies and acetylated avidin attached to highly fluorescent polymer microspheres. Biochim Biophys Acta 1983; 728:112–120.
127. Moghimi SM, Hunter AC, Murray JC. Long-circulating and target-specific nanoparticles: theory and practice. Pharmacol Rev 2001; 53:283–318.
128. Stolnik S, Illum L, Davis SS. Long circulating microparticulate drug carriers. Adv Drug Deliv Rev 1995; 16:195–214.
129. Widder KJ, Senyei AE. Magnetic microsphere: a vehicle for selective targeting of organs. In: Methods of Drug Delivery. New York: Pergamon Press, 1986:39.
130. Sezaki H, Hashida M, Muranishi S. Gelatin microspheres as carriers for antineoplastic agents. In: Bundgaard H, Hansen AB, Kofod H, eds. Optimization of Drug Delivery. Copenhagen, Denmark: Munksgaard, 1982:316.
131. Yatvin MB, Kreutz W, Horowitz BA, et al. pH-Sensitive liposomes: possible clinical implications. Science 1980; 210:1253–1255.
132. Kato T. Encapsulated drugs in targeted cancer therapy. In: Bruck SD, ed. Controlled Drug Delivery. Boca Raton: CRC Press, 1983:189.

133. Kreuter J, Liehl E. Long-term studies of microencapsulated and adsorbed influenza vaccine nanoparticles. J Pharm Sci 1981; 70:367–371.

134. Couvreur P. Polyalkylcyanoacrylates as colloidal drug carriers. Crit Rev Ther Drug Carrier Syst 1988; 5:1–20.

135. Praveen S, Sahoo SK. Polymeric nanoparticles for cancer therapy. J Drug Target 2008; 16:108–123.

136. Torchilin VP. Targeted pharmaceutical nanocarriers for cancer therapy and imaging. AAPS J 2007; 9:E128–E147.

137. Tong R, Cheng J. Anticancer polymeric nanomedicines. Polym Rev 2007; 47:345–381.

138. Couvreur P, Vanthier C. Nanotechnology; intelligent design to treat complex disease. Pharm Res 2006; 23:1417–1450.

139. Sunderland CI, Steiert M, Talmadge JE, et al. Targeted nanoparticles for detecting and treating cancer. Drug Dev Res 2006; 67:70–93.

140. Simon C. Magnetic drug targeting. New paths for the local concentration of drugs for head and neck cancer. HNO 2005; 53:600–601.

141. Chappell JC, Price RJ. Targeted therapeutic applications of acoustically active microspheres in the microcirculation. Microcirculation 2006; 13:57–70.

142. Liu J, Wong HL, Moselhy J, et al. Targeting colloidal particulates to thoracic lymph nodes. Lung Cancer 2006; 51:377–386.

143. Brioschi A, Zenga F, Zara GP, et al. Solid lipid nanoparticles: could they help to improve the efficacy of pharmacologic treatments for brain tumors? Neurol Res 2007; 29:324–330.

144. Langer R. Biodegradable long-circulating polymeric nanospheres. Science 1994; 263:1600–1603.

145. Emerich DF, Thanos CG. Targeted nanoparticle-based drug delivery and diagnosis. J Drug Target 2007; 15:163–183.

146. Duncan R. Designing polymer conjugates as lysosomotropic nanomedicines. Biochem Soc Trans 2007; 35:56–60.

147. Yang SC, Lu LF, Cai Y, et al. Body distribution in mice of intravenously injected campothecin solid lipid nanoparticles. J Control Release 1999; 59:299–307.

148. Maia CS, Mehnert W, Schafer-Korting M. Solid lipid nanoparticles as drug carriers for topical glucocorticoids. Int J Pharm 2000; 196:165–167.

149. Peracchia MT, Fattal E, Desmaele D, et al. Stealth PEGylated polycyanoacrylate nanoparticle for intravenous administration. J Control Release 1999; 60:121–128.

150. Gregoriadis G, ed. Liposome Technology. Boca Raton: CRC Press, 1984.

151. Gregoriadis G, ed. Liposome Technology. Boca Raton: CRC Press, 1993.

152. New PRC, ed. Liposome-A Practical Approach. Oxford, U.K.: IRL Press, 1990.

153. Yagi K, ed. Medical Applications of Liposomes. Tokyo, Japan, and Basel, Switzerland: Japan Scientific Press and S Karger, 1986.

154. Schmidt KH, ed. Liposomes as Drug Carriers. Stuttgart, Germany: Georg Thieme Verlag, 1986.

155. Gregoriadis G, Allison AC, eds. Liposome in Biological Systems. Chichester, U.K.: John Wiley & Sons, 1980.

156. Maruyama K, Mori A, Kennel SJ, et al. Drug delivery by organ-specific immunoliposomes. ACS Symp Ser 1991; 469:275–284.

157. Roerdnik FH, Daemen T, Bakker-Woudenberg IAJM, et al. Therapeutic utility of liposomes. In: Johnson P, Jones JGL, eds. Drug Delivery Systems and Fundamental and Techniques. Chichester, U.K.: Ellis Horwood, 1987:67.

158. Roerdink F, Regts J, Daemen T, et al. Liposomes as drug carriers to liver macrophages. In: Targeting of Drugs with Synthetic Systems. New York: Plenum Press, 1985:193.

159. Gregoriadis G, Senior J, Wolff B, et al. Fate of liposomes in vivo: control leading to targeting. In: Gregoriadis G, Poste G, Senior J, Trouet A, eds. Receptor-Mediated Targeting of Drugs. New York: Plenum Press, 1984:243.

160. Lopez-Berestein G, Juliano RL, Mehta K, et al. Liposomes in antimicrobial therapy. In: Gregoriadis G, Senior J, Poste G, eds. Targeting of Drugs with Synthetic Systems. New York: Plenum Press, 1985:193.

161. Sugarman SM, Peres-Solar R. Liposomes in the treatment of malignancy—a clinical perspective. Crit Rev Oncol Hematol 1992; 12:231–242.
162. Gregoriadis G, Florence AT. Liposomes and cancer therapy. Cancer Cells 1991; 3:144–146.
163. Gregoriadis G. Overview of liposomes. J Antimicrob Chemother 1991; 8:39–48.
164. Liliemark J. Liposomes for drug targeting in cancer chemotherapy. Eur J Surg Suppl 1991; 561:49–52.
165. Lopez-Berstein G. Liposomes as carriers of antimicrobial agents. Antimicrob Agents Chemother 1987; 31:675–678.
166. Sozaka FC Jr. The future of liposomal drug delivery. Biotechnol Appl Biochem 1990; 12:496–500.
167. Torchilin VP. Liposomes as targetable drug carriers. Crit Rev Ther Drug Carrier Syst 1985; 2:65–115.
168. Drummond DC, Meyer O, Hong K, et al. Optimizing liposomes for delivery of chemotherapeutic agents to solid tumors. Pharmacol Rev 1999; 51:691–743.
169. Hope MJ, Bally MB, Webb G, et al. Production of large unilamellar vesicles by a rapid extrusion procedure. Characterization of size distribution, trapped volume and ability to maintain a membrane potential. Biochim Biophys Acta 1985; 812:55–65.
170. Gabizon A, Dagan A, Goren D, et al. Liposomes as in vivo carriers of adriamycin: reduced cardiac uptake and preserved antitumor activity in mice. Cancer Res 1982; 42:4734–4739.
171. Mayer LD, Bally MB, Hope MJ, et al. Uptake of antineoplastic agents into large unilamellar vesicles in response to a membrane potential. Biochim Biophys Acta 1985; 816:294–302.
172. Kirby C, Gregoriadis G. Dehydration-rehydration vesicles: a simple method for high-yield drug entrapment in liposomes. Biotechnol 1984; 2:979–984.
173. Alpar O. Liposomes in drug delivery: 21 years of research. Pharm J 1991; 246:172–173.
174. Weissig V, Lasch J, Gregoriadis G. A method for preparation of liposomes with encapsulated peptide antigens and surface-linked sugar residues. Pharmazie 1991; 46:56–57.
175. Senior J, Gregoriadis G. Dehydration-rehydration vesicle methodology facilitates a novel approach to antibody-binding to liposomes. Biochim Biophys Acta 1989; 1002:58–62.
176. Andersen TL, Jensen SS, Jorgensen K. Advanced strategies in liposomal cancer therapy: problems and prospects of active and tumor specific drug release. Prog Lipid Res 2005; 44:68–97.
177. Poste G, Kirsh R, Koestler T, eds. Liposome Technology. Targeted Drug Delivery and Biological Interactions. Boca Raton: CRC Press, 1984.
178. Belchetz PE, Braidman IP, Crawly JCW, et al. Treatment of Gaucher's disease with liposome-entrapped glucocerebroside: beta-glucosidase. Lancet 1977; 2:116–117.
179. Tyrrel DA, Ryman BE, Keeton BR, et al. The use of liposomes in treating type-2 glycogenosis. Br Med J 1976; 2:88.
180. New RRC, Chance ML, Thomas SC, et al. Antileishmanial activity of antimonials entrapped in liposomes. Nature 1978; 272:55–56.
181. Alving CR, Steck EA, Chapman JWL, et al. Therapy of leishmaniasis: superior efficacies of liposome-encapsulated drugs. Proc Natl Acad Sci U S A 1978; 75:2959–2963.
182. Black CDV, Watson GJ, Ward RJ. The use of pentostam liposomes in the chemotherapy of experimental leishmaniasis. Trans R Soc Trop Med Hyg 1977; 71:550–552.
183. Bakker-Woudenberg IAJM, Lokerse AF, Roerdnik FH, et al. Free versus liposome-entrapped ampicillin in treatment of infection due to listeria monocytogenes in normal and athymic (nude) mice. J Infect Dis 1985; 151:917–924.
184. Fidler IJ. The generation of tumoricidal activity in macrophages for the treatment of established metastases. In: Nicolson GL, Milas L, eds. Cancer Invasion and Metastasis: Biologic and Therapeutic Aspects. New York: Raven Press, 1984:421.
185. Sone S, Matsura S, Ogawara M, et al. Potentiating effect of muramyl dipeptide and its lipophilic analog encapsulated in liposomes on tumor cell killing by human monocytes. J Immunol 1984; 132:2105–2110.
186. Fidler IJ, Sone S, Fogler WE, et al. Efficacy of liposomes containing a lipophilic muramyl dipeptide derivative for activating the tumoricidal properties of alveolar macrophages in vivo. J Biol Response Mod 1982; 1:43.

187. Fidler IJ, Raz A, Fogler WE, et al. The role of plasma membrane receptors and the kinetics of macrophage activation by lymphokines encapsulated in liposomes. Cancer Res 1981; 41:495–504.

188. Saiki L, Sone S, Fogler WE, et al. Synergism between human recombinant gamma-interferon and muramyl dipeptide encapsulated in liposomes for activation of antitumor properties in human blood monocytes. Cancer Res 1985; 45:6188–6193.

189. Saiki L, Fidler IJ. Synergistic activation by recombinant mouse interferon-gamma and muramyl dipeptide of tumoricidal properties in mouse macrophages. J Immunol 1985; 135:684–688.

190. Sone S, Tandon P, Utsugi T, et al. Synergism of recombinant human interferon gamma with liposome-encapsulated muramyl tripeptide in activation of the tumoricidal properties of human monocytes. Int J Cancer 1986; 38:495–500.

191. Fidler IJ, Schroit AJ. Synergism between lymphokines and muramyl dipeptide encapsulated in liposomes: in situ activation of macrophages and therapy of spontaneous cancer metastases. J Immunol 1984; 133:515–518.

192. Mayhew E, Rustum Y. Effect of liposome entrapped chemotherapeutic-agents on mouse primary and metastatic tumors. Biol Cell 1983; 47:81–85.

193. New RRC, Chance ML, Heath S. Antileishmanial activity of amphotericin and other antifungal agents entrapped in liposomes. J Antimicrob Chemother 1981; 8:371–381.

194. Rosenberg OA, Berkreneva VY, Loshakova LV, et al. An enhanced trapping of tumor cells of liposomes prepared from autologous phospholipids. Vopr Onkol 1983; 29:56–60.

195. Burkhanov SA, Kosykh VA, Repin VS, et al. Interaction of liposomes of different phospholipid and ganglioside composition with rat hepatocytes. Int J Pharm 1988; 46:31–34.

196. Abu-Dahab R, Schafer UF, Lehr CM. Lectin-functionalized liposomes for pulmonary drug delivery: effect of nebulization on stability and bioadhesion. Eur J Pharm Sci 2001; 14:37–41.

197. Bruck A, Abu-Dahab R, Borchard G, et al. Lectin-functionalized liposomes for pulmonary drug delivery: interaction with human alveolar epithelial cells. J Drug Target 2001; 9:241–251.

198. Yatvin MB, Cree TC, Tegmo-Larsson IM. Theoretical and practical considerations in preparing liposomes for the purpose of releasing drug in response to changes in temperature and pH. In: Gregoriaids G, ed. Liposome Technology. Boca Raton: CRC Press, 1984:157.

199. Weinstein JN, Magin RL, Cysyk RL, et al. Treatment of solid L1210 murine tumors with local hyperthermia and temperature sensitive liposomes containing methotrexate. Cancer Res 1980; 40:1388–1395.

200. Tacker JR, Anderson RU. Delivery of anti-tumor drug to bladder-cancer by use of phase-transition liposomes and hyperthermia. J Urol 1982; 127:1211–1214.

201. Yatvin MB, Muhensipen H, Porschen W, et al. Selective delivery of liposome-associated cis-dichlorodiamineplatinum(II) by heat and its influence on tumor drug uptake and growth. Cancer Res 1981; 41:1602–1607.

202. Roux E, Passirani C, Scheffold S, et al. Serum stable and long-circulating, PEGylated, pH-sensitive liposomes. J Control Release 2004; 94:447–451.

203. Nicolau C, Pape AL, Soriano P, et al. In vivo expression of rat insulin after intravenous administration of the liposome-entrapped gene for rat insulin I. Proc Natl Acad Sci U S A 1983; 80:1068–1072.

204. Szebeni J, Wahl SM, Betageri GV, et al. Inhibition of HIV-1 in monocyte macrophage cultures by 2′,3′-dideoxycytidine-5′triphosphate, free and in liposomes. AIDS Res Hum Retroviruses 1990; 6:691–702.

205. Phillips NC, Skamene F, Tsouka C. Liposomal encapsulation of 3′-azido-3′-deoxythymidine (AZT) results in decreased bone-marrow toxicity and enhanced activity against murine aids aids-induced immunosuppression. J Acquir Immune Defic Syndr Retrovirol 1991; 4:959–966.

206. Babincova M, Altanerova V, Lampert M, et al. Site-specific in vivo targeting of magnetoliposomes using externally applied Magnetic Field. Z Naturforsch 2000; 55:278–281.

207. Pinto-Alphandary H, Andremont A, Couvreur P. Targeted delivery of antibiotics using liposomes and nanoparticles: research and applications. Int J Antimicrob Agents 2000; 13:155–168.

208. Velpandian T, Gupta SK, Gupta YK, et al. Ocular drug targeting by liposomes and their corneal interactions. J Microencapsul 1999; 16:243–250.

209. Rogers JA, Anderson KE. The potential of liposomes in oral drug delivery. Crit Rev Ther Drug Carrier Syst 1998; 15:421–480.
210. Sun WT, Zhang N, Li AG, et al. Preparation and evaluation of N3-O-toluyl-fluorouracil-loaded liposomes. Int J Pharm 2008; 353:243–250.
211. Sun WT, Zou WW, Huang GH, et al. Pharmacokinetics and targeting property of TFu-loaded liposomes with different sizes after intravenous and oral administration. J Drug Target 2008; 16:357–365.
212. Zou WW, Sun WT, Zhang N, et al. Enhanced oral bioavailability and absorption mechanism study of N3-O-toluyl-fluorouracil-loaded liposomes. J Biomed Nanotechnol 2008; 4:90–98.
213. Taira MC, Chiaramoni NS, Pecuch KM, et al. Stability of liposomal formulations in physiological conditions for oral drug delivery. Drug Deliv Technol 2004; 11:123–128.
214. Baillie AJ, Florence AT, Muirhead LH, et al. Preparation and properties of niosomes-non ionic surfactant vesicles. J Pharm Pharmacol 1985; 37:863–868.
215. Israelachvili JN, Marcelja S, Horn RG. Physical principles of membrane organization. Q Rev Biophys 1980; 13:121–200.
216. Hunter CA, Dolan TF, Coombs GH, et al. Vesicular systems (niosomes and liposomes) for delivery of sodium stibogluconate in experimental murine visceral leishmaniasis. J Pharm Pharmacol 1988; 40:161–165.
217. Kiwada H, Nimura H, Fujisaki Y, et al. Application of synthetic alkyl glycoside vesicles as drug carriers. I. Preparation and physical properties. Chem Pharm Bull 1985; 33:753–759.
218. Echegoyen LE, Hernandez JC, Kaifer AE, et al. Aggregation of steroidal lariat liposomes (niosomes) formed from neutral crown ether compounds. J Chem Soc Chem Commun 1988; 836–837.
219. Baillie AJ. Niosomes: a putative drug carrier system. In: Gregoriadis G, Poste G, eds. Targeting of Drugs Anatomical and Physiological Considerations. New York: Plenum Press, 1988:143.
220. Azmin MN, Florence AT, Handjani-Vila RM, et al. The effect of non-ionic surfactant vesicle (niosome) entrapment on the absorption and distribution of methotrexate in mice. J Pharm Pharmacol 1985; 37:237–242.
221. Azmin MN, Florence AT, Handjani-Vila RM, et al. The effect of niosomes and polysorbate 80 on the metabolism and excretion of methotrexate in the mouse. J Microencapsul 1986; 3: 95–100.
222. Namdeo A, Jain NK. Niosomal delivery of 5-fluorouracil. J Microencapsul 1999; 16:731–740.
223. Rogerson A. (PhD). A physicochemical and biological evaluation of non-ionic surfactant vesicles. Glasgow: University of Strathclyde; 1986.
224. Baillie AJ, Coombs GH, Dolan TF, et al. Non-ionic surfactant vesicles, niosomes, as a delivery system for the anti-leishmanial drug, sodium stibogluconate. J Pharm Pharmacol 1986; 38:502–505.
225. Bijsterbosch MK, Berkel TJCV. Native and modified lipoproteins as drug delivery systems. Adv Drug Deliv Rev 1990; 5:231–251.
226. de Smidt PC, van Berkel TJ. LDL-mediated drug targeting. Crit Rev Ther Drug Carrier Syst 1990; 7:99–120.
227. Damle NS, Seevers RH, Schwendner SW, et al. Potential tumor- or organ-imaging agents XXIV: chylomicron remnants as carriers for hepatographic agents. J Pharm Sci 1983; 72:898–901.
228. Samadi-Baboli M, Favre G, Blancy E, et al. Preparation of low-density lipoprotein-9-methotxyyellipticin complex and its cyto-toxic effect against L121- and P388 leukemic cells in vitro. Eur J Cancer Clin Oncol 1989; 25:233.
229. Lestavel-Delattre S, Martin-Nizard F, Clavey V, et al. Low-density lipoprotein for delivery of an acrylophenone antineoplastic molecule into malignant cells. Cancer Res 1992; 52:3629–3635.
230. Kempen HJM, Hoes C, Boom JHV, et al. A water-soluble cholesteryl containing trisgalactoside: synthesis, properties. J Med Chem 1984; 27:1306–1312.
231. Scoazec JY, Feldman G. Both endothelial cells and macrophages of the hepatic sinusoid express the CD4 molecule—possible implications for HIV infection. Hepatology 1989; 10:627.

232. Joel DD, Laissue JD, LeFevre ME. Distribution and fate of ingested carbon particles in mice. J Reticuloendothelial Soc 1978; 72:440–451.

233. Takahashi T. Emulsion and activated carbon in chemotherapy. Crit Rev Ther Drug Carrier Syst 1985; 2:245–247.

234. Huang YN, Hagiwara A, Wang W, et al. Local injection of M-CH combined with i.p. hyperthermic hypo-osmolar infusion is an effective therapy in advanced gastric cancer. Anticancer Drugs 2002; 13:431–435.

235. Ito K, Kiriyama K, Watanabe T, et al. A newly developed drug delivery system using fine particles of activated charcoal for targeting chemotherapy. ASAIO Trans 1990; 36:M199–M202.

236. Ortner M, Taha AAM, Schreiber S, et al. Endoscopic injection of mitomycin adsorbed on carbon particles for advanced esophageal cancer: a pilot study. Endoscopy 2004; 36:421–425.

237. Nakase Y, Hagiwara A, Kin S, et al. Intratumoral administration of methotrexate bound to activated carbon particles: antitumor effectiveness against human colon carcinoma xenografts and acute toxicity in mice. J Pharmacol Exp Ther 2004; 311:382–387.

238. Roth JC, Curiel DT, Pereboeva L. Cell vehicle targeting strategies. Gene Ther 2008; 15:716–729.

239. Dean MF, Muir H, Benson PF, et al. Increased breakdown of glycosaminoglycans and appearance of corrective enzyme after skin transplants in Hunter syndrome. Nature 1975; 257:609–614.

240. Matas AJ, Sutherland DER, Steffes MW, et al. Hepatocellular transplantation for metabolic deficiencies—decrease of plasma bilirubin in gunn rats. Science 1976; 192:892–894.

241. Baum R. Combinatorial approaches provide fresh leads for medicinal chemistry. Chem Eng News 1994; 72:20–26.

242. Younoszai R, Sorenson RL, Lindal AW. Homotransplantation of isolated pancreatic islets. Diabetes 1970; 19(suppl 1):406–408.

243. Prieto J, Fernandez-Ruiz V, Kawa MP, et al. Cells as vehicles for therapeutic genes to treat liver diseases. Gene Ther 2008; 15:765–771.

244. Munguia A, Ota T, Miest T, et al. Cell carriers to deliver oncolytic viruses to sites of myeloma tumor growth. Gene Ther 2008; 15:797–806.

245. Sprandel U. Temperature-induced shape transformation of carrier erythrocytes. Res Exp Med 1990; 190:267–275.

246. Ihler GM, Tsang HC. Erythrocyte carriers. Crit Rev Ther Drug Carrier Syst 1984; 1:155–187.

247. Magnani M, Rossi L, D'ascenzo M, et al. Erythrocyte engineering for drug delivery and targeting. Biotechnol Appl Biochem 1998; 28:1–6.

248. Hamidi M, Tajerzadeh H. Carrier Erythrocytes: an overview. Drug Deliv 2003; 10:9–20.

249. Magnani M, Rossi L, Fraternale A, et al. Erythrocyte-mediated delivery of drugs, peptides and modified oligonucleotides. Gene Ther 2002; 9:749–751.

250. Magnani M, ed. Erythrocyte engineering for drug delivery and targeting. Texas and New York: Landes Bioscience and Kulwer Academic/Plenum Publishers, 2003.

251. Millan CG, Marinero MLS, Castaneda AZ, et al. Drug, enzyme and peptide delivery using erythrocytes as carriers. J Control Release 2004; 95:27–49.

252. Jaitely V, Kanaujia P, Venkatesan N, et al. Resealed erythrocytes: drug carrier potentials and biomedical applications. Indian Drugs 1995; 33:589–594.

253. Hamidi M, Zarrin A, Foroozesh M, et al. Applications of carrier erythrocytes in delivery of biopharmaceuticals. J Control Release 2007; 118:145–160.

254. Benatti U, Zocchi E, Tonetti M, et al. Enhanced antitumor activity of adriamycin by encapsulation in mouse erythrocytes targeted to liver and lungs. Pharmacol Res 1989; 21(suppl 2):27–32.

255. Leu HJ, Wenner A, Spycher MA. Erythrocyte diapedesis in venous stasis syndrome. (Electron microscopic examinations). VASA 1981; 10:17–23.

256. Price RJ, Skyba DM, Kaul S, et al. Delivery of colloidal particles and red blood cells to tissue through microvessel ruptures created by targeted microbubble destruction with ultrasound. Circulation 1998; 98:1264–1267.

257. Sprandel U, Lanz DJ, von Horsten W. Magnetically responsive erythrocyte ghosts. Methods Enzymol 1987; 149:301–312.

258. Bax BE, Bain MD, Fairbank LD, et al. In vitro and in vivo studies with human carrier erythrocytes loaded with polyethylene glycol-conjugated and native adenosine deaminase. Br J Haematol 2000; 109:549–554.

259. Rossi L, Franchetti P, Pierige F, et al. Inhibition of HIV-1 replication in macrophages by a heterodinucleotide of lamivudine and tenofovir. J Antimicrob Chemother 2007; 59:666–675.

260. Fraternale A, Casabianca A, Rossi L, et al. Inhibition of murine AIDS by combination of AZT and DDCTP-loaded erythrocytes. In: Sprandel U, Way JL, eds. Erythrocytes as Drug Carriers in Medicine. New York: Plenum Press, 1997:73–80.

261. Deloach JR, Peters S, Pinkard O, et al. Effect of glutaraldehyde treatment on enzyme-loaded erythrocytes. Biochim Biophys Acta 1977; 496:507–515.

262. Jordan JA, Alvarez FJ, Lotero LA, et al. In vitro phagocytosis of carrier mouse red blood cells is increased by band 3 cross-linking or diamide treatment. Biotechnol Appl Biochem 2001; 34(pt 3):143–149.

263. Eichler HC, Gasic S, Daum B, et al. In vitro drug release from human carrier erythrocytes. Adv Biosci (Ser) 1987; 67:11–15.

264. Kitao T, Hattori K. Erythrocyte entrapment of daunomycin by amphotericin B without hemolysis. Cancer Res 1980; 40:1351–1353.

265. Billah MM, Finean JB, Coleman R, et al. Preparation of erythrocyte ghosts by a glycol-induced osmotic lysis under isoionic conditions. Biochim Biophys Acta 1976; 433:54–62.

266. Lin PS, Wallach DFH, Mikkelsen RB, et al. Action of halothane on human erythrocytes, mechanism of cell lysis and production of sealed ghosts. Biochim Biophys Acta 1975; 401: 73–82.

267. Gordon L, Milner AJ. Blood platelets as multifunctional cells. In: Gordon JL, ed. Platelets in Biology and Pathology. Amsterdam, The Netherlands: Elsevier/North-Holland Biomedical Press, 1976:3.

268. Weiss JM. Platelet physiology and abnormalities of platelet function (Part II). N Engl J Med 1975; 293:531.

269. Ahn YS, Byrnes JJ, Harrington WJ, et al. Treatment of idiopathic thrombocytopenia with vinblastine-loaded platelets. N Engl J Med 1978; 298:1001–1007.

270. Ahn YS, Harrington WJ, Byrnes JJ, et al. Treatment of autoimmune hemolytic anemia with vinca-loaded platelets. JAMA 1983; 249:2189–2194.

271. Penney NS, Ahn YS, McKinney EC. Sinus histiocytosis with massive lymphadenopathy. A case with unusual skin involvement and a therapeutic response to vinblastine-loaded platelets. Cancer 1982; 49:1994–1998.

272. Woo SY, Klappenbach RS, McCullars GM, et al. Familial erythrophagocytic lymphohistio-cytosis: treatment with vinblastine-loaded platelets. Cancer 1986:2566–2570.

273. Segal AW, Thakur ML, Arnot RN, et al. Indium-111-labelled leucocytes for localization of abscesses. Lancet 1976; 2:1056–1058.

274. Gainey MA, McDougall IR. Diagnosis of acute inflammatory conditions in children and adolescents using In 111 oxine white blood cells. Clin Nucl Med 1984; 9:71–74.

275. Sixou S, Teissie J. In vivo targeting of inflamed areas of eletroloaded neutrophils. Biochem Biophys Res Commun 1992; 186:860–862.

276. Sezaki H, Hashida M. Macromolecule-drug conjugate in targeted cancer chemotherapy. Crit Rev Ther Drug Carrier Syst 1984; 1:1–38.

277. Staros JV, Wright RW, Swingle DM. Enhancement by N-hydroxysulfosuccinimide of water-soluble carbodiimide-mediated coupling reactions. Anal Biochem 1986:220–222.

278. Kopecek J, Duncan R. Poly(N-(2-hydroxypropyl)methacrylamide) macromolecules as drug carrier systems. In: Illum L, Davis SS, eds. Polymers in Controlled Drug Delivery. Bristol, U.K.: Wright, 1987:152.

279. Lloyd JB. Soluble polymers as targetable drug carriers. In: Johnson P, Llyod JG, eds. Drug Delivery Systems Fundamental and Techniques. Chichester, U.K., and Weinheim, Germany: Ellis Horwood and VCH Verlagsgesellschaft, 1987:95.

280. Krishenbaum K, Zuckermann RN, Dill KA. Designing polymers that mimic biomolecules. Curr Opin Struct Biol 1999; 9:530–535.

281. Blakey DC. Drug targeting with monoclonal antibodies. A review. Acta Oncol 1992; 31:91–97.

282. Hellstrom KE, Hellstrom I, Goodman GE. Antibodies for drug delivery. In: Robinson JR, Lee VH, eds. Controlled Drug Delivery: Fundamental and Applications. New York: Marcel Dekker, 1987:623.

283. Sikora K. Monoclonal antibodies and drug targeting in cancer. In: Gregoriadis G, Poste G, eds. Targeting of Drugs Anatomical and Physiological Considerations. New York: Plenum Press, 1987:69.

284. Muzykantov VR, Christofidou-Solomidou M, Balyasnikova I, et al. Streptavidin facilitates internalization and pulmonary targeting of an anti-endothelial cell antibody (platelet-endothelial cell adhesion molecule 1): a strategy for vascular immunotargeting of drugs. Proc Natl Acad Sci U S A 1999; 96:2379–2384.

285. Arano Y, Fujioka Y, Akizawa H, et al. Chemical design of radiolabeled antibody fragments for low renal radioactivity levels. Cancer Res 1999; 59:128–134.

286. Tai A, Blair AH, Ghosh T. Tumor inhibition by chlorambucil covalently linked to antitumor globulin. Eur J Cancer Clin Oncol 1979; 15:1357–1363.

287. Ghose T, Tai J, Guclu A, et al. Inhibition of a mouse hepatoma by the alkylating agent trenimon linked to immunoglobulins. Cancer Immunol Immunother 1982; 13:185–189.

288. Pimm MV, Robins RA, Embleton MJ, et al. A bispecific monoclonal antibody against methotrexate and a human tumor associated antigen augments cytotoxicity of methotrexate-carrier conjugate. Br J Cancer 1990; 61:508–513.

289. Ghosh MK, Kildsig DO, Mitra AK. Preparation and characterization of methotrexate-immunoglobulin conjugates. Drug Des Deliv 1989; 4:13–25.

290. Ding L, Samuel J, MacLean GD, et al. Effective drug-antibody targeting using a novel monoclonal antibody against the proliferative compartment of mammalian squamous carcinomas. Cancer Immunol Immunother 1990; 32:105–109.

291. Hudecz F, Ross H, Price MR, et al. Immunoconjugate design: a predictive approach for coupling of daunomycin to monoclonal antibodies. Bioconjug Chem 1990; 1:197–204.

292. Frankel AE, Powell BL, Lilly MB. Diphtheria toxin conjugate therapy of cancer. In: Giaccone G, Schilsky R, Sondel P, eds. Cancer Chemotherapy and Biological Response Modifiers. Amsterdam, The Netherlands: Elsevier Science BV, 2002:301–314.

293. Raso V, Ritz J, Basala M, et al. Monoclonal antibody-ricin A chain conjugate selectively cytotoxic for cells bearing the common acute lymphoblastic leukemia antigen. Cancer Res 1982; 42:457–464.

294. Page M, Thibeault D, Noel C, et al. Coupling a preactivated daunorubicin derivative to antibody—a new approach. Anticancer Res 1990; 10:353–358.

295. Garnett MC. Targeted drug conjugates: principles and progress. Adv Drug Deliv Rev 2001; 53:171–216.

296. Ghose T, Blair AH. The design of cytotoxic agent-antibody conjugates. Crit Rev Ther Drug Carrier Syst 1987; 3:263–359.

297. Rowland GF, Simmonds RG, Corvalan JRF, et al. Monoclonal antibodies for targeted therapy with vindesine. In: Peters H, ed. Protides of the biological fluids. Proc Colloq 1983; 30:375.

298. Ojima I, Geng X, Wu X, et al. Tumor-specific novel taxoid-monoclonal antibody conjugates. J Med Chem 2002; 45:5620–5623.

299. Griffiths GL, Mattes MJ, Stein R, et al. Cure of SCID mice bearing human B-lymphoma xenografts by an anti-CD74 antibody-anthracycline drug conjugate. Clin Cancer Res 2003; 9:6567–65671.

300. Samokhin GP, Smirnov MD, Muzykantove VR, et al. Red blood cells targeting to collagen coated surfaces. FEBS Lett 1983; 154:257–261.

301. Urdal DL, Hakomori S. Tumor-associated ganglion-trisylceramide—target for antibody-dependent, avidin-mediated drug killing of tumor cells. J Biol Chem 1980; 255:509–516.

302. Lukyanov AN, Elbayoumi TA, Chanilam AR, et al. Tumor-targeted liposomes: doxorubicin-loaded long-circulating liposomes modified with anti-cancer antibody. J Control Release 2004; 100:135–144.

303. Eichler HG, Gasic S, Bauer K, et al. In vivo clearance of antibody-sensitized human drug carrier erythrocytes. Clin Pharmacol Ther 1986; 40:300–303.

304. Glukhova MA, Domogatsky SP, Kabakov AE, et al. Red blood cell targeting to smooth muscle cells. FEBS Lett 1986; 198:155–158.

305. Cao Y, Lam L. Bispecific antibody conjugates in therapeutics. Adv Drug Deliv Rev 2003; 55:171–195.

306. Peipp M, Valerius T. Bispecific antibodies targeting cancer cells. Biochem Soc Trans 2002; 30:507–511.

307. Trouet A, Campeneere DD, Burain R, et al. Desoxyribonucleic acid as carrier of antitumor drugs. In: Gregoriadis G, ed. Drug Carriers in Biology and Medicine. London, U.K.: Academic Press, 1979:87.

308. Trouet A. Carriers for bioactive materials. In: Kostelnik RJ, ed. Polymeric Delivery Systems. New York: Gordon & Breach, 1978:157.

309. Paul C, Lliemark J, Tidefelt U, et al. Pharmacokinetics of daunorubicin and doxorubicin in plasma and leukemic-cell from patients with acute nonlymphoblastic leukemia. Drug Monit 1989; 11:140–148.

310. Trouet A, Jadin JM, Hoof FV. Lysosomotropic chemotherapy in protozoal diseases. In: Biochemistry of Parasites and Host-Parasites Relationships. Amsterdam, The Netherlands: North-Holland, 1976:519.

311. Franssen EJ, Amsterdam RG, Visser J, et al. Low molecular weight proteins as carriers for renal drug targeting: naproxen–lysozyme. Pharm Res 1991; 8:1223–1230.

312. Maack T, Johnson V, Kau ST, et al. Renal filtration, transport and metabolism of low molecular weight proteins: a review. Kidney Int 1979; 16:251–270.

313. Kok RJ, Grijpstra F, Walthuis RB, et al. Specific delivery of captopril to the kidney with the prodrug captopril-lysozyme. J Pharmacol Exp Ther 1999; 288:281–285.

314. Qian ZM, Tang PL. Mechanisms of iron uptake by mammalian cells. Biochim Biophys Acta 1995; 1269:205–214.

315. Laske DW, Youle RJ, Oldfield EH. Tumor regression with regional distribution of the targeted toxin Tf-CRM107 in patients with malignant brain tumors. Nat Med 1997; 3:1362–1368.

316. Hagihara N, Walbridge S, Olson AW, et al. Vascular protection by chloroquine during brain tumor therapy with Tf-CRM107. Cancer Res 2000; 60:230–254.

317. Meijer DKF, Sluijs PVD. Covalent and noncovalent protein binding of drugs: implications for hepatic clearance, storage, and cell-specific drug delivery. Pharm Res 1989; 6:105–118.

318. Molema G, Jansen RW, Pauwels R, et al. Targeting of antiviral drugs to T4-lymphocytes anti-HIV activity of neoglycoprotein-AZTMP conjugates in vitro. Biochem Pharmacol 1990; 40:2603–2610.

319. Roche AC, Midoux P, Pimpancau V, et al. Endocytosis mediated by monocyte and macrophage membrane lectins—application to antiviral drug targeting. Res Virol 1990; 141:243–249.

320. Chu BCF, Whiteley JM. High molecular weight derivatives of methotrexate as chemotherapeutic agents. Mol Pharmacol 1977; 13:80–88.

321. Han JH, Oh YK, Kim DS, et al. Enhanced hepatocyte uptake and liver targeting of methotrexate using galactosylated albumin as a carrier. Int J Pharm 1999; 188:39–47.

322. Chu BCF, Whiteley JM. Control of solid tumor metastases with a high molecular weight derivative of methotrexate. J Natl Cancer Inst 1979; 62:79–82.

323. Whiteley JM, Nimec Z, Galivan J. Treatment of reuber H35 hepatoma cells with carrier bound methotrexate. Mol Pharmacol 1981; 19:505–508.

324. Beijaars L, Molema G, Weert B, et al. Albumin modified with mannose 6-phosphate: a potential carrier for selective delivery of antifibrotic drugs to rat and human hepatic stellate cells. Hepatology 1999; 29:1486–1493.

325. Fiume L, Busi C, Mattioli A. Targeting of antiviral drugs by coupling with protein carriers. FEBS Lett 1983; 153:6–10.

326. Swart PJ, Beijaars L, Kuipers ME, et al. Homing of negatively charged albumins to the lymphatic system—general implications for drug targeting to peripheral tissues and viral reservoirs. Biochem Pharmacol 1999; 58:1425–1435.

327. Varga JM, Asato N. Hormones as drug carriers. In: Targeted Drugs. New York: John Wiley & Sons, 1983:73.

328. Nechusthan A, Yarkoni S, Marianvsky I, et al. Adenocarcinoma cells are taregted by the new GnRH-PE66 chimeric toxin through specific gonadotropin-release hormone binding sites. J Biol Chem 1997; 272:11597–11603.

329. Schlick J, Dulieu P, Desvoyes B, et al. Cytotoxicity activity of a recombinant GnRH-PAP fusion toxin on human tumor cell lines. FEBS Lett 2004; 472:21–246.

330. Ross AD, Angaran DM. Colloids vs crystalloids—a continuing controversy. Drug Intell Clin Pharm 1984; 18:202–212.

331. Moleteni L. Dextran as drug carriers. In: Gregoriadis G, ed. Drug Carriers in Biology and Medicine. New York: Academic Press, 1979:25.

332. Schacht E. Polysaccharide macromolecules as drug carriers. In: Illum L, Davis SS, eds. Polymer in Controlled Drug Delivery. Bristol, U.K.: IOP Publishing, Wright, 1987:131.

333. Genta I, Perugini P, Pavanetto F, et al. Microparticulate drug delivery systems. EXS 1999; 87:305–313.

334. Matsumoto S, Arase Y, Takakura Y, et al. Plasma disposition and in vivo and in vitro antitumor activities of mitomycin C-dextran conjugate in relation to the mode of action. Chem Pharm Bull 1985; 33:2941–2947.

335. Schaschke N, Assfatglvlachleidt I, Machleidt W, et al. β-Cyclodextrin/epoxysuccinyl peptide conjugates: a new drug targeting system for tumor cells. Bioorg Med Chem Lett 2000; 10: 677–680.

336. Friend DR, Pangburn S. Rationale for targeted drug delivery. Med Res Rev 1987; 7:53–106.

337. Shen WC, Ryser HJP. Poly(L-lysine) and poly(D-lysine) conjugates of methotrexate— different inhibitory effect of drug resistant cells. Mol Pharmacol 1979; 16:614–622.

338. Chu BCF, Howell SB. Differential toxicity of carrier-bound methotrexate toward human lymphocytes, marrow and tumor cells. Biochem Pharmacol 1981; 30:2545–2552.

339. Zunino F, Savi G, Giuliani F, et al. Comparison of antitumor effects of daunorubicin covalently linked to poly-L-amino acid carriers. Eur J Cancer Clin Oncol 1984; 20:421–425.

340. Hurwitz E, Wilchek M, Pitha J. Soluble macromolecules as carriers for daunorubicin. J Appl Biochem 1980; 2:25–35.

341. Campbell P, Glover G, Gunn JM. Inhibition of intracellular protein degradation by pepstatinyl, poly(L-lysine), and pepstatinyl-poly(L-lysine). Arch Biochem Biophys 1980; 203:676–680.

342. Kopecek J. The potential of water-soluble polymeric carriers in targeted and site-specific drug delivery. J Control Release 1990; 11:279–290.

343. Vasey PA, Kaye SB, Morrison R, et al. Phase I clinical and pharmacokinetic study of PK1 (N-2-hydroxypropyl)methacrylamide copolymer doxorubicin: first member of a new class of chemotherapeutic agent-drug polymer conjugate. Clin Cancer Res 1999; 5:83–94.

344. Caiolfa VR, Zamai M, Fiorino A, et al. Polymer bound camptothecin: initial biodistribution and antitumor activity studies. J Control Release 2000; 65:105–119.

345. Merum Terwogt JM, Ten Bokkel Huinink WW, Shellens JH, et al. Phase I clinical and pharmacokinetic study of PNU 166945, a novel polymer-conjugated prodrug of paclitaxel. Anticancer Drugs 2001; 12:315–323.

346. Gianasi E, Wasil M, Evagorou EG, et al. HPMA copolymer platinates as novel antitumor agents: in vitro properties, pharmacokinetics, and antitumor activity. Eur J Cancer 1999; 3:994–1002.

347. Seymour LW, O'Hare K, Duncan R, et al. 1st order and 2nd order drug targeting and hepatic melanoma. Br J Cancer 1991; 63:833.

348. Kopecek J, Rihova B, Krinick NL. Targetable photoactivatable polymeric drugs. J Control Release 1991; 16:137–144.

349. Maeda H. SMANCS and polymer-conjugated macromolecular drugs: advantages in cancer chemotherapy. Adv Drug Deliv Rev 2001; 46:169–185.

350. Maeda H, Matsumura Y. New tactics and basic mechanisms of targeting chemotherapy in solid tumors. In: Kimura K, ed. Cancer Chemotherapy: Challenge for the Future. Tokyo, Japan: Excerpta Medical, 1989:42.

351. Matsumra Y, Kimura M, Yamamoto T, et al. Involvement of the kinin-generating cascade in enhanced vascular permeability in tumor tissue. Jpn J Cancer Res 1988; 79:1327–1334.
352. Konno T, Maeda H. Targeting chemotherapy of hepatocellular carcinoma: arterial administration of SMANCS/Lipiodol. In: Okada K, Ishak KG, eds. Neoplasm in the Liver. New York: Springer-Verlag, 1987:343.
353. Konno T, Maeda H. Targeting anticancer chemotherapy for primary and secondary liver cancer using arterially administered oily anticancer agents. In: Kimura K, ed. Cancer Chemotherapy: Challenges for the Future. Tokyo, Japan: Medica, 1987:287.
354. Greish K, Fang J, Inutsuka T, et al. Macromolecular therapeutics: advantages and prospects with special emphasis on solid tumour targeting. Clin Pharmacokinet 2003; 43:1089–1105.
355. Yamamoto H, Miki T, Oda T, et al. Reduced bone marrow toxicity of neocarzinostatin by conjugation with divinyl ether–maleic acid copolymer. Eur J Cancer 1990; 26:253–260.
356. Przybylski, Fell E, Ringsdorf H, et al. Pharmacologically active polymers. 17. Synthesis and characterization of polymeric derivatives of anti-tumor agent methotrexate. Makromol Chem Macromol Chem Phys 1978; 179:1719–1733.
357. Breslow DS, Edwards EI, Newburg NR. Divinyl ether-maleic anhydride (Pyran) copolymer used to demonstrate the effect of molecular weight on biological activity. Nature 1973; 246:160–162.
358. Oh DM, Han HK, Amidon GL. Drug transport and targeting. Intestinal transport. Pharm Biotechnol 1999; 12:59–88.
359. Jia W, Li H, Zhao L, et al. Gut microbiodata: a potential new territory for drug targeting. Nature Rev 2008; 7:123–129.
360. Lenaerts V, Gurny R, eds. Bioadhesive Drug Delivery Systems. Boca Raton: CRC Press, 1990.
361. Klokkers-Bethke K, Fischer W. Development of a multiple unit drug delivery system for positioned release in the gastrointestinal tract. J Control Release 1991; 15:105–112.
362. Alia J, Arora S, Ahuja A, et al. Formulation and development of hydrodynamically balanced system for metformin: in vitro and in vivo evaluation. Eur J Pharm Biopharm 2007; 67:196–291.
363. Rajanikanth PS, Mishra B. Floating in situ gelling system for stomach site-specific delivery of clarithromycin to eradicate H-pylori. J Control Release 2008; 125:33–41.
364. Coppi G, Lannuccelli V, Cameroni R. Polysaccharide in-coating process for freely swellable hydrogels. Pharm Dev Technol 1998; 3:347–353.
365. Patel AU, Shah T, Amin A. Therapeutic opportunities in colon-specific drug-delivery systems. Crit Rev Ther Drug Carrier Syst 2007; 24:147–202.
366. Patel GN, Patel GC, Patel RB, et al. Colon-specific delivery. Oral colon-specific drug delivery: an overview. Drug Deliv Technol 2006; 6:62–72.
367. Press AG, Hauptmann IA, Hauptmann L, et al. Gastrointestinal pH profiles in patients with inflammatory bowel disease. Aliment Pharmacol Ther Drug Monit 1988; 12:673–678.
368. Fallingborg J. Intraluminal pH of the human gastrointestinal tract. Dan Med Bull 1999; 46:183–196.
369. Nugent SG, Kumar D, Rampton DS, et al. Intestinal luminal pH in inflammatory bowel disease: possible determinants and implications for therapy with aminosalicylates and other drugs. Gut 2001; 48:571–577.
370. Fallingborg J, Christensen LA, Jacobson BA, et al. Very low intraluminal pH in patients with active ulcerative colitis. Dig Dis Sci 1993; 38:1989–1993.
371. Raimundo AH, Evans DF, Rogers J, et al. Gastrointestinal pH profiles in ulcerative colitis. Gastroenterology 1992; 104:A681.
372. Sinha VR, Kumria R. Microbially triggered drug delivery to the colon. Eur J Pharm Sci 2003; 18:3–18.
373. Saffran M, Kumar GS, Savariar C, et al. A new approach to the oral administration of insulin and other peptide drugs. Science 1986; 233:1081–1084.
374. Kakoulides EP, Smart JD, Tsibouklis J. Azocrosslinked poly(acrylic acid) for colonic delivery and adhesion specificity: in vitro degradation and preliminary ex vivo bioadhesion studies. J Control Release 1998; 54:95–109.

375. Kakoulides EP, Smart JD, Tsibouklis J. Azocross-linked poly(acrylic acid) for colonic delivery and adhesion specificity: synthesis and characterization. J Control Release 1998; 52:291–300.

376. Roldo M, Barbu E, Brown JF, et al. Orally administered, colon-specific mucoadhesive azopolymer particles for the treatment of inflammatory bowel disease: an in vivo study. J Biomed Mater Res 2006; 79A:706–715.

377. Roldo M, Barbu E, Brown JF, et al. Azo compounds in colon-specific drug delivery. Expert Opin Drug Deliv 2007; 4:547–560.

378. van den Mooter G, Offringa G, Kalala W, et al. Synthesis and evaluation of new linear azo-polymers for colonic targeting. STP Pharma Sci 1995; 5:36–40.

379. van den Mooter G, Samyn C, Kignet R. In vivo evaluation of a colon-specific drug delivery system: an absorption study of theophylline from capsules coated with azopolymers. Pharm Res 1995; 12:244–247.

380. Samyn C, Kalala W, van den Mooter G, et al. Synthesis and in vitro biodegradation of poly (ester-ester) azo polymers designed for colon targeting. Int J Pharm 1995; 121:211–216.

381. Sinha VR, Kumaria R. Polysaccharides in colon-specific drug delivery. Int J Pharm 2001; 224:19–38.

382. Bronsted BH, Kopecek J. Hydrogels for site-specific drug delivery to the colon: in vitro and in vivo degradation. Pharm Res 1992; 9:1540–1545.

383. Shanta K, Ravichandran P, Rao K. Azo polymeric hydrogels for colon targeted drug delivery. Biomaterials 1995; 16:1313–1318.

384. Liu ZL, Hu H, Zhuo RX. Konjac glucomannan-graft-acrylic acid hydrogels containing azo crosslinker for colon-specific delivery. J Pharm Sci 2004; 42:4370–4378.

385. Yin Y, Yang YJ, Xu H. Hydrophobically modified hydrogels containing azoaromatic crosslinks: swelling properties, degradation in vivo and application in drug delivery. Eur Polym J 2002; 38:2305–2311.

386. Sinha VR, Bhinge JR, Kumria R, et al. Development of pulsatile systems for targeted drug delivery of celecoxib for prophylaxis of colorectal cancer. Drug Deliv 2006; 13:221–225.

387. Stevens HNE, Wilson CG, Welling PG, et al. Evaluation of pulsincap (TM) to provide regional delivery of dofetilide to the human GI tract. Int J Pharm 2002; 236:27–34.

388. Mastiholimath VS, Dandagi PM, Jain SS, et al. Time and pH dependent colon specific, pulsatile delivery of theophylline for nocturnal asthma. Int J Pharm 2007; 328:49–56.

389. Minko T. Drug targeting to the colon with lectins and neoglycoconjugates. Adv Drug Deliv Rev 2004; 56:491–509.

390. Woodley JF. Lectins for gastrointestinal targeting—15 years on. J Drug Target 2000; 7:325–333.

391. Bridges JF, Woodley JF, Duncan R, et al. Soluble N-(2-hydroxypropyl) methacrylamide copolymers as a potential oral, controlled-release, drug delivery system. I. Bioadhesion to the rat intestine in vitro. Int J Pharm 1988; 44:213–223.

392. Ito R, Machida Y, Sannan T, et al. Magnetic granules—a novel system for specific drug delivery to esophageal mucosal in oral administration. Int J Pharm 1990; 61:109–117.

393. O'Hagan DT. The intestinal uptake of particles and the implications for drug and antigen delivery. J Anat 1996; 189:477–482.

394. Wachsmann D, Klein JP, Scholler M, et al. Local and systemic immune response to orally administered liposome soluble *s-mutans* cell wall antigens. Immunology 1985; 54:189–193.

395. O'Hagan DT, Palin K, Davis SS, et al. Microparticles as potentially orally active immunological adjuvants. Vaccine 1989; 7:421–424.

396. O'Hagan DT, Palin KJ, Davis SS. Poly(butyl-2-cyanoacrylate) particles as adjuvants for oral immunization. Vaccine 1989; 7:213–216.

397. O'Hagan DT, Rahman D, McGee JP, et al. Biodegradable microparticles as controlled release antigen delivery systems. Immunology 1989; 73:239–242.

398. Challacombe SJ, Rahman D, Jeffery H, et al. Enhanced secretory IgA and systemic IgC antibody responses after oral immunization with biodegradable microparticles containing antigen. Immunology 1992; 76:164–168.

399. O'Hagen DT, Rahman D, Jeffery H, et al. Controlled-release microparticles for oral immunization. Int J Pharm 1994; 108:133–139.

400. Florence AT. Issues in oral nanoparticle drug carrier uptake and targeting. J Drug Target 2004; 12:65–70.

401. Wigness BD, Dorman FD, Rhode TD, et al. The spring-driven implantable pump. A low-cost alternative. ASAIO J 1992; 38:M454–M457.

402. Buchwald H, Rhode TD. Implantable pumps. Recent progress and anticipated future advances. ASAIO J 1992; 38:772–778.

403. Salem JL, Micossi P, Dumm FL, et al. Clinical trial of programmable implantable insulin pump for type-I diabetes. Diabetes Care 1992; 15:877–885.

404. Salem JL, Charles MA. Devices for insulin administration. Diabetes Care 1990; 13:955–979.

405. Blackshear PJ, Rhode TD. Implantable infusion pumps for drug delivery in man: theoretical and practical considerations. Horiz Biochem Biophys 1989; 9:293–309.

406. Blackshear PJ. Implantable pumps for insulin delivery: current clinical status. In: Johnson P, Lloyd-Jones JG, eds. Drug Delivery Systems, Fundamentals and Techniques. Chichester, U.K.: Ellis Horwood, 1987:139.

407. Gallo JM, Sanzgiri Y, Howerth EW, et al. Serum, cerebrospinal fluid, and brain concentrations of a new zidovudine formulation following chronic administration via an implantable pump in dogs. J Pharm Sci 1992; 81:11.

408. Boorjian SA, Milowsky MI, Kaplan J, et al. Phase 1/2 clinical trial of interferon a2b and weekly liposome-encapsulated all-trans retinoic acid in patients with advanced renal cell carcinoma. J Immunother 2007; 30:655–662.

409. Molema G, Meijer DKF. Targeting of drugs to various blood cell types using (neo)glycoproteins, antibodies and other protein carriers. Adv Drug Deliv Rev 1994; 14:25–50.

10

New Imaging Methods for Dosage Form Characterization

Colin D. Melia
Formulation Insights Group in Drug Delivery, School of Pharmacy, The University of Nottingham, Nottingham, U.K.

Barry Crean
L.B.S.A. and Formulation Insights Group in Drug Delivery, School of Pharmacy, The University of Nottingham, Nottingham, U.K.

Samuel R. Pygall and Hywel D. Williams
Formulation Insights Group in Drug Delivery, School of Pharmacy, The University of Nottingham, Nottingham, U.K.

INTRODUCTION

In the past decades in vitro assessments of dosage form performance were undertaken almost exclusively through studies of drug release kinetics. In recent years however, we have seen the introduction of a range of imaging techniques that allow the pharmaceutical scientist to investigate drug release processes and to discern more clearly the dynamic events that contribute to the underlying drug release mechanisms. This complex area of pharmaceutical research is still in its infancy and few of these techniques are in widespread use, but within this chapter we aim to provide the reader with a brief introduction to illustrate the potential of some of these new approaches. There are new microscopic and spectroscopic techniques that can provide, for example, (*i*) a topological or three-dimensional (3D) internal characterization of dose form morphology, (*ii*) surface and internal chemical imaging, (*iii*) observations of the behavior of the whole dosage form or of individual components on a macro-, micro-, or nanoscale, and (*vi*) allow real-time monitoring of product quality during the manufacturing process. It is beyond the scope of this chapter to provide descriptions of all new methods that have been applied to characterize medicinal products in this way (a non-exhaustive summary is provided in Table 1), and for explanations of theory and instrumentation the reader is directed to more specialized and authoritative reviews. This chapter will focus on the potential of a few chosen techniques that are experiencing a growing kernel of pharmaceutical application, and which the authors believe have a high potential for enhancing our future understanding of the way dosage forms behave.

Table 1 A Selection of Imaging Techniques Applied to Pharmaceutical Dosage Forms

Method	Examples of application in the characterization of solid dosage forms	References
Optical techniques		
Optical imaging	Morphological studies, dissolution, swelling, coating integrity	
Fluorescence microscopies	Diffusion, dissolution, microenvironmental pH, bioadhesion, gel development in hydrophilic matrices, drug release processes, surface roughness in tablets and pellets	5–16
Spectroscopic methodologies		
Fourier transform infrared spectroscopy	Mapping of pharmaceutical components, drug dissolution, polymer swelling, drug degradation, molecular interactions	19–31
Near-infrared spectroscopy and imaging	Analysis of intact dosage forms (tablets, capsules, lyophilized products), processing monitoring and process control (tabletting, film coating, packaging).	32–36
Raman spectroscopy	API detection, Mapping of pharmaceutical components within dosage forms, quality control, chemical analysis, polymorphism, probing the size of nanosized and nanostructured materials	37–50
Terahertz pulsed spectroscopy and imaging	Characterization of crystalline behavior in drugs and materials, measurement of coating thickness and uniformity in tablets, structural imaging, and 3D chemical imaging	51–56
Nuclear and electron methodologies		
Nuclear magnetic resonance	Hydration kinetics and patterns in extended-release and immediate-release systems, drug release mechanisms and dissolution behavior, density mapping, formulation processes	62–93
Electron paramagnetic resonance	Free radical detection, dosage form microviscosity, micropolarity, microenvironmental pH, drug release mechanisms	94–103
Scanning and transmission electron microscopies	Morphological characterization of all types of materials and solid and semisolid dosage forms.	
Energy-dispersive X-ray microanalysis	Atomic composition of surfaces in pellets tablets etc.	
Surface analytical techniques		
Scanning near-field optical microscopy	Topographical imaging technique with resolution beyond the Abbé diffraction limit	104
Scanning thermal microscopy	Mapping surface domains with different thermal properties	105–108
Atomic force microscopy	Topographical morphology and adhesion forces dispersive surface energy, nanoindentation	111–132
X-ray photoelectron spectroscopy	Surface chemistry elucidation of atomic and chemical bonding composition in solid dosage forms	133–138

Table 1 A Selection of Imaging Techniques Applied to Pharmaceutical Dosage Forms (*Continued*)

Method	Examples of application in the characterization of solid dosage forms	References
Time-of-flight secondary ion mass spectrometry	Surface chemistry determination of pharmaceutical compound and systems by mass spectrometry	139–145
Other techniques		
X-ray microcomputed tomography	Internal structures such as density distribution maps in tablets, intragranular porosity, bone biomaterials	146–160

FLUORESCENCE MICROSCOPY TECHNIQUES

Fluorescence microscopy encompasses a family of related techniques that includes (*i*) fluorescence optical microscopy, (*ii*) confocal fluorescence and spinning disc techniques, (*iii*) multiphoton microscopy, (*iv*) total internal reflection fluorescence microscopy, (*v*) single-molecule fluorescence, (*vi*) single-channel opening events, (*vii*) fluorescence resonance energy transfer, (*viii*) high-speed exposures, (*ix*) two-photon imaging, and (*x*) fluorescence lifetime imaging (1). While fluorescence techniques are highly developed in cell biology applications, few have been utilized in the context of pharmaceutical dosage forms, and only confocal laser scanning microscopy (CLSM) has a significant presence in the literature (2).

CLSM combines the sensitivity, selectivity, and versatility of fluorescence quantification with a capability for high-resolution imaging, noninvasive optical sectioning, and 3D reconstructions. In contrast to the conventional fluorescence microscope, the CLSM uses rastered laser point illumination and a pinhole aperture in an optically conjugate plane in front of the detector to ensure out-of-focus signals contribute little to the image. These features markedly improve image quality and within optically transparent samples, "optical slicing" of the specimen is possible (3). An excellent review of the fundamentals underpinning confocal fluorescence techniques has been provided by White and Errington (4) and a recent review of the pharmaceutical applications of CLSM has been provided by Pygall et al. (2).

Fluorescent signals in dosage forms may arise from the natural autofluorescence of incorporated drugs and materials or from the addition of specific fluorophore markers, and the rapidity of CLSM image acquisition allows dynamic processes to be followed at high resolution. Cutts et al. (5) have used CLSM to explore the time-dependent depletion of the autofluorescent drug minocycline from commercial pellets of Minocin SR®. The biphasic pattern of drug depletion was fitted to a mathematical model, which provided both dissolution and diffusion kinetic parameters. The effectiveness of different subcoats in conferring acid resistance to enteric-coated pellets has been studied by Guo et al. (6), with CLSM imaging demonstrating marked differences in drug concentration within the coat, which could be related to subcoating composition and eventual performance of the dosage form. A method for quantitatively mapping the pattern of internal swelling within polymer matrices using fluorescent microspheres as nondiffusing markers, has been described by Adler et al. (7). The technique revealed a progressive wave of expansion moving from the exterior of a hydrating hydrophilic matrix and toward the core, and movements within the core as a result of stress relaxation.

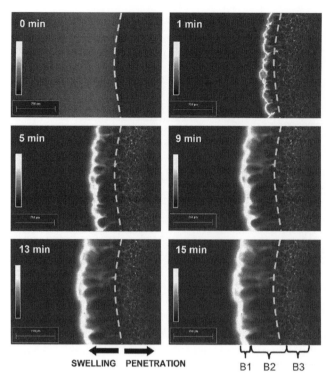

Figure 1 Confocal laser scanning microscopy. A time series of fluorescence images showing the pattern of hydration during the early stages of gel layer development in an HPMC hydrophilic matrix. The bright regions (high fluorescence) indicate regions of hydrated polymer highlighted by a penetrating cellulose-active fluorophore. The dotted line is the initial boundary of the dry matrix. B1 is a region of polymer disentanglement and dissolution at the matrix edge, B2 a region where columnar swelling of HPMC particles is forming the gel layer, and B3 is a network region of initial fluid penetration probably resulting from capillary ingress into tablet pores. Ex 488/Em >510 nm. Scale bar = 750 μm. Grayscale image ranging from pixel intensity 0 (*black*) to >256 (*white*). *Source*: From Ref. 8.

Bajwa et al. (8) have developed a real-time confocal fluorescence imaging method for examining the critical early stages of gel layer formation in hydroxypropyl methylcellulose (HPMC) matrices (Fig. 1). The images reveal the sequence of early gel layer formation and liquid ingress into the tablet network, formation of a coherent gel by outward columnar swelling of polymer particles, and eventual coalescence of the individual hydrating HPMC particles. In addition, the technique also demonstrated how increasing ionic strength suppressed gel layer growth, disrupted particle coalescence, thereby demonstrating the physical mechanisms by which salt-induced acceleration of drug release can occur.

Several studies have utilized CLSM techniques to study the distribution and release of biomolecules incorporated in microcapsules and microspheres and to measure the encapsulation efficiency (9,10). Lipophilic fluorophores have been utilized to locate oil-rich regions within mixed-phase microspheres and to examine the distribution of polymeric components with microcapsules. Encapsulated oil could be differentiated from other components, and other fluorescent markers allowed visualization of polymer distribution in the capsule wall (11). The technique has also been used to explore the relationship between drug release and drug distribution, in biodegradable poly(sebacic anhydride) microspheres containing three marker drugs with different hydrophobicity and water solubility. It was shown how preferential localization of water-soluble compounds at the microsphere surface prevented the development of extended-release properties, and the authors concluded that if a drug strongly redistributes within the solvent extraction cycle of manufacture, extended release might not be achievable (12).

The use of pH-responsive fluorophores to measure microenvironmental pH within pharmaceutical dose forms has been a particular focus of CLSM applications. The low pH microenvironment resulting from the hydrolysis of biodegradable polymers such as polylactic glycolic acid (PLGA) has been investigated using fluorescein (13). Fu et al. (14) have used entrapped dextran conjugates of pH-sensitive fluorophores to develop a ratiometric method for measuring changes in pH gradients in degrading PLGA microspheres. Li and Schwendeman (15) used this method to monitor the distribution and duration of neutral pH microclimates when acid neutralizers were incorporated in the microsphere. Cope et al. (16) have developed a ratiometric method using a single fluorophore for mapping the pH microenvironment in acid-modified extruded spheronized pellets. The method was sensitive over the range pH 2 to 6, and gave pH measurements to ± 0.1 units over the range pH 3.5 to 5.5. This range is suitable for the weak acids commonly incorporated as internal pH modifiers to accelerate release of weakly basic drugs, and it was demonstrated how the longevity of a low pH environment within the dosage form was a function of acid modifier solubility.

SPECTROSCOPIC TECHNIQUES

There has been a surge of interest in the characterization of pharmaceutical dosage forms using spectroscopic imaging techniques. Such methods offer advantages of molecular level characterization, molecular specificity, and noninvasive, nondestructive, component imaging of ingredients and microbehavior. Improved instrumentation and data-processing speeds now allow spectral information to be collected on an individual pixel basis. Listed below are pertinent examples that illustrate recent pharmaceutical imaging applications of Fourier transform infrared (FTIR) spectroscopy, Raman spectroscopy, near-infrared (NIR) spectroscopy, and terahertz pulsed spectroscopy (TPS).

Fourier Transform Infrared Spectroscopy Imaging

FTIR spectroscopy exploits infrared (IR) absorption in the mid-IR (400–4000 cm^{-1}) region and provides information on the molecular chemistry of materials and interactions (17). IR spectra in this region arise from molecular motions within a chemical bond, and a comprehensive review of the pharmaceutical applications of FTIR can be found elsewhere (18).

FTIR, in imaging mode, can be used to map sample surfaces nondestructively, at normal temperature and pressures, and in dry and wet samples. As the methodology relies on the characteristic absorbance of molecular vibrations in the sample, there is no requirement for dyes or labeling methods to aid visualization. Recent applications of FTIR imaging have included spatial and temporal maps of spectral changes during, for example, drug release from semisolid polyethylene glycol (PEG) and polyethylene oxide (PEO) formulations (19,20), diffusion in polymer films for transdermal delivery (21,22), drug solvent and drug macromolecule interactions (23,24), and drug penetration into transdermal acceptor systems, both artificial (21) and stratum corneum (25,26). In a series of papers, Kazarian and coworkers have exploited FTIR imaging to obtain chemical images that differentiate excipients in tablets (27). They have imaged hydrating matrix tablets (28) by compacting the tablet directly onto the attenuated total reflectance (ATR) crystal and, using a flow-through dissolution apparatus, correlated drug release with quantitative changes in drug, polymer, and water distribution (28). Concentration gradients and the composition of released particles have been identified (29). In a solid PEG melt dispersion, molecularly dispersed ibuprofen could be distinguished from crystalline phase–separated drug ibuprofen (20). These workers also examined the influence of moisture and compression pressure on the density and component distribution of compacted pharmaceutical tablets (30) and suggested this method as a high-throughput method of investigating changes during stress storage testing (31).

Near-Infrared Spectroscopy Imaging

The NIR region ($\sim$700–2500 nm) is located between the visible and mid-IR, and absorbance bands in this region originate primarily from the overtones of stretching vibrations of OH, CH, NH, and SH groups. NIR imaging has the important advantage of allowing direct analysis of solid samples or products without the need for specialized cells or prior preparation, and measurements can be taken rapidly and easily in air, without the need for close contact. These properties make NIR spectroscopy and imaging suitable for real-time in-process control during manufacturing processes, and this is being developed as a major application. Disadvantages of NIR include a high detection threshold (rendering it unsuitable for trace analysis) and the inherent complexity of the spectra, which include components from different vibrational energy levels, overtones, and combination bands. As a result, given suitable calibration, chemometric analysis, and validation, NIR spectra can be used to quantify individual components within a mixture, even though the molecular origin of individual absorbance bands can be difficult to identify.

NIR spectroscopy has been used for compositional analysis of a wide variety of dosage forms and has seen applications from powders to packaging (32). Imaging has allowed NIR to come to the forefront as a Process Analytical Technology (PAT) tool. Several tablet manufacture studies have described how NIR can be used for the online prediction of tablet hardness, content uniformity, and the effects of varying compression force (33–35). An example of NIR image illustrating the distribution of a drug in a tablet is shown in Figure 2. A study by Clarke (36) clearly illustrates how NIR chemical images can be used to map the distribution of different components within a tablet formulation, and has demonstrated how the cluster size of disintegrant particles within a tablet can be related to compression force and changing tablet dissolution characteristics.

Raman Spectroscopy and Imaging

Raman spectroscopy (spectral range 100–4000 cm^{-1}) also probes molecular vibrational transitions and provides information that is, in many ways, complementary to FTIR spectroscopy. Raman spectra are obtained by focusing monochromatic radiation onto the sample and determining scattered light as a function of frequency. Most light is scattered at the same wave number (Rayleigh scattering), but some light is scattered at slightly higher (anti-Stokes scattering) and lower (Stokes scattering) wave numbers. The spectrum is characteristic of the type and coordination of the molecules involved in the scattering process, and like IR spectroscopy, it provides a "molecular fingerprint" of the chemical species of interest (37). Raman spectra can be collected using dispersive or Fourier transform (FT–Raman) instruments, the choice depending on the sample being examined. In addition, confocal Raman microscopy is available where Raman signals collected through

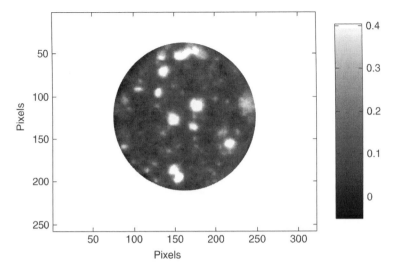

Figure 2 NIR imaging. A 2D NIR map illustrating the distribution (and aggregation) of drug particles within the surface of a compressed tablet. The image was taken in air and without sample preparation. Grayscale intensity from white (highest) to black (lowest). *Source*: Image courtesy of Professor Peter Timmins, Bristol-Myers Squibb, Moreton, U.K.

confocal optics eliminate Raman signals above and below the point of focus and, therefore, can be used spatially to probe below a sample surface, at micron-scale resolution.

The theory of Raman spectroscopy and its applications to quantitative pharmaceutical analysis are reviewed elsewhere (18,38). As a spectroscopic tool, Raman is a rapid and nondestructive technique. Spectra can be recorded directly inside packaging without interference (39), and it is possible to quantify active pharmaceutical ingredients and excipients in a variety of pharmaceutical formulations. Recently, there has been significant improvement of Raman spectrometers with cheaper lasers, better notch filters, and more sensitive detectors, allowing better detection of the weak Raman signals (40). These and other technical improvements such as fiber-optic sample probes and compact optical designs have corresponded with a significant increase in literature reporting the quantitative analysis of pharmaceutical products (41) and materials (27). Raman spectroscopy may also be used to investigate aqueous pharmaceutical formulations (such as solutions and suspensions) as water has a relatively weak Raman signal (42–44).

Recent years have seen the development of Raman techniques to image and map pharmaceutical dosage forms, in particular the spatial distribution of the constituents from characteristic Raman spectral features (45). Line or point mapping can be used and the issue of long acquisition times can be overcome through the use of multivariate analysis to remove noise from the acquired Raman maps (46–48). Drug substances often exhibit strong Raman scattering, in contrast to most other excipients used in tablet formulations, and Raman mapping can therefore be used to analyze drug distributions in dosage forms containing low drug concentrations (0.5% w/w). One study showed how the domain size of incorporated drug could be related to the particle size distribution of the raw drug material, making Raman maps good indicators of the source of active pharmaceutical ingredients used in tablet manufacturing. Multivariate analysis can be performed to simultaneously check for the presence of undesirable drug polymorphs (49). Other examples show Raman line mapping used for rapid analysis of bead formulations (47) and to quantitatively determine the spatial distribution of polymer in alginate beads (50).

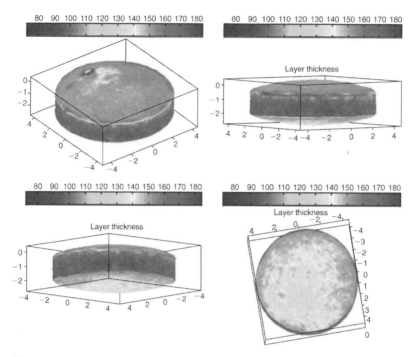

Figure 3 Terahertz imaging of tablet coating thickness. These 3D images illustrate the variability in coating thickness around a film-coated tablet and show how the coating was thinner on the upper and lower axial surfaces than on the radial surface of the tablet. The original illustration was color coded to highlight the variations in evenness of coating, and some of these can also be seen in this grayscale interpretation. The scales in the *x*, *y*, and *z* directions are in millimeter. *Source*: From Ref. 55.

Terahertz Pulsed Spectroscopy and Imaging

TPS and terahertz pulsed imaging (TPI) have only recently been applied to the physical characterization of pharmaceutical materials and dosage forms. Terahertz radiation lies in the far IR, in the range 60 GHz to 4 THz (51), and spectroscopic interrogation of this region has recently become possible through advances in detectors and laser sources (52). Terahertz radiation is of particular interest as it excites intermolecular interactions, librational and vibrational modes, as well as probing weak interactions between molecules. Reviews of terahertz technology and potential pharmaceutical applications have been provided by Pickwell and Wallace (53) and Zeitler et al. (51). TPS has been used to explore crystal structure, solvates, and polymorphism in pharmaceutical actives and excipients (38,51). An early application of TPI has been tablet coatings, where the semitransparency of many excipients to terahertz radiation allows delineation of surfaces with different refractive indices. This has enabled detailed cross-sectional information on the thickness, uniformity, quality, and structure of the tablet coat to be acquired nondestructively (51,54,55) (Fig. 3). A capability for 2D and 3D chemical mapping and the detection of buried interfaces (51) provide clear potential for future PAT applications where, as terahertz radiation is penetrating but nonionizing, TPI has been advanced as a safer alternative to X-ray tomography (56).

RESONANCE TECHNIQUES

Nuclear magnetic resonance (NMR) imaging [or magnetic resonance imaging (MRI)] and electron paramagnetic resonance (EPR) [or electron spin resonance (ESR)] utilize electromagnetic radiation emitted from magnetic species (^{1}H, ^{13}C, ^{19}F, ^{31}P nuclei or free radical probes) resonating in an external magnetic field. In the imaging modality, the intensity of this radiation is used to quantify and map the spatial distribution of these entities, and, in addition, spin-lattice (T_1) and spin-spin (T_2) relaxation times can provide insights into the local chemical and molecular environment. In the case of EPR, paramagnetic probes are introduced into the sample, and changes in the spectral shape can be interpreted to provide similar information. In both cases, advanced processing of the acquired data allows generation of 2D and 3D maps. The theoretical background of NMR and EPR imaging (57,58) and reviews of their application to pharmaceutical drug delivery systems can be found elsewhere (59–61). The principal attraction of these techniques is that they can provide noninvasive and nondestructive internal images of events inside a dosage form or living system. The limitations include a trade-off between acquisition time and resolution and image distortion artifacts, which can occur, for example, at water-air and water-solid interfaces (62,63).

Nuclear Magnetic Resonance Imaging

Extended-Release Dosage Forms

^{1}H NMR imaging has been used to investigate the role of water in dosage form behavior (59,60), and a particular focus has been internal patterns of hydration in extended-release systems. Hydrophilic matrices were an obvious target for early studies as their surface-hydrated polymer diffusion barrier is critical to their ability to maintain extended release. NMR imaging has been used to compare gel layer growth, core dimensions (64), and the measure water self-diffusion coefficient (SDC) gradients within the gel (65). The polymer concentration gradient within the gel layer has been estimated by calibrating T_1 and T_2 against standard solutions (66), and many formulation and polymer variables have been compared (67). Tritt-Goc et al. modeled water diffusion in the gel layer from SDC gradient data and examined the influence of molecular weight, ionic strength, and an incorporated tetracycline on SDC (68–70). ^{19}F NMR imaging of triflupromazine and 5-fluorouracil has been used to investigate drug transport in HPMC matrices (71) and diffusion in thermally responsive hydrogels (72). Internal mapping of water distribution has been used to examine hydration patterns in a wide variety of other extended-release devices. These include osmotic pumps (73), compression-coated tablets (74), pulsed-release capsules (75) (Fig. 4), biodegradable PLA/PLGA scaffolds (76,77), compressed inert polymethacrylate matrices (78), cross-linked high-amylose starch hydrogels, (79,80), and stimuli-responsive polymers (81). Marshall et al. (82) have used NMR imaging in conjunction with confocal microscopy to examine water and polymer concentration gradients within a developing bioadhesive bond and Dahlberg et al. (83) have recently described a method by which a hydrated polymer carrier can be imaged directly. Mikac et al. (84) have described how current density imaging can be used to map ionic species released from matrix tablets. Benchtop MRI instrumentation is now available, with lower capital and running costs than the full-scale instruments with superconducting magnets, and Strübing and coworkers (85) have acquired useful images of the swelling and internal behavior of floating matrices using this type of instrument.

Other Pharmaceutical Applications

The literature reports NMR imaging techniques being utilized in a range of other pharmaceutical applications. Often these are isolated studies, but they provide important illustrations of the potential of these techniques. For example, density distributions in

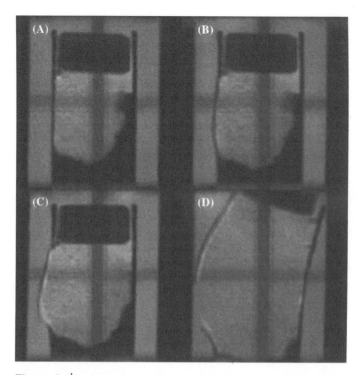

Figure 4 ^{1}H NMR microscopy images of disintegration mechanisms in a chronopharmaceutical capsule. Hydrated regions appear gray, whereas the capsule shell and unhydrated plug appear black. Sagittal planar images through the capsule after (**A**) 7 minutes, (**B**) 10 minutes, (**C**) 15 minutes, and (**D**) 28 minutes hydration illustrate how water penetrating the capsule/plug seal resulted in internal swelling and a dramatic splitting of the capsule shell, in this experimental formulation. A simple change in capsule coating subsequently obviated this problem. *Source*: From Ref. 75.

tablets, as a function of tablet shape, compression force, and lubrication have been examined by impregnating tablets with an oil-based NMR contrast medium (63,86). The disintegration of immediate-release tablets has been captured by FLASH (fast low angle shot) imaging and this has been used to compare the disintegration of commercial paracetamol tablets (87) and PEG matrices (88). The water distribution in pellet extrudates for subsequent spheronization has been examined in relation to extrusion conditions (89), and powder segregation and mixing patterns during blending have been visualized (90). Where NMR imaging does not provide the information required, an alternative option is to relate NMR measurements to imaging other types of microscopy. For example, the release of different components of a tablet polymer film coat has been followed by ^{1}H-NMR spectroscopy and related to film morphology through environmental scanning electron microscopy (ESEM) micrographs (91).

A significant future direction for NMR imaging is the assessment of dosage form behavior during in vitro dissolution testing. In an early study, Fyfe et al. (92) used a modified Sotax USP apparatus 4 within an NMR magnet to compare matrices imaged under static and flow-through conditions. Flow-through rate was shown to have significant effects on an osmotic pump and an erosion-based compressed matrix (Fig. 5). An alternative rotating disc apparatus has been designed, which mimics the hydrodynamics of dissolution testing by permitting tablet rotation at any speed, under temperature control, and sink conditions within the NMR spectrometer (93).

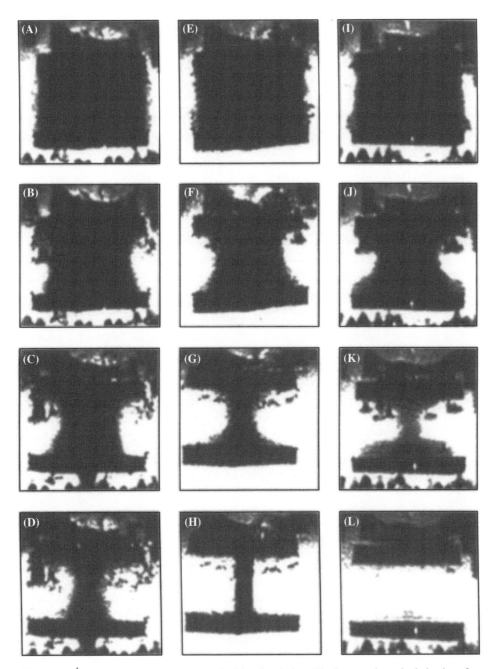

Figure 5 ¹H NMR microscopy images of tablet dissolution. The images show the behavior of an erodible matrix containing an internal scaffold, within a flow-through dissolution cell. Images **A–D** were obtained under static conditions, images **E–H** and **I–L** were obtained at 4 and 16 mL/min flow, respectively. The rows represent images taken at 0.5, 3, 6, and 10.5 hours. The full width of the image is equivalent to 16 mm in the sample. *Source*: From Ref. 92.

Electron Paramagnetic Resonance

EPR has been less widely used for dosage form characterization, but possesses some potential advantages over NMR. The greater magnetic moment exhibited by electrons requires a higher electromagnetic frequency to induce a state of resonance, and as a result, output signals are shifted from the radio to the microwave region, which results in superior signal-to-noise ratios. This feature permits introduced magnetic probes (spin probes) to be detected at low concentrations, which allows for diversity in their physiochemical properties. This introduces the potential for the spin probe to mimic drug compounds (61). An EPR approach can also retrieve information about a dosage internal environment. For example, spin probes can be chosen to explore microviscosity, micropolarity, pH, and probe concentration, in addition to mapping their spatial distribution within the sample (61).

An early application of EPR to pharmaceuticals was in the detection of free radicals after irradiation sterilization of sterile products (94–96). However Mäder et al. (97) have also highlighted the potential of EPR for noninvasively probing the internal micro-environment of drug delivery systems, both in vitro and in vivo. There have been EPR spectroscopic investigations of, for example, drug-induced changes in the microstructure of proteinaceous (98) and hydrophilic matrices (99), and EPR spectroscopy has been combined with NMR imaging, to provide information on microenvironmental pH and mobility in biodegradable polyanhydrides (97). EPR imaging has been used to map changes in microenvironmental pH and microviscosity, during hydrolytic degradation of poly orthoesters (100) and in matrix systems containing acidifying agents (101). Kroll et al. (102) have used EPR imaging to map the changing microacidity in the skin after application of acidic agents such as salicylic acid in topical creams and emulsions. In the future, we are likely to see more efficient EPR imaging tools, and high-resolution 2D and 3D imaging techniques are already under development (103).

SURFACE ANALYTICAL TECHNIQUES

Scanning Probe Microscopies

Scanning probe microscopes (SPMs) are a group of powerful, surface-sensitive instruments, which, when used complementarily with traditional analytical techniques, can provide detailed nanoscale information of raw ingredients and medicinal products. SPMs use a fine probe tip to sense the surface of a sample and obtain topographical or localized force surface profiles. Atomic force microscopy (AFM) has been the most widely used in pharmaceutical research, but scanning near-field optical microscopy (SNOM) (104) and scanning thermal microscopy (SThM) (105–108) have considerable future potential for light and thermal surface profiling of pharmaceutical samples. For example, Sanders et al. (106) have used SThM for localized thermal analysis to differentiate different polymorphic forms of cimetidine.

Atomic Force Microscopy

AFM has a resolution in the micrometer to sub-nanometer range and a theoretical force sensitivity of 10^{-15} N. Comprehensive reviews of the AFM technique are available in the literature (109,110), but the fundamental principle is of a finely tipped apex (hereinafter probe) attached to the end of a flexible cantilever, which is rastered across a substrate surface, the topography of which is described by cantilever deflection measured through a laser optical lever. Topographical images of substrate surfaces can be obtained in "tapping mode," where the cantilever oscillates at its resonant frequency, or in "contact mode," where the probe scans over the surface under a constant load (109). AFM has been used to visualize the topography of pharmaceutical materials at the nanoscale and assess their impact on medicinal product and pharmaceutical process performance (111,112). For example, tapping-mode AFM imaging has been used to visually discriminate cimetidine polymorphs in single crystals (111) and to observe the recrystallization of spray-dried amorphous lactose at high humidities (112). The ability of AFM to undertake measurements under liquid has allowed the kinetic process of surface dissolution in soluble crystalline substances to be visualized in real time and on different crystal faces (113,114).

AFM can also be used to measure surface and interfacial forces and provide information on localized material properties through indentation measurements (115). The probe-substrate interaction force is measured by the cantilever deflection as the probe approaches, contacts and then retracts from the surface. The compliance region of the force/distance curves, in which the probe indents the sample surface, may be usefully used to describe the contact mechanics of the sample (107,116,117). For instance, Ward et al. (107) have made nanomechanical measurements on sorbitol particles, and could distinguish amorphous and crystalline domains through Young's modulus values. Probe-sample adhesion can be calculated using Hooke's law, from the displacement hysteresis as the probe is withdrawn from the surface. This can be used for example to measure particle-particle interactions (118–121), to investigate the effects of humidity changes (122–124), to quantify surface free energy values (125–130), and to construct cohesive-adhesive balances (129,130). Practical applications include the design of products for inhalation therapy, where particle-particle force measurements can be used to screen formulations for adequate drug detachment from carrier particles or to screen inhalation packaging surfaces, through measurements of adhesion and friction forces between drug particles and polymer-coated canisters (131,132). Young et al. (122) have used AFM to compare the influence of humidity on the aerosolization of salbutamol sulfate, in the micronized and SEDS (solution-enhanced dispersion by supercritical fluids) form.

X-Ray Photoelectron Spectroscopy

X-ray photoelectron spectroscopy (XPS or ESCA) is a surface-specific technique for the quantitative determination of surface elemental and chemical composition. In principle, X-ray irradiation of the sample releases core-level photoelectrons, the energy of which is characteristic of the element and chemical bonding of the element from which photoelectron originated. XPS has been used to characterize the surfaces of implant systems (133), biodegradable microparticles (134,135), and to determine drug encapsulation efficiency in nanoparticles (136). Cook et al. (137) have used XPS to characterize the surface of a peptide-modified poly(lactic acid-*co*-lysine) in relation to its use as a biocompatible material to control cell behavior. The literature reports very few pharmaceutical applications of imaging XPS. However, recent advances in lateral resolution, sensitivity, and compensation for topographical signal intensity have demonstrated its potential (138).

Time-of-Flight Secondary Ion Mass Spectrometry

Time-of-flight secondary ion mass spectrometry (ToF-SIMS) uses a pulsed (<1 ns) primary ion beam to ionize a sample surface, and the emitted secondary ions are then analyzed by time of flight (which is a function of their mass to charge ratio) in a mass spectrometer. There are three different modalities of ToF-SIMS analysis: (*i*) mass spectra, which are used to determine the elemental and molecular species present, (*ii*) imaging, which provides a visual map of distribution of individual species on the surface, and (*iii*) depth profiling, which is used to determine the distribution of chemical species as a function of depth.

In the imaging modality, a ToF-SIMS image is generated by rastering a finely focused ion beam across the sample surface. Each pixel in the image provides a mass spectrum, which is then used to determine the composition and spatial distribution of sample surface constituents. Pharmaceutical applications have included surface characterization of multi-particulate controlled-release systems (139), the quantification of drug concentration and polymer degradation in drug-polymer blends (140), and the physicochemical organization of biodegradable polymer blends (141). A good illustration of chemical imaging of component distribution in a solid dosage form has been provided by Luk et al. (142).

Providing a comprehensive characterization of pharmaceutical dosage forms requires a multi-instrumental approach as no single surface analytical technique can ascertain both the chemical and morphological nature of the surfaces. To this end, SPM, XPS, and ToF-SIMS have been used as complementary techniques with which to characterize the surface nature of dosage forms (141,143–145).

TOMOGRAPHY

X-Ray Microcomputed Tomography

X-ray microcomputed tomography (XMCT or MicroCT) has relatively recently been developed for the imaging of pharmaceutical materials, granules, and solid dosage forms (146–149). It is a powerful tool for the noninvasive and 3D investigations of internal structure (150–153). The sample is rotated between a high-intensity collimated X-ray beam and a detector that measures the intensity of the transmitted X rays. These 2D "shadow" images of the object, obtained at different angles of rotation, are then reconstructed to produce a 3D map of the relative atomic density within the sample, using a Feldkamp algorithm (150, 152–156). The intensity of X rays reaching the detector is a function of the intensity of the incident radiation, the sample path length, and the X-ray linear attenuation coefficient of the intervening sample material. A longer sample path length and a greater material coefficient of attenuation lead to the detection of weakened radiation intensity owing to a greater number of diffraction and scattering events. These varying levels of signal intensity provide the contrast in the grayscale images, which, for example, can be used for calculations of sample density, volume, morphology, porosity, and pore-size distribution.

It can be anticipated that XMCT will see widespread use in probing the internal structure of solid pharmaceuticals. Recent examples in tablets have included studies of compaction process conditions (157), the mapping of tablet density and porosity (146,158), changes in structure on hydration (159) (Fig. 6), and the detection of internal fractures (160). XMCT also has the potential to provide a powerful tool for process optimization and root cause analysis in formulation development.

CONCLUSIONS

This chapter provides a short introduction of how modern imaging techniques have been applied to the characterization of pharmaceutical systems. The rapid advances in instrumentation and data processing will increasingly provide pharmaceutical scientists

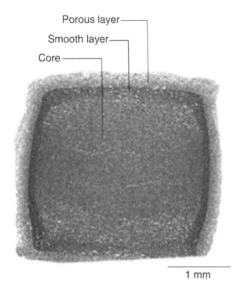

Figure 6 X-ray microcomputed tomography. An axial cross-section through a freeze-dried 15-minute swollen high-amylose starch pellet, in which variations in X-ray attenuation provide evidence of an outer surface membrane. The pellet size is 3.0 (height) × 3.3 (width). The membrane thickness is 300 μm on the right and left edges (at mid height) and 450 μm at the top and bottom sides of the pellet. The smooth layer ranges from 130 μm on the right and left edges to 200 μm on the top and bottom sides. *Source*: From Ref. 159.

with new opportunities to gain unrivalled information on many aspects of pharmaceutical dosage forms. This will include the physical and chemical attributes of dosage forms and materials, a greater understanding of composition, structure, and complexity of behavior, and an ability to assess in far greater detail the consequences of manufacturing process variables. This new knowledge will increasingly contribute to the development of optimized products and processes through understanding and design. As these techniques become increasingly sophisticated, and more fully exploited, a new age of pharmaceutical technology may emerge in which new dosage forms are developed from a position of fundamental understanding underpinned by high-resolution characterization of their complex behavior.

ACKNOWLEDGMENTS

The authors gratefully acknowledge the help, support, and advice of Prof. Peter Timmins, (Bristol-Myers Squibb, Moreton, U.K.), Prof. Karsten Mäder (Martin-Luther-University, Halle-Wittenberg, Germany), Dr. Chris Sammon (Sheffield Hallam University, Sheffield, U.K.), Prof. Martyn Davies, and Prof. Richard Bowtell (The University of Nottingham, Nottingham, U.K.) in the preparation of this chapter.

REFERENCES

1. Gumbleton M, Stephens DJ. Coming out of the dark: the evolving role of fluorescence imaging in drug delivery research. Adv Drug Deliv Rev 2005; 57(1):5–15.
2. Pygall SR, Whetstone J, Timmins P, et al. Pharmaceutical applications of confocal laser scanning microscopy: the physical characterisation of pharmaceutical systems. Adv Drug Deliv Rev 2007; 59(14):1434–1452.

3. Minsky M. Memoir in inventing the confocal scanning microscope. Scanning 1988; 10:128–138.
4. White NS, Errington RJ. Fluorescence techniques for drug delivery research: theory and practice. Adv Drug Deliv Rev 2005; 57(1):17–42.
5. Cutts LS, Hibberd S, Adler J, et al. Characterising drug release processes within controlled release dosage forms using the confocal laser scanning microscope. J Control Release 1996; 42(2):115–124.
6. Guo HX, Heinamaki J, Yliruusi J. Amylopectin as a subcoating material improves the acidic resistance of enteric-coated pellets containing a freely soluble drug. Int J Pharm 2002; 235(1–2): 79–86.
7. Adler J, Jayan A, Melia CD. A method for quantifying differential expansion within hydrating hydrophilic matrixes by tracking embedded fluorescent microspheres. J Pharm Sci 1999; 88(3): 371–377.
8. Bajwa GS, Hoebler K, Sammon C, et al. Microstructural imaging of early gel layer formation in HPMC matrices. J Pharm Sci 2006; 95(10):2145–2157.
9. Determan AS, Trewyn BG, Lin VSY, et al. Encapsulation, stabilization, and release of BSA-FITC from polyanhydride microspheres. J Control Release 2004; 100(1):97–109.
10. Volodkin DV, Petrov AI, Prevot M, et al. Matrix polyelectrolyte microcapsules: new system for macromolecule encapsulation. Langmuir 2004; 20(8):3398–3406.
11. Lamprecht A, Schäfer UF, Lehr CM. Visualization and quantification of polymer distribution in microcapsules by confocal laser scanning microscopy (CLSM). Int J Pharm 2000; 196(2): 223–226.
12. Berkland C, Kipper MJ, Narasimhan B, et al. Microsphere size, precipitation kinetics and drug distribution control drug release from biodegradable polyanhydride microspheres. J Control Release 2004; 94(1):129–141.
13. Shenderova A, Burke TG, Schwendeman SP. The acidic microclimate in poly(lactide-co-glycolide) microspheres stabilizes camptothecins. Pharm Res 1999; 16(2):241–248.
14. Fu K, Pack DW, Klibanov AM, et al. Visual evidence of acidic environment within degrading poly(lactic-co-glycolic acid) (PLGA) microspheres. Pharm Res 2000; 17(1):100–106.
15. Li L, Schwendeman SP. Mapping neutral microclimate pH in PLGA microspheres. J Control Release 2005; 101(1–3):163–173.
16. Cope SJ, Hibberd S, Whetstone J, et al. Measurement and mapping of pH in hydrating pharmaceutical pellets using confocal laser scanning microscopy. Pharm Res 2002; 19(10): 1554–1563.
17. Bugay DE. Characterization of the solid-state: spectroscopic techniques. Adv Drug Deliv Rev 2001; 48(1):43–65.
18. Wartewig S, Neubert RHH. Pharmaceutical applications of Mid-IR and Raman spectroscopy. Adv Drug Deliv Rev 2005; 57(8):1144–1170.
19. Coutts-Lendon CA, Wright NA, Mieso EV, et al. The use of FT-IR imaging as an analytical tool for the characterization of drug delivery systems. J Control Release 2003; 93(3):223–248.
20. Kazarian SG, Chan KLA. "Chemical Photography" of drug release. Macromolecules 2003; 36(26):9866–9872.
21. Bobiak JP, Koenig JL. Regions of interest in FTIR imaging applications: diffusion of nicotine into ethylene-co-vinyl acetate films. J Control Release 2005; 106(3):329–338.
22. Rafferty DW, Koenig JL. FTIR imaging for the characterization of controlled-release drug delivery applications. J Control Release 2002; 83(1):29–39.
23. Gaudreau S, Neault JF, Tajmir-Riahi HA. Interaction of AZT with human serum albumin studied by capillary electrophoresis, FTIR and CD spectroscopic methods. J Biomol Struct Dyn 2002; 19(6):1007–1014.
24. Neault JF, Benkirane A, Malonga H, et al. Interaction of cisplatin drug with Na,K-ATPase: drug binding mode and protein secondary structure. J Inorg Biochem 2001; 86(2–3):603–609.
25. Alberti I, Kalia YN, Naik A, et al. In vivo assessment of enhanced topical delivery of terbinafine to human stratum corneum. J Control Release 2001; 71(3):319–327.
26. Hanh BD, Neubert RHH, Wartewig S, et al. Penetration of compounds through human stratum corneum as studied by Fourier transform infrared photoacoustic spectroscopy. J Control Release 2001; 70(3):393–398.

27. Chan KLA, Hammond SV, Kazarian SG. Applications of attenuated total reflection infrared spectroscopic imaging to pharmaceutical formulations. Anal Chem 2003; 75(9):2140–2146.

28. van der Weerd J, Kazarian SG. Combined approach of FTIR imaging and conventional dissolution tests applied to drug release. J Control Release 2004; 98(2):295–305.

29. Van der Weerd J, Kazarian SG. Release of poorly soluble drugs from HPMC tablets studied by FTIR imaging and flow-through dissolution tests. J Pharm Sci 2005; 94(9):2096–2109.

30. Elkhider N, Chan KLA, Kazarian SG. Effect of moisture and pressure on tablet compaction studied with FTIR spectroscopic imaging. J Pharm Sci 2007; 96(2):351–360.

31. Chan KLA, Kazarian SG. High-throughput study of poly(ethylene glycol)/ibuprofen formulations under controlled environment using FTIR imaging. J Comb Chem 2006; 8(1): 26–31.

32. Reich G. Near-infrared spectroscopy and imaging: basic principles and pharmaceutical applications. Adv Drug Deliv Rev 2005; 57(8):1109–1143.

33. Blanco M, Alcala M. Content uniformity and tablet hardness testing of intact pharmaceutical tablets by near infrared spectroscopy: a contribution to process analytical technologies. Anal Chim Acta 2006; 557(1–2):353–359.

34. Cogdill RP, Anderson CA, Drennen JK. Using NIR spectroscopy as an integrated PAT tool. Spectroscopy 2004; 19(12):104–109.

35. Guo J-H, Skinner GW, Harcum WW, et al. Application of near-infrared spectroscopy in the pharmaceutical solid dosage form. Drug Dev Ind Pharm 1999; 25(12):1267–1270.

36. Clarke F. Extracting process-related information from pharmaceutical dosage forms using near infrared microscopy. Vib Spectrosc 2004; 34(1):25–35.

37. Keresztury G. Raman spectroscopy: theory. In: Chalmers JM, Griffiths PR, eds. Handbook of Vibrational Spectroscopy: Theory and Instrumentation. London: John Wiley & Sons, 2002: 71–87.

38. Strachan CJ, Rades T, Gordon KC, et al. Raman spectroscopy for quantitative analysis of pharmaceutical solids. J Pharm Pharmacol 2007; 59(2):179–192.

39. Vergote GJ, Vervaet C, Remon JP, et al. Near-infrared FT-Raman spectroscopy as a rapid analytical tool for the determination of diltiazem hydrochloride in tablets. Eur J Pharm Sci 2002; 16(1–2):63–67.

40. McCreery RL. Raman Spectroscopy for Chemical Analysis. New York: Wiley-Interscience, 2000.

41. Vankeirsbilck T, Vercauteren A, Baeyens W, et al. Applications of Raman spectroscopy in pharmaceutical analysis. Trends Anal Chem 2002; 21(12):869–877.

42. De Beer TRM, Vergote GJ, Baeyens WRG, et al. Development and validation of a direct, non-destructive quantitative method for medroxyprogesterone acetate in a pharmaceutical suspension using FT-Raman spectroscopy. Eur J Pharm Sci 2004; 23(4–5):355–362.

43. Orkoula MG, Kontoyannis CG, Markopoulou CK, et al. Quantitative analysis of liquid formulations using FT-Raman spectroscopy and HPLC: the case of diphenhydramine hydrochloride in Benadryl®. J Pharm Biomed Anal 2006; 41(4):1406–1411.

44. Tian F, Zeitler JA, Strachan CJ, et al. Characterizing the conversion kinetics of carbamazepine polymorphs to the dihydrate in aqueous suspension using Raman spectroscopy. J Pharm Biomed Anal 2006; 40(2):271–280.

45. Turrell G, Corset J. Raman Microscopy: Developments and Applications. London: Elsevier, 1996.

46. Sasic S. Raman mapping of low-content API pharmaceutical formulations. I. Mapping of alprazolam in Alprazolam/Xanax tablets. Pharm Res 2007; 24(1):58–65.

47. Sasic S, Clark DA, Mitchell JC, et al. Raman line mapping as a fast method for analyzing pharmaceutical bead formulations. Analyst 2005; 130(11):1530–1536.

48. Zhang L, Henson MJ, Sekulic SS. Multivariate data analysis for Raman imaging of a model pharmaceutical tablet. Anal Chim Acta 2005; 545(2):262–278.

49. Henson MJ, Zhang L. Drug characterization in low dosage pharmaceutical tablets using Raman microscopic mapping. Appl Spectrosc 2006; 60(11):1247–1255.

50. Heinemann M, Meinberg H, Buchs J, et al. Method for quantitative determination of spatial polymer distribution in alginate beads using Raman spectroscopy. Appl Spectrosc 2005; 59(3): 280–285.

51. Zeitler JA, Taday PF, Newnham DA, et al. Terahertz pulsed spectroscopy and imaging in the pharmaceutical setting - a review. J Pharm Pharmacol 2007; 59(2):209–223.

52. Wallace VP, Taday PF, Fitzgerald AJ, et al. Terahertz pulsed imaging and spectroscopy for biomedical and pharmaceutical applications. Faraday Discuss 2004; 126:255–263.

53. Pickwell E, Wallace VP. Biomedical applications of terahertz technology. J Phys D Appl Phys 2006; 39(17):R301–R310.

54. Fitzgerald AJ, Cole BE, Taday PF. Nondestructive analysis of tablet coating thicknesses usign terahertz pulsed imaging. J Pharm Sci 2005; 94(1):177–183.

55. Ho L, Muller R, Romer M, et al. Analysis of sustained-release tablet film coats using terahertz pulsed imaging. J Control Release 2007; 119(3):253–261.

56. Wu H, Heilweil EJ, Hussain AS, et al. Process analytical technology (PAT): effects of instrumental and compositional variables on terahertz spectral data quality to characterize pharmaceutical materials and tablets. Int J Pharm 2007; 343(1–2):148–158.

57. Callaghan PT. Principles of Nuclear Magnetic Resonance Microscopy. Oxford: Oxford University Press, 1991.

58. Weil JA, Bolton JR. Electron Paramagnetic Resonance: Elementary Theory and Practical Applications. 2nd ed. New Jersey: John Wiley & Sons, 2007.

59. Melia CD, Rajabi-Siahboomi AR, Bowtell RW. Magnetic resonance imaging of controlled release pharmaceutical dosage forms. Pharm Sci Technol Today 1998; 1(1):32–39.

60. Richardson JC, Bowtell RW, Mader K, et al. Pharmaceutical applications of magnetic resonance imaging (MRI). Adv Drug Deliv Rev 2005; 57(8):1191–1209.

61. Lurie DJ, Mader K. Monitoring drug delivery processes by EPR and related techniques - principles and applications. Adv Drug Deliv Rev 2005; 57(8):1171–1190.

62. Bowtell R, Sharp JC, Peters A, et al. NMR microscopy of hydrating hydrophilic matrix pharmaceutical tablets. Magn Reson Imaging 1994; 12(2):361–364.

63. Nebgen G, Gross D, Lehmann V, et al. ^{1}H NMR microscopy of tablets. J Pharm Sci 1995; 84(3): 283–291.

64. Rajabi-Siahboomi AR, Bowtell RW, Mansfield P, et al. Structure and behavior in hydrophilic matrix sustained-release dosage forms. 2: NMR-imaging studies of dimensional changes in the gel layer and core of HPMC tablets undergoing hydration. J Control Release 1994; 31(2): 121–128.

65. Rajabi-Siahboomi AR, Bowtell RW, Mansfield P, et al. Structure and behavior in hydrophilic matrix sustained release dosage forms. 4: Studies of water mobility and diffusion coefficients in the gel layer of HPMC tablets using NMR imaging. Pharm Res 1996; 13(3):376–380.

66. Fyfe CA, Blazek AI. Investigation of hydrogel formation from hydroxypropylmethylcellulose (HPMC) by NMR spectroscopy and NMR imaging techniques. Macromolecules 1997; 30(20): 6230–6237.

67. Baumgartner S, Lahajnar G, Sepe A, et al. Quantitative evaluation of polymer concentration profile during swelling of hydrophilic matrix tablets using ^{1}H NMR and MRI methods. Eur J Pharm Biopharm 2005; 59(2):299–306.

68. Tritt-Goc J, Kowalczuk J. Spatially resolved solvent interaction with glassy HPMC polymers studied by magnetic resonance microscopy. Solid State Nucl Magn Reson 2005; 28(2–4):250–257.

69. Tritt-Goc J, Pislewski N. Magnetic resonance imaging study of the swelling kinetics of hydroxypropylmethylcellulose (HPMC) in water. J Control Release 2002; 80(1–3):79–86.

70. Kowalczuk J, Tritt-Goc J, Pislewski N. The swelling properties of hydroxypropyl methyl cellulose loaded with tetracycline hydrochloride: magnetic resonance imaging study. Solid State Nucl Magn Reson 2004; 25(1–3):35–41.

71. Fyfe CA, Blazek-Welsh AI. Quantitative NMR imaging study of the mechanism of drug release from swelling hydroxypropylmethylcellulose tablets. J Control Release 2000; 68(3): 313–333.

72. Dinarvand R, Wood B, Demanuele A. Measurement of the diffusion of 2,2,2-trifluoroacetamide within thermoresponsive hydrogels using NMR imaging. Pharm Res 1995; 12(9): 1376–1379.

73. Shapiro M, Jarema MA, Gravina S. Magnetic resonance imaging of an oral gastrointestinal-therapeutic-system (GITS) tablet. J Control Release 1996; 38(2–3):123–127.

74. Fahie BJ, Nangia A, Chopra SK, et al. Use of NMR imaging in the optimization of a compression-coated regulated release system. J Control Release 1998; 51(2–3):179–184.

75. Sutch JCD, Ross AC, Kockenberger W, et al. Investigating the coating-dependent release mechanism of a pulsatile capsule using NMR microscopy. J Control Release 2003; 92(3): 341–347.

76. Djemai A, Gladden LF, Booth J, et al. MRI investigation of hydration and heterogeneous degradation of aliphatic polyesters derived from lactic and glycolic acids: a controlled drug delivery device. Magn Reson Imaging 2001; 19(3–4):521–523.

77. Milroy GE, Cameron RE, Mantle MD, et al. The distribution of water in degrading polyglycolide. Part II: magnetic resonance imaging and drug release. J Mater Sci Mater Med 2003; 14(5):465–473.

78. Karakosta E, McDonald PJ. An MRI analysis of the dissolution of a soluble drug incorporated within an insoluble polymer tablet. Appl Magn Reson 2007; 32(1–2):75–91.

79. Baille WE, Malveau C, Therien-Aubin H, et al. NMR imaging studies of high amylose starch tablets. Abstr Pap Am Chem Soc 2004; 228:U239.

80. Malveau C, Baille WE, Zhu XX, et al. NMR imaging of high-amylose starch tablets. 2: effect of tablet size. Biomacromolecules 2002; 3(6):1249–1254.

81. Prior-Cabanillas A, Barrales-Rienda JM, Frutos G, et al. Swelling behaviour of hydrogels from methacrylic acid and poly(ethylene glycol) side chains by magnetic resonance imaging. Polym Int 2007; 56(4):506–511.

82. Marshall P, Snaar JEM, Ng YL, et al. Localised mapping of water movement and hydration inside a developing bioadhesive bond. J Control Release 2004; 95(3):435–446.

83. Dahlberg C, Fureby A, Schuleit M, et al. Polymer mobilization and drug release during tablet swelling. A H-1 NMR and NMR microimaging study. J Control Release 2007; 122(2):199–205.

84. Mikac U, Demsar A, Demsar F, et al. A study of tablet dissolution by magnetic resonance electric current density imaging. J Magn Reson 2007; 185(1):103–109.

85. Strubing S, Metz H, Mäder K. Characterization of polyvinyl acetate based floating matrix tablets. J Control Release 2008; 126(2):149–155.

86. Djemai A, Sinka IC. NMR imaging of density distributions in tablets. Int J Pharm 2006; 319(1–2):55–62.

87. Tritt-Goc J, Kowalczuk J. In situ, real time observation of the disintegration of paracetamol tablets in aqueous solution by magnetic resonance imaging. Eur J Pharm Sci 2002; 15(4): 341–346.

88. Kwiecinski S, Weychert M, Jasinski A, et al. Tablet disintegration monitored by magnetic resonance Imaging. Appl Magn Reson 2002; 22(1):23–29.

89. Tomer G, Newton JM, Kinchesh P. Magnetic resonance imaging (MRI) as a method to investigate movement of water during the extrusion of pastes. Pharm Res 1999; 16(5):666–671.

90. Sommier N, Porion P, Evesque P, et al. Magnetic resonance imaging investigation of the mixing-segregation process in a pharmaceutical blender. Int J Pharm 2001; 222(2):243–258.

91. Strubing S, Metz H, Mäder K. Mechanistic analysis of drug release from tablets with membrane controlled drug delivery. Eur J Pharm Biopharm 2007; 66(1):113–119.

92. Fyfe CA, Grondey H, Blazek-Welsh AI, et al. NMR imaging investigations of drug delivery devices using a flow-through USP dissolution apparatus. J Control Release 2000; 68(1):73–83.

93. Abrahmsen-Alami S, Korner A, Nilsson I, et al. New release cell for NMR microimaging of tablets: swelling and erosion of poly(ethylene oxide). Int J Pharm 2007; 342(1–2):105–114.

94. Montanari L, Cilurzo F, Valvo L, et al. Gamma irradiation effects on stability of poly(lactide-co-glycolide) microspheres containing clonazepam. J Control Release 2001; 75(3):317–330.

95. Bittner B, Mader K, Kroll C, et al. Tetracycline-HCl-loaded poly(DL-lactide-co-glycolide) microspheres prepared by a spray drying technique: influence of gamma-irradiation on radical formation and polymer degradation. J Control Release 1999; 59(1):23–32.

96. Maggi L, Segale L, Machiste EO, et al. Chemical and physical stability of hydroxypropyl methylcellulose matrices containing diltiazem hydrochloride after gamma irradiation. J Pharm Sci 2003; 92(1):131–141.

97. Mäder K, Cremmilleux Y, Domb AJ, et al. In vitro in vivo comparison of drug release and polymer erosion from biodegradable P(FAD-SA) polyanhydrides - a noninvasive approach by the combined use of electron paramagnetic resonance spectroscopy and nuclear magnetic resonance imaging. Pharm Res 1997; 14(6):820–826.

98. Katzhendler I, Mäder K, Friedman M. Correlation between drug release kinetics from proteineous matrix and matrix structure: EPR and NMR study. J Pharm Sci 2000; 89(3): 365–381.

99. Katzhendler I, Mäder K, Azoury R, et al. Investigating the structure and properties of hydrated hydroxypropyl methylcellulose and egg albumin matrices containing carbamazepine: EPR and NMR study. Pharm Res 2000; 17(10):1299–1308.

100. Capancioni S, Schwach-Abdellaoui K, Kloeti W, et al. In vitro monitoring of poly(ortho ester) degradation by electron paramagnetic resonance imaging. Macromolecules 2003; 36(16): 6135–6141.

101. Siepe S, Herrmann W, Borchert HH, et al. Microenvironmental pH and microviscosity inside pH-controlled matrix tablets: an EPR imaging study. J Control Release 2006; 112(1):72–78.

102. Kroll C, Herrmann W, Stosser R, et al. Influence of drug treatment on the microacidity in rat and human skin - an in vitro electron spin resonance imaging study. Pharm Res 2001; 18(4): 525–530.

103. Blank A, Freed JH, Kumar NP, et al. Electron spin resonance microscopy applied to the study of controlled drug release. J Control Release 2006; 111(1–2):174–184.

104. Pohl DW, Fischer UC, Durig UT. Scanning near-field optical microscopy (SNOM). J Microsc (Oxf) 1988; 152:853–861.

105. Price DM, Reading M, Hammiche A, et al. Micro-thermal analysis: scanning thermal microscopy and localised thermal analysis. Int J Pharm 1999; 192(1):85–96.

106. Sanders GHW, Roberts CJ, Danesh A, et al. Discrimination of polymorphic forms of a drug product by localized thermal analysis. J Microsc (Oxf) 2000; 198:77–81.

107. Ward S, Perkins M, Zhang JX, et al. Identifying and mapping surface amorphous domains. Pharm Res 2005; 22(7):1195–1202.

108. Craig DQM, Kett VL, Andrews CS, et al. Pharmaceutical applications of micro-thermal analysis. J Pharm Sci 2002; 91(5):1201–1213.

109. Allen S, Davies MC, Roberts CJ, et al. Atomic force microscopy in analytical biotechnology. Trends Biotechnol 1997; 15(3):101–105.

110. Cappella B, Dietler G. Force-distance curves by atomic force microscopy. Surf Sci Rep 1999; 34(1–3):1–152.

111. Danesh A, Chen XY, Davies MC, et al. The discrimination of drug polymorphic forms from single crystals using atomic force microscopy. Pharm Res 2000; 17(7):887–890.

112. Price R, Young PM. Visualization of the crystallization of lactose from the amorphous state. J Pharm Sci 2004; 93(1):155–164.

113. Danesh A, Connell SD, Davies MC, et al. An in situ dissolution study of aspirin crystal planes (100) and (001) by atomic force microscopy. Pharm Res 2001; 18(3):299–303.

114. Hillner PE, Manne S, Gratz AJ, et al. AFM images of dissolution and growth on a calcite crystal. Ultramicroscopy 1992; 42:1387–1393.

115. Binning G, Quate CF, Gerber C. Atomic force microscope. Phys Rev Lett 1986; 56(9): 930–933.

116. Davies M, Brindley A, Chen XY, et al. Characterization of drug particle surface energetics and Young's modulus by atomic force microscopy and inverse gas chromatography. Pharm Res 2005; 22(7):1158–1166.

117. Perkins M, Ebbens SJ, Hayes S, et al. Elastic modulus measurements from individual lactose particles using atomic force microscopy. Int J Pharm 2007; 332(1–2):168–175.

118. Berard V, Lesniewska E, Andres C, et al. Affinity scale between a carrier and a drug in DPI studied by atomic force microscopy. Int J Pharm 2002; 247(1–2):127–137.

119. Bunker MJ, Roberts CJ, Davies MC. Towards screening of inhalation formulations: measuring interactions with atomic force microscopy. Expert Opin Drug Deliv 2005; 2(4):613–624.

120. Hooton JC, German CS, Allen S, et al. Characterization of particle-interactions by atomic force microscopy: effect of contact area. Pharm Res 2003; 20(3):508–514.

121. Hooton JC, German CS, Allen S, et al. An atomic force microscopy study of the effect of nanoscale contact geometry and surface chemistry on the adhesion of pharmaceutical particles. Pharm Res 2004; 21(6):953–961.

122. Young PM, Price R, Tobyn MJ, et al. The influence of relative humidity on the cohesion properties of micronized drugs used in inhalation therapy. J Pharm Sci 2004; 93(3):753–761.

123. Jones R, Pollock HM, Geldart D, et al. Inter-particle forces in cohesive powders studied by AFM: effects of relative humidity, particle size and wall adhesion. Powder Technol 2003; 132(2–3): 196–210.

124. Jones R, Pollock HM, Cleaver JAS, et al. Adhesion forces between glass and silicon surfaces in air studied by AFM: effects of relative humidity, particle size, roughness, and surface treatment. Langmuir 2002; 18(21):8045–8055.

125. Relini A, Sottini S, Zuccotti S, et al. Measurement of the surface free energy of streptavidin crystals by atomic force microscopy. Langmuir 2003; 19(7):2908–2912.

126. Zhang JX, Ebbens S, Chen XY, et al. Determination of the surface free energy of crystalline and amorphous lactose by atomic force microscopy adhesion measurement. Pharm Res 2006; 23(2):401–407.

127. Hooton JC, German CS, Davies MC, et al. Comparison of morphology and surface energy characteristics of sulfathiazole polymorphs based upon single particle studies. Eur J Pharm Sci 2006; 28(4):315–324.

128. Traini D, Rogueda P, Young P, et al. Surface energy and interparticle forces correlations in model pMDI formulations. Pharm Res 2005; 22(5):816–825.

129. Begat P, Morton DAV, Staniforth JN, et al. The cohesive-adhesive balances in dry powder inhaler formulations II: influence on fine particle delivery characteristics. Pharm Res 2004; 21(10):1826–1833.

130. Begat P, Morton DAV, Staniforth JN, et al. The cohesive-adhesive balances in dry powder inhaler formulations I: direct quantification by atomic force microscopy. Pharm Res 2004; 21(9):1591–1597.

131. Bunker MJ, Davies MC, Chen XY, et al. Single particle friction on blister packaging materials used in dry powder inhalers. Eur J Pharm Sci 2006; 29(5):405–413.

132. Bunker MJ, Roberts CJ, Davies MC, et al. A nanoscale study of particle friction in a pharmaceutical system. Int J Pharm 2006; 325(1–2):163–171.

133. Ma WJ, Ruys AJ, Mason RS, et al. DLC coatings: Effects of physical and chemical properties on biological response. Biomaterials 2007; 28(9):1620–1628.

134. Shakesheff KM, Evora C, Soriano I, et al. The adsorption of poly(vinyl alcohol) to biodegradable microparticles studied by x-ray photoelectron spectroscopy (XPS). J Colloid Interface Sci 1997; 185(2):538–547.

135. Evora C, Soriano I, Rogers RA, et al. Relating the phagocytosis of microparticles by alveolar macrophages to surface chemistry: the effect of 1,2-dipalmitoylphosphatidylcholine. J Control Release 1998; 51(2–3):143–152.

136. Dong YC, Feng SS. Methoxy poly(ethylene glycol)-poly(lactide) (MPEG-PLA) nanoparticles for controlled delivery of anticancer drugs. Biomaterials 2004; 25(14):2843–2849.

137. Cook AD, Hrkach JS, Gao NN, et al. Characterization and development of RGD-peptide-modified poly(lactic acid-co-lysine) as an interactive, resorbable biomaterial. J Biomed Mater Res 1997; 35(4):513–523.

138. New XPS/ESCA 2006. YKI News 2006:6.

139. Belu AM, Davies MC, Newton JM, et al. TOF-SIMS characterization and imaging of controlled-release drug delivery systems. Anal Chem 2000; 72(22):5625–5638.

140. Lee JW, Gardella JA. Simultaneous time-of-flight secondary ion MS quantitative analysis of drug surface concentration and polymer degradation kinetics in biodegradable poly(L-lactic acid) blends. Anal Chem 2003; 75(13):2950–2958.

141. Davies MC, Shakesheff KM, Shard AG, et al. Surface analysis of biodegradable polymer blends of poly(sebacic anhydride) and poly(DL-lactic acid). Macromolecules 1996; 29(6): 2205–2212.
142. Luk SY, Patel N, Davies MC. Chemical imaging of pharmaceuticals by time-of-flight secondary ion mass spectrometry. Spectrosc Eur 2003; 15(1):14–18.
143. Feng SS, Huang GF. Effects of emulsifiers on the controlled release of paclitaxel (Taxol (R)) from nanospheres of biodegradable polymers. J Control Release 2001; 71(1):53–69.
144. Leadley SR, Shakesheff KM, Davies MC, et al. The use of SIMS, XPS and in situ AFM to probe the acid catalysed hydrolysis of poly(orthoesters). Biomaterials 1998; 19(15):1353–1360.
145. Ton-That C, Shard AG, Teare DOH, et al. XPS and AFM surface studies of solvent-cast PS/PMMA blends. Polymer 2001; 42(3):1121–1129.
146. Sinka IC, Burch SF, Tweed JH, et al. Measurement of density variations in tablets using X-ray computed tomography. Int J Pharm 2004; 271(1–2):215–224.
147. Farber L, Tardos G, Michaels JN. Use of X-ray tomography to study the porosity and morphology of granules. Powder Technol 2003; 132(1):57–63.
148. Bouwman AM, Henstra MJ, Westerman D, et al. The effect of the amount of binder liquid on the granulation mechanisms and structure of microcrystalline cellulose granules prepared by high shear granulation. Int J Pharm 2005; 290(1–2):129–136.
149. Hancock BC, Mullarney MP. X-ray microtomography of solid dosage forms. Pharm Technol 2005; 29(44):92–100.
150. Morgan CL. Principles of computed tomography: combined translational-rotational scanning systems, Basic Principles of Computed Tomography. Baltimore, MD: University Park Press, 1983:19–68.
151. Hounsfield GN. Computerized transverse axial scanning (tomography). 1: description of system. Br J Radiol 1973; 46(552):1016–1022.
152. Cormack AM. Representation of a function by its line integrals, with some radiological applications. J Appl Phys 1963; 34(9):2722–2727.
153. Cormack AM. Representation of a function by its line integrals, with some radiological applications II. J Appl Phys 1964; 35(10):2908–2913.
154. Feldkamp LA, Davis LC, Kress JW. Practical cone-beam algorithm. J Opt Soc Am A Opt Image Sci Vis 1984; 1(6):612–619.
155. Flannery BP, Deckman HW, Roberge WG, et al. 3-Dimensional X-ray microtomography. Science 1987; 237(4821):1439–1444.
156. Wellington SL, Vinegar HJ. X-ray computerized-tomography. J Pet Technol 1987; 39(8): 885–898.
157. Fu XW, Elliott JA, Bentham AC, et al. Application of X-ray microtomography and image processing to the investigation of a compacted granular system. Part Part Syst Char 2006; 23(3–4): 229–236.
158. Busignies V, Leclerc B, Porion P, et al. Quantitative measurements of localized density variations in cylindrical tablets using X-ray microtomography. Eur J Pharm Biopharm 2006; 64(1):38–50.
159. Chauve G, Raverielle F, Marchessault RH. Comparative imaging of a slow-release starch excipient tablet: evidence of membrane formation. Carbohydr Polym 2007; 70(1):61–67.
160. Inman SJ, Briscoe BJ, Pitt KG. Topographic characterization of cellulose bilayered tablets interfaces. Chem Eng Res Des 2007; 85(A7):1005–1012.

11
Aspects of Pharmaceutical Physics

Göran Frenning and Göran Alderborn
Department of Pharmacy, Uppsala University, Uppsala Biomedical Center, Uppsala, Sweden

INTRODUCTION

Physical concepts, measurement techniques, and analysis methods are widely used in pharmaceutical research and development. In the area of powder technology, for instance, these include methods to characterize particles and tablets in terms of surface area, porosity, and mechanical strength.

In many cases, one does not pay attention to the physical origin of the concept, which is instead considered as common knowledge of the pharmaceutical scientist. Yet in others, the methods may only recently have found their way into the pharmaceutics laboratories and at the time of writing may thus be considered as relatively novel.

Considering the importance of the underlying physics, the purpose of this chapter is to provide a unified description of some common physical concepts that are widely used—albeit sometimes in other disciplines—to describe and/or analyze data. This chapter is not intended as a general overview of physical knowledge that is of relevance to the pharmaceutical scientist, but rather aims at discussing some of the important concepts in more depth.

Physics has been described as an economy of thought (1)—since it is able to summarize a vast number of seemingly disparate empirical phenomena in just a few basic laws. In the same spirit, we hope that this chapter will be able to connect different aspects of pharmaceutical physics, and hopefully help the reader by emphasizing general principles rather than details.

FRACTAL ANALYSIS AND PERCOLATION THEORY

General Principles

Many objects in nature exhibit self-similarity, that is, they look more or less the same regardless of the degree of magnification (at least within some limits). Examples include coastlines, mountain ridges, snowflakes, leaves, branched polymers, etc. As pointed out by Mandelbrot, such self-similar objects may generally be described as *fractals* (2). A fractal analysis is often fruitful for structurally disordered materials, in particular for (partially) amorphous solids, such as the polymers commonly used as excipient materials. Percolation theory may be used to describe transport through such disordered structures (one example is the transport of water through coffee in an ordinary coffee percolator), and it is therefore natural that percolation theory and fractals have much in common.

Fractals

Perfect fractals, which exhibit exact self-similarity on all length scales, may be constructed as a mathematical idealization by repeated application of certain generators. This procedure is illustrated in Figure 1 for two famous fractals: the von Koch curve (or snowflake) and the Sierpinski gasket (the von Koch snowflake is obtained if one starts with an equilateral triangle rather than a line and for each side performs the same operations as for the von Koch curve). The von Koch snowflake and the Sierpinski gasket may serve as illustrations of the two main types of fractals: surface fractals and mass fractals. As the name indicates, a surface fractal has a fractal surface, but the interior mass or volume (surface in two dimensions) is not fractal. Mass fractals do, on the other hand, have a fractal interior (compare with the Sierpinski gasket), and this in turn results in the surface being fractal as well. In addition to these two basic types, one may introduce a third type of fractal, referred to as a pore fractal (3). This fractal is characterized by a fractal pore space embedded in a

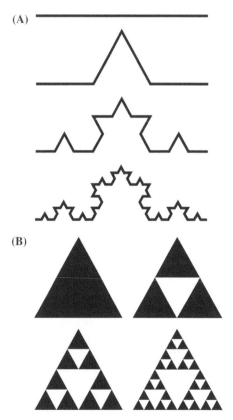

(A)

(B)

Figure 1   Generation of perfect fractals (the first four generations are shown). (**A**) The von Koch curve. (**B**) The Sierpinski gasket.

nonfractal matrix, and as a consequence of the pore space being fractal, the pore wall is fractal as well.

The name fractal stems from the fact that such self-similar objects may be characterized by a dimension that is a nonintegral (fractional) number. This may be seen from a resolution analysis: the object is measured with different resolution, and the dimension is inferred from the way the measured value *scales* with resolution (size of the yardstick). Consider, for example, the measurement of the length of a line. If one compares the value obtained using a yardstick of length L, denoted by $\mathcal{L}(L)$, with the value $\mathcal{L}(L/r)$ obtained using a yardstick of length L/r (where $r > 1$ is the resolution), one will find that they are related by $\mathcal{L}(L/r) = r^1 \mathcal{L}(L)$. Similarly, if one measures the area of a regular object using yardsticks of length L and L/r, one will find that the area scales as $\mathcal{A}(L/r) = r^2 \mathcal{A}(L)$. These results make sense, since the line and area have one and two dimensions, respectively. For a general object (fractal or not), one may therefore *define* the dimension as the exponent d_f in the *scaling relation*

$$\mathcal{M}(L/r) = r^{d_f} \mathcal{M}(L) \tag{1}$$

where $\mathcal{M}(L)$ and $\mathcal{M}(L/r)$ are the measured values using yardsticks of length L and L/r, respectively. As an example, consider the von Koch curve depicted in Figure 1. Regardless of the size of the yardstick, it will not be able to follow all turns of the fractal. However, if a yardstick of length L is able to follow one generation of the curve, a yardstick of length $L/3$ would be able to follow the next; hence the measured values are related by $\mathcal{M}(L/3) = 4\mathcal{M}(L)$. Moreover, comparison with equation (1), with $r = 3$, reveals that $3^{d_f} = 4$, and by taking the natural logarithm of both sides, we find that the fractal dimension $d_f = \ln 4 / \ln 3 \approx 1.26$. Hence, the dimension of the von Koch curve lies between the dimension of a line (of dimension 1) and the dimension of the embedding space (in this case, an area of dimension 2). The same is true also in higher dimensions, and a fractal surface thus in general has a dimension between 2 and 3.

As noted above, fractals that are exactly self-similar on all length scales are a mathematical idealization. Fractals found in nature instead are usually statistically self-similar: regardless of scale, they have the same statistical properties such as the distribution of voids, particle sizes, etc. (4). Moreover, naturally occurring fractals exhibit a fractal structure only on certain length scales. At sufficient magnification, one eventually encounters individual molecules or atoms, and hence, a lower cutoff must exist. Similarly, an upper cutoff exists, which may be the finite size of an object or a so-called correlation length (see the next section).

Percolation Theory

The basic problem in percolation theory may be described fairly easily (5). Assume that we have a regular array of squares, such as a sheet of quad-ruled paper, as indicated in Figure 2. The array is assumed to be large enough so that the influence of the boundaries is negligible. Now suppose that a fraction p of the squares are filled, whereas the remaining ones are left empty. In percolation theory, each square is called a *site*, which may be *occupied* with a certain probability p and is thus empty with probability $1-p$. We will here confine ourselves to *random percolation*, in which case each site is occupied independently of its neighbors (as usual, in probability theory, this assumption greatly simplifies the analysis of the situation). As may be seen in Figure 2, the occupied sites form *clusters* of various sizes (a single occupied site surrounded by empty sites is considered as a cluster of size 1); occupied sites that share a common edge are nearest neighbors and belong to the same cluster. Basically, percolation theory deals with the number and properties of the thus formed clusters.

Figure 2 The basic percolation problem (for clarity, the percolating cluster is shown in black and nonpercolating clusters in gray). (**A**) $p < p_c$ (**B**) $p = p_c$ (**C**) $p > p_c$.

An alternative to the *site percolation* problem described above assumes that all sites are occupied and that nearest neighbors are connected to each other by either open or closed bonds. In this case, p is the probability that a randomly selected bond is open (and thus, $1-p$ is the probability that it is closed). Sites connected to each other by open bonds belong to the same cluster (this definition makes sense if one recalls the coffee percolator; water can only flow through open pores). Since the conclusions drawn from such *bond percolation* may be understood by using site percolation, we will here focus on the latter.

The single most important concept in percolation theory is the *percolation threshold*, which may be understood as follows. First, assume that p (the probability of occupation) is very small. In this case, very few sites are occupied, and the clusters are all of finite size (each cluster is surrounded by many empty sites). Then assume that p is close to unity, so that almost all sites are occupied. Reversing the argument, it is realized that a few "holes" of finite size exist in an otherwise unbounded cluster that spans the

Table 1 Percolation Thresholds for Some Common Lattices

Lattice	Dimension	Percolation threshold	
		Site	Bond
Square	2	0.593	0.500
Honeycomb	2	0.696	0.653
Simple cubic	3	0.312	0.249
Body-centered cubic	3	0.246	0.180
Face-centered cubic	3	0.198	0.119

whole system. Somewhere in between these two extreme values, one will therefore have a situation where an infinite cluster forms. The probability at which the infinite (or *percolating*) cluster appears is called the percolation threshold, often denoted by p_c. At the percolation threshold, the infinite cluster is often referred to as the *incipient infinite cluster* since it begins to exist at this point.

The percolation threshold has many similarities with phase transitions, since the behavior of the system changes abruptly at this point. Assuming, for instance, that the occupied sites are able to conduct an electric current, whereas the empty ones are not, the conductivity σ will be zero when $p < p_c$ and nonzero when $p > p_c$. Moreover, close to the percolation threshold, the conductivity will follow a *power law*

$$\sigma \propto (p - p_c)^{\mu} \tag{2}$$

where the *conductivity exponent* μ is approximately 1.3 and 2.0 in two and three dimensions, respectively (the symbol $\propto$ is used to indicate proportionality) (5,6). Critical exponents like μ are, as a rule, independent of the lattice type used (but they do depend on the spatial dimension). Similar relations hold for other properties as well, one example being the strength of a polymer network. It should be emphasized, however, that relation (2) is valid in the vicinity of p_c only. Further away from the percolation threshold, effective-medium theory usually provides a better description (7). In addition to the square lattice discussed so far, there are of course other regular arrangements of sites in two and three dimensions. Some common lattices and their percolation thresholds are listed in Table 1 (see Ref. 5 for a more extensive list).

Although we have defined percolation in terms of occupied sites, it is clear that no principal difference exists between these sites and the empty ones, and one may therefore equally well inquire at which probability the empty sites form an infinite cluster. Evidently, this will occur when p (the probability of occupation) equals $1 - p_c$. Therefore, provided $p_c < 1/2$, there will exist a region in which both the occupied and empty sites percolate. This phenomenon cannot however occur in two dimensions since the appearance of one infinite cluster excludes the possibility of another.

Cluster structure The infinite cluster obtained for $p = p_c$ in Figure 2 is seen to have holes (that themselves often contain other clusters) on many different length scales. This observation indicates that a fractal analysis may be appropriate. A resolution analysis (see sect. "Fractals") may be performed by placing a square of size $L \times L$ (using the lattice spacing as the unit of length) on the infinite cluster and counting the number of sites within the square that belong to this cluster. Doing this for a number of lengths L, one will find that the cluster mass obeys the scaling equation (1), with $d_f \approx 1.9$, which means that the infinite cluster is indeed a fractal.

Also, when $p > p_c$, the infinite cluster is generally fractal on some, but not all, length scales. This may be understood in terms of the correlation length ξ, which, for $p > p_c$, is a measure of the largest hole in the infinite cluster. The holes in the cluster will therefore not be readily observable on length scales $L > \xi$ but will produce an average density lower than that of a completely solid object. Hence, a resolution analysis performed for $L > \xi$ will show that the cluster mass increases as L^2 (in two dimensions), not as L^{d_f}. As was the case for the conductivity discussed above, the correlation length obeys a power law close to the percolation threshold. However, whereas the conductivity vanishes at the threshold, the correlation length diverges: $\xi \propto 1/|p - p_c|^\nu$, where the exponent $\nu > 0$ (in fact, ν is assumed to equal 4/3 in two dimensions, whereas $\nu \approx 0.9$ in three dimensions) (5). This in turn implies that the incipient infinite cluster is fractal on all length scales.

As we have seen, power laws generally emerge close to the percolation threshold, when a fractal structure is obtained. This may be interpreted as a consequence of the power function being *scale invariant*: if $f(x) = x^\alpha$ (where α is a constant), then $f(cx) = (cx)^\alpha \propto x^\alpha = f(x)$ for any constant c. Alternatively, one may note that the power function may be written without introducing a length scale. This is not possible for other functions, since the argument of functions must generally be dimensionless. If x has dimension of length, we must write $e^{x/L}$ (rather than e^x), for instance, where L is a suitably selected length scale.

Diffusion as a random walk We have already mentioned that percolation theory is useful for describing transport in disordered systems, and will here illustrate this fact by using *Brownian motion*: If colloidal particles suspended in a fluid are viewed under the microscope, they are seen to undergo an erratic motion caused by random collisions with the molecules of the fluid. Brownian motion is closely connected to diffusion (see sect. "Transport as a Nonequilibrium Phenomenon") but may also be considered as a *random walk* (5,8). Suppose that time t is divided into a number of small time steps and that the particle during time step i moves a small distance Δx_i. For random motion on a one-dimensional *regular lattice*, each displacement increment Δx_i will be either $+1$ or -1 (using the lattice spacing as the unit of length), and either value is equally probable. The total displacement after n time steps is the sum of all displacement increments: $x_n = \sum_{i=1}^{n} \Delta x_i$. Assuming that each displacement increment is independent of the others, the expectation value of x_n is seen to vanish (the expectation value of a sum of independent random variables is the sum of the expectation values of each variable). To calculate the expectation value of the squared displacement (denoted by $\langle x_n^2 \rangle$), we note that x_n^2 will contain n terms $(\Delta x_i)^2$ and a number of cross terms of the form $2(\Delta x_i)(\Delta x_j)$. The expectation value of the latter is however zero since approximately half of the terms are positive and the remaining ones are negative. Moreover, since $(\Delta x_i)^2 = 1$ for all i, we find that $\langle x_n^2 \rangle = n \propto t$ (remember that n is the number of time steps). Analogous results hold for two and three dimensions, provided diffusion occurs on a regular lattice *without disorder*.

To see how disorder affects transport (in this case diffusion), we may consider a random walk on a percolation lattice, as in Figure 2. As suggested by de Gennes (9), this problem is often referred to as the "ant in the labyrinth." Again, it is instructive to consider the two extreme cases that the probability p is very small and close to unity. In the first case (and in fact always as long as $p < p_c$), all clusters are of finite size, which means that the distance an "ant" situated on a randomly selected cluster can move is bounded. Since it will take some time for the ant to move along the winding extent of the cluster, $\langle x^2(t) \rangle$ is expected to increase with time, but it will be bounded when time tends to infinity. When p is close to 1, the situation will, on the other hand, not differ significantly from that described in the preceding paragraph for a lattice without disorder, and therefore, $\langle x^2(t) \rangle \propto t$. It is therefore realized that a *crossover* between these two behaviors must occur when p increases past the percolation threshold. We have seen that the cluster is a fractal in the vicinity of p_c, and it is therefore perhaps not surprising that the squared distance in this case will follow a power law, of the form $\langle x^2(t) \rangle \propto t^{2/d_w}$, where $d_w > 2$ is the fractal dimension of the walk. In other words, diffusion is *anomalous*.

Pharmaceutical Applications

Drug Transport and Release
Drug release from matrix systems generally occurs by diffusion through a disordered polymer matrix, and percolation concepts are therefore useful for describing this process. It is in this regard interesting to note that one of the most commonly used semiempirical models of drug release from such systems is indeed the Korsmeyer–Peppas *power law* (10,11).

The systematic study of percolation effects on drug release was initiated by Bonny and Leuenberger, who investigated the release of the readily soluble drug caffeine from ethyl cellulose matrices (12). All surfaces of the matrix except one were covered with paraffin, which ensured that drug release occurred in one direction only. Therefore, the amount of released drug would follow the Higuchi square-root-of-time law (13) for ordinary (as opposed to anomalous) diffusion. The porosity of the fully extracted matrix was considered as the equivalent of the occupation probability p in the abstract percolation model, and this probability was varied by using different amounts of drug (10–90% w/w). In agreement with theoretical predictions, a lower percolation threshold was observed, below which drug release was incomplete. In addition, an upper threshold was identified, above which the matrix collapsed into separate fragments upon drug release. The described study has been followed by many others who have focused on various aspects of the process, such as the fractal dimension of pore system (14) (see later in the text), the effects of particle size and drug/excipient particle size ratio (15,16), and three-dimensional release (17).

In addition, Monte Carlo simulations of drug release from fractal and nonfractal matrices have been performed, and in the light of these, it has been suggested that the Weibull function is able to describe the entire release process (18). According to the Weibull model, the amount of released drug M increases with time as $M = M_\infty[1 - \exp(-at^b)]$, where M_∞ is the total amount present in the matrix and a and b are constants. In other words, the amount of drug remaining in the matrix decays as $\exp(-at^b)$, which may be compared to the decay of the dielectric polarization according to the Kolrausch–Williams–Watts (KWW) relaxation function mentioned in section "Nonexponential Relaxation."

Powder Compaction

The formation of a tablet has been described as a site and bond percolation phenomenon (19), and percolation theory may undoubtedly provide valuable insights into the compaction process. The application is however less straightforward than for drug release since the particles in a powder are in contact also before a coherent tablet has formed, and in this sense, the system thus percolates from the outset. In compaction applications, particles are therefore instead considered to belong to the same cluster if they are connected by a bond of nonzero strength (20). Nevertheless, the relative density (or solid

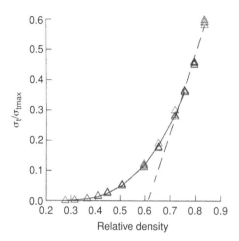

Figure 3 Tensile strength of tablets formed from microcrystalline cellulose as a function of relative density. In agreement with percolation theory, a power-law behavior was observed close to the percolation threshold (*solid line*), and a crossover to an effective-medium behavior was seen for larger relative density (*dashed line*). *Source*: From Ref. 20.

fraction) is usually assumed to correspond to the occupation probability of the abstract percolation model. To clearly see percolation effects, one needs to investigate the strength of tablets at relatively low relative densities. Nice results have been obtained for microcrystalline cellulose, an excellent tablet former, for which the tensile strength was indeed found to closely follow a power law in the vicinity of the percolation threshold (Fig. 3) (20). Further above the percolation threshold, the tensile strength was found to increase linearly with relative density, which may be understood in terms of effective-medium theory (21). Similar concepts were used by Alderborn, who suggested that the tensile strength increases approximately linearly with applied pressure in a region above the critical formation pressure (the pressure required to form a coherent tablet) (22,23).

Pore Structure

As mentioned above, disordered materials such as the polymer matrices often used for drug delivery usually exhibit a fractal structure on some length scales (typically in the submicrometer region). The fractal dimension may be determined by a number of techniques, including small-angle scattering of X rays and neutrons (24), gas adsorption (25), and mercury intrusion (26). In the pharmaceutical field, mercury intrusion and gas adsorption appear to be most common, although the fractal dimension has also been inferred from atomic force microscopy (27) and imaging techniques (28). Mercury intrusion has been used to investigate the fractal structure of pores in tablets (14) and pellets (29).

Gas adsorption is a suitable method for a fractal analysis because it is sensitive to the fine structure of the pores and has negligible adverse affects on the pore system. The results are usually analyzed by using fractal generalizations of the Brunauer–Emmett–Teller (BET) isotherm (30) or of the Frenkel–Halsey–Hill (FHH) isotherm (31). The latter may also be seen as a fractal generalization of the Kelvin equation and is therefore also applicable in the capillary condensation regime (32). It has been claimed that the fractal BET theory is more appropriate for *mass fractals* (see sect. "Fractals"), whereas *surface fractals* are to be analyzed using the fractal FHH theory (33). These methods have been applied to cellulose powders (34) and tablets (35).

COMPUTATIONAL MECHANICS

General Principles

The mechanical response of systems of distinct particles is often adequately described by Newton's laws, which constitute the bases of classical mechanics (36) (see sect. "The Discrete Element Method"). However, additional concepts are needed for deformable matter, such as stress and strain, which will be described here (37). We will focus on solid materials, but remark that the same principles are also valid for fluids (in which case the field is usually referred to as computational fluid dynamics).

Deformation and Strain

Consider uniaxial compression of a powdered material and assume that die-wall friction may be neglected (Fig. 4A). Since the radial motion is constrained by the die wall, it is realized that the motion of the powder will then be along the compression direction only. This motion results in a *deformation* of the powder, that is, the particles are *displaced* from their initial positions to their final positions. A deformation may be thought of as a transformation from an initial *reference configuration* to the deformed *current configuration*.

Most deformations result in the material being strained, for instance, elongated or compressed (exceptions occur when the material is translated or rotated as a whole, without changing shape). In the uniaxial powder compression example, the deformation decreases the height of the powder from the initial value H_0 to the current value H (Fig. 4A). Often used measures of uniaxial strain include the *engineering strain*

$$\varepsilon^{\text{eng}} = \frac{H - H_0}{H_0} \tag{3}$$

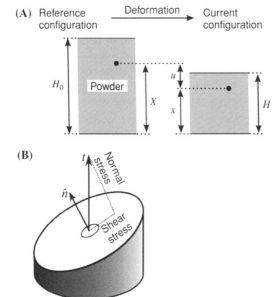

(A) Reference configuration → Deformation → Current configuration

(B)

Figure 4 Illustration of the basic mechanical concepts. (**A**) Deformation and strain. (**B**) Stress.

and the *natural strain*

$$\varepsilon^{\text{nat}} = \ln\left(\frac{H}{H_0}\right) \tag{4}$$

also referred to as the logarithmic strain. As seen, both of these strain measures vanish for the undeformed material (when $H = H_0$) and are negative for compression and positive for elongation. Moreover, the difference between the two strain measures is significant only for relatively large strains. As equations (3) and (4) indicate, the strain in general depends on the choice of reference configuration (initial height in this case). For elastic materials (see later in the text), which assume well-defined shapes when unloaded, the reference configuration is usually taken to coincide with the unloaded state and is therefore well defined. However, for materials that also undergo inelastic straining, the reference configuration is to some extent arbitrary.

In general, the strain in the material is usually expressed in terms of the gradient of the displacement u with respect to the reference placement of particles. In the one-dimensional case, this yields

$$\varepsilon = \frac{\partial u}{\partial X} \tag{5}$$

where X is the coordinate of the particle in the reference configuration. That equation (5) indeed produces a reasonable result may be seen from the powder compression example. Let us to this end assume that the powder is uniformly strained (i.e., that the strain is independent of the particular location in the powder) and that the lower punch is stationary, whereas the upper one is mobile (as usually is the case in tableting). When the powder is compressed from the initial height H_0 to the final height H, a particle will be displaced from its initial position X to its current position $x = HX/H_0$ (both X and x are measured as distances above the lower punch). In other words, the displacement may be calculated as the difference $u = x - X = HX/H_0 - X$. Finally, application of equation (5) shows that the resulting strain $\varepsilon = \partial u/\partial X = H/H_0 - 1$, a result that is seen to exactly coincide with the engineering strain in equation (3).

For more general deformations, it is necessary to represent the strain as a tensor (a matrix), with components ε_{ij}, where i and j both go from 1 to 3 (in the three-dimensional case). The diagonal elements (the ones for which $i = j$) still represent normal strain (elongation or compression) as in the uniaxial case [compare with equation (3)]. The off-diagonal elements (obtained when $i \neq j$) represent shear strains, which may be interpreted in terms of the angle change of two directions that are perpendicular in the reference configuration.

Stress

Straining of a material generally produces a stress. In the uniaxial compression example, the upper and lower punch experience a pressure, which may be regarded as a normal stress. In fact, if one introduces an imaginary cut through any point of the powdered material, whose orientation is specified by the outward unit normal $\hat{n}$, one will find that the powder on one side of the cut affects the powder on the other side via a surface force, a *traction* (Fig. 4B). As the pressure, the traction is defined as the force per unit area, but this force need not be directed along the normal of the cut but may also have a tangential component; the traction is a vector, with three components in the three-dimensional case. Moreover, the traction depends on the orientation of the cut (the normal $\hat{n}$), and since this normal may be directed along the x-, y-, and z-axes of a three-dimensional Cartesian coordinate system, we are thus led to the conclusion that nine components are required to specify the stress at a certain point of the material. In fact, an argument based on the balance of linear momentum (see later in the text), or force in the static case, reveals that the stress σ may be considered as a linear transformation between the direction of the cut (the unit normal $\hat{n}$) and the traction, of the form $\sigma \cdot \hat{n} = t$, which means that stress is a tensor.

The stress tensor may be represented as a 3×3 matrix, with components σ_{ij}, where i and j both go from 1 to 3. The diagonal elements represent normal stresses, whereas the off-diagonal ones represent shear stresses. Positive normal stresses are tensile, while negative ones are compressive (but an opposite sign convention is sometimes used, most notably in the soil mechanics literature). Finally, from the balance of angular momentum (or torque in the static case), it follows that the stress tensor and its matrix representation are symmetric ($\sigma_{ij} = \sigma_{ji}$), meaning that only six out of the nine components are in fact independent.

Not to burden the presentation with unnecessary mathematical complexities, we will, in what follows, nevertheless, mostly restrict ourselves to one-dimensional examples. In this case, the stress tensor has only one component, which represents a normal stress (a pressure), and the indices may be omitted.

Balance Laws

General physical laws often state that quantities like mass, energy, and momentum are conserved. In computational mechanics, the most important of these balance laws pertains to *linear momentum* (when reckoned per unit volume, linear momentum may be expressed as the material density ρ times velocity v). The balance equation for linear momentum may be considered as a generalization of Newton's second law, which states that mass times acceleration equals total force. As we saw in the previous section, stresses in a material produce tractions, which may be considered as internal forces. In addition, external forces such as gravity may contribute to the total force. These are commonly reckoned per unit mass and are usually referred to as *body forces* to distinguish them from tractions, which may be considered as *surface forces*. For a one-dimensional motion, balance of linear momentum requires that (37,38)

$$\rho a = \frac{\partial \sigma}{\partial x} + \rho b \tag{6}$$

where a is the acceleration and b is the body force. This equation closely resembles Newton's second law if one thinks of $\partial \sigma / \partial x$ as an internal force (reckoned per unit volume).

In addition to the momentum balance equation (6), one generally needs an equation that expresses conservation of mass, but no other balance laws are required for so-called purely mechanical theories, in which temperature plays no role (as mentioned, balance of angular momentum has already been included in the definition of stress). If thermal effects are included, one also needs an equation for the balance of energy (that expresses the first law of thermodynamics: energy is conserved) and an entropy inequality (that follows from the second law of thermodynamics: the entropy of a closed system cannot decrease). The entropy inequality is, strictly speaking, not a balance law but rather imposes restrictions on the material models.

Material Models

The balance laws described in the previous section are assumed to be valid for all materials. They do not, however, completely specify the mechanical response in the sense that there are more unknowns than equations. To obtain a complete description, it is thus necessary to complement the balance laws with certain material-specific equations. These describe the material constitution and are therefore often called *constitutive equations*. Although a large number of constitutive models exist, they may be classified as being of three main types: elastic, elastoplastic, and viscoelastic/viscoplastic (viscoelastic and viscoplastic models are both characterized by a rate-dependent response and are therefore often described as one entity). Although it perhaps may appear more natural to consider the strain to be a function of the applied stress, it turns out to be more convenient to describe the constitutive models using a strain-driven format, that is, to consider strain as the independent variable (38).

Elastic materials For elastic materials, the stress and strain are related by a unique functional relationship, which may be linear (linearly elastic material) or nonlinear (hyperelastic materials). The function between stress and strain may generally be assumed to be linear for small strains, and in the one-dimensional case, one obtains Hooke's law (37,38)

$$\sigma = E\varepsilon \tag{7}$$

where E is the Young's modulus. The deformation history does not influence the stress in an elastic material in any way, and thus, the material has no memory of previous configurations. As indicated in Figure 5A, a deformed elastic material will hence recover its initial shape when unloaded. Since the stress in an elastic material is a unique function of the strain, so is the strain energy. Therefore, elastic deformation is completely nondissipative, that is, all applied mechanical work is converted to strain energy.

Elastoplastic materials Elastoplastic materials deform elastically for small strains, but start to deform plastically (permanently) for larger ones. In the small-strain regime, this behavior may be captured by writing the total strain as the sum of elastic and plastic parts (i.e., $\varepsilon = \varepsilon^e + \varepsilon^p$, where ε^e and ε^p are the elastic and plastic strains, respectively). The stress in the material is generally assumed to depend on the elastic strain only (not on the plastic strain or the strain rate), and hence, no unique functional relationship exists between stress and strain. This fact also implies that energy is dissipated during plastic deformation. The point at which the material starts to deform plastically (the yield locus) is usually specified via a yield condition, which for one-dimensional plasticity may be stated as (38)

$$f(\sigma) = |\sigma| - \sigma_y = 0 \tag{8}$$

where $f(\sigma)$ is called the yield function, σ_y is the yield stress, and $|\sigma|$ indicates the magnitude of σ. The material deforms elastically as long as the yield function is negative but starts to deform plastically when the yield locus is reached [at which point $f(\sigma) = 0$]. A typical loading-unloading sequence of an elastoplastic material may thus appear as in Figure 5B.

Visoelastic/viscoplastic materials The distinguishing mark of viscoelastic and viscoplastic materials is a response that depends on the rate of straining. Viscoelastic and viscoplastic strains are, however, not equivalent since the former is completely recoverable, whereas the latter is not. In other words, the undeformed configuration is eventually recovered when a viscoelastic material is unloaded, whereas a permanent deformation may persist for viscoplastic materials.

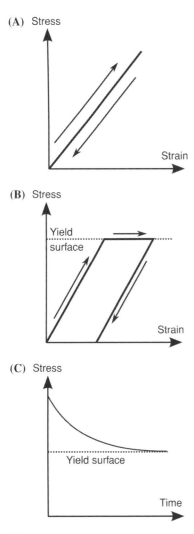

Figure 5 Schematic illustration of the behavior of elastic, elastoplastic, and viscoplastic materials. A loading-unloading sequence is shown in (**A**) and (**B**), whereas stress relaxation following straining past the yield point is depicted in (**C**). (**A**) Elastic. (**B**) Elastoplastic. (**C**) Viscoplastic.

Viscoplastic materials, therefore, share many features with elastoplastic materials but, in addition, exhibit a dependence on the rate of straining. Again, a decomposition of the total strain is convenient, this time into elastic and viscoplastic parts (i.e., $\varepsilon = \varepsilon^{e} + \varepsilon^{vp}$, where ε^{e} and ε^{vp} are the elastic and viscoplastic strains, respectively). In analogy with the elastoplastic case, the boundary of the elastic region may be specified in terms of a yield function. However, whereas the region outside the yield surface was inadmissible in the elastoplastic case, the stress is allowed to lie outside the yield surface in the viscoplastic one. Hence, straining beyond the yield point generally results in the creation of an excess (or extra) stress σ^{ex} that decays toward zero with time, typically as (38)

$$\sigma^{ex}(t) = \sigma_0^{ex} e^{-t/\tau} \qquad (9)$$

where the relaxation time $\tau = \eta/E$, with η being the viscosity of the material (E is the Young's modulus, as before). This behavior is illustrated in Figure 5C.

A General Example: Propagation of Waves

Although the main applications of the outlined theory will be discussed in section "Pharmaceutical Applications" below, we present here one particular example: propagation of longitudinal (sound) waves through a material. Propagation of sound waves forms the basis of many important techniques, such as ultrasonic testing of tablets and ultrasonic imaging. The starting point is the momentum balance equation (6), with zero body force. If we let u represent the displacement of particles, we may, for small strains, compute the acceleration as the second derivative $a = \partial^2 u/\partial t^2$. For small displacements, it is not necessary to make a distinction between the reference coordinates X and the current coordinates x, and thus, $\varepsilon = \partial u/\partial x$, according to equation (5). Assuming a linearly elastic behavior (which is reasonable for small displacements), the stress becomes $\sigma = E \partial u/\partial x$, according to equation (7). Inserting these expressions in equation (6) and dividing both sides by ρ finally produces

$$\frac{\partial^2 u}{\partial t^2} = \frac{E}{\rho} \frac{\partial^2 u}{\partial x^2}. \tag{10}$$

This equation describes propagation of sound waves, with wave speed $c_s = \sqrt{E/\rho}$, and is therefore usually referred to as the wave equation. In fact, the general solution may be expressed as $u(x,t) = f_R(x - c_s t) + f_L(x + c_s t)$, where the first term represents a wave traveling to the right and the second, a wave traveling to the left. Here, f_R and f_L are arbitrary functions of the indicated arguments. Although this particular derivation pertains to sound waves, *all* wave motions are in fact described by equations of the same form.

Computational Methods

With some exceptions (such as the analysis of propagation of small-amplitude waves in section "Propagation of Waves"), it is generally not possible to solve (continuum) mechanical problems analytically. The reason for this is that the governing equations are typically nonlinear, with the nonlinearity resulting either from the material model (material nonlinearity) or from large strains (geometric nonlinearity). Instead, the solution is obtained by using approximate *numerical methods*, also called *computational methods*. Here we describe the two most important numerical methods in computational mechanics: the finite and the discrete element (DE) method. Sometimes, however, other methods may be preferable for specific processes [granulation is, for instance, conveniently described using population balance models (39)].

The Finite Element Method

The finite element (FE) method is a very versatile numerical method that may be used to solve almost any problem, provided that the solution may be considered as a continuously varying function of position and time (40,41). At first sight, it may appear that the FE method would therefore have limited applicability for powders, since quantities such as density, stress, and strain do not vary continuously on the particle scale. However, a sufficiently fine powder may be idealized as a hypothetical continuous material, formally obtained by averaging over representative volume elements (42,43). These volume elements must be much larger than the particle size and at the same time much smaller than macroscopic dimensions of interest (such as the tablet height or diameter), and hence, other methods are required for coarse powders or granular materials (see later in the text).

(A)

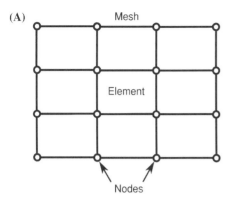

(B)

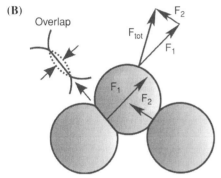

Figure 6 Basic principle of the (**A**) FE and (**B**) DE methods. (**A**) FE. (**B**) DE. *Abbreviations*: FE, finite element; DE, discrete element.

The basic principle of the FE method is illustrated in Figure 6A. The problem domain (the region in space occupied by the powder) is first subdivided into a number of *finite elements*, collectively referred to as the FE *mesh*. The mesh is commonly constructed in such a way that no material exchange occurs between elements, which instead change their form as a result of the deformation (Lagrangian meshes). Sometimes, however, a mesh fixed in space (an Eulerian mesh) is more useful, especially in fluid mechanical applications. In each element, the unknown quantity (the displacement u) is *interpolated* using FE basis functions. In this way, the problem of finding the variation in u within the element is reduced to that of finding its value at certain points, referred to as *nodes*, located at the element boundaries. Since u is assumed to be continuous, this placement of the nodes implies that the nodal values are shared between neighboring elements. An equation system for the unknown nodal values of u may therefore be obtained from the requirement that the governing equation [the three-dimensional analogue of the momentum balance equation (6)] be satisfied in each element (in an average or *weak* sense). As indicated above, this equation system will generally be nonlinear, and hence, iterative methods are used in its solution. We refer the reader to the many good books on the FE method for a more exhaustive discussion, in particular the ones by Hughes (40) and Bonet and Wood (44).

The Discrete Element Method

Contrary to the FE method, the DE method (45) retains a description in terms of individual, interacting particles. This fact makes the DE method fairly straightforward conceptually. Basically, Newton's laws are used to determine the motion of each particle from a consideration of the forces it experiences (Fig. 6B). Interparticle contact forces dominate for compression simulations, but other forces—due to gravity or electrostatic interactions, for instance—may be of importance in other applications. Usually, a simplified contact description is used, with forces essentially being determined from the particle "overlap" (Fig. 6B) using contact mechanics (46). The particle motion is typically determined using an explicit solution scheme (40,47), without the need to solve any equations.

Although straightforward in principle, large-scale DE simulations pose some computational challenges. The first of these is related to *contact detection*. To determine which particles are in contact, it would perhaps be tempting to calculate the distance between all particle pairs and to conclude that two particles are in contact whenever this distance is smaller than the particle diameter (assuming monodisperse spherical particles for simplicity). However, such a "brute force" contact detection algorithm would not work except for systems of very few particles, since the number of particle pairs is proportional to the number of particles squared (for a typical powder containing $\sim 10^6$ particles, the number of particle pairs would be $\sim 10^6 \times 10^6 = 10^{12}$, which is indeed a very large number). Instead, contact detection algorithms based on a spatial search are typically employed (47). In fact, algorithms have been devised (48,49), whose computational time scales linearly with the number of particles (rather than quadratically as for the brute force method). The second challenge is related to the fact that explicit algorithms are stable only if sufficiently small time steps are used. The maximal (or *critical*) time step is typically proportional to $\sqrt{m/k}$, where m is the particle mass and k its stiffness, expressed in terms of the Young's modulus. Therefore, a prohibitively small time step is sometimes needed for stiff particles.

In some applications, most notably powder compression, the simplified contact description of the DE method may lead to inaccurate results. For this reason, a combined FE/DE method has been proposed (47,50). The FE/DE method describes each particle as a deformable body (as per the standard FE method) and uses the DE method to handle its motion. Combined FE/DE simulations are therefore realistic but at the same time very time consuming. For this reason, application of the method has hitherto been restricted to two-dimensional systems (51–55). With increasing computer power, the combined FE/DE method is nevertheless expected to be of great value in the future.

Pharmaceutical Applications

Many important pharmaceutical unit operations handle and process powders in various ways, and these unit operations may be analyzed and modeled by using computational mechanics. Examples include powder compression and compaction, powder flow, fluidization, mixing and segregation, packing, and milling.

Powder Compression

Tablets are generally formed by confined compression of powders, and much effort has therefore been devoted to understanding and optimizing this unit operation. In this work, FE and DE simulations play an important role.

In other disciplines, the FE method has been used to model powder compression for a relatively long time, but the first FE analysis of pharmaceutical powder compression appeared in 2002 (56). Since then, the method has been used by a number of researchers focusing on the behavior of commonly used excipient materials such as lactose (56–58) and microcrystalline cellulose (59–63). The data obtained from FE simulations are typically related to the variation in density and stress in a powder or compact. The effects of friction and compact shape on the variation in density may be determined (60–63). The distribution of stress may give insights into common failure mechanisms of tablets. Some investigations have, for instance, observed strain localization during unloading, that is, the occurrence of localized plastic deformation and concurrent stress relief. This may be seen as a narrow region characterized by a large stress gradient, the position of which appears to coincide with the failure surface in capping (Fig. 7A) (57,58).

The DE and combined FE/DE methods are interesting, since they are able to provide complementary information on the particle scale (54,64). In particular, the relationship between particle properties (such as Young's modulus and yield stress) and powder properties may be elucidated. In this manner, it has been shown that the Heckel's parameter (65) (also referred to as the yield pressure) indeed reflects the yield stress of individual particles *provided that* the ratio between the Young's modulus and yield stress is sufficiently high (Fig. 7B) (64). For lower ratios, the Heckel's parameter rather reflects the Young's modulus.

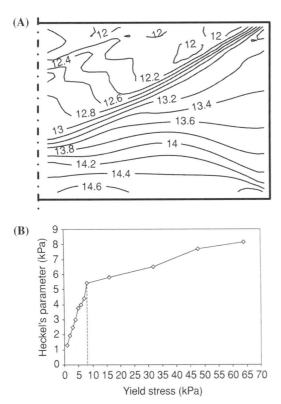

Figure 7 Application of the FE and DE methods. (**A**) Pressure distribution (MPa) in a lactose tablet during unloading obtained from FE simulations. A cross section of half the tablet is shown, with a dashed-dotted symmetry line. (**B**) Relationship between the Heckel's parameter and yield stress of individual particles obtained from DE simulations. The Young's modulus was kept constant at 250 kPa. *Abbreviations*: FE, finite element; DE, discrete element. *Source*: From Refs. 58 and 64.

Other Applications

Computational mechanics, and in particular the DE method, may be successfully used to analyze a wide range of operations involving powders and granular materials. Of particular relevance in a pharmaceutical context are applications related to flow of powders in hoppers (66), fluidized beds (67), and mixers (68,69). The method has been applied in the analysis of ball mills (70) and may be used to look more deeply into certain processes such as vibration-induced size segregation of granular materials (71) and packing (72).

TRANSPORT PROCESSES

General Principles

Transport as a Nonequilibrium Phenomenon

Physical processes related to transport of a substance (matter, heat, charge, etc.) from one location to another are often collectively referred to as transport processes. Familiar examples include chemical diffusion, air flow through porous materials, and flow of electric currents though resistors. As these examples indicate, transport is generally a nonequilibrium phenomenon, and, as such, is usually analyzed within the realm of nonequilibrium thermodynamics or statistical mechanics (73–77), often using the Boltzmann equation (78) as the starting point. Here we briefly describe two important general results that emerge from such an analysis. The first is related to the mathematical form of transport equations and the second to the close relationship that exists between transport—a nonequilibrium phenomenon—and fluctuations that are present in the system in thermal equilibrium.

The analysis of transport produces a fairly intuitive result: the flux $\mathcal{J}$ (an extensive property) depends on a driving force $\mathcal{F}$, which in turn may generally be expressed as the *gradient* of an appropriate intensive quantity (chemical potential, temperature, electric potential, etc.). We use a calligraphic font to indicate that these are generalized quantities; the driving force may, for instance, be an electric field or a stress. It is realized that the driving force vanishes if the intensive quantity in question does not depend on location, which is the case for a system in global thermodynamic equilibrium. Moreover, since the flux must vanish whenever the driving force vanishes, it must, in the linear regime, be possible to express the relation between the driving force and the resulting flux as

$$\mathcal{J} = \mathcal{L}\mathcal{F} \qquad (11)$$

where $\mathcal{L}$ is a linear transport coefficient. Equation (11) is the prototype for many often used transport equations, some of which are summarized in Table 2.

We remark that sometimes more general transport equations are also needed in the linear regime. The reason for this is twofold: simultaneous fluxes may interact, and in a

Table 2 Particular Instances of the General Linear Transport Equation (11)

Name	Driving force	Transport coefficient
Fick's law	Concentration gradient	Diffusivity
Fourier's law	Temperature gradient	Thermal conductivity
Ohm's law	Electrical potential gradient	Electrical conductivity
Darcy's law	Pressure gradient	Permeability

binary system, diffusion of one species may thus in general be influenced not only by the concentration gradient of the same species but also by that of the other. Such more general transport processes were analyzed by Onsager, who derived the famous reciprocal relations that bear his name (79,80). Moreover, sometimes memory effects are important (see later in the text).

The relationship between transport and fluctuations alluded to above is most easily introduced by using Brownian motion as an example. Brownian motion is clearly a random or stochastic process, and if we follow a particular particle, initially located at the origin, we may consider its position $x(t)$ at time t as a random variable (for simplicity, here we assume that the particle may move along one dimension only). In the section above, we considered Brownian motion as a random walk and found that the average squared distance traveled by a particle is proportional to time. Here we reinvestigate this process by using the diffusion equation. In fact, an argument due to Einstein reveals that

$$\langle x^2(t) \rangle = 2Dt \tag{12}$$

where D is the diffusion coefficient (similar equations hold in two and three dimensions, but the proportionality constant is then $4D$ and $6D$ rather than $2D$). This is the Einstein–Smoluchowski equation, derived by Einstein in one of his famous 1905 papers (81) and independently rederived by Smoluchowski (82). [For the interested reader, we remark that the derivation of equation (12) proceeds as follows: the so-called causal Green's function, defined as the solution to the diffusion equation (Fick's second law) that initially corresponds to a delta function at the origin, may be written as $e^{-x^2/(4Dt)}/\sqrt{4\pi Dt}$. The causal Green's function may be interpreted as the conditional probability of finding a particle at location x at time t that was at the origin at time zero. Calculation of the second moment of this function produces equation (12).]

Einstein pointed out that the same random forces that produce Brownian motion are also in operation when the particle is dragged through the medium. Whereas diffusion is characterized by the diffusion coefficient, drag is usually quantified in terms of a mobility μ, a proportionality constant between the applied force F and the terminal velocity v, where $v = \mu F$. In fact, the diffusion coefficient and mobility are related by

$$D = \mu k_B T \tag{13}$$

where k_B is the Boltzmann constant and T is the absolute temperature. The Einstein relation (13) is an example of fluctuation-dissipation theorems, which generally relate the systematic and random parts of a microscopic force (83). Another well-known fluctuation-dissipation theorem is that of Nyquist, which shows that the thermal noise in a resistor may be expressed solely in terms of its resistance and the absolute temperature (84). General fluctuation-dissipation theorems may be derived using linear response theory, to be discussed next.

Memory Effects: Hereditary Integrals and Linear Response Theory

Whereas the general linear transport equation (11) usually provides an adequate description of transport processes, there are cases of practical interest where a generalization is needed: Since the transport coefficient $\mathcal{L}$ is a constant, equation (11) implies that the response—the flux $\mathcal{J}$—momentarily follows the driving force $\mathcal{F}$, which is not always the case. Consider, for example, the response of a viscoelastic material (such as a gel) to an applied stress or the response of a dielectric material to an applied electric field, both of which generally lag behind the driving force. Such delayed responses may be interpreted as resulting from the system having a *memory* of previously applied forces but do not imply that the system is necessarily nonlinear. In fact, provided the driving force is small enough, delayed responses may be successfully analyzed by using hereditary integrals (see Ref. 85 and references therein) or linear response theory, originally developed by Kubo (86). Moreover, using the relationship between transport and fluctuations described in the previous section, it is possible to derive general expressions for transport coefficients in terms of certain correlation functions [often referred to as the Kubo or the Green–Kubo formulas (86–88)].

In practical applications of the linear-response formalism, it is often more convenient to express the response in terms of a displacement $\mathcal{D}$ rather than a flux $\mathcal{J}$, and we will therefore focus on this case here. The response of a gel to an applied stress is, for instance, conveniently expressed as a strain, and likewise, the response of a dielectric material to an applied electric field is often expressed as a polarization [which is closely related to the so-called electric displacement field (89)]. As a mechanical analogue would indicate, a flux is generally proportional to a velocity, and the displacement is therefore computed as the time integral of the flux.

Time-domain response To introduce the general ideas, let us investigate the response of an electric circuit consisting of a resistor (resistance R) in series with a capacitor (capacitance C), as illustrated in Figure 8A. This electric circuit, in fact, gives rise to the same response as the Debye model, originally proposed to describe the dielectric response of systems containing noninteracting dipoles (90). In rheology, an essentially equivalent response is obtained from the Kelvin–Voigt model (37), consisting of a parallel arrangement of a spring and a dashpot (Fig. 8A). In our example, the driving force is the applied electric potential $U(t)$, and the response is the charge $Q(t)$ on the capacitor. The applied potential is assumed to be zero in the far past (in the limit $t \rightarrow -\infty$), but otherwise, no assumptions are made on the time evolution of $U(t)$. Since the time derivative of the charge equals the electric current, the voltage across the resistor may be expressed as $R\,dQ/dt$ (by Ohm's law), whereas the voltage across the capacitor equals Q/C (by the definition of capacitance). The applied voltage is the sum of these two contributions, and thus, the time evolution of Q is governed by the ordinary differential equation

$$\frac{dQ}{dt} + \frac{1}{\tau}Q = \frac{C}{\tau}U \tag{14}$$

where we have introduced the *relaxation time* $\tau = RC$. Equation (14) may be readily solved by using the method of integrating factor. Multiplication of the equation by $e^{t/\tau}$ and integration from $-\infty$ to t shows that

$$Q(t) = \int_{-\infty}^{t} \frac{C}{\tau} e^{-(t-t')/\tau} U(t')\,dt'$$
$$= \int_{0}^{\infty} \frac{C}{\tau} e^{-s/\tau} U(t-s)\,ds \tag{15}$$

Notice that the factor $e^{-t/\tau}$ is a constant in the first integral, which allowed us to write it as part of the integrand. The second integral is obtained from the first by making the substitution $s = t - t'$ (s is often referred to as the *time lapse*). As seen from equation (15), the response of the system is completely characterized by the function $\psi(t) = (C/\tau)e^{-t/\tau}$, which is therefore called the *response function* (or sometimes the *aftereffect function* to highlight the fact that the response is delayed). Moreover, it is seen that the (delayed) response may be expressed as a convolution or hereditary integral.

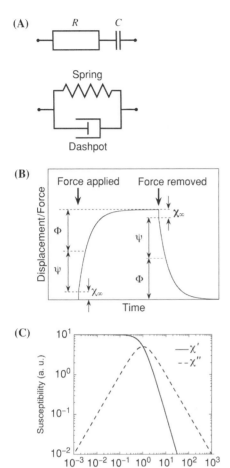

Figure 8 Linear response. (**A**) Analogous models. (**B**) Time-domain response. (**C**) Frequency-domain response.

Although the response function will generally differ from the one obtained in the example considered above, the description of delayed responses has general validity. In addition to delayed responses, many systems also exhibit instantaneous responses (on the time scale of the experiment). In the electric example, an instantaneous response would result from a capacitor in parallel with the described circuit (or a spring in series with the Kelvin–Voigt element). The total response may be expressed as the sum of the instantaneous and the delayed responses, and thus, the relation between the driving force and the resulting displacement may generally be expressed as

$$\mathcal{D}(t) = \chi_\infty \mathcal{F}(t) + \int_0^\infty \psi(s)\mathcal{F}(t-s)\,ds \qquad (16)$$

where the proportionality constant for the instantaneous response is written as χ_∞ because short times correspond to high frequencies. The response function $\psi(t)$ is often written as the derivative of the creep function $\Psi(t)$ [commonly denoted by $J(t)$ in the rheological literature (91,92)]. Alternatively, the response function may be written as the negative derivative of the relaxation function $\Phi(t)$. The creep function describes the response of a system following the application of a constant force at time zero (assuming that the system was previously in equilibrium). The relaxation function, on the other hand, describes the response of the system following a sudden removal of the force at time zero (assuming that the force was previously applied for sufficiently long time so that a steady state could be reached). The creep and relaxation functions are illustrated in Figure 8B.

Before proceeding to the frequency-domain response, we remark that it is sometimes useful to consider the force to be a function of the displacement (and not the other way round). This is particularly true for mechanical applications, and analogous developments to those outlined above show that stress may be related to strain by an equation of the same form as equation (16).

Frequency-domain response It is often convenient to characterize the linear response of systems in the frequency rather than in the time domain. If one applies a periodic loading with angular frequency ω [circular frequency $f = \omega/(2\pi)$], one will obtain a periodic response of the same frequency, but the response will generally be out of phase.

$$\mathcal{F}(t) = \mathcal{F}_0 \cos \omega t \rightarrow \mathcal{D}(t) = \mathcal{D}_0 \cos(\omega t - \delta) \tag{17}$$

In these expressions, $\mathcal{F}_0$ and $\mathcal{D}_0$ are amplitudes and δ is the phase shift. In general, $\mathcal{D}_0$ and δ are functions of ω. The response may be resolved into in-phase ($\cos \omega t$) and out-of-phase ($\sin \omega t$) components by using the trigonometric identity $\cos(\omega t - \delta) = \cos \delta \cos \omega t + \sin \delta \sin \omega t$.

An alternative, and often more convenient, representation of periodic responses utilizes complex numbers. In fact, since the real part of $e^{-i\omega t}$ is $\cos \omega t$, the response indicated in equation (17) is equivalent to

$$\mathcal{F}(t) = \mathcal{F}_0 e^{-i\omega t} \rightarrow \mathcal{D}(t) = \mathcal{D}_0 e^{-i(\omega t - \delta)} = \mathcal{D}_0^* e^{-i\omega t} \tag{18}$$

where $\mathcal{D}_0^* = \mathcal{D}_0 e^{i\delta}$ is a complex amplitude. Since $e^{i\delta} = \cos \delta + i \sin \delta$ (Euler's formula), it is seen that the in-phase component of the response in equation (17) corresponds to the real part of the response in equation (18), whereas the out-of-phase component corresponds to the imaginary part. The reader is cautioned that an alternative sign convention is also in widespread use, resulting from a representation of harmonic quantities as $e^{+i\omega t}$ rather than as $e^{-i\omega t}$.

Mathematically, the time and frequency-domain responses are connected via Fourier–Laplace transforms, but the same conclusions may be reached by inserting the complex force from equation (18) in equation (16). In this manner, one obtains the expression

$$\mathcal{D} = [\chi_\infty + \chi^*(\omega)]\mathcal{F} \tag{19}$$

where

$$\chi^*(\omega) = \int_0^\infty \psi(s)e^{i\omega s}\, ds \tag{20}$$

is a complex frequency-dependent susceptibility. The latter is often decomposed into real and imaginary parts, $\chi^*(\omega) = \chi'(\omega) + i\chi''(\omega)$, where

$$\chi'(\omega) = \int_0^\infty \psi(s)\cos \omega s\, ds \quad \text{and} \quad \chi''(\omega) = \int_0^\infty \psi(s)\sin \omega s\, ds \tag{21}$$

as seen by using Euler's formula mentioned above. The real (in-phase) part corresponds to energy storage and the imaginary (out-of-phase) part to energy loss. For this reason, χ' (or $\chi_\infty + \chi'$) and χ'' are sometimes referred to as the storage and loss moduli, respectively. [To the benefit of the interested reader, we mention that this assertion may be verified as follows. As in mechanics, work may be expressed as the product of force and the displacement over which the force is acting. The instantaneous power (work per unit time) may therefore be computed as the product of force and the time derivative of the displacement: $\mathcal{F}dD/dt$. The energy imparted on the system per cycle is finally obtained by integrating this expression over one cycle. For the in-phase component, $\mathcal{F}dD/dt \propto \cos\omega t \sin\omega t \propto d(\cos^2 \omega t)/dt$, which means that the integral over one cycle vanishes. For the out-of-phase component, $\mathcal{F}dD/dt \propto \cos^2 \omega t$, and a nonzero result is obtained, which corresponds to the dissipated energy.]

Let us, at this point, return to the example described above (Fig. 8A), for which an exponentially decaying response function was obtained. This response function is here written as $\psi(t) = (\Delta\chi/\tau)e^{-t/\tau}$, where τ is the relaxation time and $\Delta\chi$ is a constant that may be interpreted as the maximal change in χ', hence the notation. As equation (20) shows, the corresponding complex frequency-dependent susceptibility is

$$\chi^*(\omega) = \frac{\Delta\chi}{1 - i\omega\tau} \tag{22}$$

and this susceptibility is readily decomposed into real and imaginary parts

$$\chi'(\omega) = \frac{\Delta\chi}{1 + (\omega\tau)^2} \quad \text{and} \quad \chi''(\omega) = \frac{\Delta\chi\omega\tau}{1 + (\omega\tau)^2} \tag{23}$$

respectively (multiply both the numerator and denominator by $1 + i\omega\tau$ and use the conjugate rule in the latter). The same result is of course obtained by using equation (21). This frequency-domain response is illustrated in Figure 8C, which shows the real and imaginary parts of the susceptibility as functions of angular frequency on a log-log scale [for reasons that will become apparent in the next section, a log-log representation is often preferable (93)]. As seen in Figure 8C, the imaginary part exhibits a peak centered around $\omega = 1/\tau$. Such loss peaks are a common feature in dielectric and rheological spectra, but their shape often deviates from that predicted by exponential relaxation (see later in the text). In fact, all changes in the storage modulus are invariably connected with losses in some frequency range. This follows from a global relationship between χ' and χ'' referred to as the Kramers–Krönig relations (94).

Nonexponential Relaxation

As indicated above, exponential relaxation does not generally provide a satisfactory description of experimental data. The response of dielectric materials is instead generally found to be characterized by certain power laws, both in the time and frequency domains (95,96). As observed by Curie and von Schweidler, a long time ago (97,98), the polarization current following the application of a constant electric field typically decays as a power function of time. The same is true for the dielectric response function, since it is proportional to the current: $\psi(t) \propto 1/t^\alpha$, where α is a positive constant. This response corresponds to a power law also in the frequency domain, of the form $\chi^*(\omega) \propto (i\omega)^{\alpha-1}$. Also when the response is characterized by more than one power law (as is usually the case for real systems), the imaginary part $\chi'' \propto \omega^{\alpha-1}$ in the appropriate frequency interval (the result for the real part is somewhat more complicated, since it also involves an additive constant).[a] Although the underlying physics is not fully understood, it is clear that the dielectric response thus generally exhibits fractal characteristics (99).

These observations underlie many of the empirical functions commonly used to describe dielectric loss peaks, for instance, the ones proposed by Cole and Cole (100), Davidson and Cole (101), and Havriliak and Negami (102). In the time domain, the empirical KWW relaxation function $\Phi(t) \propto \exp[-(t/\tau)^{\alpha}]$ often provides a reasonable description of experimental data (103). Since the response function is calculated as the negative derivative of $\Phi(t)$, it behaves as a power law for short times. Moreover, the ubiquitous occurrence of power laws in (dielectric) spectra explains why log-log representations often are preferable: power laws present themselves as straight lines when a log-log scale is used.

Depending on the appearance of the spectrum when the angular frequency ω approaches zero, dielectric responses of materials are often classified as being either dipolar in nature or carrier dominated. In the first case, the polarization is attributed to the reorientation of permanent dipoles, and in the latter to the displacement of partially mobile charge carriers. These two behaviors may be interpreted as being manifestations of different values of the exponent α in a power law of the form $\chi'' \propto \omega^{\alpha-1}$ at low frequencies: when ω approaches zero, χ'' tends to zero whenever the exponent $\alpha > 1$ but increases indefinitely when $\alpha < 1$. Likewise, the real part χ' approaches a finite value when $\alpha > 1$ but increases indefinitely in the same way as the imaginary part when $\alpha < 1$. Since no finite value is approached when $\alpha < 1$, this case usually is referred to as low-frequency dispersion (104,105).

It is interesting to contrast low-frequency dispersion with direct currents. To elucidate the effect of a nonzero direct-current (dc) conductivity σ_0 on the frequency-domain response, let us assume that a driving force $\mathcal{F} = \mathcal{F}_0 e^{-i\omega t}$ is applied, as in equation (18), and consider the situation for small angular frequencies ω. When ω approaches zero, the flux/current $\mathcal{J} \simeq \sigma_0 \mathcal{F}$, because the driving force varies so slowly that any delay in the response may be neglected, which in effect means that the transport equation (11) is recovered. The flux/current is computed as the time derivative of the displacement, and for a time dependence of the form $e^{-i\omega t}$, we thus find that $-i\omega\mathcal{D} = d\mathcal{D}/dt = \mathcal{J}$. Comparing the expressions for $\mathcal{J}$ (using the fact that $-1/i = i$), it is seen that $\mathcal{D} \simeq i(\sigma_0/\omega)\mathcal{F}$. A nonzero dc conductivity therefore results in a contribution to the imaginary part of the susceptibility that increases without bound as ω^{-1} when ω approaches zero. This behavior is similar to that obtained for low-frequency dispersion, especially when the exponent α is close to zero, and low-frequency dispersion is therefore sometimes also called quasi-dc conduction. Note, however, that the real part of the susceptibility is unaffected by a nonzero dc conductivity, whereas it increases in the same way as the imaginary part for low-frequency dispersion.

Even though the described behavior is rather universal for the dielectric response, it is not certain to what extent the same is true for the rheological response. It, however, seems to be applicable in the vicinity of the gel point (106), and experimental evidence in favor of a more general applicability appears to accumulate (107).

---

[a] If the response function were to decay as the same power law for all times, convergence of the integral in equation (20) would require that the exponent α be smaller than 1, but exponents larger than 1 are permitted in some time intervals.

Pharmaceutical Applications

Many processes in pharmaceutics are related to transport, and the applications of the outlined theory are therefore numerous. Notwithstanding their practical importance, the special instances of the general transport equation (11) listed in Table 2 are assumed to be relatively familiar, and will therefore not be discussed further in this chapter. Instead, we focus our attention on applications of hereditary integrals and linear response theory, in particular on *dynamic mechanical analysis* (DMA) and *impedance spectroscopy*.

Dynamic Mechanical Analysis

In DMA, a sinusoidal stress (or strain) is applied on a sample, and the resulting strain (or stress) is determined, typically for frequencies between 0.01 and 100 Hz (108). Since experiments are commonly performed at different temperatures, this technique is alternatively referred to as dynamic mechanical thermal analysis (DMTA). The basic information obtained from a DMA experiment is the storage and loss moduli, and their dependence on frequency and/or temperature. When applied to polymeric systems, DMA may in particular be used to quantify glass transitions, rate and extent of curing, gelation (e.g., sol-gel transitions), polymer morphology/compatibility, and interactions between polymers or between drug molecules and polymeric excipients (109). Pharmaceutical applications of DMA are numerous, and here we mention just a few examples. In one study, dynamic rheological properties of gels intended for ocular delivery were determined and correlated with the residence time in the eye (110). In another, polymer films were investigated, and glass transition temperatures and the degree of miscibility of the polymers were determined (111). In addition, DMA has been used to investigate compacts (112) as well as uncoated (113) and coated (114) pellets.

Impedance Spectroscopy

In impedance spectroscopy [IS; also referred to as dielectric spectroscopy (DS)], a sinusoidal electric field is applied across a sample, and the resulting polarization (or electric displacement) is determined as a function of frequency. The frequency sweep typically ranges from about 1 MHz down to about 1 mHz, but measurement may be performed at higher frequencies by using special equipment.

The beauty of the technique is its generality: all matter contains charges that produce a measurable dielectric response, and the technique may therefore be applied to solids, semisolids, and liquids. In pharmaceutical applications, however, the dielectric properties are seldom of interest in their own right (115,116), but useful information may often be extracted from the spectrum. Loss peaks of the type described above are generally associated with relaxation times, which may be related to the motion of polymer segments (117). The dc conductivity may be extracted from the spectrum and used as an indicator of the creation of bonding surfaces during tableting (118). In a similar manner, IS has been used to investigate mucoadhesion of gels (119). Moreover, information about the transport of charged drug substances (for instance in gels) may be obtained (120), which makes a determination of the diffusion coefficient possible via the Einstein relation (13). Since the permittivity of water is substantially higher than that of most other substances, dielectric measurements may be used to monitor the water content during granulation, which may be of great practical value in a process analytical technology context (121). IS also enables directed measurements of charge transport or dipolar reorientation, and may therefore be used to investigate anisotropy in paper and tablets, for instance (122).

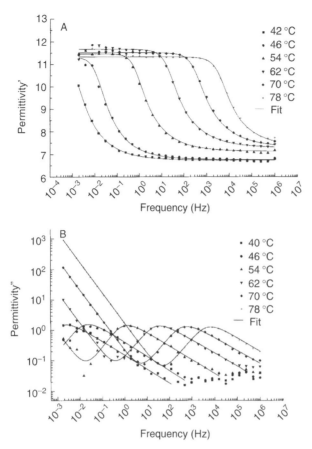

Figure 9 Real and imaginary parts of the permittivity obtained from impedance spectroscopy for amorphous indometacin at different temperatures. *Source*: From Ref. 123.

As was the case for DMA, IS measurements may be performed at different temperatures and may, for instance, be used to characterize the thermal behavior of amorphous drugs. One example is given in Figure 9, which shows the real and imaginary parts of the dielectric permittivity for amorphous indometacin at different temperatures (123). The spectra are seen to exhibit an evident relaxation peak, the position of which changes with temperature. The corresponding relaxation time was found to drastically decrease with increasing temperature of the amorphous material and to increase by ~ 6 orders of magnitude at the onset of crystallization. Moreover, a contribution from dc conduction may be clearly seen in the imaginary part of the permittivity for low frequencies (especially at higher temperatures).

These examples by no means exhaust the possibilities, but, nevertheless, indicate the usefulness of IS. More examples of the application of IS in a pharmaceutical and generic context may be found in Refs. 124 and 125, respectively.

CONCLUDING REMARKS

Our intention with this chapter has been to provide a unified description of some important physical concepts that are widely used to describe and/or analyze data. Rather than aiming at a complete literature overview, we have discussed a few selected areas in more depth. It is foreseen that the application of physical concepts is going to play an important role in pharmaceutical science in the future, and pharmaceutical physics is therefore expected to be a growing field.

REFERENCES

1. Duhem PMM. The Aim and Structure of Physical Theory. Princeton: Princeton University Press, 1991. [Translated from the French by Philip P. Wiener.]
2. Mandelbrot BB. The Fractal Geometry of Nature. Rev. ed. San Francisco: W. H. Freeman and Company, 1982.
3. Pfeifer P, Ehrburger-Dolle F, Rieker TP, et al. Nearly space-filling fractal networks of carbon nanopores. Phys Rev Lett 2002; 88:115502.
4. Cusack NE. The Physics of Structurally Disordered Matter: An Introduction. Bristol: Adam Hilger, 1987.
5. Stauffer D, Aharony A. Introduction to Percolation Theory. 2nd ed. London: Taylor & Francis, 1992.
6. Sahimi M. Applications of Percolation Theory. London: Taylor & Francis, 1994.
7. Kirkpatrick S. Percolation and conduction. Rev Mod Phys 1973; 45:574–588.
8. Havlin S, Ben-Avraham D. Diffusion in disordered media. Adv Physics 1987; 36:695–798.
9. de Gennes PG. La percolation: un concept unificateur. La Recherche 1976; 7:919–927.
10. Korsmeyer RW, Gurny R, Doelker E, et al. Mechanisms of solute release from porous hydrophilic polymers. Int J Pharm 1983; 15:25–35.
11. Peppas NA. Analysis of Fickian and non-Fickian drug release from polymers. Pharm Acta Helv 1985; 60:110–111.
12. Bonny JD, Leuenberger H. Matrix type controlled release systems. I. Effect of percolation on drug dissolution kinetics. Pharm Acta Helv 1991; 66:160–164.
13. Higuchi T. Rate of release of medicaments from ointment bases containing drugs in suspension. J Pharm Sci 1961; 50:874–875.
14. Bonny JD, Leuenberger H. Determination of fractal dimensions of matrix-type solid dosage forms and their relation with drug dissolution kinetics. Eur J Pharm Biopharm 1993; 39:31–37.
15. Caraballo I, Millán M, Rabasco AM. Relationship between drug percolation threshold and particle size in matrix tablets. Pharm Res 1996; 13:387–390.
16. Millán M, Caraballo I, Rabasco AM. The role of the drug/excipient particle size ratio in the percolation model for tablets. Pharm Res 1998; 15:216–220.
17. Brohede U, Valizadeh S, Stromme M, et al. Percolative drug diffusion from cylindrical matrix systems with unsealed boundaries. J Pharm Sci 2007; 96:3087–3099.
18. Kosmidis K, Argyrakis P, Macheras P. A reappraisal of drug release laws using Monte Carlo simulations: the prevalence of the Weibull function. Pharm Res 2003; 20:988–995.
19. Leuenberger H, Leu R. Formation of a tablet: a site and bond percolation phenomenon. J Pharm Sci 1992; 81:976–982.
20. Kuentz M, Leuenberger H, Kolb M. Fracture in disordered media and tensile strength of microcrystalline cellulose tablets at low relative densities. Int J Pharm 1999; 182:243–255.
21. Kuentz M, Leuenberger H. Modified Young's modulus of microcrystalline cellulose tablets and the directed continuum percolation model. Pharm Dev Technol 1998; 3:13–19.
22. Eriksson M, Alderborn G. The effect of particle fragmentation and deformation on the interparticulate bond formation process during powder compaction. Pharm Res 1995; 12: 1031–1039.
23. Alderborn G. A novel approach to derive a compression parameter indicating effective particle deformability. Pharm Dev Technol 2003; 8:367–377.
24. Bale HD, Schmidt PW. Small-angle X-ray-scattering investigation of submicroscopic porosity with fractal properties. Phys Rev Lett 1984; 53:596–599.
25. Pfeifer P, Avnir D. Chemistry in noninteger dimensions between two and three. I. Fractal theory of heterogeneous surfaces. J Chem Phys 1983; 79:3558–3565.

26. Friesen WI, Mikula RJ. Fractal dimensions of coal particles. J Colloid Interface Sci 1987; 120: 263–271.
27. Li T, Park K. Fractal analysis of pharmaceutical particles by atomic force microscopy. Pharm Res 1998; 15:1222–1232.
28. Fini A, Garuti M, Fazio G, et al. Diclofenac salts. I. Fractal and thermal analysis of sodium and potassium diclofenac salts. J Pharm Sci 2001; 90:2049–2057.
29. Schroder M, Kleinebudde P. Structure of disintegrating pellets with regard to fractal geometry. Pharm Res 1995; 12:1694–1700.
30. Pfeifer P, Wu YJ, Cole MW, et al. Multilayer adsorption on a fractally rough surface. Phys Rev Lett 1989; 62:1997–2000.
31. Avnir D, Jaroniec M. An isotherm equation for adsorption on fractal surfaces of heterogeneous porous materials. Langmuir 1989; 5:1431–1433.
32. Yin Y. Adsorption isotherm on fractally porous materials. Langmuir 1991; 7:216–217.
33. Pfeifer P, Obert M, Cole MW. Fractal BET and FHH theories of adsorption: a comparative-study. Proc R Soc Lond A 1989; 423:169–188.
34. Strømme M, Mihranyan A, Ek R, et al. Fractal dimension of cellulose powders analyzed by multilayer BET adsorption of water and nitrogen. J Phys Chem B 2003; 107:14378–14382.
35. Nilsson M, Mihranyan A, Valizadeh S, et al. Mesopore structure of microcrystalline cellulose tablets characterized by nitrogen adsorption and SEM: the influence on water-induced ionic conduction. J Phys Chem B 2006; 110:15776–15781.
36. Goldstein H, Poole CP, Safko JL. Classical Mechanics. 3rd ed. Upper Saddle River: Pearson Education, 2002.
37. Malvern LE. Introduction to the Mechanics of a Continuous Medium. Englewood Cliffs, NJ: Prentice Hall, 1969.
38. Simo JC, Hughes TJR. Computational Inelasticity. New York: Springer, 1998.
39. Hounslow MJ, Ryall RL, Marshall VR. A discretized population balance for nucleation, growth, and aggregation. AIChE J 1988; 34:1821–1832.
40. Hughes TJR. The Finite Element Method: Linear Static and Dynamic Finite Element Analysis. Mineola, NY: Dover Publications, 2000.
41. Belytschko T, Liu WK, Moran B. Nonlinear Finite Elements for Continua and Structures. Chichester: Wiley, 2000.
42. Hassanizadeh SM, Gray WG. General conservation equations for multiphase systems. 1. Averaging procedure. Adv Water Resour 1979; 2:131–144.
43. Hassanizadeh SM, Gray WG. General conservation equations for multiphase systems. 2. Mass, momenta, energy and entropy equations. Adv Water Resour 1979; 2:191–208.
44. Bonet J, Wood RD. Nonlinear Continuum Mechanics for Finite Element Analysis. Cambridge: Cambridge University Press, 1997.
45. Cundall PA, Strack ODL. A discrete numerical model for granular assemblies. Geotechnique 1979; 29:47–65.
46. Johnson KL. Contact Mechanics. Cambridge: Cambridge University Press, 1985.
47. Munjiza A. The Combined Finite-Discrete Element Method. Chichester: Wiley, 2004.
48. Munjiza A, Andrews KRF. NBS contact detection algorithm for bodies of similar size. Int J Numer Methods Eng 1998; 43:131–149.
49. Williams JR, Perkins E, Cook B. A contact algorithm for partitioning N arbitrary sized objects. Eng Comput 2004; 21:235–248.
50. Munjiza A, Owen DRJ, Bicanic N. A combined finite-discrete element method in transient dynamics of fracturing solids. Eng Comput 1995; 12:145–174.
51. Ransing RS, Gethin DT, Khoei AR, et al. Powder compaction modelling via the discrete and finite element method. Mater Des 2000; 21:263–269.
52. Gethin DT, Ransing RS, Lewis RW, et al. Numerical comparison of a deformable discrete element model and an equivalent continuum analysis for the compaction of ductile porous material. Comput Struct 2001; 79:1287–1294.
53. Gethin DT, Lewis RW, Ransing RS. A discrete deformable element approach for the compaction of powder systems. Model Simul Mater Sci Eng 2003; 11:101–114.

54. Lewis RW, Gethin DT, Yang XSS, et al. A combined finite-discrete element method for simulating pharmaceutical powder tableting. Int J Numer Methods Eng 2005; 62:853–869.

55. Gethin DT, Yang X-S, Lewis RW. A two dimensional combined discrete and finite element scheme for simulating the flow and compaction of systems comprising irregular particulates. Comput Methods Appl Mech Eng 2006; 195:5552–5565.

56. Michrafy A, Ringenbacher D, Tchoreloff P. Modelling the compaction behaviour of powders: application to pharmaceutical powders. Powder Technol 2002; 127:257–266.

57. Wu C-Y, Ruddy OM, Bentham AC, et al. Modelling the mechanical behaviour of pharmaceutical powders during compaction. Powder Technol 2005; 152:107–117.

58. Frenning G. Analysis of pharmaceutical powder compaction using multiplicative hyperelasto-plastic theory. Powder Technol 2007; 172:103–112.

59. Sinka IC, Cunningham JC, Zavaliangos A. The effect of wall friction in the compaction of pharmaceutical tablets with curved faces: a validation study of the Drucker–Prager Cap model. Powder Technol 2003; 133:33–43.

60. Cunningham JC, Sinka IC, Zavaliangos A. Analysis of tablet compaction. I. Characterization of mechanical behavior of powder and powder/tooling friction. J Pharm Sci 2004; 93:2022–2039.

61. Sinka IC, Cunningham JC, Zavaliangos A. Analysis of tablet compaction. II. Finite element analysis of density distributions in convex tablets. J Pharm Sci 2004; 93:2040–2053.

62. Michrafy A, Dodds JA, Kadiri MS. Wall friction in the compaction of pharmaceutical powders: measurement and effect on the density distribution. Powder Technol 2004; 148:53–55.

63. Kadiri MS, Michrafy A, Dodds JA. Pharmaceutical powders compaction: experimental and numerical analysis of the density distribution. Powder Technol 2005; 157:176–182.

64. Hassanpour A, Ghadiri M. Distinct element analysis and experimental evaluation of the Heckel analysis of bulk powder compression. Powder Technol 2004; 141:251–261.

65. Heckel RW. Density-pressure relationships in powder compaction. Trans Metal Soc AIME 1961; 221:671–675.

66. Langston PA, Tüzün U, Heyes DM. Discrete element simulation of granular flow in 2D and 3D hoppers: dependence of discharge rate and wall stress on particle interactions. Chem Eng Sci 1995; 50:967–987.

67. Mikami T, Kamiya H, Horio M. Numerical simulation of cohesive powder behavior in a fluidized bed. Chem Eng Sci 1998; 53:1927–1940.

68. Stewart RL, Bridgwater J, Zhou YC, et al. Simulated and measured flow of granules in a bladed mixer—a detailed comparison. Chem Eng Sci 2001; 56:5457–5471.

69. Kuo HP, Knight PC, Parker DJ, et al. The influence of DEM simulation parameters on the particle behaviour in a V-mixer. Chem Eng Sci 2002; 57:3621–3638.

70. Cleary PW. Predicting charge motion, power draw, segregation and wear in ball mills using discrete element methods. Miner Eng 1998; 11:1061–1080.

71. Rosato AD, Blackmore DL, Zhang N, et al. A perspective on vibration-induced size segregation of granular materials. Chem Eng Sci 2002; 57:265–275.

72. Siiria S, Yliruusi J. Particle packing simulations based on Newtonian mechanics. Powder Technol 2007; 174:82–92.

73. Prigogine I. Non-equilibrium Statistical Mechanics. Vol 1. New York: Interscience, 1962.

74. Prigogine I. Introduction to Thermodynamics of Irreversible Processes. 3rd ed. New York: Interscience, 1967.

75. Kubo R, Toda M, Hashitsume N. Statistical Physics II: Nonequilibrium Statistical Mechanics. 2nd ed. Berlin: Springer, 1991.

76. Kondepudi D, Prigogine I. Modern Thermodynamics: From Heat Engines to Dissipative Structures. Chichester: Wiley, 1998.

77. Zwanzig R. Nonequilibrium Statistical Mechanics. Oxford: Oxford University Press, 2001.

78. Boltzmann L. Lectures on Gas Theory. New York: Dover Publications, 1995. [Reprinted from Vorlesungen über Gastheorie.2nd ed. Leipzig: Barth, 1912.]

79. Onsager L. Reciprocal relations in irreversible processes. I. Phys Rev 1931; 37:405–426.

80. Onsager L. Reciprocal relations in irreversible processes. II. Phys Rev 1931; 38:2265–2279.

81. Einstein A. Über die von der molekularkinetischen Theorie der Wärme geforderte Bewegung von in ruhenden Flüssigkeiten suspendierten Teilchen. Ann Phys 1905; 17:549–560.
82. von Smoluchowski M. Zur kinetischen Theorie der Brownschen Molekularbewegung und der Suspensionen. Ann Phys 1906; 21:756–780.
83. Kubo R. The fluctuation-dissipation theorem. Rep Prog Phys 1966; 29:255–284.
84. Nyquist H. Thermal agitation of electric charge in conductors. Phys Rev 1928; 32:110–113.
85. Gurtin ME, Sternberg E. On the linear theory of viscoelasticity. Arch Rat Mech Anal 1962; 11:291–356.
86. Kubo R. Statistical-mechanical theory of irreversible processes. I. General theory and simple applications to magnetic and conduction problems. J Phys Soc Jpn 1957; 12:570–586.
87. Green MS. Markoff random processes and the statistical mechanics of time-dependent phenomena. J Chem Phys 1952; 20:1281–1295.
88. Green MS. Markoff random processes and the statistical mechanics of time-dependent phenomena. II. Irreversible processes in fluids. J Chem Phys 1954; 22:398–413.
89. Jackson JD. Classical Electrodynamics. 3rd ed. New York: Wiley, 1999.
90. Debye P. Polar Molecules. New York: Dover Publications, 1945.
91. Barnes HA, Hutton JF, Walters K. An Introduction to Rheology. Amsterdam: Elsevier, 1989.
92. Ferry JD. Viscoelastic Properties of Polymers. 3rd ed. New York: Wiley, 1980.
93. Jonscher AK. Presentation and interpretation of dielectric data. Thin Solid Films 1978; 50: 187–204.
94. Jonscher AK. Dielectric Relaxation in Solids. London: Chelsea Dielectrics Press, 1983.
95. Jonscher AK. The 'universal' dielectric response. Nature 1977; 267:673–679.
96. Jonscher AK. Universal Relaxation Law. London: Chelsea Dielectrics Press, 1996.
97. Curie MJ. Recherches sur le pouvoir inducteur spécifique et la conductibilité des corps cristallisés. Ann Chim Phys 1889; 17:385–434.
98. von Schweidler ER. Studien über die Anomalien in Verhalten der Dielektrika. Ann Phys 1907; 24:711–770.
99. Niklasson GA. Fractal aspects of the dielectric response of charge carriers in disordered materials. J Appl Phys 1987; 62:R1–R14.
100. Cole KS, Cole RH. Dispersion and absorption in dielectrics. I. Alternating current characteristics. J Chem Phys 1941; 9:341–351.
101. Davidson DW, Cole RH. Dielectric relaxation in glycerol, propylene glycol, and n-propanol. J Chem Phys 1951; 19:1484–1490.
102. Havriliak S, Negami S. A complex plane analysis of α-dispersions in some polymer systems. J Polym Sci C 1966; 14:99–117.
103. Williams G, Watts DC, Dev SB, et al. Further considerations of non symmetrical dielectric relaxation behaviour arising from a simple empirical decay function. Trans Faraday Soc 1971; 67:1323–1335.
104. Jonscher AK. Low-frequency dispersion in carrier-dominated dielectrics. Philos Mag B 1978; 38:587–601.
105. Dissado LA, Hill RM. Anomalous low-frequency dispersion: near direct current conductivity in disordered low-dimensional materials. J Chem Soc Faraday Trans 2, 1984; 80:291–319.
106. Winter HH, Chambon F. Analysis of linear viscoelasticity of a cross-linking polymer at the gel point. J Rheol 1986; 30:367–382.
107. Sollich P, Lequeux F, Hébraud P, et al. Rheology of soft glassy materials. Phys Rev Lett 1997; 78:2020–2023.
108. Craig DQM, Johnson F. Pharmaceutical applications of dynamic mechanical thermal analysis. Thermochimica Acta 1995; 248:97–115.
109. Jones DS. Dynamic mechanical analysis of polymeric systems of pharmaceutical and biomedical significance. Int J Pharm 1999; 179:167–178.
110. Edsman K, Carlfors J, Petersson R. Rheological evaluation of poloxamer as an in situ gel for ophthalmic use. Eur J Pharm Sci 1998; 6:105–112.
111. Lafferty SV, Newton JM, Podczeck F. Dynamic mechanical thermal analysis studies of polymer films prepared from aqueous dispersion. Int J Pharm 2002; 235:107–111.

112. Hancock BC, Dalton CR, Clas S-D. Micro-scale measurement of the mechanical properties of compressed pharmaceutical powders. 2: The dynamic moduli of microcrystalline cellulose. Int J Pharm 2001; 228:139–145.

113. Bashaiwoldu AB, Podczeck F, Newton JM. Application of dynamic mechanical analysis (DMA) to determine the mechanical properties of pellets. Int J Pharm 2004; 269:329–342.

114. Bashaiwoldu AB, Podczeck F, Newton JM. Application of Dynamic Mechanical Analysis (DMA) to the determination of the mechanical properties of coated pellets. Int J Pharm 2004; 274:53–63.

115. Craig DQM. Applications of low-frequency dielectric-spectroscopy to the pharmaceutical sciences. Drug Dev Ind Pharm 1992; 18:1207–1223.

116. Craig DQM. Dielectric spectroscopy as a novel analytical technique within the pharmaceutical sciences. STP Pharma Sci 1995; 5:421–428.

117. Einfeldt J, MeiÞner D, Kwasniewski A. Polymerdynamics of cellulose and other polysaccharides in solid state-secondary dielectric relaxation processes. Prog Polym Sci 2001; 26:1419–1472.

118. Nilsson M, Frenning G, Grasjo J, et al. Conductivity percolation in loosely compacted microcrystalline cellulose: an in situ study by dielectric spectroscopy during densification. J Phys Chem B 2006; 110:20502–20506.

119. Hägerstrom H, Edsman K, Strømme M. Low-frequency dielectric spectroscopy as a tool for studying the compatibility between pharmaceutical gels and mucous tissue. J Pharm Sci 2003; 92:1869–1881.

120. Brohede U, Bramer T, Edsman K, et al. Electrodynamic investigations of ion transport and structural properties in drug-containing gels: dielectric spectroscopy and transient current measurements on catanionic carbopol systems. J Phys Chem B 2005; 109:15250–15255.

121. Gradinarsky L, Brage H, Lagerholm B, et al. In situ monitoring and control of moisture content in pharmaceutical powder processes using an open-ended coaxial probe. Meas Sci Technol 2006; 17:1847–1853.

122. Ek R, Hill RM, Newton JM. Low frequency dielectric spectroscopy characterization of microcrystalline cellulose, tablets and paper. J Mater Sci 1997; 32:4807–4814.

123. He R, Craig DQM. An investigation into the thermal behaviour of an amorphous drug using low frequency dielectric spectroscopy and modulated temperature differential scanning calorimetry. J Pharm Pharmacol 2001; 53:41–48.

124. Craig DQM. Dielectric Analysis of Pharmaceutical Systems. London: Taylor & Francis, 1995.

125. Barsoukov E, Macdonald JR, eds. Impedance Spectroscopy: Theory, Experiment, and Applications. 2nd ed. Hoboken, NJ: Wiley-Interscience, 2005.

12

Pharmaceutical Aspects of Nanotechnology

Alexander T. Florence
Centre for Drug Delivery Research, The School of Pharmacy, University of London, London, U.K.

INTRODUCTION

Nanotechnology is the science that deals with particles or constructs which have dimensions ranging from several nanometers to around 100 to 150 nm (Fig. 1), although more commonly the upper limit is stretched to 200 nm. It is not possible to cover the whole gamut of nanotechnology or even only the pharmaceutical aspects of the subject in all its manifestations in one chapter. As a discipline, nanotechnology has already spawned several journals dealing with the physics, biology, toxicology, engineering, and pharmaceutical applications; many books (1–4); chapters and reviews; and a rapidly growing number of scientific papers and consensus reports (5,6). However, a treatise on modern pharmaceutics could hardly ignore the subject of pharmaceutical nanotechnology, which shows such promise, even though the field may be tainted somewhat with the hype from which it suffers (7). Elsewhere in the book, other chapters consider the topic: chapter 1, volume 1 suggests that many aspects of nanotechnology will feature in future paradigms of pharmaceutical research and has discussed some of the unsolved issues; chapter 9, volume 2 addresses target-oriented drug delivery including nanoparticulate carrier systems; and chapter 13, volume 1 on disperse systems draws attention to nanosuspensions. The thrust of this chapter is the use of nanoparticles as drug carriers and targeting agents, and it also points to the potential use of nanoparticles as excipients and as part of new, often hybrid materials. Its emphasis is on the pharmaceutics of these nanosystems. The chapter does not address liposome technology or solid lipid nanoparticle (SLN) systems. Liposomes are exhaustively covered in the three volumes edited by Gregoriadis and published in 2006 (8). SLNs have a large literature and are the subject of a recent review (9).

Scheme 1 illustrates the domains of nanomedicine. These can be considered to cover nanodevices, nanocarriers [which include nature's own vehicles such as low-density lipoprotein (LDL) particles (10,11)], viruses, and transmitter vesicles. Nanotoxicology is of course a primary consideration, but is outside the scope of this chapter. Diagnostic devices and imaging techniques employing nanoparticles are being developed rapidly.

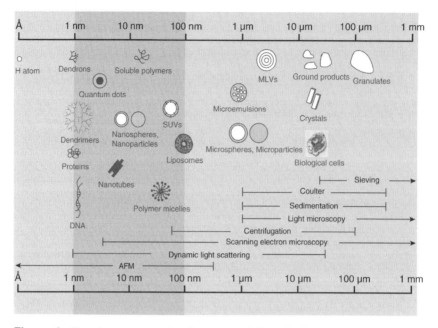

Figure 1 The size spectrum showing nanoparticle and other nanosystems in the context of microparticulates and macrosystems. Also shown are the methods employed to measure the particle size and size distribution of this range of materials. *Abbreviations*: MLV, multilamellar vesicle; SUV, single unilamellar vesicles. *Source*: From Ref. 13.

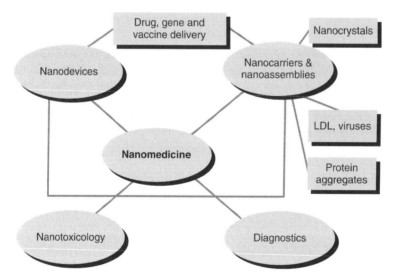

Scheme 1 The domains of nanomedicine including aspects of pharmaceutical nanotechnology. There are of course no strict boundaries between the subdomains. The links shown here are deliberate. Drug nanocrystals, for example, could be considered, like aggregates of therapeutic peptides and proteins, to be their own carriers systems, predominantly without additives.

Nanopharmacy, or pharmaceutical nanotechnology, comprises, but is not limited to, the topics shown in Scheme 2. These encompass the manipulation and processing of nanosystems in the 2 nm–150 nm size range, their physicochemical characterization, applications and biological evaluation.

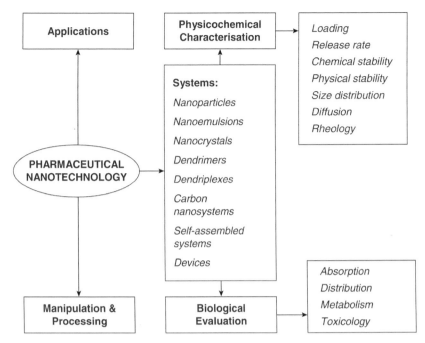

Scheme 2 Pharmaceutical nanotechnology's main areas of focus, namely, the manipulation and processing; the physicochemical characterization of a variety of systems in relation to their application; their biological evaluation. The last involves an understanding of the interaction between their physicochemical properties and biological barriers and environments. Absorption, distribution, metabolism, and toxicology refer to both the drug once released from the delivery system and the delivery system itself, while being aware of possible synergistic effects of the two.

Typical pharmaceutical carrier systems in the domain of nanotechnology include nanoparticles, nanosuspensions, nano (micro) emulsions, nanocrystals, dendrimers and dendriplexes, and carbon nanotubes (CNTs) as well as the smallest liposomes. Scheme 2, which suggests the main areas of focus in pharmaceutical nanotechnology, summarizes, for example, the wide range of means of characterizing nanosystems through investigation of their drug loading (rate and capacity), release rate, the chemical and physical stability of both drug and carrier, the crucial particle size and particle size distribution, surface charge and character (hydrophilic, hydrophobic), and nanoparticle diffusion and rheology. Shape features in nanosystems composed of CNTs. Biological evaluation of nanosystems involves knowledge of the absorption of both the drug and the carrier with its encapsulated or attached drug, carrier and drug distribution, excretion, and metabolism. Indeed, in vivo there are three potential aspects of biodistribution: that of drug released from the carrier, drug still encapsulated within the carrier, and the distribution of drug-depleted carriers.

The whole topic, however, is in a way defined by the size and size range of the systems concerned. Small size takes the particular object or structure in question within the realms of nanotechnology, as seen in Figure 1. It brings with it certain advantages and disadvantages, which we will discuss. Figure 1 illustrates the size spectrum of different systems from the macroscopic range, through the microscopic to the nanoscopic and the modes of measurement of particle size distribution. It can be inferred that dendrimers, small spherical or quasi-spherical synthetic polymers, are both particles and molecules and represent irreducibly small delivery agents. Quantum dots are a form of stabilized nanocrystal made from semiconductor materials such as zinc sulfide and cadmium selenide, which have applications in sensors and tracking (imaging) at the nanoscale (12).

NANOPARTICLES IN PHARMACY

Although the descriptor *nanotechnology* came to the fore in the late 1980s, it has a somewhat longer pedigree in pharmacy, in fact since Professor Peter Speiser and his colleagues (14–16) in Zurich prepared and investigated "nanoparts" and "nanocapsules" in the 1970s as laid out in a historical perspective written by Kreuter (17). Surfactant micelles (18), which have diameters of some 1 to 3 nm, have also been studied for many decades as solubilizers of poorly water-soluble drugs (19,20) and would be considered to be nanosystems in today's parlance. Microemulsions, a descriptor coined by Schulman in 1959 (21), are like the Neoral™ ciclosporin formulation, mainly nanoemulsions with droplets in the size range of 10 to 100 nm. It is claimed that the first commercial microemulsion, although not described as such, was introduced in 1928. Micelles and other surfactant-based systems are covered in chapter 14, volume 1.

COLLOIDS

Nanoparticles come within the field of colloidal systems. Colloids such as gold sols have been used in research since Faraday's time (22). Gold sols are used today as "novel" vectors (23). The science of colloids dates from the moment Thomas Graham (24) defined the term in 1861. Wolfgang Ostwald described the size range that colloids inhabit as the "world of neglected dimensions." Thus the topic is not new, but there have been many advances in the technology of size measurement and surface characterization of these systems that allows greater insight into how nanoparticles behave as carriers of drugs in vivo, so that this submicron world has indeed become visible and certainly not neglected. Given the large number of materials from which nanoparticles can be fabricated and their different surface properties and other characteristics, it is impossible to generalize about nanoparticles as applied to drug delivery; to do so would be like generalizing about polymers or indeed chemistry. The remainder of this chapter should be read with this truism in mind: not all nanosystems do everything.

MATERIALS BASED ON NANOPARTICLES

Apart from using nanosystems of a variety of designs and materials as carriers of drugs, there is a second aspect of the topic, which we will discuss briefly. That is the application of nanotechnology and nanoparticles in the design and fabrication of new systems, systems that as a result of their precise nanometer-sized building blocks have precise dimensions and controllable properties. A related topic, using biomolecules to template and mold the formation of especially inorganic materials, is considered in a review by Zhou (25). There is also the possibility of using nanoparticles of suitable materials as excipients, for example, as lubricants (26) for small devices. Both these topics are covered later.

NANOPARTICLES AS DRUG CARRIERS

The rationale for the encapsulation of drugs in nanoparticles, or in some cases the adsorption of drugs on their surface, is twofold. First, the drug is protected from the external environment until such time as it is released. Once released of course the drug behaves as free drug, although it might be deposited in different organs at different levels compared with administered free drug. Second, the nanoparticles rather than the characteristics of the drug itself determine the fate of the drug. It is important to distinguish between the *pharmacokinetics* of a drug when released from a carrier and the kinetics of the particles, which have been given the descriptor *particokinetics* (27). Clearly, the fate and distribution of the particles affect the behavior of the drug, modifying the locus, pattern, and rate of its release.

Small size is of course one of the defining features which distinguishes nanoparticles from microparticles and microparticles from fine powders. Size is particularly important in determining the ability of nanoparticles to access sites that are out of bounds to larger particles. There is, however, often a continuum of diameters, and one of the great challenges in drug targeting is the production of nanosystems with a narrow size distribution. Nature achieves this almost to perfection as with one example, the carriers of cholesterol—LDLs—have a mean diameter of 26.7 nm and a range of 25.8 to 28.2 nm in young healthy females and 25.5 to 28.1 nm in males (28). Another challenge is the maintenance of that size distribution after administration of the nanosuspensions by any route. Nanosystems have the potential for several advantageous effects, which include protection of drug or other active from harsh biological environments, slow release of contents, acting as adjuvants in vaccine delivery, and achieving drug delivery to specific regions of the body (e.g., liver, spleen, tumors, and inflamed sites). Attached ligands increase the probability of interaction with specific receptors in drug targeting but cannot be assumed, as we discuss later, lead to quantitative (complete) interactions, uptake, or activity.

Nanoparticles or other nanoconstructs have the special advantage that their small diameters allow penetration into tissues, translocation, and diffusion in the body where microparticles may be hindered. Small size at the limit (where the drug molecules approach the size of the carrier as with dendrimers) however, often means low loading capacity of individual particles and, at the limit, a large carrier/drug ratio. At the other end of the scale, some nanoparticles consist only of active, as in drug nanosuspensions or aggregates of therapeutic proteins.

Although there is the theoretical opportunity to reach hidden targets because of their small size, it does not mean that all can or do, as size alone is not sufficient. Surface characteristics are often the key, whether the particles are charged or they carry surface ligands; the nature of the material from which the nanoparticles are fabricated is relevant especially to the mode of degradation and release of the encapsulated therapeutic agent. The relative affinity of the drug for the nanoparticle and the medium in which the nanoparticle finds itself is another factor dependent on material and drug properties. Small diameters mean large surface areas/unit weight and hence a large surface for decoration with specific ligands, although, as will be recognized, both the percentage coverage and the orientation or heterogeneity of the surface ligands can be factors in the success of uptake in vivo. Multifunctionality may be the key to improved success of nanoparticle-receptor interactions, for example, in cancer chemotherapy (29). New materials will provide new opportunities for ingenuity in the design and manufacture of these materials.

Already, a wide variety of materials have been used in the preparation of nanosystems, both organic (mainly polymeric) and inorganic, as seen in Table 1: polymers, lipids, phospholipids, metals, CNTs, and ceramics have all been employed to date.

Viruses are a prime example of natural nanoparticles; attenuated viral particles have been used in gene transfection and virus-based nanoparticles (VNP) studied as targeting systems (51,52).

Table 1 Nanoparticles with Medical Uses

System	Uses	References
Dendrimers	Targeting of cancer cells, drug delivery, imaging.	31, 32
Ceramic nanoparticles	Passive targeting of cancer cells	33
Lipid-encapsulated perfluorocarbon nanoemulsions	Passive targeting of cancer cells	34
Magnetic nanoparticles	Specific targeting of cancer cells, tissue imaging	35, 36
LH-RH-targeted silica-coated lipid micelles	Specific targeting of cancer cells	35
Thiamine-targeted nanoparticles	Directed transfer across Caco-2 cells	37
Liposomes	Specific targeting of cancer cells, gene therapy, drug delivery	38–40
Nanoparticle-aptamer bioconjugate	Targeting of prostate cancer cells	41
Anti-Flk antibody-coated ^{90}Y nanoparticles	Anti-angiogenesis therapy	42
Gold nanoshells	Tissue imaging, thermal ablative cancer therapy	43, 44
Anti-HER2 antibody-targeted gold/silicon nanoparticles	Breast cancer therapy	45
CLIO paramagnetic nanoparticles	Imaging of migrating cells	46
Quantum dots	Tissue imaging	47
Silicon-based nanowires	Real-time detection and titration of antibodies, virus detection, chip-based biosensors	48
CNTs	Electronic biosensors	49
Transfersomes	Noninvasive vaccine delivery, drug delivery	50

Table in the main has been taken from Ref. 30 with the original references, but with some substitutes.
Aptamer: an oligonucleotide or peptide that bind specific target molecules.
Flk: vascular endothelial growth factor receptor.
HER2 receptor, which when overexpressed, is associated with breast cancer and stomach cancer
Abbreviations: CLIO, cross-linked iron oxide; CNTs, carbon nanotubes.

Lacerda et al. (53) summarize in Figure 2 the factors of import in drug delivery with nanoparticles (a term used in this chapter to cover the gamut of systems). Particles administered intravenously will be recognized and removed by the reticuloendothelial system after the adsorption of opsonins, plasma proteins that can determine recognition of the coated particles by mononuclear phagocytes. Such opsonin adsorption, or opsonization can be prevented to a greater or lesser extent by the transformation of a hydrophobic surface of the circulating particle to one covered by hydrophilic (polyoxyethylene)-based surfactants such as the block copolymer poloxamers. Blood flow dynamics (discussed later) control the distribution of the particles in the circulation, except those that extravasate. Uptake into cells after passage through the tissues and endothelium is itself a complex navigational process involving factors such as interstitial pH, hydrostatic pressure differences, lymphatic flow, and particle diffusion. We will discuss diffusion later, directly dependent $[D = f(1/r)]$ on the inverse of the particle radius, r, and on the viscosity and other features of the medium in which they move.

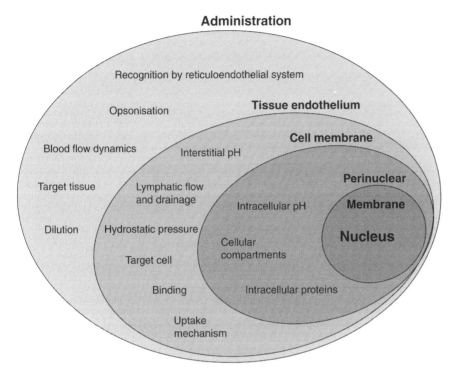

Figure 2 The multiple factors involved in the administration and targeting of nanosystems in the tissue endothelium, cell membrane, and cytoplasm. *Source*: From Ref. 53.

One pressing pharmaceutical problem is to design and formulate systems that are stable in vitro but which can also survive their dilution in blood, mixing, shearing forces in flow, and the many changes in their environment as they passage through tissues, and also their change in surface characteristics brought about by protein absorption in vivo. The schematic below (Fig. 3) develops the theme of Figure 2, showing the complex pathway between design intent and action.

The first key point is the compatibility of drug and carrier, which influences the active's distribution in the carrier and its release profile. The particles must flow in the blood, and there they suffer shear forces; particle opsonization by blood proteins affect their uptake by the reticuloendothelial system (RES). Escape from the blood through extravasation is but the first step in the movement of the systems toward extravascular targets.

APPLICATION OF NANOPARTICLES IN DRUG DELIVERY

Nanoparticles can, in principle, be used to deliver drugs, genes, and radiolabels by a variety of routes listed below. References to individual papers, which apply to the route in question, are cited here as examples only. Routes include

- Ocular (54)
- Oral (55)
- Intravenous (56), intraperitoneal (57), intraluminal (58), subcutaneous (59), or intramuscular (60)

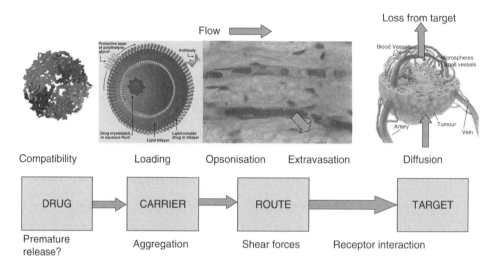

Figure 3 Diagrammatic illustration of the issues associated with the presentation of drugs in carrier systems designed for targeting: compatibility, loading, opsonization, extravasation, and diffusion are the main parameters that determine arrival at the target site. Premature release of drug, aggregation of the particles, and shear forces in capillary flow affect receptor interaction and uptake.

- Nasal (61)
- Inhalation (62)
- Intratumoral (63)

Delivery to the brain (64) and the lymphatics (65) can also employ nanoparticles.

In ocular delivery to the cul-de-sac of the eye, nanoparticles in suspension can prolong the action of the drug both by slow release and their slower escape by way of the punctae compared to a solution, and perhaps the adhesive qualities of some nanosystems (66) also assist.

Oral delivery is a potential means of delivering vaccines, to provide slow release of drugs, or through bioadhesive nanoparticles to achieve uptake for systemic activity, although to date the evidence for significant (>5%) uptake is limited (67). Bioadhesive nanoparticles have been advocated to assist adhesion of the carriers to the mucosa and thus increase the probability of arrest, as well as to provide time for the transfer of drug from the carriers or the particles themselves into the gut wall. Knowledge of the importance of the gut-associated lymphoid tissue (GALT) is crucial to the understanding of some of these possibilities. The M-cells and lymphoid tissues of other anatomical regions can be important in particle delivery; for example, the nasal associated lymphoid tissue (NALT), the bronchial associated lymphoid tissue (BALT), and other sites such as the omentum associated lymphoid tissue (OALT) provide the possibility of access of particles in small quantities. Such small quantities may be sufficient for immunization with oral vaccines or with very potent drugs. Oral uptake of nanoparticles (68) is determined by their diameter (small sizes are absorbed to a greater extent than larger particles); particles coated with nonionic surfactants show reduced uptake and charged particles, being hydrophilic, are also less well absorbed than hydrophobic particles.

Intravenous delivery allows the particles to enter the circulation immediately, but the fate of the particles so administered is not necessarily simple, as the flow properties of the particles and their interactions with blood components can be complex. As particle size is key in the delivery of particulates to the lung, there are possibilities for using

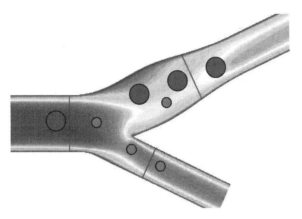

Figure 4 Diagrammatic representation of size-dependent particle route differentiation as well as fluid flow in branching network. In this schematic, larger particles are prevented from entering the lower branch by their size while the main vessel branch accommodates both large and smaller particles. The base diagram is from a simulation of carotid bifurcation and complex flows by L. Fatone and P. Gervasio, Ecole Polytechnique de Lausanne (which is used here simply to illustrate not only geometrical complexities but also flow complexities that will occur to a greater or lesser in smaller vessels also).

nanoparticles, although their size range lies below those derived for microparticulates for optimal deposition in the bronchial tree; deposition of nanoparticles of C60 fullerene has been found to be some 50% greater than that of microparticles (69).

This chapter cannot deal with the biological fate of particles per se but will rather concentrate on some of their physical and chemical aspects, which determine fate and activity. To be successful in therapeutics, systems must have optimal size, surface characteristics with preferably high loading capacity and efficiency, a high degree of stability (chemical and physical), appropriate release characteristics at the target site, and in addition be biodegradable and biocompatible. Not all drug/active-polymer/carrier combinations can be readily formulated, some because of the low affinity of the drug for the carrier. Incompatibility between drug and carrier is demonstrated by protein drugs which do not always mix with polymers without phase separation. Formulations where drug and carrier material phase separate, that is, do not produce an isotropic mixture, or during the production process, there is movement of drug toward the surface of the particles usually lead to burst release effects. Herein lies the difficulty of always comparing systems produced in different laboratories. Polydispersity of size and failure to achieve optimal size during preparation can also lead to ambiguous biological outcomes. It is clear that polydispersity complicates the achievement of targeting as it can lead to differentiation of the fate of the particles, as demonstrated in Figures 3 and 4. Figure 5 reiterates the importance of particle size over a range of physical and biological factors.

Particle size may be directly or indirectly implicated in all the areas shown in Figure 5. For example, the relationship between diffusion coefficient and radius is a directly inverse one; drug release, which is surface area related, is dependent on the erosion process in some nanosystems.

Size is of course not unrelated to other features and factors as Figure 5 shows. While size defines all nanosystems, they can differ in their material properties, chemistry, and physics.

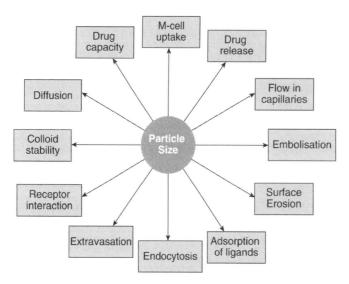

Figure 5 The key position of particle size in determining directly or indirectly the behavior and fate of nanoparticles.

HARD AND SOFT SYSTEMS

It is useful, for reasons which are apparent in relation to movement of nanoparticles in vivo, to divide nanosystems into two types, "hard" and "soft," although there are obviously intermediate situations. Hard systems, for example, polymeric nanoparticles and nanocapsules, nanosuspensions or nanocrystals, dendrimers, and carbon nanotubes are neither flexible nor elastic. Hard systems can block capillaries and fenestrae that have dimensions similar to the particles, whereas soft systems can deform and reform to varying degrees. Erythrocytes and many liposomes fall into this category and are thus better able to navigate capillary beds and tissue extracellular spaces. Soft systems include nanoemulsions (microemulsions) and polymeric micelles.

MANUFACTURING CHALLENGES

Clearly, the issue of particle diameter and distribution of particle sizes is very important in nanoparticulate systems for therapeutic or diagnostic use. Few systems are truly monodisperse, and there must be precise measurement and recording of size distributions in relation to the scope and limitations of the chosen mode of measurement. There is the requirement for the production of consistent particle size systems. Solvents used in production must be removed, and removal of impurities from surfaces carried out, and the ability to incorporate labile drugs without degradation into the particulate carrier are but some aspects of handling and preparing nanoparticulates. The selection of the material which will form the basis of the nanoparticle, will depend on the inherent properties of the drug, including its solubility and stability, the surface characteristics required of the system, degrees of biodegradability and biocompatibility, assuming of course nontoxic substances, and the drug release profile that is sought. Last, but not the least, protection of workers due to nanoparticle aerosol formation during handling has to be considered.

MANUFACTURING METHODS

There are a large number of methods (Table 2) to prepare nanoparticulate systems. These depend to a large extent on the material (polymer, protein, metal, ceramic) that will form the basis of the carrier. One can, in essence, consider three approaches to their production: (*i*) by comminution (in the case of solids, milling, and in the case of liquids, high pressure emulsification); (*ii*) molecular self-assembly, such as that occurs with polymeric surfactants to form polymeric micelles or with dendrons to form dendrimeric aggregates; and (*iii*) precipitation from a good solvent as shown in Figure 6.

Table 2 addresses methods of preparation of polymeric or protein-carrier particles while Table 3 deals with nanocrystal or nanosuspension-production methods. These are discussed in turn.

Table 2 Methods of Manufacturing Polymeric or Protein Nanoparticles

Method
Solvent displacement
Salting out
Emulsion diffusion
Emulsion-solvent evaporation
SCF technology
Complexation/coacervation
Reverse micellar methods
In situ polymerization

Abbreviation: SCF, supercritical fluid.

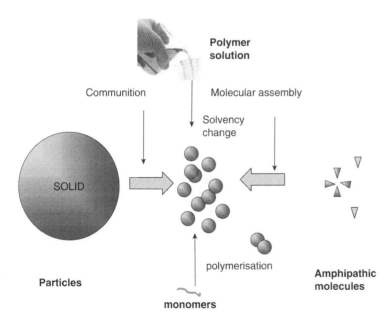

Figure 6 The main broad avenues of nanoparticle production. Comminution or size reduction (say by high-pressure homogenization or critical solution technology), precipitation methods by salting out or other solvency changes in solutions of drug-polymers mixtures and molecular assembly of amphipathic components. Methods are listed in Table 2.

Table 3 Modes of Preparation of Nanocrystalline Suspensions

Precipitation methods
   Hydrosol (developed by Sucker, Sandoz)
   Amorphous particle [NanoMorph™ Soliqs (Abbott)]

Homogenization methods
   Microfluidisation technology (SkyePharma, Canada)
   Piston-gap method (Dissocubes™, SkyePharma ∼500 nm)
   Nanopure technology (PharmaSol, Germany)

Combination technologies
   Microprecipitation™ and High shear (NANOEDGE™)
   Nanopure™ XP technology

Sonochemical methods (e.g., for azithromycin) (70)

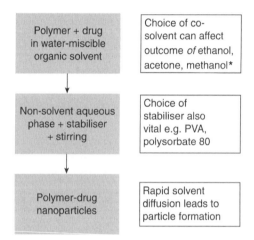

Scheme 3 A summary of the solvent-displacement method by which the particles in Figure 7 were prepared. *See, for example, Ref. 71.

Solvent Displacement Methods

These methods, shown in Scheme 3, are perhaps the simplest means of preparing polymeric nanoparticles, provided that the polymer and drug can be solubilized in ethanol, acetone, or methanol as water-miscible solvents. The polymer, in the presence of the aqueous phase of appropriate stabilizers such as polyvinyl alcohol (PVA) or polysorbate 80, forms remarkably narrow distribution nanoparticles.

Figure 7 shows a photomicrograph of ciclosporin A nanoparticles prepared by this method. The ciclosporin in these particles is most likely to be formed in the amorphous state on first manufacture. After a period of time, the ciclosporin crystallizes and its oral absorption from the nanoparticles is greatly reduced (72).

Salting Out

A variant on this technique is the one illustrated in Scheme 4, where a polymer is dissolved in a water-miscible organic solvent, which is added to a stirred aqueous gel containing a salting-out agent and a stabilizer.

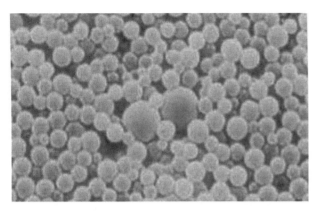

Figure 7 Ciclosporin A nanoparticles number average diameter ~ 200 nm, prepared by a solvent displacement method (see Scheme 3). *Source*: From Ref. 72.

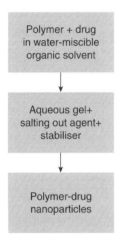

Scheme 4 Schematic of the salting-out method in which a polymer and drug are dissolved in a water-miscible organic solvent before addition to an aqueous gel with a salting-out agent and stabilizer.

Emulsion Diffusion

The use of a partly water-miscible solvent in which the drug and polymer is dissolved is shown in Scheme 5. An emulsion is formed on addition of the polymer-drug solution to an aqueous phase containing a stabilizer. Because of the partial miscibility of the first solvent, solvent diffuses from the dispersed droplets into the bulk to provide after some time polymer nanoparticles containing drug.

Emulsion-Solvent Evaporation

Scheme 6 illustrates a different approach. It involves the dissolution of the drug-polymer mix in an organic solvent, which is immiscible with water, so that on addition to an aqueous phase, an emulsion is formed in the presence of appropriate emulsifiers. On heating, the internal organic phase can be evaporated in a controlled fashion leaving the

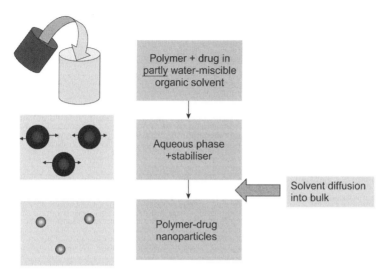

Scheme 5 Schematic of the emulsion technique where the drug and polymer are dissolved in a partly water-miscible solvent, which is then added to an aqueous phase where emulsion particles are formed. The solvent, being partly miscible in the water phase, diffuses from the droplets eventually leaving the nanoparticles as the droplets shrink.

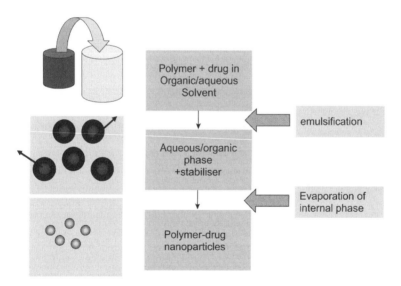

Scheme 6 Similar to the process in Scheme 5, where emulsification of the polymer/drug organic solution takes place forming an oil-in-water system. The alternative is the dissolution of the polymer and drug in an aqueous phase, which is added to an organic phase to form a water-in-oil emulsion. In both cases, the internal phase is then evaporated leaving the polymer-drug particles.

polymer-drug nanoparticles, whose size is dependent on the properties of the emulsion. In a variant of this process, if the drug and the polymer or protein (e.g., albumin) are dissolved in water this would be added to an organic phase. A water-in-oil emulsion would be formed initially from which the water would be removed by evaporation. The oily phase would later be "washed" off.

Super Critical Fluid Technologies

A supercritical fluid (SCF) is any substance at a temperature and pressure above its thermodynamic critical point. Such a fluid can diffuse through solids such as a gas and dissolve materials such as a liquid. Carbon dioxide and water are the most commonly used SCFs.

SCF technologies deserve a special mention as they have been less commonly applied on a laboratory scale in the preparation of nanoparticles (73). Scheme 7 and Figures 8 and 9 summarize the approach used. A drug and polymer mixture is dissolved in an organic solvent or carbon dioxide. Under certain conditions of pressure and temperature, the liquid phase is transformed into the supercritical state as seen in Figure 8. Here the supercritical state is found at pressures >74 bar (atmospheric pressure = 1.013 bar) and at temperatures >31°C. The rapid expansion of this supercritical solution on exposure to atmospheric pressure causes the formation of microspheres or nanospheres; Figure 9 on the other hand illustrates the use of a solvent, which can be formed into a

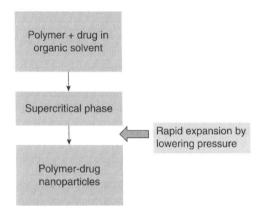

Scheme 7 (**A**) Schematic of the process of producing nanoparticles using supercritical fluid technology. See, for example, Ref. 73.

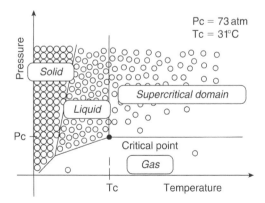

Figure 8 Pressure versus temperature phase diagram for a liquid, showing the solid/liquid/gas phase boundaries and above a T_c and a P_c, the supercritical domain. *Abbreviations*: T_c, critical temperature; P_c, critical pressure.

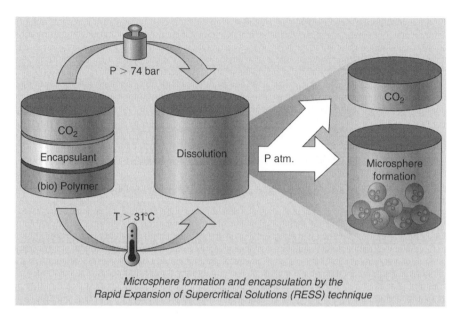

Figure 9 Diagrammatic representation of microsphere formation. After dissolution of the polymer and drug in admixture with CO_2, a process of rapid expansion takes place. Adjusting the parameters can lead to nanoparticle formation.

supercritical state, to which CO_2 is infused; particles are formed because of a decreased solubility of the polymer.

Rapid Expansion of Supercritical Solutions

Rapid expansion of supercritical solutions (RESS) processing is used to prepare microspheres. Microencapsulation takes place when a pressurized supercritical solvent containing the shell material and the active ingredient is released through a small nozzle; the abrupt pressure drop causes the desolvation of the shell material and the formation of a coating layer around the active ingredient (74). A prerequisite for this technology is that the compounds effectively dissolve in the SCF, which limits its application.

Gas-Antisolvent and Supercritical Fluid Antisolvent Method

An SCF can be used as an *antisolvent*, which will cause precipitation of a dissolved substrate from a liquid solvent. This approach, called the SAS (supercritical fluid antisolvent) or GAS (gas antisolvent) method, results in a pronounced volume expansion greater than with RESS, leading to supersaturation and then precipitation of the "solutes." (Fig. 10).

In each of the methods discussed, there is considerable scope for changing process parameters to achieve nanoparticles with different characteristics. To date, there are few comprehensive systematic studies that allow any fine degree of prediction of outcomes.

Reverse Micellar or Microemulsion Method

Figure 11 illustrates the formation of metallic nanoparticles using reverse microemulsions as an example of growing particles within individual dispersed phases or molecular containers. In this process, a metal salt is solubilized in the aqueous interior of

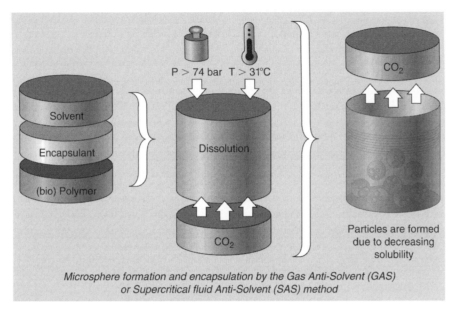

Figure 10 This GAS or SAS variant involves taking the solvent, drug, and polymer dissolution and then using an SCF as an antisolvent to produce the particles. *Abbreviations*: GAS, gas antisolvent; SAS, supercritical fluid antisolvent; SCF, supercritical fluid. *Source*: From Ref. 74.

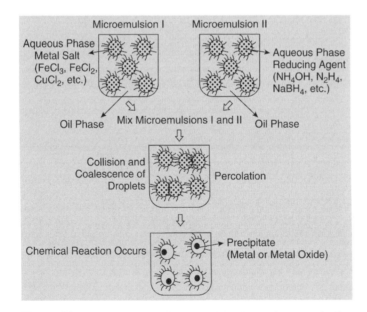

Figure 11 The preparation of nanoparticles by the inverse micelle process in which a chemical reaction between microemulsion or inverse micelles after collision and perhaps fusion converts the soluble salt into an insoluble metal or metal oxide as shown. *Source*: From Ref. 75.

microemulsion I. The aqueous phase of microemulsion II contains a reducing agent. When mixed, collision and coalescence of the droplets allow the chemical reaction to proceed, thus producing the precipitate of the metal or metal oxide within the confines of the droplet. Thus, droplet size determines to an extent nanoparticle size. Vesicles can be used for producing nanoparticles by acting as a template in a similar manner. Dendrimers (see later in the chapter) have also been used to form nanoparticles.

Coacervation and Complexation Techniques

Coacervation has been a process used in the fabrication of microparticles for many decades since Bungenberg de Jong and Kruyt described the phenomenon ca. 1932. A coacervate is a gel-like liquid state of matter, which can be treated to produce solid microparticles or nanoparticles. There are several ways to form coacervates. One is in *complex coacervation* in which positively charged macromolecules I are mixed with negatively charged macromolecules; under certain conditions of temperature and relative concentration and ionic strength, there will be a phase separation where particles of a coacervate form. An example is shown of a phase diagram in Figure 12. It is also possible in the process of *simple coacervation* with one macromolecule type of whatever charge to create coacervate particles with the device of solvent change and salting out. Albumin nanoparticles prepared by coacervation have been employed in oligonucleotide delivery (76).

In Situ Polymerization

In this mode of synthesis of polymeric nanoparticles (e.g., of polybutylcycanoacrylates), monomeric materials (e.g., butylcyanoacrylate) are dispersed in a suitable solvent and emulsified. An initiator is generally added to the system and the monomers condense to form a polymeric matrix, although in the case of the alkyl cyanoacrylates no initiator is required as the aqueous medium acts as the initiator of polymerization. As one example (78) isobutylcyanoacrylate dissolved in ethanol can be mixed with an oil plus an oil-soluble drug to constitute one phase; the second phase is an aqueous solution of 0.5% Pluronic F68 (poloxamer 118). The two phases are mixed and the polyisobutylcyanoa-crylate is formed at the interface between the oil and the water. The formation of alkylcyanoacrylate films at oil/water interfaces was investigated over 30 years ago (79).

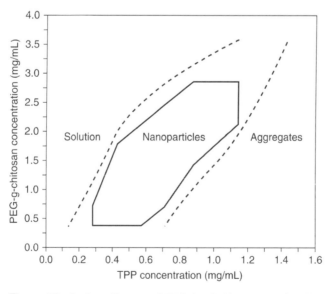

Figure 12 A phase diagram of PEGylated chitosan as a function of TPP concentration showing the region where "nanogel" nanoparticles form. *Abbreviations*: PEG, polyoxyethylene glycol; TPP, tripolyphosphate. *Source*: From Ref. 77.

NANOCRYSTALS

The interest in the production of nanocrystals of insoluble drugs is twofold: reduced particle size of any solid increases the surface area per unit weight of drug and hence increases the rate of dissolution of the drug, all things being equal. According to the Noyes–Whitney equation relating the weight change, dw, with time, dt

$$\frac{dw}{dt} = \left[\frac{DA}{\delta}\right][c_s - c]$$

where A is the surface area of the material, D is the diffusion coefficient, δ is the diffusion layer thickness and c_s is the saturation solubility, c being the concentration of drug in the solution at any given time t. There may be, as a result, supersaturation, but the equilibrium solubility remains the same, that is, until critical small particles sizes in the nanometer range are reached, as shown in Figure 13. The combination of increased intrinsic solubility and increased surface area has the potential to change solution properties dramatically. If the absorption of the drug is dissolution rate limited, this will assist in the rate of absorption; enhanced solubility has the potential to increase concentration gradients across the biological membrane. Comminution increases A but does not change c_s until the dimensions are reduced to the levels shown in Figure 13.

Surface energies of a sample of drugs are as follows (81): ibuprofen, 52 dyne/cm; naproxen, 42 dyne/cm; nifedipine, 38 dyne/cm; hydrocortisone acetate 37 dyne/cm; and itraconazole 36 dyne/cm (82).

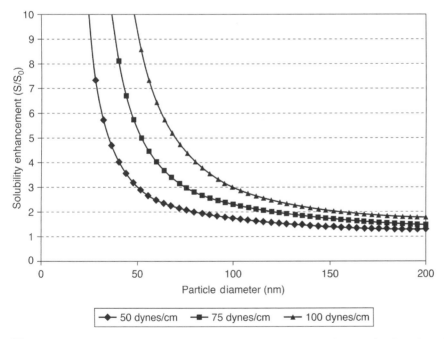

Figure 13 The solubility enhancement as a function of particle diameter for three hypothetical compounds with surface energies of 50, 75, and 100 mN/m (dynes/cm). It can be seen that where S_0 is the solubility of a large crystal, and S is the solubility of the crystal of a specific size, the solubility enhancement (S/S_0) does not increase significantly until particle diameters reach below ∼75 nm for drugs with a surface energy of 50 mN/m. *Source*: From Ref. 80.

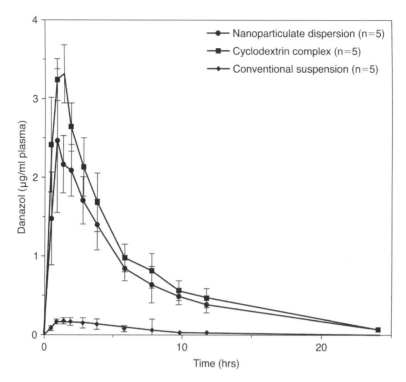

Figure 14   Danazol is a drug with an aqueous solubility of 10 μg/mL. Here danazol plasma levels are plotted as a function of time after administration of three forms of the drug including a nanoparticle dispersion and a hydroxypropyl-β-cyclodextrin complex, using a suspension with a mean particle size of 10 μm as a comparator. *Source*: From Ref. 83.

Figure 14 demonstrates the advantage in the case of danazol of the use of nanoparticulate dispersions compared with conventional suspensions. The saturation solubility (25°C) of danazol in water has been found to range from ∼0.58 μg/mL to the 10μg/mL cited in reference 83.

Dendrimers

The first synthesis of dendrimers or hyperbranched polymers in the 1980s by Tomalia introduced after a period of skepticism a new class of nanoparticles. Recently, they have gained prominence in pharmaceutical nanotechnology as drug and gene vectors because of their precise chemistry, predictable physical architecture, and ability to be synthesized in a uniform size with diameters in 2 to 10 nm size range. Dendrimers are spherical or quasi-spherical polymeric molecules, which are synthesized by divergent or convergent methods. While they are indeed single molecules, they are also nanoparticles, some of which are biodegradable to a greater or lesser extent.

Figure 15 shows both a 2D representation of a lipophilic dendrimer based on lysines, with terminal alkyl groups (84) and a polyamidoamine (PAMAM) dendrimer, now widely used experimentally. The versatility of almost endless variations in internal and external groups makes this a fascinating field of nanotechnology. The unreacted version of lysine-based dendrimer will have terminal amine groups and hence be cationic

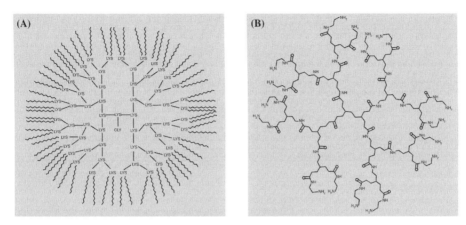

Figure 15 (**A**) A hydrophobic poly(lysine)-based dendrimer with 64 alkyl surface groups and a glycine core, as synthesized by T. Sakthivel. (**B**) a PAMAM dendrimer showing the terminal amine groups. *Abbreviation*: PAMAM, polyamidoamine.

Generation	G0	G1	G2	G3	G4
# of surface groups	3	6	12	24	48
Diameter (nm)	1.4	1.9	2.6	3.6	4.4
2D graphical representation					
3D chemical structure view					

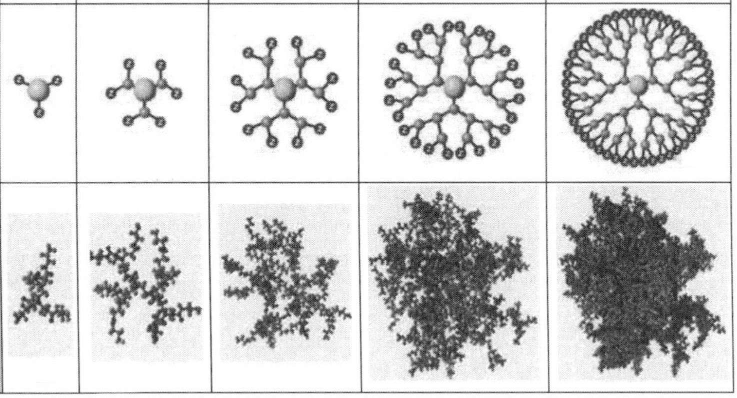

Figure 16 Representation of the synthetic process building up dendrimers from a multivalent core (Generation 0) through the first generation, G1, to G4 with a diameter of 4.4 nm and 48 surface groups. Both the 2D and 3D representations are given. *Source*: Courtesy of Dendritic Nanotechnologies.

and freely soluble. Where the terminal amine groups are reacted, the resulting dendrimers can be water insoluble. They can be converted into anionic systems too. Drug can be incorporated in small amounts in the core or in the outer hydrophobic layer if the dendrimer possesses one, or on the surface of charged dendrimers, electrostatically or covalently. Figure 16 shows a representation of the "generations" of dendrimer, G0 to G4, the number of surface groups ranging from 3 to 48 with the further generation product and their diameters from 1.9 to 4.4 nm. The divergent method of synthesis follows the route from G0 to G4 or above as shown in the figure by addition sequentially of branched reactive molecules to the core.

There are a number of textbooks dealing with dendrimers in medicine and pharmacy, including *Dendrimer Based Nanomedicines* (85), *Dendrimers and Other Dendritic Polymers* (86), and a series on dendrimer chemistry, the latest of which is *Dendrimers V* (87).

Dendrimers have the potential, in many cases, to act in a wide range of functions, as

- Drug carriers (88)
- Gene delivery vectors (89)
- Stabilizers (e.g., of DNA) (90)
- Solubilizers (91)
- Building blocks for new materials

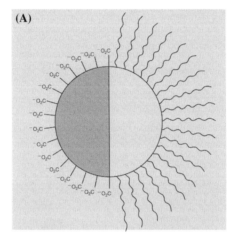

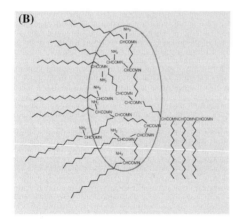
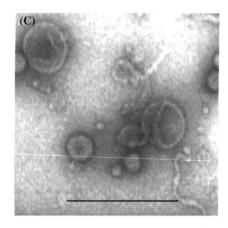

Figure 17 (**A**). A two-dimensional representation of an amphipathic dendrimer, with both carboxylic acid groups and alkyl chains, resulting in a hydrophilic and hydrophobic hemisphere each. In solution, this feature will encourage self-association. (**B**). An amphipathic polyalkyl dendron prepared by Al-Jamal et al. (97), which forms dendrisomes, vesicular structures, shown in (**C**), capable of solubilizing drugs. In the diagram the hydrophilic interior comprising branched lysine chains is shown. The bar represents 200 nm.

- Gel-formers (92)
- Lubricants (93)
- Film formers (94)

and in some cases, like a good number of polymers can be considered to have biological activity of their own (95,96).

Dendrons are partial dendrimers, which are used in their own right and can also be employed to construct complete dendrimers by convergent processes. The dendrimer shown in Figure 17A might have been constructed from two hydrophobic dendrons and two anionic dendrons covalently attached to a core molecule. The resulting structure is itself amphipathic and will have a tendency to aggregate in an aqueous environment.

HIGHER-ORDER DENDRIMER STRUCTURES

A variety of secondary structures can be formed from dendrimer or dendron primary units (98). We have prepared dendrisomes (vesicles) from amphipathic dendrons (Fig. 16). Dendriplexes can be formed by interactions between anionic macromolecules and cationic dendrimers or dendrons, for example. Hydrophobic dendrimers whose surface groups are reacted to form an alkyl surface will aggregate and can be formulated as so-called dendrimer-derived nanoparticles some 200 nm in diameter (99).

Dendrimeric "micelles" shown in Figure 18 were formed by spontaneous association of surface-active partial dendrimers, in this case lysine-based systems with one, two, or three alkyl (C_{10}–C_{18}) chains. Amphipathic dendrons with three C_{14} chains and eight terminal NH_2 groups form aggregates with a molecular weight of 52,700 (aggregation number 33); the C_{18} analogue has an aggregation number of 78 (100). In the presence of 0.1% NaCl, the aggregates grow to 50 nm as seen in Figure 18.

Five different generations of amphiphilic dendrimers based on poly(propyleneimine) also form small spherical aggregates at pH 1 with diameters ranging from 20 to 200 nm. Under some conditions, asymmetric aggregates are formed with axial ratios of up to 1:8 (101).

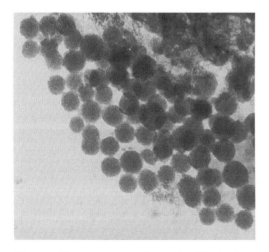

Figure 18 Aggregates of amphipathic dendrons in 0.1% NaCl, each of these micelle-like structures being about 50 nm in diameter. *Source*: From Ref. 100.

(A)   (B)

(C)   (D)

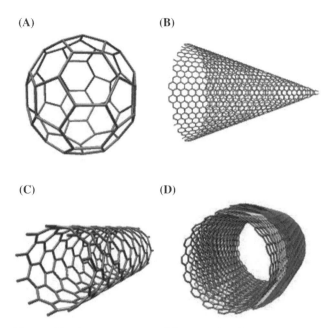

Figure 19 Computer-generated images of carbon nanostructures showing (**A**) a spherical C60 fullerene "Buckyball" structure, (**B**) a conical form, (**C**) a SWNT and (D) a cylindrical multiwalled CNT MWNT. *Abbreviations*: SWNT, single-walled nanotube; MWNT, multiwalled nanotube. *Source*: From Ref. 102.

CARBON NANOTUBES

Fullerenes are carbon molecules, which can be prepared in the form of hollow spheres, ellipsoids or tubes. Computer generated images of carbon nanostructures have been published (102) and are shown in Figure 19.

Drugs can be sequestered inside the nanotubes and the surface of the tubes can be derivatized (103). Typical dimensions of SWNT are 1 to 3 nm in diameter and 0.5 to 2 μm in length. The inner diameter is from 0.6 to 2.4 nm, and the length of the tubes may vary up to 100 μm. With multiple walls, the separation between the layers is of the order of 0.3 to 0.4 nm. Foldvari and Bagonluri (104) have discussed drug delivery and compatibility issues. The asymmetry of CNTs may have consequences in their biodistribution as well as toxicity.

HYBRID SYSTEMS

There is an increasing trend to consider nanoparticles as part of other delivery systems to create what are in effect hybrid systems. Dendrimers and dendrons can thus be found as particles in emulsions or vesicles. Macromolecular-dendrimer complexes (dendriplexes) may be incorporated in polylactic-co-glycolic acid (PLGA) nanoparticles (105). Dendrimers may also be grafted to linear polymers (as shown in Fig. 20).

In the "graft to" route, a reactive polymer is reacted with complete dendrons/dendrimers as shown in Figure 20A. In the "graft-from" method (Fig. 20B), the polymer is reacted with low-generation dendritic species, which are further reacted to produce grafted dendrimers of higher generations. The macromonomer route employs a polymerizable dendrimer (the macromonomer), which is polymerized to form the dendronized polymer as shown in Figure 20C.

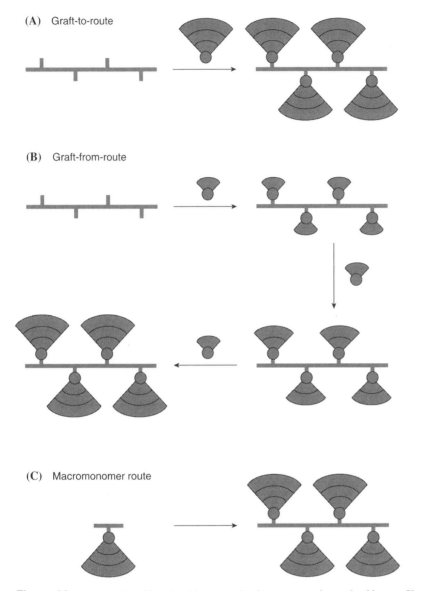

(A) Graft-to-route

(B) Graft-from-route

(C) Macromonomer route

Figure 20 Modes of grafting dendrimers or dendrons onto polymer backbones. Shown here are (**A**) the *graft-to* route, (**B**) the *graft-from* method, and (**C**) the *macromonomer* route. *Source*: From Ref. 106.

Nanoparticles of all descriptions can be used not only as suspensions but also as freeze-dried powders for reconstitution, incorporated into liposomes, as aerosols, in gels and microspheres (e.g., gelatin), adsorbed onto microparticles, dispersed in soft-gelatin capsules [e.g., in polyoxyethylene glycols (PEGs)], or as mini-depot tablets.

TEMPLATING WITH DENDRIMERS

Dendrimers can be used for tasks other than drug delivery. As dendrimers can incorporate in their fixed spherical constructs metals as well as other materials such as dyes and drugs, it is reasonable that they should be able to act as templates for growing crystals when the

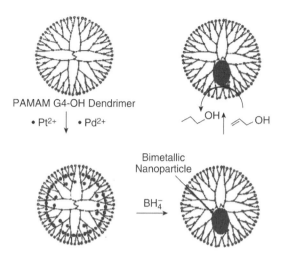

PAMAM G4-OH Dendrimer

• Pt²⁺ ↓ • Pd²⁺

Figure 21 Schematic diagram of the use of a G4 PAMAM dendrimer as a template for the formation of bimetallic (palladium/platinum) nanoparticles. *Abbreviation*: PAMAM, polyamido-amine. *Source*: From Ref. 107.

reaction takes place within the confines of the dendrimer itself. A nonpharmaceutical example is shown in Figure 21 in which palladium and platinum salts are reacted in a PAMAM dendrimer to form bimetallic particles.

Nanoparticle Flow

In experimental work on drug targeting with nanoparticulate carriers, little attention has been paid to the question of the flow of nanoparticles in the blood and interstitial spaces (108). This is unfortunate because the theoretical advantage of nanosystems is their small size, allowing freer movement than microspheres in the circulation, including the lymph and in tissues. Flow rates are important not least in the determination of the possibility of nanoparticle interaction with endothelial receptors prior to internalization, or indeed in the decoupling of carriers and receptors due to shear forces. Flow of nanoparticles is a vital element in extravasation and in the enhanced permeation and retention (EPR) effect. What is the influence of nanoparticle size on particle flow in the circulation? And, with the advent of CNTs in particular, what is the influence of shape on flow and fate? CNTs certainly behave differently in the blood from spherical C60 fullerenes. CNTs activate human platelets and induce them to aggregate, whereas their spherical analogues do not (109), but there is little information on other physical differences. The question has been asked: what are the differences between the spheres and nanotubes that underlie these different interactions? Shape is an obvious parameter and surface characteristics too. All the systems tended to self-aggregate, forming assemblies of some 10 μm in diameter in some cases, but there is no clear-cut relationship between aggregate size and biological effect. The jury is still out. Flow is affected by shape. Asymmetry leads to higher viscosity compared with spherical objects in suspension. There are indeed reports of flow-induced alignment of CNTs to form macroscopic fibers and ribbons (110) and also of polystyrene lattices (111).

There are many reasons why more attention needs to be paid to the flow behavior of nanoparticles. Figure 22 shows some of the events prior to and at attachment. First, nanoparticles in vivo are driven by the blood flow to distant sites. Second, particle

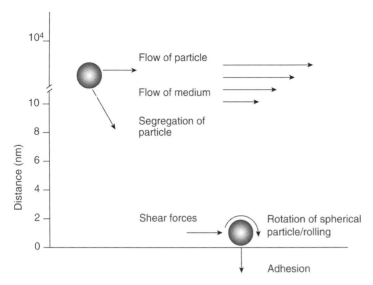

Figure 22 A (not to scale) reminder that interaction forces leading to adhesion of particles to biological surfaces compete with particle flow, medium flow, and shear forces but, most importantly, it should be noted that attractive forces come into play at very small distances, that is, <10 nm. For those particles which adhere, there are shear forces which act to detach the nanoparticles, and there is the potential for particles to roll if they are spherical.

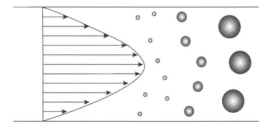

Figure 23 Diagram showing the velocity pattern in a tube of flowing liquid, depicting particles of different size, separating in flow according to their diameter. The large particles, being unable to approach close to the capillary wall, experience the faster fluid streamlines toward the center, hence they move more rapidly, as described by Silebi and DosRamos (112,113).

velocities can be size dependent because the flow rates across the diameter of the vessels is not constant and hence particle segregation in polydisperse systems might occur as shown in Figure 23. Third, flow results in shearing forces at the point of interaction between nanoparticles and the target receptors; smaller particles suffer lower forces than larger particles to dislodge them from receptor surfaces. This is illustrated in Figure 23. And any aggregation of particles, which might even be flow induced, will alter flow patterns and of course interactions with receptors.

Segregation of particles shown in Figure 23 perhaps complicates quantitative access to distant targets in polydisperse systems. Fluid velocity in tubes is not constant throughout the diameter of the tube, as Figure 22 indicates, a feature important when we consider the interaction of nanoparticles with epithelial cells or capillary walls.

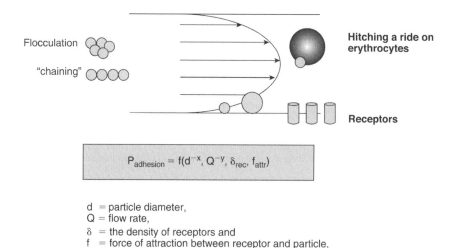

d = particle diameter,
Q = flow rate,
δ = the density of receptors and
f = force of attraction between receptor and particle,
     itself dependent on particle ligand coverage

Figure 24 There is only a probability of adhesion of nanoparticles even when decorated with specific ligands for endothelial receptors in flow conditions. This figure illustrates effects such as flocculation, chain formation and adsorption to erythrocytes (see text).

Figure 24 illustrates possible flocculation and chaining of particles in flow conditions. Larger particles close to the walls of the vessels experience greater shearing forces because of the nature of the flow patterns shown. Particles that adhere to erythrocytes move with them until detachment, often prolonging their own circulation times. Adhesion, seen as a prerequisite to cellular uptake from blood and interstitial fluids is not a foregone conclusion. The probability of adhesion, $P_{adhesion}$ can be written phenomenologically as in Figure 24. The factors include particle diameter, flow rate, the density of receptors, and the force of attraction between particle and receptor.

Some particles adhere to erythrocytes and move with them (114). Flocculation and chaining of particles can occur, and these events will alter the interactive possibilities with receptors. Ding and Wen (115) formulated a theoretical model examining particle migration in nanoparticle suspensions flowing through a pipe. It considers particle migration due to spatial gradients in viscosity and shear rate as well as Brownian motion. Particle migration due to these effects results in nonuniformity in particle concentration over the cross-section of the pipe, in particular for larger particles. Three mechanisms were proposed for migration in such nonuniform shear flow: (*i*) shear-induced migration, where particles move from regions of higher shear rate to regions of lower shear rate; (*ii*) viscosity gradient–induced migration, where particles move from regions of higher viscosity to regions of lower viscosity; and (*iii*) self-diffusion due to Brownian motion.

Figure 25 reinforces previous diagrams and considers in greater detail the forces involved in nanoparticle interaction with biological surfaces at close approach. Physical adsorption of ligands to the surface of nanoparticles or covalent attachment of ligands changes the nature of the primary surface and will influence each of the forces referred to here.

One strategy that has been adopted to enhance the possibility of surface contact has been through the use of superparamagnetic nanoparticles (117) and a 0.5-T magnet placed close to the flow chamber.

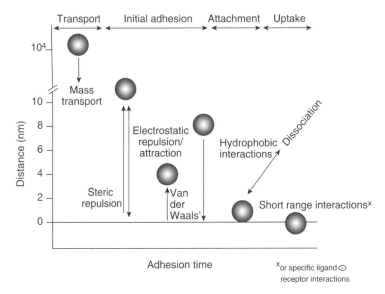

Figure 25 Processes occurring in the deposition of nanoparticles in flow conditions as a function of the range of interaction of forces (nm) and adhesion times. At the start, mass transport to the surface occurs, initial adhesion following through electrostatic attraction and van der Waals' forces. Hydrophobic interactions can play their part as well as specific receptor-ligand interactions, which are short-range interactions. *Source*: From Ref. 116.

AGGREGATION

Given their large surface to volume/weight ratios, nanoparticles are prone to aggregate. The formulation of a stable nanoparticle suspension in the laboratory is one thing, the maintenance of the monodisperse state in vivo is another. Particles in blood, gut, nose, or lungs have moved from an aqueous-based medium to a more complex biological situation, as in blood. There are biological consequences as opsonins adsorb from the plasma onto the surface of the nanoparticles, which leads to uptake by the RES if not checked. But in terms of the pharmaceutics of the nanosystems, the potential of the particles to aggregate is the key. Aggregation changes the hydrodynamic size of the particles, affects their diffusion and extravasation, and reduces the effective surface area for interactions with receptors. PEGylation of course creates a hydrated surface on hydrophobic particles, which exerts both steric and enthalpic stability, and reduces opsonin adsorption, leading to increased circulation times and enhanced possibility of nanoparticle uptake after multiple passages.

PEGYLATED NANOPARTICLES

The process of PEGylation involves covalent attachment of PEG chains to the hydrophobic surface of the particles. PEGylation clearly changes the nature of the surface, turning often a very hydrophobic nanoparticle surface into a hydrophilic one, forming a "protective" layer, which is a barrier to flocculation and perhaps interaction with cell surfaces. This effect of PEG depends on its chain length (118). PEG 5000 has a greater effect than PEG 2000 or PEG 750 as predicted by calculations of enthalpic and entropic stabilization, not dissimilar to the estimates of the effect of ethylene oxide chain length on nonionic stabilized emulsions (119). The polymer chains provide in addition a physical and thermodynamic barrier with its attached water molecules.

NANOPARTICLE DIFFUSION

Clearly, particle radius is a key parameter in the diffusion of particles from a region of high concentration to one of low concentration. Because of the paramount importance in most applications of particle size and the need to evaluate data from different laboratories, there has been some scrutiny recently of the results cited in papers for particle diameters of nanoparticle samples (120,121). The former (120) lists the methods available and the optimal size ranges for each: light scattering for the range 50 nm to 1 μm, laser light diffraction (1–1000 μm), scanning electron and transmission electron microscopy (50 nm–100 μm), field flow fractionation 20 nm to 1 μm. These two papers (120,121) should be read closely.

The Stokes–Einstein equation relates the diffusion coefficient, D, to continuous phase viscosity η and the radius of the particle, r thus:

$$D = \frac{kT}{6\Pi\eta r}$$

Hence in the same medium, for example., in water, the diffusion coefficient of spherical particles is inversely related to radius. This alone is important in thinking of the translocation of nanoparticles, say toward their targets in tissues. Diffusion occurs in free solution, in cell culture media, in the gel-like interior of cells, perhaps in the cell nucleus and in the extracellular matrix. In the brain, for example, diffusion of drugs from nanoparticles or implants is slow, and the radius of spread of a drug like paclitaxel after release from implants or nanoparticles is of the order of only millimeters (122). Gels have been used as models for diffusion of nanoparticles in complex media: the Stokes–Einstein equation applies and the ratio of diffusion in the gel (D) to diffusion in water (D_o) can be calculated. In gels, the viscosity relevant to the equation is not the bulk viscosity but the so-called microscopic viscosity (123), η_o, which is actually close to that of water, as it is the viscosity of the medium in which nanoparticles move between the entangled chains of the macromolecular gels. When the diameter of the particles approach 10 to 20 nm in hydroxypropyl methylcellulose (HPMC) gels diffusion ratios (D/D_0) asymptote to zero.

Diffusion within cells is even more complex than within simple gels; first the cytoplasm is a molecularly crowded zone, a complex gel with structural obstacles such as actin and myosin fibers and strands. There is the additional tortuosity that occurs in gels as the moving particle avoids the regions of the macromolecular chains and the obstruction effects from the impenetrable regions of the cytoplasm. If we designate D_e as the effective diffusion coefficient and D_0 the coefficient in water, we can write where τ is the tortuosity factor and ε is the void fraction available to the diffusing solute:

$$\frac{D_e}{D_0} = \frac{\varepsilon}{\tau}$$

where $\varepsilon = (1-\varphi_p)$, and where φ_p is the volume fraction of the polymer or other materials. Tortuosity is defined as $\tau = \sqrt{(D_o/D_e)}$, where D_o (cm^2/s) is the free (aqueous) diffusion coefficient of the molecule and D_e (cm^2/s) is the effective (apparent) diffusion coefficient in brain tissue. Tortuosity is related to the hindrance imposed on a diffusing particle by

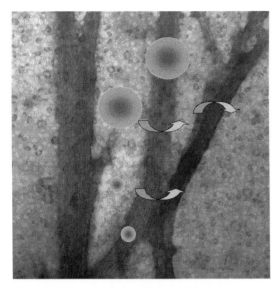

Adsorption

Obstruction/
Entrapment

Obstruction

Adsorption

Figure 26 An electron photomicrograph of an actin gel in vitro with added dendrimers and superimposed spheres representing (not to scale) dendrimer and nanoparticles. *Source*: From Ref. 123.

the cellular elements, and possibly the extracellular matrix is then the diffusion coefficient in the gel, D_G as a ratio of the coefficient in water is given by (124).

$$\frac{D_G}{D_0} = \frac{(1 - \phi_p)^2}{(1 + \phi_p)^2}$$

and

$$\frac{D_e}{D_0} = \frac{(1 - \phi_p)^3}{(1 + \phi_p)^2}$$

The diffusion coefficient of 6-nm dendrimers in the cytoplasm of Caco-2 cells and SK/MES-1 cells (125) has been determined to be 9.8×10^{-11} cm^2/s and $\sim 6 \times 10^{-11}$ cm^2/s^{-1}, respectively, some 1000× lower than that in water. Not only is there a tortuous path to navigate in cells but also physical barriers such as the actin-myosin network to bypass, as shown in Figure 26.

The 6-nm dendrimers under study also adsorbed to an extent onto the actin fibrils, thus further reducing diffusion. Superimposed on the photomicrograph are nanoparticles to illustrate the problems in diffusion through such a medium: adsorption, obstruction, and entrapment. The overall effect is to markedly reduce diffusion; at a certain particle radius diffusion virtually ceases. These few descriptions simply underline the supreme importance of nanoparticle diameter. This is one reason why to generalize about nanoparticles is somewhat difficult when not only are the substance of nanoparticles and their surface coatings different but the fundamental property of size varies over such a wide range. This in turn means that dependent properties such as surface area and volume vary even more.

NANOPARTICLE AND MATERIALS

Nanoparticles should not be considered only as drug delivery vectors. New materials and systems can be obtained, for example, using nanoparticles to form new structures, using

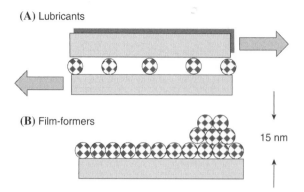

Figure 27 (**A**) Diagrammatic representation of the potential lubricant effect of adsorbed dendrimers between two flat surfaces, and (**B**) the formation of monolayers and multilayers of dendrimers. *Source*: From Ref. 93.

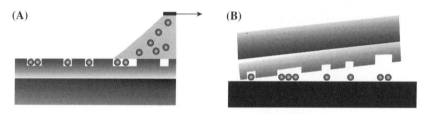

Figure 28 A schematic representation of so-called nanostructuring by way of a soft-lithography process. (**A**) Filling of depressions in the polymer plate; (**B**) imprinting on a solid surface (see text) *Source*: Courtesy of *Nature*.

nanoparticles to coat materials, using hybrid systems, such as cellulose fibers, and nanoparticles (126) or nanoparticles as part of processes, for example, with imprinting technologies. Figure 27 diagrammatically illustrates how dendrimers, for example, might be used as lubricants or film-forming agents.

Defined patterns of nanoparticles on surfaces—nanostructuring—can be achieved by processes shown in Figure 28 involving (*i*) the controlled deposition or patterning of nanoparticles and (*ii*) their imprinting on another surface. Figure 28A shows the depressions in a semirigid polymer plate being filled with gold nanoparticles by sweeping a liquid dispersion of the particles across the surface. The particles are pressed together by the receding meniscus. Figure 28B shows the polymer plate used to deposit the gold nanoparticles onto another surface, the pattern of deposition being determined by the lithographed patterns in the original.

The final examples, taken from a range of possibilities, illustrate first the use of nanoparticles (in Fig. 29, dendrimers of two generations) on the morphology of calcium carbonate particles prepared in their presence. The larger dendrimer has a greater effect on the product whose particles size is much smaller than that prepared with the lower generation dendrimer.

Second, the use of CNTs embedded in a membrane matrix to provide nanochannels for precise separations (Fig. 30). The last example illustrates the influence of processing on the morphology of spherical silica particles produced by variation of the conditions particles can be produced as "onion rings" or with a hexagonal internal structure. "Carbon onions" can be produced and are found to have durable tribological properties (128) (Fig. 31).

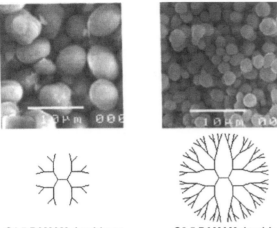

G1.5 PAMAM dendrimer   G3.5 PAMAM dendrimer

Figure 29 Scanning electron micrographs of calcium carbonate formed in the presence of two dendrimers, G1.5 PAMAM and G3.5 PAMAM. *Abbreviation*: PAMAM, polyamidoamine. *Source*: From Ref. 127.

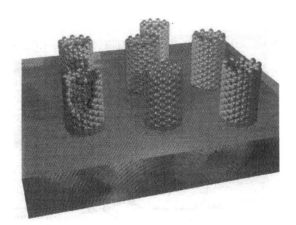

Figure 30 CNTs embedded in a membrane matrix create novel filters with controlled pores. *Source*: From Ref. 129.

REGULATORY CHALLENGES: CHARACTERIZATION

Regulatory challenges are not artificial standards but have generally evolved for good reasons to ensure reproducibility and quality in vitro and in vivo, as for any pharmaceutical. Regulators will have the same problems as all scientists have in developing rational standards and reasonable measures of the quality and safety of nanosystems, with a preference for tests that are predictive of behavior in vivo. Some of the parameters, which must be closely defined, would include those in Table 4. This is a rapidly developing field. Not only is there the issue of nanoparticles of varying modes of degradation, surface properties, and surface ligands, but also targeted systems. Targeted systems by definition congregate in specific organs hence can alter the toxicological

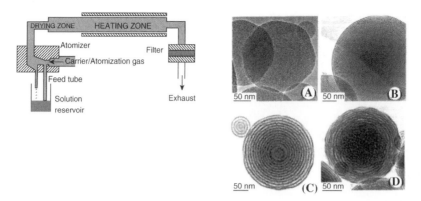

Figure 31 Aerosol-assisted self-assembly of mesostructured spherical silica nanoparticles with hexagonal and cubic morphology as well as layered structures. The method relies of evaporation-induced interfacial self-assembly confined to spherical aerosol droplets. *Source*: From Ref. 130.

Table 4 Parameters and Questions Which Must be Addressed Before Clinical Use of Nanosystems

Particle size determination is key: can there be a standardized procedure for measuring mean particle diameter and size distribution?
Is there assurance of stability of size in vitro, that is, lack of aggregation/flocculation?
Standardization of surface characteristics: what specific methodology is used? ζ-Potential measurements may be nonspecific.
The distribution and properties of ligands on the surfaces of targeted systems
Determination or prediction of stability in vivo (esp. of particle diameter)
Measurement and validation of the release rate of active from the systems and the choice of suitable experimental media
Biocompatibility: is the system compatible with blood?
Biodegradability: is there evidence of biodegradation of the system to nontoxic products?
Toxicity of nanosystems: what are reasonable predictive animal or tissue culture tests?

balance of a drug; their slow temporal and changed spatial release may have implications for the toxic effects of a drug. The role of dissolution in the fate and effect of nanoparticles has been addressed by Borm and colleagues (131).

CONCLUSIONS

This chapter has not only given a flavor of some of the issues, which relate to the use of nanoparticles and dendrimers in drug delivery and targeting, but it has also drawn attention to the potential to use these nanometer objects as excipients and building blocks for new devices and materials. It has stressed the fact that nanoparticles are in fact colloidal systems subject to the same laws of stability and interactions as other subdivided material in suspension. It has not been appropriate to discuss nanotoxicology here, but we need to be vigilant with any systems studied to examine the possibility of toxic effects, discussed by the Oberdörsters (132). Uptake of nanoparticles by the oral route whether by swallowing or by inhalation and then swallowing, is a route by which particles may gain entry to the systemic circulation and certain organs such as the lymph nodes and spleen.

REFERENCES

1. Thassu D, Deleers M, Pathak Y, eds. Nanoparticulate Drug Delivery Systems. New York: Informa Healthcare, 2007.
2. Torchilin VP, ed. Nanoparticulates as Drug Carriers. London: Imperial College Press, 2006.
3. Ozin GA, Arsenault AC. Nanochemistry:A Chemical Approach to Nanotechnology. Royal Society of Chemistry: Cambridge, 2005.
4. Drexler KE. Nanosystems. Molecular Machinery, Manufacturing and Computation. New York: John Wiley & Sons, 1992.
5. Nanomedicine. Nanotechnology for Health. European Technology Platform: Strategic Agenda for Nanomedicine. November 2006.
6. Roco MC. The US National Nanotechnology Initiative after 3 years 2001–2003. J Nanopart Res 2004; 6:1–10.
7. Drexler EK. Engines of Creation: the Coming Era of Nanotechnology. New York: Anchor Books, 1986.
8. Gregoriadis G, ed. Liposome Technology. Volumes I, II, and III, 3rd. ed. New York: Informa Healthcare, 2006.
9. Muchow M, Maincent P, Müller RH. Lipid nanoparticles with a solid matrix (SLN(R), NLC (R), LDC(R) for oral drug delivery. Drug Dev Ind Pharm 2008; 34:1394–1405.
10. Florence AT, Halbert GW. Lipoproteins and microemulsions as carriers of therapeutic and chemical agents. In: Shaw JM, ed. Lipoproteins as Carriers of Pharmacological Agents. London: CRC Press, 1991:141 et seq.
11. Corbin IR, Li H, Chen J, et al. Low-density lipoprotein nanoparticles as magnetic resonance imaging contrast agents. Neoplasia 2006; 8:488–498.
12. Dubertret B, Skourides P, Norris DJ, et al. In vivo imaging of quantum dots encapsulated in phospholipid micelles. Science 2002; 298:1759–1762.
13. Ruenraroengsak P. PhD thesis, The School of Pharmacy, University of London 2007.
14. Birrenbach G, Speiser P. Polymerised micelles and their use as adjuvants. J Pharm Sci 1976; 65:1763–1766.
15. Kreuter J. Nanoparticles and nanocapsules—new dosage forms in the nanometer size range. Pharm Acta Helv 1978; 53:33–39.
16. Couvreur P, Tulkens P, Roland M, et al. Nanocapsules: a new type of lysosomotropic carrier. FEBS Lett 1977; 84:323–326.
17. Kreuter J. Nanoparticles—a historical perspective. Int J Pharm 2007; 331:1–10.
18. Hartley GS. Aqueous Solutions of Paraffin-Chain Salts. A Study in Micelle Formation. Paris: Hermann & Cie, 1936.
19. McBain MEL, Hutchinson E. Solubilization and Related Phenomena. New York: Academic Press, 1955.
20. Elworthy PH, Florence AT, Macfarlane CB. Solubilization by Surface Active Agents. London: Chapman and Hall, 1968.
21. Schulman JH, Stoeckenius W, Prince LM. Mechanism of formation and structure of microemulsions by electron microscopy. J Phys Chem 1959; 63:1677–1680.
22. Faraday M. The Bakerian Lecture: Experimental relations of gold (and other metals) to light. Philos Trans R Soc 1857; 147:145–181.
23. Paciottis GF, Myer L, Weinreich D, et al. Colloidal gold: a novel nanoparticle vector for tumour directed drug delivery. Drug Deliv 2004; 11:169–183.
24. Graham T. Liquid diffusion applied to analysis. Phil Trans R Soc (Lond) 1861; 151:183–224.
25. Zhou Y. Recent progress in biomolecule-templated nanomaterials. Curr Nanosci 2006; 2:123–134.
26. Martin JM, Ohmae N. Nanolubricants. New York: Wiley, 2008.
27. Teeguarden JG, Hinderliter PM, Orr G, et al. Particokinetics in vitro: dosimetry considerations for in vitro nanoparticle toxicity assessments. Toxicol Sci 2007; 95:300–312.
28. Ambrosch A, Dierkes J, Mühlen I, et al. LDL size distribution in relation to insulin sensitivity and lipoprotein patterning in young and healthy subjects. Diabetes Care 1998; 21:2077–2084.

29. Ferrari M. Cancer nanotechnology : opportunities and challenges. Nat Rev Cancer 2005; 5:161–171.

30. McNeil SE. Nanotechnology for the biologist. J Leukoc Biol 2005; 78:585–594.

31. Quintana A, Raczka E, Piehler L, et al. Design and function of a dendrimer-based therapeutic nanodevice targeted to tumor cells through the folate receptor. Pharm Res 2002; 19:1310–1316.

32. Wang SJ, Brechbiel M, Wiener EC. Characteristics of a new MRI contrast agent prepared from polypropyleneimine dendrimers, generation 2. Invest Radiol 2003; 38:662–668.

33. Roy I, Ohulchanskyy TY, Pudavar HE, et al. Ceramic-based nanoparticles entrapping water-insoluble photosensitizing anticancer drugs: a novel drug-carrier system for photodynamic therapy. J Am Chem Soc 2003; 125:7860–7865.

34. Lanza GM, Winter P, Caruthers S, et al. Novel paramagnetic contrast agents for molecular imaging and targeted drug delivery. Curr Pharm Biotechnol 2004; 5:495–507.

35. Bergey EJ, Levy L, Wang XP, et al. DC magnetic field induced magnetocytolysis of cancer cells targeted by LH-RH magnetic nanoparticles in vitro. Biomed Microdevices 2002; 4:293–299.

36. Jirak D, Kriz J, Herynek V, et al. MRI of transplanted pancreatic islets. Magn Reson Med 2004; 52:1228–1233.

37. Russell-Jones GJ, Arthur L, Walker H. Vitamin B12-mediated transport of nanoparticles across Caco-2 cells. Int J Pharm 1999; 179:247–255.

38. Dubey PK, Mishra V, Jain S, et al. Liposomes modified with cyclic RGD peptide for tumor targeting. J Drug Target 2004; 12:257–264.

39. Reszka RC, Jacobs A, Voges J. Liposome-mediated suicide gene therapy in humans. Methods Enzymol 2005; 391:200–208.

40. ten Hagen TL. Liposomal cytokines in the treatment of infectious diseases and cancer. Methods Enzymol 2005; 391:125–145.

41. Farokhzad OC, Jon S, Khademhosseini A, et al. Nanoparticle-aptamer bioconjugates: a new approach for targeting prostate cancer cells. Cancer Res 2004; 64;7668–7672.

42. Li L, Wartchow CA, Danthi SN, et al. A novel antiangiogenesis therapy using an integrin antagonist or anti-Flk-1 antibody-coated 90Y-labeled nanoparticles. Int J Radiat Oncol Biol Phys 2004; 58:1215–1227.

43. Voura EB, Jaiswal JK, Mattoussi H, Simon SM. Tracking metastatic tumor cell extravasation with quantum dot nanocrystals and fluorescence emission-scanning microscopy. Nat Med 2004; 10:993–998.

44. Loo C, Lowery A, Halas N, et al. Immunotargeted nanoshells for integrated cancer imaging technology. Nano Lett 2005; 5:709–711.

45. Hirsch LR, Stafford RJ, et al. Nanoshell-mediated near-infrared thermal therapy of tumors under magnetic guidance. Proc Natl Acad Sci U S A 2003; 100:13549–13554.

46. Lewin M, Carlesso N, Tung CH, et al. Tat peptide-derivatized magnetic nanoparticles allow in vivo tracking and recovery of progenitor cells. Nat Biotechnol 2000; 18:410–414.

47. Medintz IL, Mattoussi H, Clapp AR. Potential clinical applications of quantum dots. Int J Nanomedicine 2008; 3:151–167.

48. Patolsky F, Zheng G, Leiber CM. Nanowire sensors for medicine and the life sciences. Nanomedicine 2006; 1:51–65.

49. Bianco A, Kostarelos K, Prato M. Applications of carbon nanotubes in drug delivery. Curr Opinion Chem Biol 2005; 9:674–679.

50. Cevc G, Blume G. Biological activity and characteristics of triamcinolone acetonide formulated with the self-regulating drug carriers, transfersomes. Biochim Biophys Acta 2003; 1614;156–164.

51. Manchester M. Targeted therapy using virus-based nanoparticles (VNPs). Nanomedicine 2006; 2:294.

52. Manchester M, Singh P. Virus based nanoparticles (VNPs): platform technologies for diagnostic imaging. Adv Drug Deliv Rev 2006; 58:1505–1522.

53. Lacerda L, Bianco A, Prato M, et al. Carbon nanotubes as nanomedicines: from toxicology to pharmacology. Adv Drug Deliv Rev 2006; 58:1460–1470.

54. Sanchez A, Alonso MJ. Nanoparticulate carriers for ocular drug delivery. In: Torchilin VP, ed. Nanoparticles as Drug Carriers. Imperial College Press: London 2006:649–673.

55. Jung T, Kamm W, Breitenbach A, et al. Biodegradable nanoparticles for oral delivery of peptides: is there a role for polymers to affect mucosal uptake? Eur J Pharm Biopharm 2000; 50:147–160.

56. Lu W, Sun Q, Wan J, et al. Cationic albumin-conjugated pegylated nanoparticles allow gene delivery into brain tumors via intravenous administration. Cancer Res 2006; 66:11878–11887.

57. Maincent P, Thouvenot P, Amicabile C, et al. Lymphatic targeting of polymeric nanoparticles after intraperitoneal administration in rats. Pharm Res 1992; 9:1534–1539.

58. Guzman LA, Labhasetwar V, et al., Local intraluminal infusion of biodegradable polymeric nanoparticles. Circulation 1996; 94:1441–1448.

59. Pandey R, Khuller GK. Subcutaneous nanoparticle-based antitubercular chemotherapy in an experimental model. J Antimicrob Chemother 2004; 54:266–268.

60. Zhou X, et al. The effect of conjugation to gold particles on the ability of low molecular weight chitosan to transfer DNA vaccine. Biomaterials 2007; 29:111–117.

61. Allemann E, Gurny R, Doelker E, et al. Distribution, kinetics and elimination of radioactivity after intravenous and intramuscular injection of 14C savoxepine loaded poly(D,L-lactic acid) nanospheres in rats. J Control Release 1994; 29:97–104.

62. Sham J.O-H, Zhang Y, Finlay WH, et al. Formulation and characterization of spray-dried powders containing nanoparticles for aerosol delivery to the lung. Int J Pharm 2004; 269: 457–467.

63. Oyewumi MO, Yokel RA, Jay M, et al. Comparison of cell uptake, biodistribution and tumor retention of folate coated and PEG-coated gadolinium nanoparticles in tumor-bearing mice. J Control Release 2004; 95:613–626.

64. Kreuter J. Nanoparticulate carriers for drug delivery to the brain. In: Torchilin VP, ed. Nanoparticles as Drug Carriers. Imperial College Press: London, 2006:527–547.

65. Phillips W. Nanoparticles for targeting lymphatics. In: Torchilin VP, ed. Nanoparticles as Drug Carriers. Imperial College Press: London, 2006:598–608.

66. De TK, Bergey EJ, Chung JS, et al. Polycarboxylic acid nanoparticles for ophthalmic drug delivery: an ex vivo evaluation with human cornea. J Microencapsul 2004; 21:841–855.

67. Florence AT. Nanoparticle uptake by the oral route: fulfilling its potential? Drug Discov Technol 2005; 2:75–81.

68. Florence AT. Oral particle uptake; irrefutable and significant. J Pharm Sci (in press).

69. Baker GL, Gupta A, Clark ML, et al. Inhalation toxicity and lung toxicities of C60 fullerene nanoparticles and microparticles. Toxicol Sci 2008; 101:122–131.

70. Pi Z, Zhao X-Y, Yang C, et al. Preparation of ultrafine particles of azithromycin by sonochemical method. Nanomedicine 2007; 3:86–88.

71. Peltonen L. The effect of cosolvents on the formulation of nanoparticles. AAPS PharmSciTech 2002; 3(4):art 32.

72. Ford J, Woolfe J, Florence AT. Nanospheres of cyclosporin A; poor oral absorption in dogs. Int J Pharm 1999; 183:3–6.

73. Byrappa K, Ohara S, Adschiri T. Nanoparticles synthesis using supercritical fluid technology – towards biomedical applications. Adv Drug Deliv Rev 2007; 60:299–327.

74. Gate2Tech. Available at www.gate2tech.com.

75. Eastoe J, Hollamby MJ, Hudson L. Recent advances in nanoparticle synthesis with reversed micelles. Adv Colloid Interface Sci 2006; 128–130:5–15.

76. Arnedo A, Espuelas S, Irache JM. Albumin nanoparticles as carriers for a phosphodiester oligonuclotide. Int J Pharm 2002; 244:59–72.

77. Wu Y, et al. Chitosan nanoparticle formation by ionic interaction between PEG-Chitosan and tripolyphosphate. Int J Pharm 2005; 295:235–245.

78. Al-Khouri N, Roblot-Truepel L, Fessi H, et al. Development of a new process for the manufacture of polyisobutylcyanoacrylate nanocapsules. Int J Pharm 1986; 28:125–132.

79. Florence AT, Haq ME, Johnson JR. Some properties of films of polyalkylcyanoacrylates formed at oil-water interfaces. J Pharm Pharmacol 1975; 27(Suppl):7P.
80. Kipp JE. The role of solid nanoparticle technology in the parenteral delivery of poorly water soluble drugs. Int J Pharm 2004; 284:109–122.
81. Choi J-Y, Yoo JY, Kwak H-S, et al. Role of polymeric stabilizers for drug nanocrystal dispersions. Curr Appl Phys 2005; 5:472–474.
82. Rabinow BE. Nanosuspensions in drug delivery. Nat Rev Drug Discov 2004; 3:785–796.
83. Liversidge GG, Cundy KC. Particle size reduction for improvement of oral bioavailability of hydrophobic drugs: absolute oral bioavailability of nano-crystalline danazol in beagle dogs. Int J Pharm 1995; 125:91–97.
84. Sakthivel T, Toth I, Florence AT. Synthesis and physicochemical properties of lipophilic polyamide dendrimers. Pharm Res 1998; 15:776–782.
85. Majoros IJ, Baker JR, eds. Dendrimer-based Nanomedicine. New Jersey: World Scientific Publishing 2008.
86. Fréchet JMJ, Tomalia DA. Dendrimers and other Dendritic Polymers. New York: Wiley and Sons, 2002.
87. Schalley CA, Vögtle F, eds. Dendrimers V: Functional and Hyperbranched Building Blocks, Photophysical properties, applications in Materials and Life Science. Topics in Current Chemistry. Springer, 2003.
88. Gillies ER, Fréchet JMJ. Dendrimers and dendritic polymers in drug delivery. Drug Discov Today 2005; 10:35–43.
89. Dufès C, Uchegbu IF, Schätzlein A. Dendrimers in gene delivery. Adv Drug Deliv Rev 2005; 57:2177–2202.
90. Bielinska AU, Kukouska-Lattalo JF, Baker JR Jr. The interaction of plasmid DNA with polyamidoamine dendrimers: mechanism of complex formation and analysis of alterations induced in nuclease sensitivity and transcriptional activity of the complexed DNA. Biochim Biophys Acta 1997; 1353:180–190.
91. Yiyun C, Tongwen X. Dendrimers as potential drug carriers. I. Solubilization of non-steroidal anti-inflammatory drugs in the presence of polyamidoamine dendrimers. Eur J Med Chem 2005; 40:1188–1192 [Epub September 8, 2005].
92. Marmillon C, Gauffre F, Gulik-Krzywicki T, et al. Organophosphorus dendrimers as new gelators for hydrogels. Angew Chem Int Ed Engl 2001; 113:2696–2699.
93. Li X, Curry M, Zhang J, et al. Nanotribological studies of dendrimer mediated metallic thin films. Surf Coating Tech 2004; 177–178, 504–511.
94. Xu F, Thaler SM, Barnard JA. Structural and mechanical properties of dendrimer-mediated thin films. J Vac Sci Technol 2005; 23:1234–1237.
95. Shaunak S, Thomas S, Gianasi E, et al. Polyvalent dendrimer glucosamine conjugates prevent scar tissue formation. Nat Biotechnol 2004; 22:977–984.
96. Dufès C, Keith WN, Bilsland A, et al. Synthetic anticancer gene medicine exploits intrinsic antitumor activity of cationic vector to cure established tumors. Cancer Res 2005; 65:8079–8084.
97. Al-Jamal KT, Sakthivel T, Florence AT. Solubilisation and transformation of amphipathic lipid dendron vesicles (dendrisomes) into mixed micelles. Colloids Surf A Physicochem Eng Asp 2005; 268:52–59.
98. Al-Jamal KT, Ramaswamy C, Florence AT. Supramolecular structures from dendrons and dendrimers. Adv Drug Deliv Rev 2005; 57:2238–2270.
99. Singh B, Florence AT. Hydrophobic dendrimer-derived nanoparticles. Int J Pharm 2005; 298:348–353.
100. Ramaswamy C, Florence AT. Self-assembly of some amphipathic dendrons. J Drug Deliv SciTech 2005; 15:307–311.
101. Schenning APH, Elissen-Román C, Weener J-W, et al. Amphiphilic dendrimers as building blocks in supramolecular assemblies. J Am Chem Soc 1998; 120:8199–8208.
102. Foldvari M, Bagonluri M. Carbon nanotubes as functional excipients for nanomedicines: I Pharmaceutical properties. Nanomedicine 2008; 4:173–182.

103. Bianco A, Kostarelos K, Partidos CD, et al. Biomedical applications of functionalised carbon nanotubes. Chem Commun (Camb) 2005; 5:571–577.

104. Foldvari M, Bagonluri M. Carbon nanotubes as functional excipients for nanomedicines: II Drug delivery and biocompatibility issues. Nanomedicine 2008; 4:183–200.

105. Ribiero S, Hussain N, Florence AT. Release of DNA from dendriplexes encapsulated in PLGA microspheres. Int J Pharm 2005; 298:354–360.

106. Frauenrath H. Dendronized polymers—building a new bridge from molecules to nanoscopic objects. Prog Polym Sci 2005; 30:325–384. Available at: ETH D-MATL. www.polychemc. mat.ethz.ch/frauenrath/index/.

107. Scott RW, Datye AK, Crooks RM. Bimetallic palladium-platinum dendrimer encapsulated catalysts. J Am Chem Soc 2003; 125:3708–3709.

108. Florence AT. Nanoparticle flow: implications for drug delivery. In: Torchilin VP, ed. Nanoparticulates as Drug Carriers. London: Imperial College Press, 2006.

109. Radomski A, Jurasz P, Alonso-Escolano D, et al. Nanoparticle-induced platelet aggregation and vascular thrombosis. Br J Pharmacol 2005; 146:882–893.

110. Vigolo B, Pénicaud A, Coulon C, et al. Macroscopic fibers and ribbons of oriented carbon nanotubes. Science 2000; 290:1331–1334.

111. Oles V. Shear-induced aggregation and breakup of polystyrene latex particles. J Colloid Interface Sci 1992; 154:351–358.

112. Silebi CA, Dosramos JG. Axial dispersion of submicron particles in capillary hydrodynamic fractionation. AIChE J 1989; 35:1351–1364.

113. Silebi CA, Dosramos JG. Separation of submicrometer particles by capillary hydrodynamic fractionation (CHDF). J Colloid Interface Sci 1989; 130:14–24.

114. Chambers E, Mitrigotri S. Prolonged circulation of large polymeric nanoparticles by non-covalent adsorption on erythrocytes. J Control Release 2004; 100:111–119.

115. Ding Y, Wen D. Particle migration in a flow of nanoparticle suspensions. Powder Technol 2005; 149:84–92.

116. Vacheethanasee K, Marchant RE. Non-specific Staphylococcus epidermidis adhesion: contributions of bacterial hydrophobicity and charge. In: An YH, Friedman RJ, eds. Handbook of Bacterial Adhesion: Principles, Methods and Applications. Totowa NJ: Humana Press, 2000:73–90.

117. Darton NJ, Hallmark B, Huan X, et al. The in-flow capture of superparamagnetic nanoparticles for targeted therapeutics. Nanomedicine 2008; 4:19–29.

118. Mori A, Klibanov AL, Torchilin VP, et al. Influence of the steric barrier of amphipathic poly (ethyleneglycol) and ganglioside GM1 on the circulation time of liposomes and on the target binding of immunoliposomes in vivo. FEBS Lett 1991; 284:263–266.

119. Florence AT, Rogers JA. Emulsion stabilization by non-ionic surfactants: experiment and theory. J Pharm Pharmacol 1971; 23:153–169, 233–251.

120. Gaumet M, Vargas A, Gurny R, et al. Nanoparticles for drug delivery: the need for precision in reporting particle size parameters. Eur J Pharm Biopharm 2008; 69:1–9.

121. Keck C, Müller R. Size analysis of submicron particles by laser diffractometry—90% of the published measurements are false. Int J Pharm 2008; 355:150–163.

122. Siepmann J, Siepmann F, Florence AT. Local controlled drug delivery to the brain: mathematical modeling of the underlying mass transport mechanisms. Int J Pharm 2006; 314:101–119.

123. Ruenraroengsak P, Florence AT. The diffusion of latex nanospheres and the effective (microscopic) viscosity of HPMC gels. Int J Pharm 2005; 298:361–366.

124. Mackie JS, Meares P. The diffusion of electrolytes in a cationic membrane. I Theoretical. Proc R Soc London A 1955; 232:498–509.

125. Ruenraroengsak P, Al-Jamal K, Hartell N, et al. Cell uptake, cytoplasmic diffusion and nuclear access of a 6.5nm diameter dendrimer. Int J Pharm 2007; 331:215–219.

126. Small AC, Johnston JH. Novel hybrid materials of cellulose fibres and nanoparticles. NSTI Nanotech Abstract 2008.

127. Naka K, Chujo Y. Effect of anionic dendrimers on the crystallisation of calcium carbonate in aqueous solution. C R Chimie 2003; 6:1193–1200.

128. Joly-Pottuz L, Vacher B, Ohmae N, et al. Anti-wear and friction reducing mechanism of carbon nano-onions as lubricant additives. Tribol Lett 2008; 30:69–80.
129. Majumder M, Chopra N, Andrews R, et al. Nanoscale hydrodynamics: enhanced flow in carbon nanotubes. Nature 2005; 438:44.
130. Lu Y, Fan H, Stump FA, et al. Aerosol-assisted self-assembly of mesostructured spherical nanoparticles. Nature 1999; 398:223–226.
131. Borm P, Klaesigg FC, et al. Research strategies for safety evaluation of nanomaterials. Part V: Role of dissolution in biological fate and effects of nanoscale particles. Toxicol Sci 2006; 90:23–32.
132. Oberdörster G, Oberdörster E, Oberdörster J. Nanotoxicology: an emerging discipline evolving from studies of ultrafine particles. Environ Health Perspect 2005; 113:823–839.

13

Dosage Forms for Personalized Medicine: From the Simple to the Complex

Alexander T. Florence
Centre for Drug Delivery Research, The School of Pharmacy, University of London, London, U.K.

Juergen Siepmann
Department of Pharmaceutical Technology, College of Pharmacy, Université Lille Nord de France, Lille, France

INTRODUCTION

The basic ambition of personalized medicines is for patients to receive medications, which if not tailored for them as individuals, will be designed more specifically for them as part of a group of genetically, physiologically, or pathologically similar patients. This is in contrast to the current and frequently applied modus, which involves most patients receiving the same drug at the same dose and at the same frequency as others. There are of course exceptions to this. The postgenomic era in which we are purported to live has promised much, but has delivered less. The promise is that through a better understanding of pharmacogenetics and pharmacogenomics and through genetic profiling of patients especially those involved in clinical trials, more valuable data will become available to support the treatment of individuals and groups who are first likely to respond to the medication and/or be unlikely to suffer adverse reactions from its administration.

DRUG AND DOSAGE FORM IN PERSONALIZED MEDICINE

Attention directed toward this promised land has so far been largely on the drug itself, rather than on modes of delivery. A recent report on *Personalised Medicines* from the United Kingdom's Royal Society (1) does not mention delivery systems at all. This is perhaps understandable because the emphasis has been not only on the drug but also on its suitability for a given group or subgroup of patients. However, given that dosage forms can influence both pharmacokinetic and pharmacodynamic outcomes and the quality of effect, the role that delivery systems will or should play in personalized medicine should be addressed. The discipline of pharmaceutics (as well as pharmacokinetic analysis) has a key part to play in ensuring that appropriate formulations are available for appropriate drugs for appropriate patients, and of course, in affordable forms. The United Kingdom's Medicines and Health Regulatory Agency (MHRA) (2) has recognized the need for a multiplicity of dosage forms, even if only to deliver different doses of active substance. They state:

> Personalised medicine can occur on the basis of dose adjustment for side effects, dose adjustment for efficacy, dose adjustment for concomitant medication, metabolising rate and renal excretion, drug choice due to allergic potential, drug choice due to resistance profile of the infecting organism, drug choice due to biological target, and drug choice according to the personal wishes of a patient.

> Increasingly accurate and specific medical information on each individual patient is becoming available to provide prescribers with more and more information from increasingly sensitive physical methods and the wider application of biomarkers (for instance to identify drug metabolising characteristics of each individual patient). This will result in future medicines needing to be available to provide a greater range of doses for prescribers; there will be fewer numbers of patients in the target indication at the time of product registration due to better use of inclusion and exclusion criteria.

The MHRA's optimistic hope is that "medicines will be safer, more effective and have fewer side effects as the dose will be adjusted to ensure that the most appropriate dose is prescribed to each patient."

It would be wrong to assume that improvements in medication safety and quality of effect will occur solely through new drugs, new understanding modes of action, interaction and adverse reactions, and novel means of drug delivery. One of the greatest barriers to successful therapy is nonadherence or noncompliance with prescribed medication. The other is medication error (3). In 2000, the U.S. Institute of Medicine's report *To Err is Human: Building a Safer Health System* states that nearly 100,000 individuals in the United States die each year from medication errors in the hospital setting. A recent paper points out that fatal medication errors in the home have risen 360% over the period 1983 to 2004 (4). There are thus larger issues than can be discussed here where there are perhaps not technological solutions at the point of administration or taking the medicine, but control at the locus of prescribing and dispensing. Even in highly computerized hospitals it has been claimed that adverse drug events can still be at an unacceptable level (5). Compliance or adherence (the latter being the preferred but not perfect term) is a challenge; Osterberg and Blaschke (6) recall C. E. Koop's dictum: "Drug don't work in patients who don't take them." Because patients can react emotionally to a drug product (children to injections, patients reported dislike of the Exubera™ bulky inhaler), or perceive tablets and capsule color as signifying a relationship with activity—red for analgesics and pastel shades for anxiolytics—drug delivery systems can be important in determining the degree of adherence. This is an important aspect of personal medicine. The rate of adherence decreases with the increased frequency of dosing, according to Claxton (7). Once-daily dosing achieves a mean rate of compliance of just under 80%, while four-times-a-day dosing results in a decrease to 50%. The complexity of treatment is similarly a factor as is the occurrence of side effects. Hence the design of combination dose forms and more flexible dosing systems, apart from any pharmacogenetic input, can improve matters. Osterberg and Rudd (8) suggest that the use of more "forgiving" medications such as those with long half-lives, sustained-release systems, or transdermal patches might assist in this. They define forgiving as "drugs whose efficacy will not be affected by delayed or missed doses." The role of formulations in both moderating and causing adverse events is also a factor (9).

One of the technological solutions might be greater utilization of the many products now available for assisting patients in taking their medications at the right time and in the correct quantities. TalkingRx[TMa] is a device attached to a medication container, which has a microrecorder, which enables physician, pharmacist, and carers to record specific information to the individual patient. The Med-eMonitor[TM] system includes a medicine adherence device linked to a secure Internet site, which captures and reports in real time the patient's "interaction with the device."[b] There are many other such devices available.

Improved adherence—focused on the individual—has been shown, not surprisingly, to improved suppression of HIV RNA in AIDS patients (10). Nonadherence in antimicrobial therapy may lead to resistance (11). His extensive research into adherence has led Urquhart to suggest that it is a discipline itself: "the study of how ambulatory patients use prescription drugs" or pharmionics (12).

The remaining elements of this chapter do not address adherence per se but the types of dose form that may be valuable in personalized medicine, from the very simple fast-dissolving tablets and buccal films to more complex electronically driven microdevices. Some delivery systems can take the patient side of variability out of the equation. It is suggested that intelligent inhalers (13) reduce the dependence of inhaled dose of the patient's inspiratory flow, for example.

NEGLECTED DISEASES, NEGLECTED TECHNOLOGIES

A comprehensive report on *Priority Medicines for Europe and the World* by Kaplan and Laing (14) published by the World Health Organization in 2004 highlights many of the issues in the war against neglected diseases such as malaria where insufficient research and development efforts worldwide has led, and still leads to, loss of life on an unthinkable scale. In a chapter of the report dealing with "cross-cutting themes," there is a reminder of the importance of drug delivery mechanisms. The authors conclude that "there is a wide range of existing evidence-based, very often off-patent technologies that are heavily underutilized. Such technologies could be used to improve the 'patient-friendly' performance of a number of existing medicines." These, then, one might say, are neglected technologies, invented but discarded because in many cases funding bodies or the market will not pay for them, or as is sometimes the case, a fitting application has not been found.

NEGLECTED PATIENTS

In all parts of the world, two disparate patient groups for which personalized medicines (or personalized formulations) are sorely needed include children and the elderly, neither of which even comprise homogeneous sets, as discussed in chapter 6 in this volume. This will sound strangely familiar to pharmacists of a generation used to preparing medicines

---

[a]See www.talkingrx.com.

[b]See www.informedix.com.

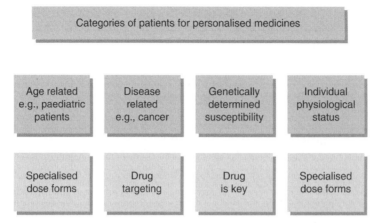

Scheme 1   Categories of patients who are candidates for personalized medicines: (*i*) those who by virtue of their age require specialized dosage forms and dose regimens, for example, the very young and the very old; (*ii*) those who share the same disease state and who require specialized delivery systems and regimens; (*iii*) those with genetically determined susceptibility to the individual drugs and who might benefit from treatment and not suffer adverse reactions; and (*iv*) those whose physiological status is similar, for example, obese patients. Different solutions are required for each of these, albeit simplified, categories: perhaps specialized dosage forms or drug-targeting systems. In the genetically determined responders, the drug is the key and the delivery system is generally secondary.

extemporaneously for individual patients. Children suffer rapid changes in metabolism and physiological function in the progression from the neonatal stage through infancy and early and late childhood. In older patients there are changes in body fat, renal clearance, and gastrointestinal function to contend with, but often there are issues because of concomitant pathologies. These groups then could be considered to be neglected patients, but there are others.

Scheme 1 illustrates the categories of patients for whom personalized medicines are or will be designed. One might include everyone if the true meaning of the personalized medicines is considered, but this is unrealistic. We can categorize patient groups according to whether they suffer from age-related, disease-related, genetically determined, or other complaints.

Formulation approaches for pediatric and geriatric patients have been discussed in this volume by Tuleu and Breitkreutz (chap. 6, vol. 2). Some of the points they make are reiterated here as these patient groups are those for which personalized medicine comes into its own. Issues relating to medicines in childhood are dealt with in a paper by Ernest et al. (15) and in more general terms by Wong et al. (16). Pediatric cardiovascular medications have been discussed (17), and general pediatric formulations in practice are dealt with (18) in the text *Paediatric Drug Handling* (19). It is not necessarily a question of high technological solutions to problems of delivery and dose. One of the most distressing consequences of the use of adult dosage forms is the necessity for large dilutions, which clearly introduces the opportunity of error. Errors of 10-fold excess or underdosing are often the root cause of serious adverse events in practice. It should not be beyond our wit to devise foolproof devices with electronic dispensing valves (say), which makes such errors difficult to commit. An simpler alternative might simply be the availability of more appropriate formulations, which contain doses relevant for the patient group in question: To be realistic, this requires dosage platforms that are readily adapted and are amenable to short production runs. For economic and practical reasons, many of these "flexible" delivery systems will be simple but not less safe or robust. The materials available for the preparation of dose forms is now extensive and should have transformed the preparation of specialized dose forms.

It could be argued that individualized medicine is available now through specialized dose forms for the very young, although in many cases this is not always so (20). We have not as a community risen to the challenge to devise and market systems suitable for children and the elderly, and certainly have not solved the issue of the safety of dosing in these cases. In pediatric medicine, Miller et al. report (21) the rather discomfiting statistics of relative error types of prescribing (3–37%), dispensing (5–58%), administering (72–75%), and documentation (17–21%). Some of these figures are difficult to accept, but surely pharmaceutical innovation, new dose forms, and modes of delivery have a part to play in rectifying the major issues? Tuleu (personal communication) argues that in addition to legislative and formulary developments, innovations in pharmaceutical formulations should improve the ease in which children can have access to more suitable medicines. Innovative modified-release preparations, she suggests, is one area among several considered "ripe" for future developments and research along with (*i*) use of less common routes of administration such as oral-transmucosal (buccal strips), intranasal, and transdermal products (for neonates mainly); (*ii*) more research into alternative safe excipients for children such as the cyclodextrins to mask the taste of drugs, or to improve solubility or to protect drugs or patient; and (*iii*) in agreement with the statements on adherence earlier in this chapter, research into children's ability to swallow, and their preferences of modes of administration and dose forms is needed. Future formulation research should explore further a range that includes mini-tablets, chewable and dispersible tablets, or more oral liquids.

Although new and innovative formulations are urgently needed, work on extemporaneous formulations should not be disregarded, as this is still an activity of vital importance in many hospital pharmacies that collaborate with physicians in trials and who also work with orphan drugs. Hence the principles of formulation and manufacture espoused in this book are clearly relevant not only to those who work in industry but also to those who practice closer to the patient.

There is a danger that complex solutions are sought for the provision of personalized medicines. True nanotechnology may one day provide new systems for delivery and new materials with which to construct vectors. But the provision of flexible-dose products is one key development. In the 21st century, splitting tablets designed for adults hardly seems a reasonable approach and is inappropriate for a multitude of adult dose forms; the use of mini-tablets, which can be administered in defined multiples, can have a role. What other roles can dosage forms have? We speculate in Scheme 2 of some of the approaches that can be taken, which we will treat here. One can think of self-regulating and pulsatile delivery systems as well as means of delivering variable doses of drugs. An important development might be the reintroduction of pharmacy-based product manufacture. This must be a development whose time has come. There have been technological advances, which might allow this in specialized pharmacies. One of these developments, three-dimensional printing (3DP), is discussed below.

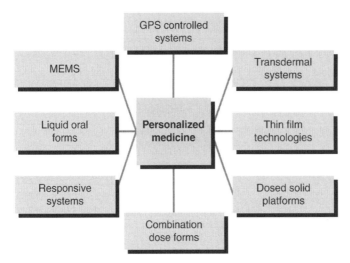

Scheme 2 Some possibilities for the pharmaceutical technologies and approaches to be used in personalized medicine, ranging from simple liquid oral dose forms where the dose can be varied by volume, through responsive systems, micro-electromechanical systems (MEMS), GPS-directed systems (see text) transdermal systems, thin film technologies with passive or active release mechanisms, combination tablet or capsule dose forms, and what we term dosed solid platforms, for example, aqueous dispersible polymer, solid gel or matrix material into which precise doses of drug can be absorbed.

LOW- AND FLEXIBLE-DOSE PRODUCTS

Products with readily variable dose levels are required. Methods for depositing drugs in solution onto biosoluble and biodegradable matrices also offer the possibility of ready and accurate fabrication in hospital and community pharmacies. A matrix platform for such products is required. Developments in bubble jet devices (22) suggest the possibility of the deposition and the adsorption of the smallest doses onto and into suitable matrices for delivery, say, to neonates by oral or buccal routes.

FAST-DISPERSING, FAST-DISSOLVING, OR FAST-MELTING TABLETS

Technologies do not always have to be complex. Probably most suitable for the very young and the elderly who might have difficulty in swallowing conventional tablets or capsules, a large number of fast-dispersing tablets are now available. They have a place in psychiatric medicine (23) where olanzapine and risperidone have been administered in fast-dissolving forms. These are produced by several methods, conventional tabletting processes suitably modified, for example, in the production of the Frosta^{TM} system (24), by freeze drying (25) and a "floss" method, which, as its name suggests, involves a fibrous matrix made from a mix of excipients (26). Table 1 shows a list of some of the products available. Not only do these products act as fast-disintegrating forms with their attendant advantages, but with selegiline used in the treatment of Parkinson's disease, the Zydis^{TM} dose form has been shown to provide higher bioavailability and a reduced concentration of active metabolites (27).

Oral film technology also offers similar advantages. Novartis Consumer Health Care has launched two products Theraflu and Triaminic Thin Strips^{TM} said to be the first

Table 1 Oral Fast-Dispersing Tablet Technologies

Technology	Company
Conventional tablet processes	
WOWTAB®	Yamanouchi
ORASOLV®	Cima Labs
EFDAS®	Elan Corp
FLASHTAB®	Prographarm
FROSTA®	Akina
Freeze-drying methods	
ZYDIS®	R. P. Scherer
LYOC®	Farmalyoc
QUICKSOLV®	Janssen Pharmaceutica
Floss formation	
FLASHDOSE®	Fuisz Technologies

Source: Adapted from Ref. 26.

systemic medicines to be delivered in this (thin strip) form (28), which is used widely in consumer products.

COMBINATION DOSE SYSTEMS

For many years, combination products were discouraged by the FDA and other regulatory authorities. The treatment of AIDS has highlighted the need for combination tablets, which have advantages as well as disadvantages. If the drug dose ratio required depends on the pharmacogenetics, then this is the opportunity for 3DP approaches or other forms of production flexibility.

According to one commentator (29), the FDA defines a combination product as one "composed of two or more regulated components—any combination of a drug and device; biological product and device; drug and biological product; or drug, device, and biological product." The FDA's definition is quite inclusive, encompassing "drug-coated devices, drugs packaged with delivery devices in medical kits, and drugs and devices packaged separately but intended to be used together." The FDA developed a categorization scheme for combination products. Under this scheme, a product is placed into one of several categories, which include

- a prefilled drug (or biological) delivery device/system;
- a device coated, impregnated, or otherwise combined with drug or biological;
- a drug/biological combination; and
- possible combination products based on mutually conforming labeling of separate products.

It is interesting with the widespread use of tablets and capsules over many decades that the difficulty of making stable combination products has been addressed recently in a commentary in *Nature Reviews. Drug Discovery* (30), which makes the point that "making a tablet out of one drug is an underrated problem in itself, so making a tablet out of multiple active pharmaceutical ingredients is a much tougher proposition." Typical combination products for HIV treatment include Combivir™ (GSK) (zidovudine and lamivudine) and Atripla™ (Gilead, Bristol Myers Squibb) (emtricitabine/tenovir and efavirenz). Pfizer's Caduet™ (amlodipine and atorvastatin) is another example. It is, in a way, encouraging, that the traditional pharmaceutics of tablet manufacture is recognized as a complex and underrated task.

MINI-TABLETS

Matrix mini-tablets based on starch/microcellulose wax mixtures have been described (31,32). The possibility with these and other mini-tablets is that different dose levels can be administered by changing the number of mini-tablets within a capsule for adults or using single units for children. It is also possible to utilize fast-dissolving mini-tablets to prepare liquid dosages extemporaneously.

THREE-DIMENSIONAL PRINTING

With the advent of 3DP, the possibility probably now exists for the return to pharmacy production of specialized dose forms, either implants (33) or oral tablets (34). The basis of the technique of 3DP was developed in Cima's laboratory in MIT, as shown in Figure 1. The key point is that the design of the finished product is elaborated on a computer so that the design is transformed into the product item by item by a modification of the bubble jet printer where inks have been replaced by drug active in suspension or solution along with binders, fillers, or polymers. If pharmaceutical tablets or implants are the desired dose form, much depends on the particle size of active, and the nature of the binder such as its viscosity. Once the product is fabricated, there is some potential for diffusion of drug molecules between layers and subsets of the structure, but research continues into such problems. The dose forms can be complex, but need not be so: the principle advantage is the ability to titrate dose and perhaps release patterns. In effect the release rate and pattern of the active(s) can be predetermined by the possibility of placing the active in different regions of the structure (Fig. 2). Figure 2A shows an experimental geometry of tablets, which can allow predetermined release patterns, in vitro at least, which could be manufactured by the technique. A "breakaway" tablet prepared by 3DP is proposed (Fig. 3), which breaks up into two parts after the dissolution of the fixative joining the parts together and is useful in combination therapy where the relative doses need to be varied according to the patient.

There are still problems to be overcome with 3DP, such as the diffusion of drugs between layers and interactions, but these can be solved by appropriate barrier layers. As these forms can be manufactured at will, the need for longer-term stability is one that perhaps will need recasting.

MICRODOSE SYSTEMS

Microdose systems can be devised where potent drugs are to be administered. Either liquid or solid drug forms can be used, the latter if incorporated into microparticles or nanoparticles. If the drug can be formed into a solution in a volatile solvent, microdoses can be applied to the matrix accurately. Such systems would lend themselves to extemporaneous dispensing. Films such as RapidFilm™ (35) (which employ water-soluble polymers such as HPMC, HPC, and PVP) are manufactured with drugs incorporated into the system, but the matrix could form the platform for the loading of drugs at will. Drug release would be passive through dissolution of the matrix or dissolution of the drug or a combination of processes. If the drug is solid, preloaded

(A)

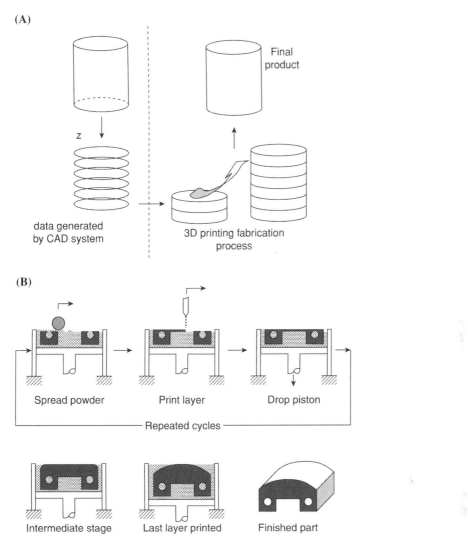

Figure 1 3DP: the principles. A schematic illustration of (**A**) the involvement of the CAD system and the printing process; (**B**) the principle of the 3DP process in which a three-dimensional structure is built up from polymer/ceramic materials from a bubble jet nozzle. *Abbreviation*: 3DP, three-dimensional printing. *Source*: From Ref. 33.

micro- or nanoparticles could be dispersed into platform vehicles for administration, the dosage dictated by the amount and drug load of the particles. These would be useful for drugs that are insufficiently stable or soluble in the liquid form.

IMPLANTED DEVICES

An implantable drug delivery system based on microactuation devices has been developed (36) (Fig. 4) by which doses can be controlled to an accuracy of 5 μL. One form of the invention can dispense solid drug, which of course is a more complex task, because of the

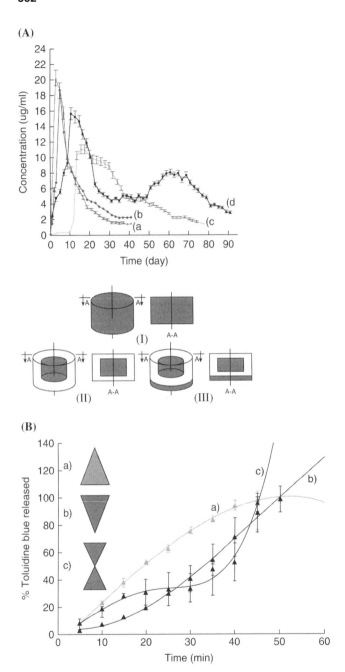

Figure 2 (**A**) Release profiles of levofloxacin from three implants I, II, and III, with the structures shown below. Implant I prepared by three-dimensional printing gives the profile labeled a, while b represents the behavior of implant I made by a conventional process; implant II gives plot c, while implant III gives plot d. (**B**) Experimental (two-dimensional) geometrical structures as shown. These allow entrance of solvent from one (*upper* or *lower*) face and produces the release patterns as shown. *Source*: Part A from Ref. 33, and part B from A.T. Florence (unpublished).

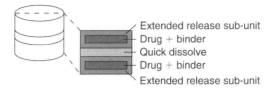

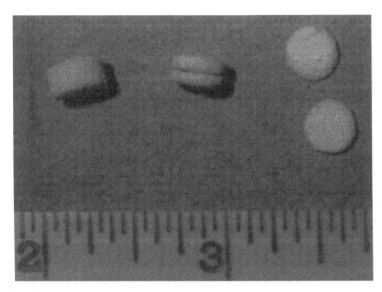

Figure 3 Breakaway tablets prepared by three-dimensional printing technology, showing in *upper* figure the principle and in the *lower* actual tablets at an intermediate stage of separation and in finally separated form.

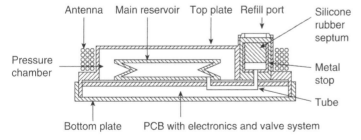

Figure 4 The design of the implantable drug delivery system based on shape memory alloy microactuation, showing the main reservoir, pressure chamber, and the printed circuit board (PCB) with electronics and valve system. The basic concept is to have a reservoir under constant pressure pushing liquid through a calibrated flow channel and valve system. Dimensions are 50 mm with a height of 15 mm. *Source*: From Ref. 36.

potential for particle jamming and blockage. Many of the issues of flow of suspensions in microfluidic devices are dealt with by Bitsch (37).

PUMPS

Patient-operated analgesic pumps are a prime example of existing tailoring of dose of drug to an individual's needs. There are a variety of opportunities with micropumps for other uses. Microfabricated electrokinetic pumps can be used to deliver water, polar organic solvents, biomacromolecules as discussed by Chen et al. (38). A new delivery system for inner ear infections involves a microcatheter delivering gentamicin driven by an electronic micropump (39). A reciprocating perfusion system has also been used for the inner ear (40). A novel electrostatic peristaltic pump described by Teymoori and Abbaspour-Sani (41), $7 \times 4 \times 1$ mm^3, is intended for medical applications. Such devices have the potential to provide accurate low doses at predetermined time intervals, which has obvious advantages in some cases.

MICROFLUIDIC DEVICES AND MICROCHIP-BASED TECHNOLOGIES

A delivery technology based on silicon microchips proposed by Langer and coworkers (42–44) involves loading nanoliter reservoirs on a microchip with one or more drugs. Figure 5A shows a schematic representation of such a device. The drug(s) is (are) filled into the reservoirs, which are square pyramidal in shape and have, for example, a volume of approximately 25 nL. They can be filled from the side with the larger opening (bottom side in Fig. 5A) using, for example, inkjet printing techniques. The drug can be in the solid, liquid, or semisolid state. The other opening of the reservoir (upper side in Fig. 5A) is sealed with a thin gold layer (e.g., 50×50 μm^2 and 0.3 μm in thickness). This thin gold layer serves as an anode. The microchip also contains a cathode (Fig. 5A). Applying a potential of +1.04 volts results in the electrochemical dissolution of the gold membrane and subsequent drug release. Figure 5B shows photographs of such a microchip device: on the left the front side and on the right the back side are illustrated. For comparison, a coin is shown on the same scale. As numerous drug reservoirs can be located on one single microchip and as each reservoir can be activated individually, this type of technology can virtually provide any type of drug release patterns, even in the case of complex drug combinations. Different administration routes can be envisaged, for instance subcutaneous implantation or swallowing. Not only drugs but also diagnostic agents and/or biosensors may be contained in the reservoirs.

Microfluidic systems now used as microlaboratories (lab-on-a-chip) have potential to deliver drugs. An electrokinetic microfluidic device is described by Chung and coworkers (45). They have studied the factors that govern the release time and also the important feature in all such systems, the dispersal pattern of the drug after release. The devices have an upper silicon structure where the drug is stored and a lower electrically polydimethylsiloxane (PDMS) backing, not unlike the device of Santini et al. (42). In their experiments 1.9-μm fluorescent polystyrene microspheres were used to follow the ejection patterns of the "load." The radius of the dispersed fluorescence increases with increasing applied voltage up to 4 V; in 40 seconds, for example, the fluorescence has dispersed to a radius of 230 μm. The reservoirs empty over periods of minutes, at 3 V in

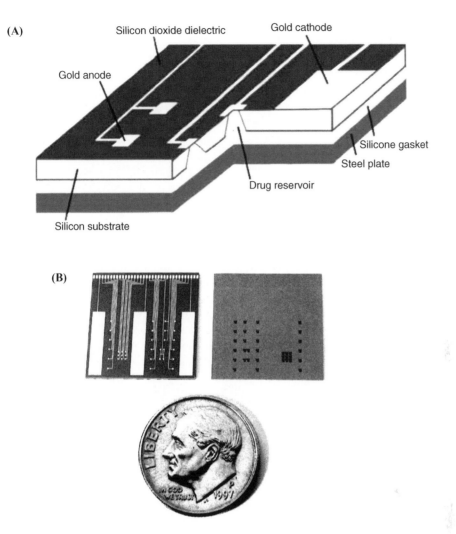

Figure 5 Microchip-based drug delivery systems: **(A)** Schematic presentation of the device structure with cathodes, anodes, and drug reservoirs. **(B)** Photographs of the front and back sides of a microchip, the coin serves as a reference for the dimensions of the system. *Source*: From Refs. 43 and 44.

10 minutes and at 4 V in around 150 seconds, important in relation to power consumption. Finite element analysis of the release patterns shows the differences between electro-osmotic and electrophoretic and electroosmotic ejection processes. These studies, among others, demonstrate that such systems have to be investigated in great detail before becoming routine, but they also make clear that the potential for the control of drug release rate and patterns of release are significant. In this work, the fluorescent markers used to trace patterns of release were as stated 1.9-μm polystyrene particles, illustrating the possibility of utilizing such devices for microparticle and nanoparticle delivery.

A combination of such a sophisticated drug delivery system with an appropriate biosensor and control unit might one day lead to an autonomous (i.e., not dependent on external triggers) "pharmacy-on-a-chip" (46–48). If a particular type of drug or drug combination could be released "on demand" in an appropriate quantity, this would allow real personalized medication.

The in vitro and in vivo performance of this type of controlled-release microchip technology has been demonstrated with the anticancer drug BCNU [1,3-bis (2-chloroethyl)-1-nitrosourea, carmustine] (49). The reservoirs were filled either with pure BCNU, or with binary BCNU:poly(ethylene glycol) (PEG) blends. Figure 6A shows the experimentally determined drug release profiles in phosphate buffer pH 7.2. The dashed lines indicate the time points of activation: at $t = 0$ and $t \approx 120$ hours, 50% of the reservoirs were opened using a potentiostat. As can be seen, the pure BCNU is only slowly released upon device activation, which can probably be attributed to the fact that this drug is highly lipophilic and that the reservoir openings are only 50 μm in size. Importantly, the addition of PEG significantly increased the release rate upon device activation (Fig. 6A), which can at least partially be explained by facilitated water imbibition into the opened reservoirs. For the studies in rats, microchips loaded with 50:50 BCNU:PEG blends and containing 0.67, 1.2, and 2.0 mg drug were implanted subcutaneously next to tumors in rat flanks. The devices were administered 10 days after tumor implantation. Half of the reservoirs were opened one day later, and the other half, six days later. For reasons of comparison, also microchips containing the maximal drug dose (2 mg) were implanted, but not activated. One group of rats was not treated at all and three groups received the same amounts of BCNU and PEG via subcutaneous injection. Figure 6B shows the experimentally determined evolution of the tumor volumes in these groups. Clearly, the performance of the activated microchips was comparable to that of the equipotent subcutaneous drug: PEG injections, proving the efficacy of this type of advanced drug delivery system. In contrast, the nonactivated device as well as the untreated group showed significant tumor growth. Importantly, the microchips offer the possibility to load different types of anticancer drugs and to engineer different release patterns to maximize therapeutic effect. This is where the knowledge of drug behavior in the targets is available and how drug when free diffuses through tissues.

Another major advantage of this type of microchip technology is that the incorporated drugs can effectively be protected against degradation. For instance BCNU is known to rapidly degrade in aqueous media (half-life = 10–20 minutes) (50), whereas it is much more stable in 95% ethanol, which has a half-life of 74 days (51). The reservoirs in the microchip can be filled with appropriate media assuring optimal stability of the incorporated drugs. Furthermore, the drugs can effectively be protected against external stress (e.g., water, enzyme) as long as the reservoirs are closed.

A review of micro-electromechanical systems (MEMS)-based delivery systems provides more detailed information of present and future possibilities (52). This covers both micropumps [electrostatic, piezoelectric, thermopneumatic, shape memory alloy bimetallic, and ionic conductive polymer films (ICPF)] and nonmechanical micropumps [magnetohydrodynamic (MHD), electrohydrodynamic (EHD), electroosmotic (EO), chemical, osmotic-type, capillary-type, and bubble-type systems]. The biocompatibility of materials for MEMS fabrication is also covered. The range of technologies available is very large and bodes well for the future.

To overcome the drawback of nondegradability of silicon-based microchips, completely degradable microchip devices have also been proposed (53). They consist of poly(lactic acid) (PLA)-based disks, containing drug-filled microreservoirs. The latter are covered with poly(lactic-co-glycolic acid) (PLGA) membranes. It was shown that these membranes are significantly deformed upon contact with aqueous media and that crack formation occurs. Recently, the performance of this type of degradable microchip was demonstrated in a rat tumor model (54). Importantly, the devices showed similar

(A)

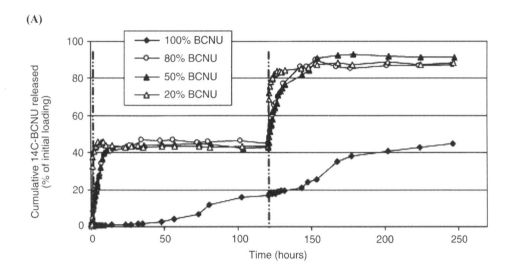

(B)

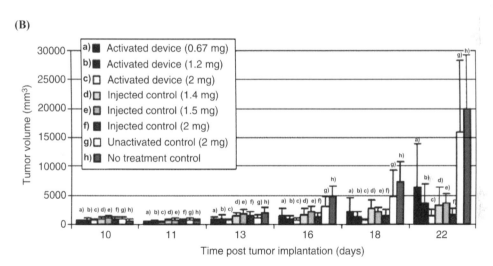

Figure 6 In vitro and in vivo performance of an anticancer drug-loaded microchip delivery system: (**A**) In vitro release of BCNU into phosphate buffer pH 7.2. The reservoirs contained either pure BCNU or binary BCNU:PEG blends. The dashed lines indicate the time points of device activation (opening 50% of the reservoirs). (**B**) Evolution of the tumor size in rat flanks upon SC implantation of BCNU:PEG-loaded microchips, containing 0.67, 1.2, or 2.0 mg drug and being activated 11 and 16 days post tumor implantation (50% of the reservoirs being opened at each time), or upon SC injection of the same amounts of BCNU and PEG, or upon SC implantation of a microchip containing 2 mg BCNU, but which was not activated. For reasons of comparison, also a nontreated control group is included. *Source*: From Ref. 49.

pharmacodynamic efficacy as Gliadel™, a marketed product based on a biodegradable polymer disk loaded with the same drug (BCNU) at the same dose. Compared with Gliadel, the degradable microchip can be expected to more easily provide complex drug release patterns, in particular in the case of drug combinations.

ELECTROACTIVE CONTROLLED-RELEASE FILMS

A promising development is that of electroactive controlled-release films (55). These may be fabricated from Prussian Blue, an FDA-approved material, which can be engineered to release precise doses of drug or other chemicals on application of a small voltage (~ 1.25 V). The film, in one example, is about 150 nm in thickness and is made from two outer negatively charged Prussian Blue layers enclosing a positively charged drug-containing layer. On application of the electrical potential, the Prussian Blue loses its charge, according to the researchers at MIT, and the film disintegrates, releasing the drug. The device can be activated remotely. The possibilities of this development are manifold, as the device can be made so small. The same group (56) describe the fabrication layer by

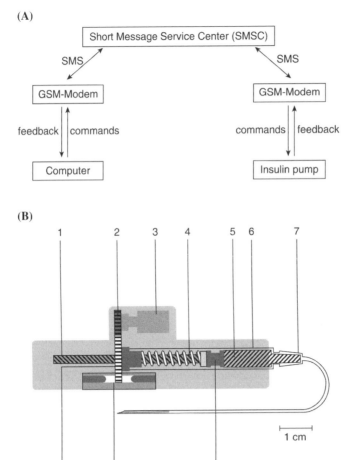

Figure 7 (**A**) The functional principle of the computer-based insulin pump controlled via GSM. (**B**) A schematic diagram of the spring-powered insulin pump devised by Gröning et al. 1, piston rod; 2, gear; 3, stepping motor; 4, spring; 5, insulin reservoir, volume 300 µL; 6, acryl glass; 7, infusion set; 8, gear; 9, infrared detector; and 10, piston. *Source*: From Ref. 57.

layer through Langmuir–Blodgett techniques and the problem of, and solution to, interlayer diffusion of the drug, an issue that occurred with three-dimensionally printed systems.

TELEPHARMACY

Another remotely activated device has been described by Gröning et al. (57). They demonstrated in a model the remote control of a device to delivery insulin (Fig. 7). This possibility of external programming and monitoring of insulin pumps is possible for continuous subcutaneous infusion. The use of SMS allows "immediate transfer of commands to the pump." There are many pitfalls to overcome: the ethics of taking control away from the patients and their carer is but one, and there are safety issues, should the GPS system fail, and presumably if in error the pump is activated by the physician or indeed by individuals accidentally. But there is no doubt that telepharmacy will impact on future medicine, whether personalized or not. The personal element could come simply as a result of automated reminders to patients to take their medications also discussed above, but the more sophisticated systems described by Gröning et al. will also have their place.

CONCLUSIONS

This short chapter gives only our personal views of some of the systems that might be used in the future when personalized medicines become more routine, once it is recognized by the whole health care community that continuing in the manner we have to date is not the way forward. But there needs to be the will to enter the arena, to pay for the systems and devices that are developed to deliver the drugs that need such special care. Pharmaceutics has a role to play through its potential to devise novel delivery solutions to difficult problems, to harness materials to build new and more precise dosage forms, and to be innovative. Academics must be courageous enough to pursue simple solutions as well as blue-sky objectives in drug delivery and targeting. And we must devise delivery devices that are appealing to individuals. If patients do not take their medicines, or there are no appropriate systems with which to deliver them, all pharmacogenetic, pharmacokinetic, and pharmacodynamic knowledge is for naught.

The pharmaceutics elaborated on in the two volumes of this text detailing progress in basic and applied knowledge suggest that we are on the cusp of improving the quality of the medication process for all.

REFERENCES

1. Personalised Medicines: Hopes and Realities. A report by The Royal Society. London: The Royal Society, 2005.
2. The potential regulatory challenges of personalised medicine. Available at: www.mhra.gov.uk.
3. Dying for drugs—at home. Lancet 2008; 372:419.
4. Phillips DP, Baker GEC, Eguchi MM. Increase in fatal medication errors. Arch Intern Med 2009; 168:1561–1566.
5. Nebeker JR, Hoffman JM, Weir CR, et al. High rates of adverse drug events in a highly computerized hospital. Arch Intern Med 2005; 165:1111–1116.
6. Osterberg L, Blaschke T. Adherence to medication. N Engl J Med 2005; 353:487–497.
7. Claxton AJ, Cramer J, Pierce C. A systematic review of the associations between dose regimens and medication compliance. Clin Ther 2001; 23:1296–1310.

8. Osterberg LG, Rudd P. Medication adherence for antihypertensive therapy. In: Oparil S, Weber MA, eds. Hypertension: A Companion to Brenner and Rector's The Kidney. 2nd ed. Philadelphia: Elsevier Mosby, 2005.

9. Florence AT, Salole EG, eds. Formulation Factors in Adverse Reactions. London: Wright, 1990.

10. Low-Beer S, Yip B, O'Shaughnessy MV, et al. Adherence to triple therapy and viral load response. J Acquir Immune Defic Syndr 2000; 23:360–361.

11. Vrijens B, Urquhart J. Patient adherence to prescribed antimicrobial drug dosing regimens. J Antimicrob Chemother 2005; 55:616–627.

12. Urquhart J, Vrijens B. New findings about patients adherence to prescribed drug dosing regimens: an introduction to pharmionics. Eur J Hosp Pharm Sci 2005; 11:103–106.

13. Tobin M, Staniforth JN, Morton D, et al. Active and intelligent inhaler device development. Int J Pharm 2004; 277:31–37.

14. Kaplan W, Laing R. Priority Medicines for Europe and the World. Geneva: WHO, 2004.

15. Ernest TB, Elder DP, Martini LM, et al. Developing paediatric medicines: identifying the needs and recognising the challenges. J Pharm Pharmacol 2007; 59:1043–1055.

16. Wong I, Sweis D, Cope J, et al. Paediatric medicines. Drug Saf 2003; 26:529–537.

17. Standing JF, Tuleu C. Paediatric formulations: getting to the heart of the matter. Int J Pharm 2005; 300:56–66.

18. Tuleu C. Paediatric formulations in practice. In: Costello I, et al., eds. Paediatric Drug Handling. London: Pharmaceutical Press, 2007.

19. Costello I, Long PF, Wong EK, et al. Paediatric Drug Handling, ULLA Postgraduate Series. London: Pharmaceutical Press, 2007

20. Florence AT. Neglected diseases, neglected devices, neglected patients? Int J Pharm 2008; 350:1–2.

21. Miller MR, Robinson KA, Lubomski LH, et al. Medication errors in paediatric care: a systematic review of epidemiology and an evaluation of evidence supporting reduction strategy recommendations. Qual Saf Health Care 2007; 16:116–126.

22. Hamamatsu Photonics KK, Japan. Micro-droplet technology. Available at: http://jp.hamamatsu.com/en/rd/publication.

23. Keith S. Advances in psychotropic formulations. Prog Neuropsychopharmacol Biol Psychiatry 2006; 30:996–1008.

24. Jeong SH, Fu Y, Park K. Frosta: a new technology for making fast-melting tablets. Expert Opin Drug Deliv 2005; 2:1107–1116.

25. Seager H. Drug-delivery products and the Zydis fast-dissolving dosage form. J Pharm Pharmacol 1998; 50:375–382.

26. Sastry SV, Nyshadham JR, Fix JA. Recent technological advances in oral drug delivery. A review. Pharm Sci Tech Today 2000; 3:138–145.

27. Poston KL, Waters C. Zydis selegiline in the management of Parkinson's disease. Expert Opin Pharmacother 2007; 8:2615–2614.

28. Vondrak B, Barnhart S. Dissolvable films for flexible product format in drug delivery. Pharm Technol Suppl 2008 (April) (see: www.pharmtech.com).

29. Ford C. Overcoming challenges on the path to combination product development. Pharmaceutical International. Available at: http://www.pharmaceutical-int.com. Accessed April 2008.

30. Franz S. The trouble with making combination drugs. Nat Rev Drug Discov 2006; 5:881–882.

31. De Brabander C, Vervaet C, Fiermans L, et al. Matrix minitablets based on starch/microcellulose wax mixtures. Int J Pharm 2000; 199:195–203.

32. De Brabander C, Vervaet C, Remon JP. Development and evaluation of sustained release mini-matrices by hot melt extrusion. J Control Release 2003; 89:235–244.

33. Huang W, Zheng Q, Sun W, et al. Levofloxacin implants with predetermined microstructure fabricated by three dimensional printing. Int J Pharm 2007; 339:33–38.

34. Rowe CW, Katstra WE, Palazzolo RD, et al. Multimechanisms oral dosage forms fabricated by three dimensional printing. J Control Release 2000; 66:11–17.

35. Vollmer U, Galfetti P. RapidFilm: oral thin films (OTF) as an innovative drug delivery system and dosage form. Drug Delivery Report Spring/Summer 2006.

36. Reynaerts D, Peirs J, Van Brussel H. An implantable drug-delivery system based on shape memory alloy micro-actuation. Sens Actuators 1997; A61:455–462.

37. Bitsch L. Critical Components in Microfluidic Systems for Drug Delivery [PhD thesis, s960370]. Denmark: Technical University of Denmark, June 27, 2006.

38. Chen L, Choo J, Yan B. The microfabricated electrokinetic pump: a potential promising drug delivery technique. Expert Opin Drug Deliv 2007; 4:119–129.

39. Thomsen J, Charabi S, Tos M. Preliminary results of a new delivery system for gentamicin to the inner ear in patients with Meniere's disease. Eur Arch Otorhinolaryngol 2000; 257:362–365.

40. Chen Z, Kujawa SG, McKenna MJ, et al. Inner ear delivery via a reciprocating perfusion system in the guinea pig. J Control Release 2007; 110:1–19.

41. Teymoori MM, Abbaspour-Sani E. Design and simulation of a novel electrostatic peristaltic micromachined pump for drug delivery applications. Sens Actuators A 2005; 117:222–229.

42. Santini JT, Cima MJ, Langer R. A controlled-release microchip. Nature 1999; 397:335–338.

43. Wang PP, Frazier J, Brem H. Local drug delivery to the brain. Adv Drug Deliv Rev 2002; 54:987–1013.

44. Li Y, Shawgo RS, Tyler B, et al. In vivo release from a drug delivery MEMS device. J Control Release 2004; 100:211–219.

45. Chung AJ, Kim D, Erikson D. Electrokinetic microfluidic devices for rapid low power delivery in autonomous microsystems. Lab Chip 2008; 8:330–338.

46. Grayson ACR, Shawgo RS, Li Y, et al. Electronic MEMS for triggered delivery. Adv Drug Deliv Rev 2004; 56:173–184.

47. Hilt JZ, Peppas NA. Microfabricated drug delivery devices. Int J Pharm 2005; 306:15–23.

48. Peppas NA. Intelligent therapeutics: biomimetic systems and nanotechnology in drug delivery. Adv Drug Deliv Rev 2004; 56:1529–1531.

49. Li Y, Duc HLH, Tyler B, et al. In vivo delivery of BCNU from a MEMS device to a tumor model. J Control Release 2005; 106:138–145.

50. Levin VA, Hoffman W, Weinkam RJ. Pharmacokinetics of BCNU in man: a preliminary study of 20 patients. Cancer Treat Rep 1978; 62:1305–1312.

51. Montgomery JA, James R, McCaleb GS, et al. The modes of decomposition of 1,3-bis (2-chloroethyl)-1-nitrosourea and related compounds. J Med Chem 1967; 10:668–674.

52. Tsai N-C, Sue C-Y. Review of MEMS-based drug delivery and dosing systems. Sens Acuators A 2007; 134:555–564.

53. Grayson ACR, Cima MJ, Langer R. Molecular release from a polymeric microreservoir device: influence of chemistry, polymer swelling, and loading on device performance. J Biomed Mater Res A 2004; 69A:502–512.

54. Kim GY, Tyler BM, Tupper MM, et al. Resorbable polymer microchips releasing BCNU inhibit tumor growth in the rat 9L flank model. J Control Release 2007; 123:172–178.

55. Wood KC, Zacharia NC, Schmidt DJ, et al. Electroactive controlled release thin films. Proc Natl Acad Sci U S A 2008; 105:2280–2285.

56. Wood KC, Chuang HF, Batten RD, et al. Controlling interlayer diffusion to achieve sustained multiagent delivery from layer-by-layer thin films. Proc Natl Acad Sci U S A 2006; 103: 10207–10212.

57. Gröning R, Remmerbach S, Jansen AC. Telemedicine: insulin pump controlled by the Global System for Mobile Communications (GSM). Int J Pharm 2007; 339:61–65.

Index

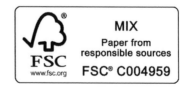